HEALTH AND HEALTHCARE SYSTEMS

Thomas Foley, MPH (HP), is a clinical assistant professor in the Public Health Division at State University of New York at Binghamton, Decker College of Nursing and Health Sciences. He is the public health representative for interprofessional education (IPE) at SUNY Binghamton, the chair of the IPE Curriculum and Assessment Committee, founding faculty advisor of the SUNY Binghamton Interprofessional Education Consortium, and the allied health representative for the Decker College of Nursing and Health Sciences' Culture of Belonging Committee. He teaches courses in global public health, health systems, social and behavioral health, interprofessional health, experiential public health, and public health biology. He earned an MPH in Health Promotion from George Washington University in Washington, DC, and completed community health doctorate course work at the Oregon Health and Science University, Portland State University in Portland, Oregon. He has over 15 years of experience in disease prevention and health promotion, primarily focusing on prevention and rehabilitation of chronic diseases through physical activity and nutrition. He integrates person-centeredness, the stages of change, and the social ecological model into his examination and translation of prevention and treatment of chronic diseases through health behaviors. He is a former U.S. Peace Corps volunteer and grass-roots community organizer.

Anna Foucek Tresidder, PhD, is a leader in health systems and program evaluation with over two decades of experience in academia and applied public health. She currently serves as the vice president of Research and Evaluation for Excelsior Wellness in Spokane, Washington, where she leads quality improvement analytics, fosters collaborations with academic institutions, and develops data-driven decision-making systems to improve healthcare outcomes. Additionally, she serves as a clinical associate professor at Washington State University's Elson S. Floyd College of Medicine, where she mentors medical students in community-based learning and research projects in collaboration with local organizations. Dr. Tresidder's academic career spans multiple institutions, where she has taught courses in healthcare policy and law, international and domestic health systems, process improvement, program evaluation, epidemiology, and research methods. For over 20 years, she has also worked as an independent consultant in evaluation and research, specializing in international health and social service programs. Her global health experience includes serving as a community development and program manager with the U.S. Peace Corps in Siansundu, Zimbabwe, where she implemented community-driven health initiatives focused on sustainable, equity-based interventions. This international perspective continues to shape her work as she collaborates with global organizations and presents on public health systems and evaluation in international forums, including recent engagements in Tokyo, Vienna, and Vancouver.

Leslie A. Bozeman, PhD, is the director of internationalization and senior international officer at Georgia Gwinnett College in Lawrenceville, Georgia. She leads the institution's internationalization efforts including global learning at home and abroad, faculty development, international partnerships, and external fundraising. Her areas of expertise include comprehensive internationalization, curricular and cocurricular internationalization, virtual exchange, and global leadership development. She is the recipient of Fulbright-Hays Summer Seminar and Fulbright International Education Administrators awards and serves on the Board of Directors of the Eiteljorg Museum in Indianapolis, Indiana. Leslie earned a doctorate in higher education administration, with a concentration in international higher education from Boston College, and an MA in teaching from American University in Washington, DC.

HEALTH AND HEALTHCARE SYSTEMS

A Global View

Editors

Thomas Foley, MPH (HP)
Anna Foucek Tresidder, PhD
Leslie A. Bozeman, PhD

SPRINGER PUBLISHING

Springer Publishing Company, LLC
902 Carnegie Center/Suite 140, Princeton, NJ 08540
www.springerpub.com
connect.springerpub.com

Acquisitions Editor: David D'Addona
Development Editor: Libby Ornstein
Production Editor: Diana Osborne
Compositor: Amnet Systems

ISBN: 978-0-8261-7473-4
eBook ISBN: 978-0-8261-7474-1
DOI: 10.1891/9780826174741

SUPPLEMENTS:

A robust set of instructor resources designed to supplement this text is located at http://connect.springerpub.com/content/book/978-0-8261-7474-1. Qualifying instructors may request access by emailing textbook@springerpub.com.

Instructor Materials:
Instructor's Manual ISBN: 978-0-8261-7475-8
Instructor Test Bank ISBN: 978-0-8261-7476-5
Instructor Chapter PowerPoints ISBN: 978-0-8261-7477-2
Instructor Sample Syllabus ISBN: 978-0-8261-7839-8

25 26 27 28 / 5 4 3 2 1

Library of Congress Cataloging-in-Publication Data is available.

Printed in the United States of America.

CONTENTS

PART IV. Health and Healthcare in South America

PART V. Health and Healthcare in the Caribbean

PART VI. Health and Healthcare in Europe and North Asia

PART VII. Health and Healthcare in North and West Africa

PART XV. Global Health Moving Forward

CONTRIBUTORS

Nadira Aitambayeva, PhD candidate Senior Lecturer, Department of Health Management, Kazakhstan Medical University "KSPH," Almaty City, Kazakhstan

Sarah Al-Aubaidy Undergraduate Student, Department of Biological Sciences, State University of New York at Binghamton, Binghamton, New York

Reethee Madona Antony, PhD, CCC-SLP Assistant Professor, Division of Speech and Language Pathology, Decker College of Nursing and Health Sciences, State University of New York at Binghamton, Binghamton, New York

Ammcise Apply, MPH, PhD candidate Graduate Research Assistant, College of Community and Public Affairs, Community Research and Action Program, State University of New York at Binghamton, Binghamton, New York

L. Esther Aranda, DrPH, MPH, MCP Research Consultant, Department of Global Health, Milken Institute School of Public Health, The George Washington University, Washington, DC

Victor Bassey Archibong, PhD, MSc Lecturer, Department of Human Anatomy, University of Rwanda, Huye, Southern Province, Rwanda

Joshua Ojodale Aruwa, DSLT, BSc.SLT, PGDE, MSc Laboratory Technologist and Researcher, School of Biomedical Sciences/Pharmacy, Kampala International University, Uganda

Serdar Atav, PhD Professor, Health Policy and Research, Decker College of Nursing and Health Sciences, State University of New York at Binghamton, Binghamton, New York

Janell Kayla Atkins, MS candidate Graduate Student, State University of New York at Binghamton, Binghamton, New York

Kellan E. Baker, PhD, MPH, MA Executive Director, Whitman-Walker Institute, Washington, DC

Imran Bari, BDS, MSc, MPH Senior Research Associate, Department of Global Health; Manager, Center on Commercial Determinants of Health, Milken Institute School of Public Health, The George Washington University, Washington, DC

Aida Barrera, MD, MSc, MSCE Research Professor, Centro de Investigaciones de las Ciencias de la Salud-CICS, Universidad de San Carlos de Guatemala, Guatemala City, Guatemala

Adugnaw Berhane, PhD Assistant Professor in Public Health, Department of Preventative Medicine, School of Public Health, Addis Ababa University, Addis Ababa, Ethiopia

Amit Bhandari, MPH, MBBS Independent Expert, Health, Nutrition and Development, Lalitpur, Nepal

Leslie A. Bozeman, PhD Director of Internationalization, Senior International Officer, Georgia Gwinnett College, Lawrenceville, Georgia

Maryellen D. Brisbois, PhD, RN, PHCNS-BC Associate Professor, Community Nursing Department, University of Massachusetts-Dartmouth, Dartmouth, Massachusetts

Parisa Broomandkhoshbacht, MPH Medical Student, Kansas City University, Kansas City, Missouri

Sharon Bryant, PhD, MPH Associate Dean of Diversity, Equity, and Inclusion, Decker College of Nursing and Health Sciences, State University of New York at Binghamton, Binghamton, New York

Itzel Eguiluz Cárdenas, PhD, MSc Adjunct Professor, Tecnológico de Monterrey, Monterrey, Mexico

Ramon Abel Castano, MD, PhD, MPH Health Systems Consultant and Researcher, Research Center for Social Protection and Health Economics (PROESA), Icesi University, Cali, Columbia

Diya Mariam Chacko, PhD candidate Research Scholar, Department of Psychology, Christ University, India

Rituparna Chakraborty, PhD, MA Assistant Professor, Department of Psychology, Christ University, India

Mei-Hsiu Chen, PhD Director of Statistical Consulting Services, Department of Mathematics and Statistics, State University of New York at Binghamton, Binghamton, New York

Jorge Colina, MA Chief Economist at Instituto para el Desarrollo Social Argentino (IDESA); External Professor at Faculty of Economics, Universidad Católica Argentina (UCA) and at Center for Interdisciplinary Studies in Health Management and Economics (CEGES), Universidad Austral, Argentina

Carl Condé, MD, MS, MPH candidate COE Scholar, LEND Fellow, SUNY Downstate Health Sciences University, Brooklyn, New York

Jeancarlo Cordoba, PhD School of Public Health, University of Costa Rica, San Pedro, Costa Rica

Anika Daniels-Osaze, EdD, MPH Associate Dean for Education, Clinical Associate Professor, Health Policy and Management, SUNY Downstate Health Sciences University, School of Public Health, Brooklyn, New York

Amy Dawson, MD, MPH, FAAFP Physician, Amwell, Instructor, Indiana Tech University, Fort Wayne, Indiana

Daniel C. Ehlke, PhD Associate Professor, Department of Health Policy and Management, SUNY Downstate School of Public Health, Brooklyn, New York

Anthony Seth Eshun, MGCPS, MWACS Surgeon Specialist, Our Lady of Grace Hospital, Breman Asikuma, Central Region, Ghana, West Africa

Fouzia Farooq, PhD, MPH Assistant Professor Department of Global Health, Milken Institute School of Public Health, The George Washington University, Washington, DC

Thomas Foley, MPH (HP) Clinical Assistant Professor, Public Health Division, Decker College of Nursing and Health Sciences, State University of New York at Binghamton, Binghamton, New York

Anna Foucek Tresidder, PhD Vice President of Research and Evaluation, Excelsior Wellness; Clinical Associate Professor, Washington State University, Elson S. Floyd College of Medicine, Spokane, Washington

Antoinette Francher-Donald, MBA Assistant Professor and Director of Experiential Learning, Keith Busse School of Business and Entrepreneurship Leadership, University of Saint Francis, Fort Wayne, Indiana

Irieleth Gallo, MS Researcher, PROESA, Universidad ICESI, Cali, Columbia

Dilli R. Gautam, MPH President, Bhutanese Community of Michigan, Grand Rapids, Michigan

James Giallella Department of History, Harpur College of Arts and Sciences, State University of New York at Binghamton, Binghamton, New York

Katherine Gilbert, LLB, MPP, MSc (Public Health) Honorary Fellow, Nossal Institute for Global Health, Melbourne, Australia

Sarah Ratkovich González, PhD, MSc, QFB Professor, Tecnológico de Monterrey, Monterrey, Mexico

Irma Marcela González-Treviño, PhD, MSc Director of Academic Development, Professor, Tecnológico de Monterrey, Monterrey, México

Heather Harewood, MBBS, MPH, DrPH Department of Preclinical and Health Sciences, The University of the West Indies, Bridgetown, Barbados

Kimberly D. Harry, PhD, MS Assistant Professor, Systems Science and Industrial Engineering Department, State University of New York, Vestal, New York

Akiko S. Hosler, PhD Associate Professor, Department of Epidemiology and Biostatistics, State University of New York at Albany, Albany, New York

Thet Su Htwe, BS, MB Visiting Assistant Professor, Decker College of Nursing and Health Sciences, State University of New York at Binghamton, Binghamton, New York

Mary Hu, MPH candidate Division of Public Health, Decker College of Nursing and Health Sciences, State University of New York at Binghamton, Binghamton, New York

Adnan A. Hyder, MD, PhD, MPH Dean and Robert A. Knox Professor, Boston University School of Public Health, Boston, Massachusetts

Taufique Joarder, DrPH, MPH, MBBS Associate Professor, Sing Health Duke-NUS Global Health Institute, Singapore

Courtney Jost, PhD, MPH Instructor, IMPACT Program Coordinator, School of Exercise, Sport, and Health Sciences, College of Health Oregon State University, Corvallis, Oregon

Suk-Young Kang, PhD, MSSW Associate Professor, Department of Social Work, State University of New York at Binghamton, Binghamton, New York

Mishalle Kayani, MPH candidate Global Health Epidemiology, Milken Institute School of Public Health, The George Washington University, Washington, DC

Uzma Rahim Khan, MBBS, MSc Assistant Professor (Research) and Research Director, Department of Emergency Medicine, Aga Khan University, Karachi, Pakistan

Sunil K. Khanna, PhD Professor, Director of the Center for Global Health, Oregon State University, Corvallis, Oregon

Lyazzat Kosherbayeva, PhD Professor, Asfendiyarov Kazakh National Medical University, Almaty City, Kazakhstan

Olivier Kubwimana, MD, MMED, FCS(ECSA) Orthopedic Surgeon, Department of Surgery, University Teaching Hospital of Butare, Huye, Rwanda; Lecturer, Department of Human Anatomy, University of Rwanda, Huye, Southern Province, Rwanda

Wesley D. Kufel, PharmD, BCPS, BCIDP Clinical Associate Professor, Department of Pharmacy Practice, Binghamton University School of Pharmacy and Pharmaceutical Sciences, Binghamton, New York; Clinical Associate Professor, Department of Medicine, Division of Infectious Diseases, State University of New York Upstate Medical University, Syracuse, New York

Maksut Kulzhanov, PhD Professor, Asfendiyarov Kazakh National Medical University, Almaty City, Kazakhstan

Linh Le, MD, MPH Chief Informatics Officer, New York State Department of Health, Assistant Professor, Russell Sage College, Troy, New York

Katelyn Lee, MPH candidate Medical Assistant, UHS Wilson Medical Center, Binghamton, New York; Research Assistant, Division of Public Health, Decker College of Nursing and Health Sciences, State University of New York at Binghamton, Binghamton, New York

Daniel F. López-Cevallos, PhD, MPH Associate Professor, Department of Health Promotion and Policy, School of Public Health and Health Sciences, University of Massachusetts, Amherst, Massachusetts

Megan MacDonald, PhD Professor and School Head, School of Exercise, Sport, and Health Sciences, College of Health, Oregon State University, Corvallis, Oregon

Alison Macintyre, MPH Senior Technical Advisor, Equitable Systems for Health, Nossal Institute for Global Health, University of Melbourne, Melbourne, Australia

Sheena Malla, MPH Research Assistant, Division of Public Health, Decker College of Nursing and Health Sciences, State University of New York at Binghamton, Binghamton, New York

Florence Mandebvu, DNP Assistant Professor, College of Nursing, SUNY Upstate Medical University, Syracuse, New York

Sara Mar, MPH Advocacy and Communications Strategist, Whitman-Walker Institute, Policy Department, Washington, DC

Samantha Mason, BA, DPT candidate Graduate Assistant, Interprofessional Education, Decker College of Nursing and Health Sciences, State University of New York at Binghamton, Binghamton, New York

Keri A. Mastro Dwyer, PharmD Clinical Assistant Professor, Department of Pharmacy Practice, Binghamton University School of Pharmacy and Pharmaceutical Sciences, Binghamton, New York

Pamela Mischen, PhD Chief Sustainability Officer, Faculty Advisor to the President Professor of Environmental Studies, Binghamton University of the State University of New York, Binghamton, NY

Abdullahi Abiodun Mohammed, PhD, MSc Lecturer, Department of Human Anatomy, University of Rwanda, Huye, Southern Province, Rwanda

Sharapat Moiynbayeva, PhD candidate Deputy Director of the Department of Science and Consulting, Kazakhstan Medical University "KSPH," Almaty City, Kazakhstan

Pablo Montero-Zamora, PhD Assistant Professor, Department of Kinesiology and Health Education, The University of Texas at Austin, Austin, Texas

Thomas C. Muller, AB Co-Editor (Retired), *Political Handbook of the World*, Binghamton University, Binghamton New York

Wolfgang Munar, SM, MD Director, Gill-Lebovic Center, Co-Director and Associate Professor, Global Health Systems Program; Department of Global Health, Milken Institute School of Public Health, The George Washington University, Washington, DC

Nazerke Narymbayeva, PhD candidate Senior Lecturer, Department of Health Management, Kazakhstan Medical University "KSPH," Almaty City, Kazakhstan

Sharifa Nasreen, PhD, MPH, MBBS Assistant Professor, SUNY Downstate Health Sciences University, Brooklyn, New York

Laila Nazarova, PhD candidate Lecturer, Department of Public Health, Asfendiyarov Kazakh National Medical University, Almaty City, Kazakhstan

Jenny K. Nielsen, MPH Navigation Services Program Manager, Refugee Education Center, Grand Rapids, Michigan

Paul Ndebele, PhD Assistant Director, Office of Research Excellence, Department of Global Health, George Washington University, Milken Institute School of Public Health, Washington, DC

Jerome A. Nenger, LLM, BL, LLB, FIPMD Research and Teaching Assistant, Community Research and Action, State University of New York at Binghamton, Binghamton, New York

Trang Nguyen, MD, DrPH, MPH Research Professor, School of Public Health, State University of New York at Albany, Albany, New York

Cathy F. Nickels-Herndon, MS, CHES, CWP Lecturer, Indiana University, School of Health and Human Sciences, Departments of Health Science and Kinesiology, Indianapolis, Indiana

Ardak Nurbakyt, PhD Professor, Asfendiyarov Kazakh National Medical University, Almaty City, Kazakhstan

Samson Ehindero Olorunnado, PhD, MSc Lecturer, Department of Human Anatomy, University of Rwanda, Huye, Southern Province, Rwanda

Luke Orgo Undergraduate Research Assistant, State University of New York at Binghamton, Binghamton, New York

Nino Paichadze, MD, MPH Assistant Research Professor, Milken Institute School of Public Health, The George Washington University, Washington, DC

Alejandra Paniagua-Avila, MD, DrPH, MPH Psychiatric Epidemiology Postdoctoral Fellow, Mailman School of Public Health, Columbia University, New York, New York

Helder Rocha Pereira, PhD, MEd, CHN, RN Coordinating Professor, School of Health, University of the Azores, Ponta Delgada, Portugal

Mariana Pinto-Alvarez, MD, MPH Graduate Research Assistant, Department of Health Promotion and Policy, School of Public Health and Health Sciences, University of Massachusetts, Amherst, Massachusetts

G. S. Prakasha, PhD, MEd, MSc, PGDGC, MPhil Associate Professor, Department of Psychology, Christ University, India

Victor Puac-Polanco, MD, DrPH, MSCE Assistant Professor, Department of Health Policy and Management, Downstate Health Sciences University, Brooklyn, New York

Dorian Ramirez-Flores, MD, MSCE, MPH Coordinador, Centro de Investigaciones de las Ciencias de la Salud -CICS, Universidad de San Carlos de Guatemala, Guatemala City, Guatemala

Benjamin Roberts, MS Graduate Teaching Assistant, School of Nutrition and Public Health, College of Health, Oregon State University, Corvallis, Oregon.

Pablo Rodríguez del Pozo, MD, JD, PhD Associate Professor of Medical Ethics in Medicine (Education), Weill Cornell Medical College, Qatar; Senior Associate External Researcher, Instituto para el Desarrollo Social Argentino (IDESA), Buenos Aires, Argentina

Daniel Romero-Alvarez, MD, PhD Associate Professor, Facultad de Ciencias de la Salud–Ciencias Biomédicas, Universidad Internacional SEK, Quito, Ecuador

Jean Paul Rugambwa, MMED General Medicine General Surgeon at the University Teaching Hospital of Butare (CHUB); Lecturer, Department of Human Anatomy, University of Rwanda, Huye, Southern Province, Rwanda

Mathias Ruhosha, MMED Surgery Consultant General Surgeon at University Teaching Hospital of Butare; Lecturer, Department of Human Anatomy, University of Rwanda, Huye, Southern Province, Rwanda

Roger Sealy, MBBS, MPH Health Sciences Lecturer and Bachelor of Health Sciences Program Coordinator, Department of Preclinical and Health Sciences, The University of the West Indies, Bridgetown, Barbados

Marwa Mamdouh Shaban, PhD, RN Lecturer at Community Health Nursing Department, Faculty of Nursing, Cairo University, Cairo, Egypt

Mostafa Shaban, RN Lecturer of Geriatric Nursing Department, Faculty of Nursing, Cairo University, Cairo, Egypt

Gurpreet Singh, PhD, PT Assistant Professor, Division of Physical Therapy, Decker College of Nursing and Health Sciences, State University of New York at Binghamton, Binghamton, New York

Victoria Eugenia Soto, PhD Director of PROESA, Universidad ICESI, Cali, Colombia

Dinara Sukenova, PhD candidate Lecturer, Department of Public Health, Asfendiyarov Kazakh National Medical University, Almaty City, Kazakhstan

Jia Sun, PhD, MPH, MS Assistant Professor, Department of Epidemiology and Biostatistics, School of Public Health, SUNY Downstate Health Sciences University, Brooklyn, New York

Shnara Svetlanova, PhD candidate Lecturer, Department of Nursing, Kazakhstan Medical University "KSPH," Almaty City, Kazakhstan

Inijesu Taiwo, MD, MPH Research Scholar, Global Health Institute, SUNY Upstate Medical University, Syracuse, New York

Brigitte Tenni, PhD, MPH Co-Head, Equitable Systems for Health, Nossal Institute for Global Health, University of Melbourne, Melbourne, Australia

Irene Torres, PhD Technical Director, Fundación Octaedro, Quito, Ecuador

Thuy Tran, MD, PhD Retired Director, Department of Medical Service Administration, Viet Nam Ministry of Health, Hanoi, Vietnam

Johnathan D. Tremblay, MPH, RPCV Independent Consultant, Kalamazoo, Michigan

Sundeep Venkatesan, MS, CCC-SLP Assistant Professor, Division of Speech and Language Pathology, Decker College of Nursing and Health Sciences, State University of New York at Binghamton, Binghamton, New York

Jiahao Wang, MPH candidate Research Assistant, Department of Public Health, Decker College of Nursing and Health Sciences, State University of New York at Binghamton, Binghamton, New York

Kathleen Visovatti Weaver, JD, MPA, MA, RN Senior Faculty Emeritus, Health Sciences, Indiana University Indianapolis, Indianapolis, Indiana

Sophie Whittington, MS Student Success Navigator, Office of Academic Programs, College of Agriculture and Life Sciences, Cornell University, Ithaca, New York

Maiya Zhakupova, MD, PhD Associate Professor, Asfendiyarov Kazakh National Medical University, Almaty City, Kazakhstan

PREFACE

We live in times when solidarity and international cooperation are needed more than ever.

—Andrej Plenkovic, Prime Minister of Croatia, February 23, 2021

By the end of the 21st century, the world's population is predicted to be greater than 10 billion (United Nations, n.d.). To protect the quality of life of our rapidly growing global community, it is imperative to view health from a global perspective. The COVID-19 pandemic and an alarming increase in catastrophic events resulting from climate change reinforce the need for a global approach to health, an approach that must include an international understanding of health inequities and disparities that span the regions and countries of the world. Too often, however, countries from certain regions of the world are not equitably included in the global comparative health literature, favoring a more Eurocentric viewpoint. *Health and Healthcare Systems: A Global View* addresses the historical injustice of a lack of international diversity in the global comparative health literature.

We strategically divided the core parts of this book into 13 regions that span the globe. Each region includes a brief regional overview chapter, which provides a snapshot of health and contextual factors such as history, geography, and social determinants derived from all countries within the region. Each region also includes two to four country profile chapters, which describe key health outcomes, health determinants, and health systems within the profiled countries in greater detail. By sampling two to four countries in each of the 13 regions, we ensure equitable representation from across the world. Importantly, a majority of the country profile chapters are written by people living in or who are originally from the profiled countries. In addition, the contributing writers in this book come from a wide breadth of academic programs and health professions. This textbook is a tremendous international and interprofessional collaboration, with contributors from across the regions of the world and disciplines of health. The following is a summary of the 13 regions and the sampled countries from each region that form the core content of *Health and Healthcare Systems: A Global View*:

- North America (Canada, Mexico, United States)
- Central America (Costa Rica, El Salvador, Guatemala)
- South America (Argentina, Colombia, Ecuador)
- The Caribbean (Barbados, Dominican Republic, Haiti, Trinidad and Tobago)
- Europe (Georgia, Great Britain, Portugal, Spain)
- North and West Africa (Egypt, Ghana, Nigeria)
- East Africa (Ethiopia, Tanzania, Uganda)
- Middle and Southern Africa (Botswana, Rwanda, Zimbabwe)
- West and Central Asia (Iran, Iraq, Kazakhstan, Turkey)
- South Asia (Bangladesh, India, Nepal, Pakistan)
- East Asia (China, Japan, South Korea, Thailand)
- Southeast Asia (Myanmar, Vietnam)
- Oceania (Australia, Papua New Guinea)

Through the strategic division of global regions and selection of multiple countries within each region, we promote cultural humility and a broader awareness of different cultural beliefs and practices, etiological factors of health and disease, approaches to and innovations in the structure and delivery of healthcare, and health outcomes and concerns across the world. As learners progress through this book, they will garner a better understanding of historical international health inequities, where and why health disparities occur, and what needs to be done to ameliorate global health. The countries featured in this book are a mix of countries with the following characteristics:

- high- to low-income
- densely and sparsely populated
- rural and urban majority
- rapidly aging and youthful
- organized with and without centralized and universal healthcare
- mainland and island nations

Health and Healthcare Systems: A Global View also includes introductory chapters centered on foundational concepts of global health and a concluding part that focuses on global health moving forward. The introductory part consists of three chapters: "Global Healthcare," "Global Health," and "Global Determinants of Health." These three introductory chapters provide definitions of terms that will be used throughout the book and a framework on how to approach reading the book. The concluding part consists of six chapters: "Global Health Moving Forward: Overview," "Climate Change," "Communicable Diseases," "Population Aging," "Mental Health," and "Forced Migration." These concluding chapters describe key issues that require focus from the global community to ameliorate global health and mitigate international health inequities and disparities.

The structure of *Health and Healthcare Systems: A Global View* allows easy organization of a course around the 15 strategic parts. The first week of the course should focus on the three introductory chapters in order for learners to garner an appreciation for global health and to be able to define key global health concepts. The core weeks of the course should be organized by the 13 regions. From each region, instructors should cover the regional overview and approximately two of the country profiles. Do not feel obligated to study all of the country profiles within each region; an à la carte approach to the country profiles included in this book allows flexibility in the learning experience. The final week should focus on global health moving forward. Learners should engage in robust discussions around etiology, distribution, inequities, and interventions regarding the crucial health issues that will have profound effects on the global community over the next several decades.

The strategic division of *Health and Healthcare Systems: A Global View* into 15 parts also allows for the integration of learner-centered assignments. We encourage educators to reserve at least 1 week of their course to allow presentations by learner teaching teams on countries not profiled in this book. This will help learners build essential global health skills and promote even greater international diversity and inclusivity by profiling more countries across the world. It is our hope that learners using this book build cultural humility skills to be better prepared for careers in global health and to advocate for health equity across the wide breadth of cultures spanning the regions and countries of the world.

Thomas Foley
Anna Foucek Tresidder
Leslie A. Bozeman

REFERENCE

United Nations. (n.d.). *Population*. https://www.un.org/en/global-issues/population

ACKNOWLEDGMENTS

There are far too many people essential to this textbook to mention everyone by name. Therefore, we are going to acknowledge the contributions of groups of people. First, we want to thank all of the authors who contributed to the chapters and ancillary items in this book. Without you, the book does not exist. You were all the collective key to the foundational purposes of this book: diversity and inclusiveness. Your involvement allowed for equitable representation across the world. Your diligent work resulted in chapters that are both highly informative and a joy to read. Next, we would like to thank our publishing team at Springer Publishing. You made this experience extremely rewarding. Your insights, support, and flexibility are truly appreciated. We would also like to thank our employers, colleagues, friends, and family for additional support. A project like this is time-consuming. Your understanding while this textbook was being completed is not taken for granted. Lastly, we would like to thank all the people who work toward promoting health equity on a global scale. It is challenging work but becoming more and more necessary as the years pass.

INSTRUCTOR RESOURCES

SPRINGER PUBLISHING CONNECT™

A robust set of instructor resources designed to supplement this text is located at http://connect.springerpub.com/content/book/978-0-8261-7474-1. Qualifying instructors may request access by emailing textbook@springerpub.com.

- **Instructor's Manual** with chapter summaries, outlines, key terms, discussion questions, and more.
- **Instructor Test Bank** with 350 multiple-choice questions
- **Instructor Chapter PowerPoints**
- **Instructor Sample Syllabus** containing a sample course syllabus with course descriptions, course objectives, recommended and additional readings, course requirements, course schedules, and more.

SPRINGER PUBLISHING

Visit https://connect.springerpub.com and look for the "**Show Supplementary**" button on the **book homepage**.

HEALTH AND HEALTHCARE SYSTEMS

PART I: Introduction to Global Health and Healthcare

CHAPTER 1

GLOBAL HEALTHCARE

Anna Foucek Tresidder and Thomas Foley

Global health is a multidisciplinary field that seeks to improve health and achieve health equity (fairness and justice) for all people worldwide. It transcends national boundaries by addressing health issues that affect populations globally, emphasizing the need for collective action to tackle these challenges (Koplan et al., 2009). Global health adopts a holistic approach, integrating health's social, economic, environmental, and political determinants. For example, ameliorating health outcomes often requires strategies that include improving education systems, promoting sustainable environmental practices, and fostering economic policies that reduce poverty. Comprehensive approaches such as these aim to enhance the health outcomes of all citizens in the population (Beaglehole & Bonita, 2010).

While often used interchangeably, global and international health differ in scope and focus. Global health focuses on challenges that transcend borders, such as pandemic response, antimicrobial resistance, and climate-related health risks. These issues emphasize equity, collaboration, and the shared responsibility of all nations (Frenk et al., 2014). International organizations, such as the World Health Organization (WHO), are pivotal in shaping global health agendas, coordinating efforts, and setting health standards worldwide. Conversely, **international health** traditionally emphasizes the health needs of low- and middle-income countries and the role of developed nations in addressing these issues through aid and technical support.

Global health addresses a broad spectrum of concerns, including infectious diseases such as HIV/AIDS and tuberculosis, noncommunicable diseases (NCDs) such as cardiovascular diseases and cancer, and health disparities and inequities. The globalization of trade, travel, and communication has significantly impacted health systems and outcomes, necessitating innovative approaches to address the interconnected nature of modern health challenges (Kickbusch et al., 2013). Moreover, global health efforts are integral to achieving the **United Nations (UN) Sustainable Development Goals** (SDGs), particularly Goal 3, which aims to ensure healthy lives and promote well-being. The UN adopted 17 SDGs in 2015 to end poverty, protect the planet, and promote peace and prosperity for the entire global community (United Nations Development Programme [UNDP], 2024). A full list of the SDGs is shown in Figure 1.1.

FUNDAMENTALS OF HEALTH SYSTEMS

DEFINITION AND PURPOSE OF HEALTH SYSTEMS

Health systems are the organized structures and processes through which health services are delivered, financed, and governed to meet a population's health needs. A well-functioning health system is essential for improving health outcomes, reducing disparities, and enhancing social well-being (WHO, 2010). Key components of a health system include financing, insurance, and delivery.

Healthcare financing is the management of money to cover the health needs of people within the system. The main goal of health financing is to allocate funding to ensure all people within the system have access to public and/or private health services. The funds for health services primarily come from taxation and employer/employee contributions (WHO, 2010). In a **multipayer system**, healthcare is financed by more than one entity, such as the government and employers/employees. In a **single-payer system**, healthcare is financed and paid for by one

FIGURE 1.1 United Nations Sustainable Development Goals (SDGs).

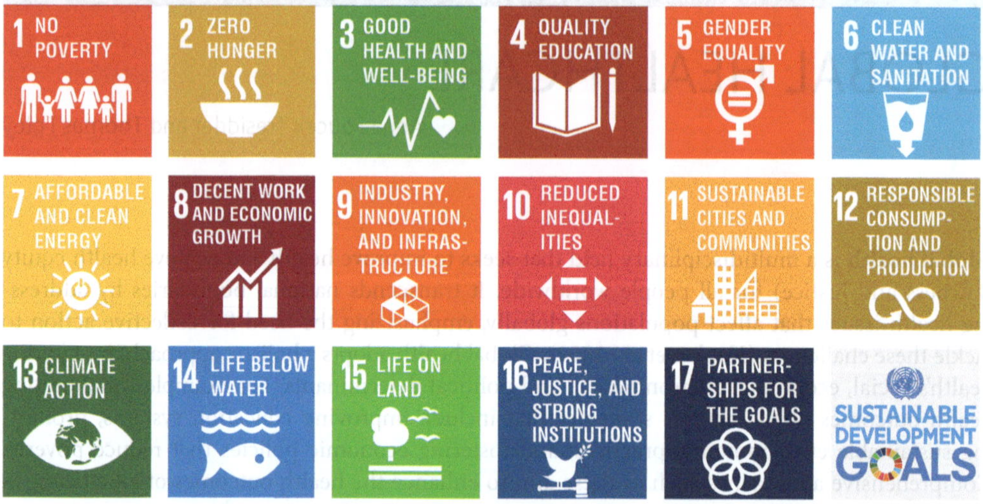
1 NO POVERTY
2 ZERO HUNGER
3 GOOD HEALTH AND WELL-BEING
4 QUALITY EDUCATION
5 GENDER EQUALITY
6 CLEAN WATER AND SANITATION
7 AFFORDABLE AND CLEAN ENERGY
8 DECENT WORK AND ECONOMIC GROWTH
9 INDUSTRY, INNOVATION, AND INFRAS-TRUCTURE
10 REDUCED INEQUAL-ITIES
11 SUSTAINABLE CITIES AND COMMUNITIES
12 RESPONSIBLE CONSUMP-TION AND PRODUCTION
13 CLIMATE ACTION
14 LIFE BELOW WATER
15 LIFE ON LAND
16 PEACE, JUSTICE, AND STRONG INSTITUTIONS
17 PARTNER-SHIPS FOR THE GOALS
SUSTAINABLE DEVELOPMENT GOALS

Source: United Nations. (n.d.). *Sustainable development goals (SDGs) and disability*. https://social.desa.un.org/issues/disability/sustainable-development-goals-sdgs-and-disability

single entity, which is the government (Donnelly et al., 2019). **Healthcare insurance** is a contract that specifies how services will be paid under a health plan. The health plan determines how service providers are reimbursed, what costs the insurers are responsible for, and what costs the insured need to pay based on where they receive services and which services they use. The main objectives of health insurance are to make health services more affordable and to protect the insured from financial risk when using necessary **healthcare** services. There are public health insurance schemes coordinated and financed by governments and private not-for-profit and for-profit health insurance coverage schemes that fund health service delivery through contributions of employers and employees (Centers for Medicare & Medicaid Services [CMS], n.d.). **Health delivery** is the provision of health services, and includes services from medical professionals, nurses, health service administrators, allied health professionals such as physical therapists and social workers, as well as facilities and equipment (WHO, 2010). Health service delivery is enabled by health financing and insurance. The strategic coordination and regulation of these three key components can improve the accessibility and quality of a health system while containing its expenses. A global health goal is the expansion of **universal health coverage (UHC)**; that is, when all people within a health system can obtain the health services they need without risk of financial hardship (Evans et al., 2013). To achieve UHC, a system needs adequate funding, health insurance schemes that cover all people, and a robust, widespread delivery system. While universal healthcare access is theoretical in nature, countries that provide universal health insurance make health services more affordable for people living in or near poverty. Universal health insurance is used synonymously to UHC; however, it is important to note that accessibility gaps can still persist.

WHO's Framework for Health Systems Strengthening expands on these three central components by highlighting six building blocks of a health system: service delivery, health workforce, health information, medical products and technologies, health financing, and leadership/governance (Figure 1.2). These components interact dynamically; for example, a strong health workforce supported by efficient health information systems can improve service delivery, ensuring better health outcomes, responsiveness, financial risk protection, and equity (WHO, 2017). Effective health systems require robust resources, precise functions, and coordinated outputs to achieve their objectives.

FIGURE 1.2 Major interdependent health system building blocks.

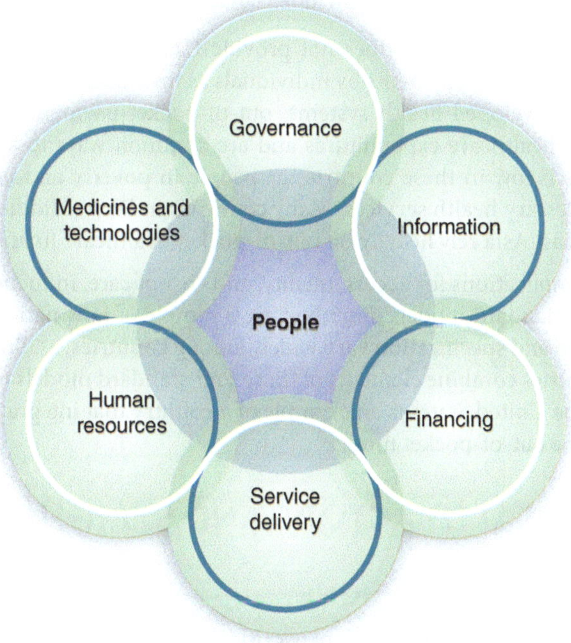

Source: de Savigny, D., & Taghreed, A. (Eds). (2009). *Systems thinking for health systems strengthening.* Alliance for Health Policy and Systems Research.

TYPES OF HEALTH SYSTEMS

Globally, health systems vary widely in structure and function. The following are four standard models (Reid, 2009):

1. ***Beveridge model:*** This single-payer, UHC system is financed by the government via taxes. Services are free at the point of service. Many health service facilities are owned by the government, and many health service providers are government employees. Countries that use this model tend to have high universal access as insurance is universal and the cost of care is contained via government involvement in finance, insurance, and delivery. Examples of countries that use the Beveridge model are the United Kingdom and Cuba.

2. ***Bismarck model:*** This multipayer, UHC system is primarily financed by employer and employee contributions, which are referred to as sickness funds. Through taxation, the government finances a smaller percentage of health services for people not covered under employment. Health services are mostly provided in the private sector; however, public **healthcare delivery** plays a small yet important role. Insurance companies are not-for-profit. Their main goal is not to make a profit, but rather to ensure that people can obtain quality healthcare without financial hardship. The Bismarck model is often referred to as socialized health insurance. Costs are contained through not-for-profit insurers and government oversight. Universal healthcare access tends to be high because insurance coverage is universal. Countries that use the Bismarck model include Germany and France.

3. ***National health insurance model:*** This single-payer, UHC system combines elements of the Beveridge and Bismarck models. Government-run health insurance plans are funded through taxation. Health services are primarily provided in the private sector, while public sector

health services play a small yet significant role. Government management of finances and regulation of insurance promotes high accessibility while containing costs. Countries that use the National Health Insurance model include Canada and South Korea.

4. *Out-of-pocket model:* This model does not provide UHC. It is a market-driven, multipayer system that relies on direct payments by individuals as insurance coverage is limited. In countries lacking well-developed health systems, out-of-pocket payments tend to account for a higher portion of healthcare expenditures and are common ways to secure health services. Healthcare access is low in these countries as people in poverty and of lower income often cannot afford necessary health services. Many countries in West, Middle, and East Africa and South and Southeast Asia rely heavily on out-of-pocket healthcare financing.

Each model has implications for access, quality, and cost of care, influencing health outcomes and equity. The four standard models described are a sample of how nations finance health services; implementation and specification vary widely among countries, as illustrated in subsequent chapters. Many countries combine elements of these four standard models to finance the delivery of health services. The United States is an example of a country that integrates aspects of all these systems, including the out-of-pocket model.

KEY GLOBAL HEALTH ACTORS AND STAKEHOLDERS

INTERNATIONAL ORGANIZATIONS

Organizations like WHO and World Bank play critical roles in global health governance. **WHO** is an agency of the UN that is responsible for global public health. **World Bank** is a global international partnership focused on ending poverty and promoting sustainable development. Key global organizations such as World Bank and WHO develop policies, set health standards, and coordinate international efforts to address health crises. For example, WHO's leadership during the COVID-19 pandemic demonstrated the importance of global cooperation in managing health emergencies.

Initiatives such as the COVID-19 Vaccines Global Access (COVAX) program exemplify coordinated efforts to ensure equitable vaccine distribution, highlighting the role of global partnerships in addressing disparities (Gostin et al., 2020). **COVAX** is a global initiative co-led by the Global Alliance for Vaccines and Immunizations (Gavi), the Coalition for Epidemic Preparedness Innovations (CEPI), and WHO to ensure equitable access to COVID-19 vaccines. It aims to accelerate vaccine development, production, and distribution by providing doses to low- and middle-income countries. By the end of 2022, COVAX had delivered more than 1.8 billion vaccine doses to 146 countries, significantly contributing to global vaccination efforts and reducing the disparity in vaccine access (Gavi, 2022).

NONGOVERNMENTAL ORGANIZATIONS AND CIVIL SOCIETY

Nongovernmental organizations (NGOs), such as Doctors Without Borders and The Gates Foundation, contribute significantly to global health through service delivery, advocacy, and funding. They often address gaps in government services, particularly in resource-limited settings, and influence policy development at national and international levels. **Doctors Without Borders**, also known as Médecins Sans Frontières (MSF), has significantly impacted global health systems by delivering critical healthcare services in regions affected by crises. During the 2014 to 2016 West Africa Ebola outbreak, MSF was instrumental in providing frontline care, setting up treatment centers, and training local healthcare workers. Their rapid response helped manage the epidemic, while their advocacy highlighted gaps in global epidemic preparedness, prompting systemic reforms such as establishing WHO's Emergencies Programme. This demonstrates how

MSF not only provides immediate medical aid but also influences long-term improvements in global health systems (MSF, n.d.; WHO, 2017).

GOVERNMENTS AND POLICYMAKERS

National governments shape global health outcomes through policies, resource allocation, and participation in bilateral and multilateral collaborations. Initiatives such as Gavi and the **Global Fund** (a partnership of international stakeholders who finance efforts to mitigate disease and promote global health equity) exemplify the impact of coordinated efforts in addressing significant health challenges (WHO, 2022). In collaboration with global initiatives, nations can achieve significant health gains. For example, Rwanda, following the 1994 genocide, rebuilt its healthcare infrastructure through partnerships with organizations like the Global Fund and Gavi. These collaborations funded programs to combat HIV/AIDS, tuberculosis, and malaria while also supporting initiatives like the introduction of the HPV vaccine, which achieved high coverage and reduced cervical cancer rates. By prioritizing universal health coverage, community-based care, and data-driven policies, Rwanda transformed its health system, showcasing the power of coordinated national and global efforts in improving health outcomes.

PRIVATE SECTOR AND PHILANTHROPY

The private sector, including pharmaceutical companies and private health providers, plays a vital role in global health financing, innovation, and service delivery. Philanthropic contributions, such as those from The Gates Foundation, have advanced research and development for diseases like malaria and HIV/AIDS. The Gates Foundation has significantly advanced global efforts to reduce malaria through funding, research, and advocacy. Since its inception, the Foundation has invested more than $2 billion in malaria prevention and treatment programs, supporting initiatives such as developing new insecticide-treated bed nets, antimalarial drugs, and innovative vaccines. Collaborating with global partners like the Global Fund and WHO, the foundation has helped reduce malaria mortality rates by more than 50% in many regions, particularly sub-Saharan Africa (The Gates Foundation, n.d.; WHO, 2021b). Their continued focus on eradication aims to achieve a malaria-free world by addressing drug resistance and improving healthcare delivery in **endemic regions** (areas where a disease regularly occurs; O'Neill, 2016).

GLOBAL HEALTH CHALLENGES

INFECTIOUS AND CHRONIC DISEASES

Global health faces numerous interconnected challenges that threaten the well-being of populations worldwide. Infectious diseases such as COVID-19, malaria, measles, dengue fever, HIV, and tuberculosis remain persistent threats, exacerbated by vaccine, testing, and treatment inequities and antimicrobial resistance (Institute for Health Metrics and Evaluation [IHME], 2024). Chronic diseases, including diabetes mellitus and cardiovascular conditions, are rising sharply due to aging populations, urbanization, and unhealthy lifestyles. Chronic diseases contribute to more than 70% of deaths worldwide (WHO, 2021a). Addressing infectious and chronic diseases requires multisectoral approaches integrating public health, education, agriculture, and economic policies alongside robust and accessible health systems capable of delivering preventive, diagnostic, and treatment services. For instance, Brazil has implemented innovative policies through its Unified Health System (Sistema Único de Saúde; SUS) to address chronic diseases. These include community-based interventions like health promotion campaigns and the Family Health Strategy, which provide primary care services and chronic disease management to underserved populations (Victora et al., 2011).

HEALTH DISPARITIES AND INEQUITIES

Health disparities are differences in health outcomes. They are caused and/or exacerbated by health inequities. **Health inequities** are structural differences in the opportunity for people to achieve full health potential. Health inequities result in avoidable differences in health status experienced by specific population groups. Health inequities profoundly and multifacetedly impact global health. These inequities are rooted in social, economic, environmental, and political determinants of health and manifest as differences in access to quality healthcare, exposure to health risks, and vulnerability to disease. Consequently, health inequities contribute significantly to the global burden of preventable morbidity and mortality, perpetuating cycles of poverty and disadvantage. Health inequities and disparities persist across and within countries, influenced by the social **determinants of health** such as poverty, lack of access to education, and gender inequality. Addressing these inequities necessitates targeted interventions and systemic reforms to promote health equity. **Health equity** is a fair and just state in which all people can achieve their full health potential (Rural Health Information Hub, 2024; Office of Disease Prevention and Health Promotion, 2024).

ENVIRONMENTAL HEALTH AND CLIMATE CHANGE

The intertwined climate change and environmental degradation crises represent a profound and multifaceted challenge to global health security. These crises act as threat multipliers, exacerbating existing health vulnerabilities and creating new ones through a complex interplay of direct and indirect pathways. Rising temperatures and altered precipitation patterns are expanding the geographic range and breeding seasons of disease vectors, increasing the risk of vector-borne diseases like malaria, dengue, Zika, and chikungunya. Concurrently, extreme weather events such as droughts, floods, and heat waves disrupt agricultural production, damage critical infrastructure, and contaminate water supplies, leading to food insecurity, malnutrition, and increased risk of waterborne diseases (Figure 1.3). These impacts are disproportionately felt by marginalized and vulnerable communities, particularly in low- and middle-income countries, further exacerbating existing health disparities and inequities. Addressing these challenges requires a comprehensive and integrated approach encompassing aggressive mitigation of greenhouse gas emissions, investments in climate change adaptation strategies, strengthening of health systems' resilience, and robust international cooperation based on principles of equity and solidarity.

SUMMARY

Global health, as an inherently interdisciplinary and equity-driven field, addresses health challenges that transcend national boundaries and demand collective action. This chapter outlines the foundational elements of global health systems, emphasizing the interplay between health outcomes, determinants of health, health systems models, and the global actors shaping policies and responses. The interconnectedness of infectious and chronic disease health disparities and environmental health justice underscores the need for integrated and innovative approaches that leverage resources across sectors and nations. Addressing global health challenges also requires recognizing their root causes in social, economic, and environmental contexts, highlighting the urgency of addressing inequities and building resilient systems to adapt to changing global dynamics, such as climate change and urbanization. Ultimately, achieving sustainable improvements in health outcomes relies on partnerships rooted in shared responsibility, innovation, and a commitment to equity. Building on this foundation, subsequent chapters delve deeper into the strategies and frameworks that drive progress in improving the health and well-being of countries across the world. The chapters in this book are written by authors with lived experience in countries often underrepresented in traditional global health textbooks.

FIGURE 1.3 How climate change affects health.

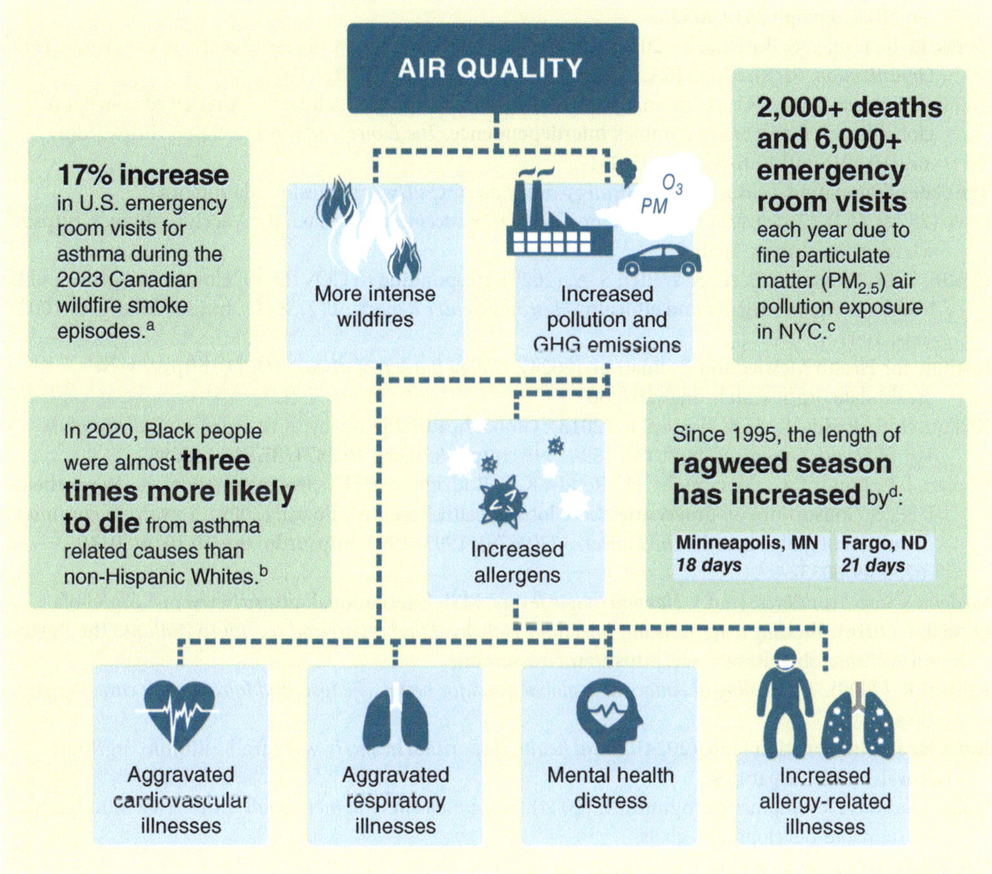

[a] https://www.cdc.gov/mmwr/volumes/72/wr/mm7234a5.htm
[b] https://minorityhealth.hhs.gov/asthma-and-african-americans
[c] https://a816-dohbesp.nyc.gov/IndicatorPublic/beta/data-stories/aq2/4
[d] https://www.epa.gov/climate-indicators/climate-change-indicators-ragweed-pollen-season

GHG, greenhouse gasses; O_3, ground-level ozone; $PM_{2.5}$, particulate matter with a diameter of 2.5 micrometers or smaller.

Source: American Public Health Association. (n.d.). *How climate change affects your health.* https://www.apha.org/news-and-media/multimedia/infographics/how-climate-change-affects-your-health

LEARNING ACTIVITIES

CourseConnect

To access self-assessment questions and interactive, competency-based learning activities for this chapter, visit www.springerpub.com/courseconnect. See inside front cover and tear-out for CourseConnect details.

REFERENCES

Beaglehole, R., & Bonita, R. (2010). What is global health? *Global Health Action, 3*(1), 5142. https://doi.org/10.3402/gha.v3i0.5142

Centers for Medicare & Medicaid Services. (n.d.). *Health insurance basics.* https://www.cms.gov/files/document/nsa-health-insurance-basics.pdf

Donnelly, P. D., Erwin, P. C., Fox, D. M., & Grogan, C. (2019). Single-payer, multi-payer, and state-based financing of health care. *American Journal of Public Health, 109*(11), 1482–1483. https://doi.org/10.2105/ajph.2019.305353

Evans, D. B., Hsu, J., & Borema, T. (2013). Universal health coverage vs. access. *Bulletin of the World Health Organization, 91*(8), 546–546A. https://doi.org/10.2471/BLT.13.125450

Frenk, J., Gomez-Dantes, O., & Moon, S. (2014). From sovereignty to solidarity: A renewed concept of global health for an era of complex interdependence. *The Lancet, 383*(9911), 94–97. https://doi.org/10.1016/S0140-6736(13)62561-1

The Gates Foundation. (n.d.). *Malaria strategy overview*. https://www.gatesfoundation.org

Gavi. (2022). *COVAX delivers over 1.8 billion COVID-19 vaccine doses*. Gavi, the Vaccine Alliance. https://www.gavi.org/covax-facility

Gostin, L. O., Friedman, E. A., & Wetter, S. A. (2020). Responding to COVID-19: How to navigate a public health emergency legally and ethically. *Hastings Center Report, 50*(2), 8–12. https://doi.org/10.1002/hast.1090

Institute for Health Metrics and Evaluation. (2024). *Global burden of disease (GBD)*. https://www.healthdata.org/research-analysis/gbd

Kickbusch, I., Reddy, K. S., & Horton, R. (2013). Global health diplomacy: Five years on. *Bulletin of the World Health Organization, 91*(3), 159–159A. https://doi.org/10.2471/BLT.13.118596

Koplan, J. P., Bond, T. C., Merson, M. H., Reddy, K. S, Rodriguez, M. H., Sewankambo, N. K., Wasserheit, J. N., & Consortium of Universities for Global Health Executive Board. (2009). Towards a common definition of global health. *The Lancet, 373*(9679), 1993–1995. https://doi.org/10.1016/S0140-6736(09)60332-9

Médecins Sans Frontières. (n.d.). *Haemorrhagic fevers*. MSF International. https://www.msf.org/ebola

O'Neill, J. (2016). *Tackling drug-resistant infections globally: Final report and recommendations*. The Review on Antimicrobial Resistance. https://amr-review.org

Reid, T. R. (2009). *The healing of America: A global quest for better, cheaper, and fairer health care*. Penguin Press.

Rural Health Information Hub. (2024). *Rural health disparities*. https://www.ruralhealthinfo.org/topics/rural-health-disparities

United Nations Development Programme. (2024). *Sustainable development goals*. https://www.undp.org/sustainable-development-goals

U.S. Office of Disease Prevention and Health Promotion. (2024). *Healthy People 2030*. https://odphp.health.gov/our-work/national-health-initiatives/healthy-people/healthy-people-2030

Victora, C. G., Barreto, M. L., do Carmo Leal, M., Monteiro, C. A., Schmidt, M. I., Paim, J., Bastos, F. I., Almeida, C., Bahia, L., Travassos, C., Reichenheim, M., Barros, F. C., & *Lancet* Brazil Series Working Group. (2011). Health conditions and health-policy innovations in Brazil: The way forward. *The Lancet, 377*(9782), 2042–2053. https://doi.org/10.1016/S0140-6736(11)60055-X

World Health Organization. (2010). *Monitoring the building blocks of health systems: A handbook of indicators and their measurement strategies*. https://iris.who.int/bitstream/handle/10665/258734/9789241564052-eng.pdf

World Health Organization. (2017). *WHO Health Emergencies Programme: Strengthening global preparedness and response to health emergencies*.

World Health Organization. (2021a). *Noncommunicable diseases*. https://www.who.int/news-room/fact-sheets/detail/noncommunicable-diseases

World Health Organization. (2021b). *World malaria report 2021*. WHO. https://www.who.int

World Health Organization. (2022). *Rwanda's primary health care strategy improves access to essential and life-saving health services*. https://extranet.who.int/uhcpartnership/story/rwandas-primary-health-care-strategy-improves-access-essential-and-life-saving-health

CHAPTER 2

GLOBAL HEALTH

Thomas Foley

INTRODUCTION

On November 15, 2022, the world's population reached 8 billion (United Nations [UN], n.d.). Keeping the ever-growing global population healthy involves monitoring key health outcome data such as morbidity and mortality from communicable and noncommunicable diseases (NCDs), infant and maternal mortality, life expectancy at birth, and the incidences of mental health disorders. Monitoring where and why these outcomes differ, such as within and between countries and regions worldwide, is essential to understanding the **etiology** (causes) of preventable morbidity and premature mortality. Socioeconomic, environmental, behavioral, and political determinants of health significantly impact these key health outcomes. Utilizing the work of **epidemiologists**, who study the occurrence and distribution of health and disease and the factors that influence health and disease, allows evidence to guide decisions intended to improve healthcare systems, health promotion programs, and public health policy and infrastructure.

COMMUNICABLE AND NONCOMMUNICABLE DISEASES

OVERVIEW

The global population is aging. In 2000, older adults (adults 65 years or older) accounted for less than 7% of the world's population. By 2023, 10% of the global population was 65 or older. It is estimated that by 2050, 16.5% of the world's population will be 65 or older, which means that the percentage of the total population that older adults account for will more than double between the start of the 21st century and 2050 (UN Data Portal, n.d.). The demographic transition to an older population is accompanied by a shift in the leading causes of morbidity (disease) and mortality (death). As nations develop and people live longer, there is a decrease in morbidity and mortality from communicable diseases and an increase in morbidity and mortality from chronic (long-lasting) **noncommunicable diseases**.

NONCOMMUNICABLE DISEASES

NCDs are long-lasting diseases that aren't directly transmitted from one person to another. NCDs are often slow in their development and not caused by acute (short-duration) infections (Pan American Health Organization [PAHO], 2022). Globally, NCDs are the leading cause of mortality. They cause more than 41 million deaths per year and approximately three out of four deaths worldwide. The NCDs that cause the most mortality from a global perspective are cardiovascular diseases (such as heart disease and stroke), chronic obstructive pulmonary disease (COPD), lung cancer, Alzheimer disease, diabetes mellitus, chronic kidney disease, and colorectal cancer. Cardiovascular diseases are the number one cause of global mortality, resulting in more than 17 million deaths per year (Piovani et al., 2022). Refer to Figure 2.1 for a list of the leading causes of global mortality.

High-income countries experience greater mortality from NCDs due to a decrease in mortality from communicable diseases and **neonatal** (newborn) disorders, an increase in life expectancy,

FIGURE 2.1 World Health Organization leading causes of global mortality in 2000, 2019, and 2021.

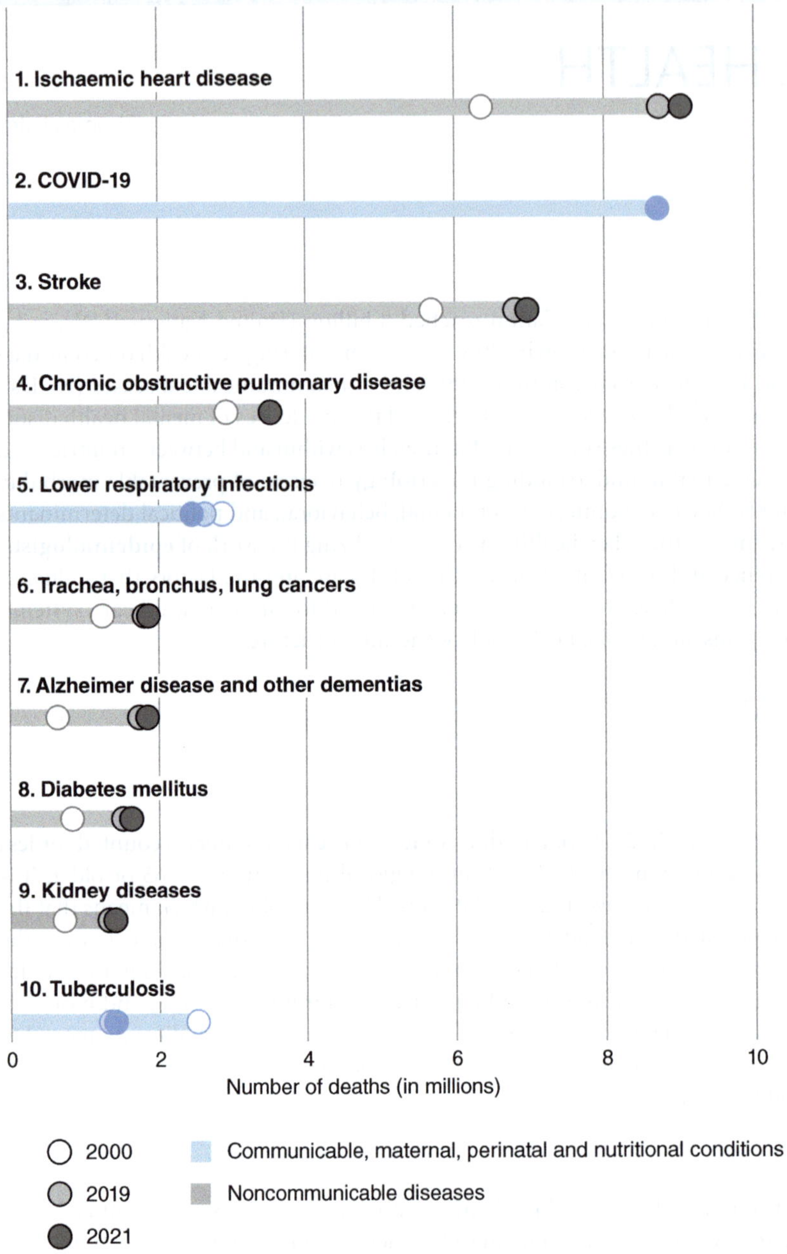

Source: World Health Organization. (2024). *The top 10 causes of death*. https://www.who.int/news-room/fact-sheets/detail/the-top-10-causes-of-death

and the health transition. The **health transition** is the societal shift from a high level of physical activity to increased sedentariness (too much time being seated) and from traditional, well-balanced whole food diets to highly processed, calorie-dense, and nutrient-deficient diets. The health transition occurs along with the **demographic transition**, which is the shift from a younger to an older population, and the **epidemiologic transition**, which is a shift from communicable to NCD mortality. As the world develops, the global community should expect increased mortality from NCDs; however, much of the global morbidity and mortality burden from NCDs is preventable.

It is estimated that approximately 80% of the burden from several common NCDs, such as cardiovascular disease and diabetes, is preventable. Addressing the underlying causes of NCDs is of the utmost importance, including among low- and middle-income countries that are beginning to undergo aging and experiencing rapid increases in incidences of preventable NCDs (Piovani et al., 2022).

Tertiary prevention (i.e., treating) of NCDs is expensive and places immense stress on individuals; families; and local, country, regional, and global healthcare systems. Global public health needs to emphasize **primary prevention** (preventing the onset) that addresses the socioeconomic, environmental, and behavioral aspects of NCD development. Effective global health promotion that intervenes on the following behavioral risk factors would significantly decrease the incidences of NCDs (Piovani et al., 2022):

- tobacco use
- unhealthy diets
- alcohol abuse
- physical inactivity

Several biological markers, which are highly correlated with the aforementioned health behaviors, are among the leading global morbidity and mortality risk factors (Institute for Health Metrics and Evaluation [IHME], n.d.), including hypertension (chronic high blood pressure), hyperglycemia (high blood sugar), hypercholesterolemia (high cholesterol), and high body mass index (BMI). Healthcare providers, in collaboration with public health, play an important role in mitigating the prevalence of NCDs through **secondary prevention** efforts, which include screenings for early detection and subsequent health education, lifestyle, and pharmaceutical interventions to abate disease progression.

COMMUNICABLE DISEASES

Communicable diseases are infectious diseases considered contagious or capable of being transmitted from one individual or species to another (Pennsylvania Department of Health, n.d.). Examples of communicable diseases include COVID-19, influenza (flu), measles, tuberculosis, syphilis, HIV, dengue, malaria, polio, cholera, and shingles. While the global morbidity and mortality from common communicable diseases have declined over the past several decades, they still pose a tremendous threat to global health and well-being and disproportionately affect less developed regions and lower-income countries around the world. In much of Africa, particularly West Africa, communicable diseases such as malaria, HIV, diarrheal diseases, and tuberculosis are among the leading causes of mortality. Some countries are regional exceptions, such as Haiti in the Caribbean, that are less developed economically and have greater communicable disease morbidity and mortality when compared to other nations within their region (UN Data Portal, n.d.). In addition, novel communicable disease outbreaks such as COVID-19, a dearth of adequate resources in highly susceptible regions, and alarming unvaccinated rates, particularly among children, are cause for grave concern for the entire global community. Continued innovation, surveillance, prevention, and preparedness are necessary to prevent future **pandemics** (global outbreaks) and mitigate the frequency and effects of epidemics (regional outbreaks).

LIFE EXPECTANCY

As the global population ages, there have been significant gains in **life expectancy at birth**; that is, the average number of years a newborn can expect to live. Before 1955, global life expectancy at birth was less than 50 years. By 2000, global life expectancy at birth was 66.43 years. In 2023, life expectancy at birth was 73.17 years, an increase of nearly 7 years since the start of the 21st century and more than 23 years since the mid-20th century (UN Data Portal, n.d.).

While life expectancy at birth is improving worldwide, there are significant intercountry and interregional life expectancy disparities (UN Data Portal, n.d.). Refer to Table 2.1 for a list of global and regional life expectancies at birth during 2000 and 2023. Less-developed regions and low-income countries with higher incidences of mortality from communicable diseases and NCDs and higher infant and maternal rates experience lower life expectancy. The countries with the highest life expectancy at birth during 2023 were Monaco (Europe) with an average of 86.37 years, San Marino (Europe) with an average of 85.71 years, Japan (East Asia) with an average of 84.71 years, South Korea (East Asia) with an average of 84.33 years, and Saint Barthelemy (Caribbean) with an average of 84.29 years. The countries with the lowest life expectancy at birth during 2023 were Nigeria (West Africa) with an average of 54.46 years, Chad (Middle Africa) with an average of 55.07 years, Lesotho (Southern Africa) with an average of 57.34 years, Central African Republic (Middle Africa) with an average of 57.41 years, and South Sudan (Middle Africa) with an average of 57.62 years.

It is disheartening to see a gap of more than 30 years of life expectancy at birth between Monaco and Nigeria. Understanding where and why low life expectancy occurs is essential to addressing global health disparities and promoting global health equity. The etiology of life expectancy disparities is multifaceted and rooted in historical injustices that manifest into present-day socioeconomic, environmental, and behavioral determinants of health. The chapters of this book will delve deeper into why there are such drastic differences between the regions and countries of the world.

TABLE 2.1 GLOBAL AND REGIONAL LIFE EXPECTANCY AT BIRTH (IN YEARS) DURING 2000 AND 2023

REGION	LIFE EXPECTANCY IN 2000	LIFE EXPECTANCY IN 2023
North America	77.04	79.64
Oceania	75.22	79.15
Europe	73.44	79.06
East Asia	73.20	78.89
South America	70.68	76.21
West Asia	70.04	75.41
Central America	71.59	74.96
World	66.43	73.17
Caribbean	69.33	73.13
Central Asia	64.41	72.63
Southeast Asia	67.40	72.13
North Africa	66.43	71.99
South Asia	62.78	71.70
Southern Africa	57.31	65.95
East Africa	51.23	65.59
Middle Africa	50.80	62.02
West Africa	49.83	58.25

Source: Adapted from UN Data Portal. (n.d.). *UN population division data portal*. United Nations. https://population.un.org/dataportal/home/

INFANT AND MATERNAL MORTALITY

Improved maternal and child healthcare has been paramount to gains in life expectancy at birth. While infant and maternal health have improved across the world, significant intercountry and regional disparities still exist. Less developed regions and low-income countries that experience higher rates of communicable disease morbidity and mortality and lower life expectancy at birth also have higher maternal mortality ratios and infant mortality rates.

The **maternal mortality ratio (MMR)** is the number of maternal deaths per 100,000 live births (UN Population Fund, 2025). In 2020, the global MMR was 223.5 maternal deaths per 100,000 live births. In North America, during 2020, the MMR was 20.2 maternal deaths per 100,000 live births. In West Africa, the MMR was 754 maternal deaths per 100,000 live births. The countries with the highest MMRs during 2020 were from West and Middle Africa: South Sudan (1,225), Chad (1,063), and Nigeria (1,047). The countries with the lowest MMRs were in Europe: Belarus (1.1), Norway (1.7), and Poland (2).

The **infant mortality rate (IMR)** is the number of infant deaths (before the first birthday) per 1,000 live births. In 2023, the global IMR was 27.3 infant deaths per 1,000 live births. Compared to the start of the 21st century, IMR worldwide has declined by nearly 50%. In 2000, the global IMR was 53.7 infant deaths per 1,000 live births. Regionally, Europe has an exceptionally low IMR. In 2023, Europe's IMR was 3.4 infant deaths per 1,000 live births. Although the IMR in West Africa has significantly decreased over the past several decades, it remains extremely high. In 2023, West Africa's IMR was 60.3 infant deaths per 1,000 live births (UN Data Portal, n.d.). Refer to Table 2.2 for a list of global and regional IMRs during 2000 and 2023. The countries with the lowest IMRs

TABLE 2.2 GLOBAL AND REGIONAL INFANT MORTALITY RATES (PER 1,000 LIVE BIRTHS) DURING 2000 AND 2023

REGION	INFANT MORTALITY RATE IN 2000	INFANT MORTALITY RATE IN 2023
Europe	8.5	3.4
East Asia	26.2	5.1
North America	7.0	5.2
Central America	25.9	11.5
South America	26.9	12.3
Central Asia	47.5	14.3
Oceania	23.8	15.4
Western Asia	33.8	17
Southeast Asia	36.8	18
North Africa	43.7	21.1
World	*53.7*	*27.3*
Caribbean	40.2	27.5
South Asia	66.9	29
Southern Africa	49.1	29.2
East Africa	86.6	35.9
Middle Africa	101.8	50.4
West Africa	101.1	60.3

Source: Adapted from UN Data Portal (n.d.). *UN population division data portal*. United Nations. https://population.un.org/dataportal/home/

during 2023 were Iceland (Europe) with 1.0 IMR, San Marino (Europe) with 1.1 IMR, Cayman Islands (Caribbean) with 1.1 IMR, Estonia (Europe) with 1.4 IMR, and Japan (East Asia) with 1.6 IMR. The countries with the highest IMRs during 2023 were Sierra Leone (West Africa) with 71.6 IMR, Nigeria (West Africa) with 69.5 IMR, Central African Republic (Middle Africa) with 68.5 IMR, Somalia (East Africa) with 66.3 IMR, and Guinea (West Africa) with 65.4 IMR.

Continued development of maternal and child healthcare, particularly in rural and low-income regions worldwide, is essential to promoting global health equity by decreasing disparities in IMR, MMR, and life expectancy at birth. Socioeconomic conditions such as access to education and healthcare and equal rights for women are key underlying causes that must be integrated into tailored, community-driven interventions focusing on improving maternal and child healthcare. One example is *Kay Manmito,* Haitian Creole for Mother's House, at the University Hospital in Mirebalais, Haiti. **Kay Manmito** serves women with at-risk pregnancies and provides free maternal–child health education, resources like food and blankets, and a kangaroo care center. **Kangaroo care** promotes skin-to-skin contact between mothers and infants, especially important for babies with preterm and low birth weight (Partners in Health, 2018). However, political instability and the resulting violence in Haiti threaten the ability of healthcare facilities, such as Kay Manmito, to operate and serve women and infants in need.

MENTAL HEALTH

Mental health is the state of an individual's cognitive, behavioral, and emotional well-being and ability to function within the social environment (World Health Organization [WHO], 2022). There is a growing need to expand the mental healthcare infrastructure on a global scale as awareness about mental health increases. Approximately 14% of the global population experienced a mental health disorder in 2021. Countries with the highest age-standardized rates of mental health disorders were Portugal, Iran, and Lebanon (IHME, n.d.) On a global scale, common mental health disorders are depression, anxiety, schizophrenia, bipolar, and suicidal ideation (WHO, 2022).

While there are efforts to standardize the diagnoses of mental illnesses, mental health is profoundly influenced by social context. Best practices in mental healthcare call for more community-based mental healthcare that utilizes the strengths of communities and the individuals within communities. Building strong social and mental healthcare infrastructure across the world, as well as addressing the socioeconomic and behavioral factors that influence mental health, are necessary to mitigate the global incidences of mental health disorders.

SUMMARY

The world's population is rapidly aging, which has resulted in NCDs being the leading causes of death worldwide. Much of the morbidity and mortality caused by NCDs is preventable. Health policies and health promotion programs that intervene on tobacco use, sedentariness, alcohol abuse, and poor nutrition can result in significant mitigation of preventable NCDs. While communicable diseases and maternal and infant mortality are declining worldwide, low-income countries and less-developed regions experience higher rates of communicable disease morbidity and mortality and infant and maternal mortality. Mental health is also growing as a global concern, likely due to increased awareness of its importance and the lack of mental healthcare infrastructure across the world.

The chapters of this book explore these key health outcomes, along with their determinants, in great depth in order to promote a better understanding as to where and why health disparities occur and what needs to be done to ameliorate global health. In addition to chapters that focus on specific regions and countries across the world, this book contains chapters that focus on specific topics such as communicable diseases and mental health.

LEARNING ACTIVITIES

CourseConnect

To access self-assessment questions and interactive, competency-based learning activities for this chapter, visit www.springerpub.com/courseconnect. See inside front cover and tear-out for CourseConnect details.

REFERENCES

Institute for Health Metrics and Evaluation. (n.d.). *Health research by location: Country profiles.* University of Washington. https://www.healthdata.org/research-analysis/health-by-location/profiles

Pan American Health Organization. (2022). *Noncommunicable diseases.* https://www.paho.org/en/topics/noncommunicable-diseases

Partners in Health. (2018). *New maternal waiting home in Haiti offers "priceless" care.* https://www.pih.org/article/new-maternal-waiting-home-haiti-offers-priceless-care

Pennsylvania Department of Health. (n.d.). *Communicable diseases.* https://www.pa.gov/agencies/health/health-statistics/communicable-diseases.html

Piovani, D., Nikolopoulos, G. K., & Bonovas, S. (2022). Non-communicable diseases: The invisible epidemic. *Journal of Clinical Medicine, 11*(9), 5939. https://doi.org/10.3390/jcm11195939

UN Data Portal. (n.d.). *UN population division data portal.* https://population.un.org/dataportal/home/

United Nations. (n.d.). *Global issues: Population.* https://www.un.org/en/global-issues/population

United Nations Population Fund. (2025). *Trends in maternal mortality 2000–2023: Estimates by WHO, UNICEF, UNFPA, World Bank Group and UNDESA/population division.* https://www.unfpa.org/publications/trends-maternal-mortality-2000-2023

World Health Organization. (2022). *Mental disorders.* https://www.who.int/news-room/fact-sheets/detail/mental-disorders

CHAPTER 3

GLOBAL DETERMINANTS OF HEALTH

Kathleen Visovatti Weaver

INTRODUCTION

When one thinks about maintaining a good health status or seeking help for a health condition or problem, one generally thinks about services from a clinic or hospital in the healthcare system. We tend to think that having health insurance is the answer to staying healthy or getting healthy. However, there are other factors that reside internal and external to the healthcare system that determine one's health and which can have an equal or greater impact on whether someone stays healthy or becomes healthier. Those factors or determinants are known as health determinants.

Some of the health determinant elements can have more of an impact on a person's health than other elements do. Some health determinant elements may have less effect on whether a person becomes unhealthy, stays healthy, or improves their health; some have a combining influence to impact health (Knickman & Elbel, 2019); and some are modifiable, and others are not.

This chapter explains the five health determinants and how they influence staying healthy, can cause someone to be unhealthy, or how making changes in a health determinant's elements can improve health over time.

Through this discussion we will consider how the health determinants contribute to healthy or unhealthy conditions. However, before we delve into the discussion of the health determinants, we first want to review how we define "health" to gain an understanding of how various health determinant elements impact the definitions and understanding of health.

REVIEW DEFINITION OF "HEALTH"

"Health starts in our homes, schools, workplaces, neighborhoods, and communities" (U.S. Department of Health and Human Services, 2018). There are both intrinsic factors and extrinsic factors to one's body that affect one's health status (Jacobsen, 2019, p. 3). An intrinsic factor can be the genes a person inherits. An extrinsic factor can be an acquired bacterial or viral infection, or one's work environment, or where one lives, and one's income in order to afford to buy healthy food.

The important consideration, though, is how we determine or define a person's health status. The World Health Organization (WHO) defines health as, "a resource for every day life. . . . Health is a positive concept emphasizing social and personal resources, as well as physical capacities" (1986). It is important to focus on the word "resource" in this definition. Consider as well WHO's gold-standard definition for health: "Health is a state of complete physical, mental, and social well-being and not merely the absence of disease or infirmity" (1948–1986). The *Merriam-Webster Dictionary* (n.d.) applies terms like "fitness," "wholesomeness," and "wellness." Other sources define health as having the ability to perform daily activities, feel well, free from disease, have optimal functioning, or being a dynamic balance. The *Mosby Medical Dictionary* goes beyond those definitions and states that health is not static, it constantly changes, and it seeks homeostasis (Mosby, 2009). Finally, the Institute of Medicine defines health as, "a state that allows the individual to adequately cope with all demands of daily life; a balance, an equilibrium" (Sartorius, 2006).

So, taking into consideration those various definitions of health, what if someone lives with an amputated limb and also qualifies for the para-Olympics; is that individual considered "unhealthy" because of their limb amputation? Or, if someone is designated legally blind, yet is gainfully employed by a high-tech company, works out every day with a personal trainer, and has a good body mass index, would we still classify that individual as "unhealthy" due to their physical blindness? Therefore, it is relevant to consider not just the physical condition of a person to decide if they are healthy or unhealthy but to remember the other definitions of health or being healthy. Thus, we need to consider by whose standards is someone considered to be in a state of "well-being" or "healthy" or "not healthy"? Is it only the biological elements which determine a state of being healthy?

WHAT IS A "DETERMINANT?"

Before we study the elements that compose the five health determinants, we first need to consider what is a "determinant." Why do we refer to certain factors as determinants of health? A determinant is something that contributes to an outcome, whether that outcome is related to health status, financial status, or education status. It is that thing, that element, or that factor that determines, causes, is the source of, or influences how somethings or someone will function. For health, it is those factors, intrinsic or extrinsic, to a person's daily life which determine whether or not they stay healthy.

WHY STUDY HEALTH DETERMINANTS?

The health determinants make a difference in a person's life, health, and lifespan. They also impact the health and economic status of a country. In 2022, the United States spent $4.5 trillion on healthcare, which is about 17.3 % of the gross domestic product (GDP; Hartman et al., 2023). The average cost of healthcare per person in the United States is about $13,500 (American Medical Association, 2024). Thus, we want to zero in on and understand how the health determinant elements play a role not just in a person's health and health status; we also want to understand how they impact the healthcare system in a country, how the finance of a country is affected, how the social culture contributes to health, why people die prematurely, and why there are many factors beyond diseases and infections which influence a country's healthcare system and the health of its population. We also want to control how much of the country's total GDP is spent on health so that some of that money can be devoted to a country's infrastructure, education, and national security.

Each health determinant, both individually and collectively, affects the health of each citizen in every country. Each health determinant also affects their life expectancy. Thus, the health of the population impacts how well a country's healthcare system will function. The health determinant elements influence how an individual or a population can stay healthy or become ill, injured, or experience an untimely death. According to the Centers for Disease Control and Prevention in 2022, life expectancy at birth in the United States was estimated to be approximately 77.5 years (Rakshit et al., 2025). "The average life expectancy at birth among comparable countries was 82.5 years in 2023" (Rakshit, 2025).

WHAT ARE THE FIVE HEALTH DETERMINANTS?

The five health determinants (Figure 3.1) are

- biological determinants,
- behavioral determinants,
- social determinants,
- environmental determinants (sometimes referred to the physical environment), and
- access determinants (Turnock, 1997, 2020).

FIGURE 3.1 Categories of health determinants and macrodeterminants.

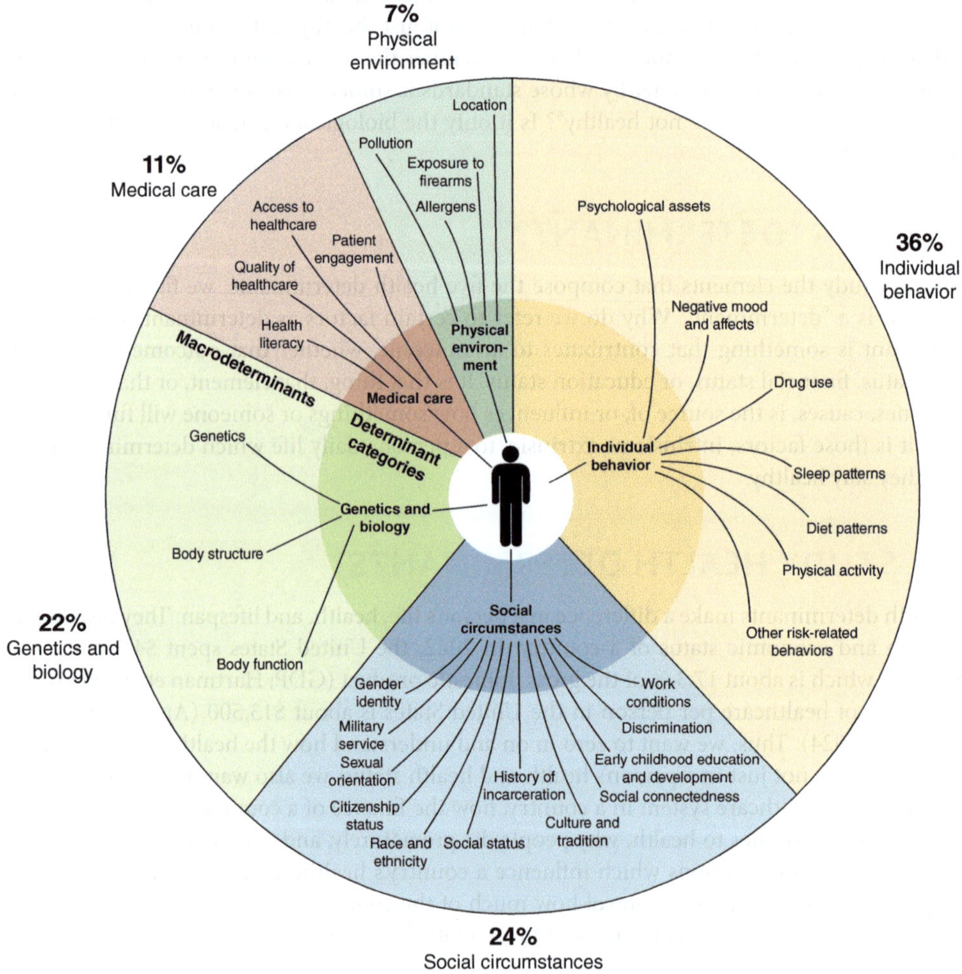

Source: Choi, E. (n.d.). *Determinants of health*. https://www.edchoi.com/assets/home/home_doh.jpg

BIOLOGICAL OR BODY DETERMINANTS

The elements that make up the biological determinant are: (a) microorganisms which cause the body to misfunction; (b) products such as vaccines and medications, which either protect the body or help to treat, cure, or relieve pain; (c) "good" bacteria in a symbiotic relationship with the human body; (d) genes which are inherited; and (e) age, race, and gender.

The elements categorized in the biological determinant are associated with approximately 20% of premature deaths. In other words, if some of the elements were controlled, less of the population would die at a younger age. "The three primary biological determinants that play a role in the health and illness of individuals are race, sex, and age" (Kyruus Health, 2022). Although there is no medical or human control over the race, age, genetics, and gender biological elements, there are other biological determinant elements which can affect one's health and life expectancy.

For some diseases, regular vaccinations or taking prescribed medication correctly can enhance one's health under the biological health determinant. Vaccinations or medications can possibly prevent an early death due to diseases and infections. However, in some developing countries of the world, neither vaccines nor medications are available in sufficient quantities to impact health status and prevent early deaths.

Application of Biological Health Determinants

An example of the biological health determinant impacting the health of a population is HIV/AIDS. It has a high incidence of occurrence and death in places like the sub-Saharan African countries of Botswana, Zimbabwe, Kenya, and Zambia (Goliber, 2002; World Factbook, 2022). Its occurrence is also due to the behavioral health determinant exhibited in certain sexual practices and professions.

BEHAVIORAL DETERMINANTS

The basic elements that define the behavioral determinant are: (a) substance use (e.g., alcohol, tobacco, drugs); (b) sexual behaviors; (c) risk taking (e.g., such as not wearing a seat belt or bike helmet); (d) nutrition (e.g., eating habits, food consumption); (e) physical activity; and (f) handwashing.

The elements associated with the behavioral determinants can account for 50% of premature deaths. "One study concluded that approximately 40% of all deaths in the United States are associated with four health behaviors: tobacco use, unhealthy diet, physical inactivity, and problem drinking (Committee on Population, 2015; National Library of Medicine, n.d.). That means the choices a person makes regarding certain lifestyle behaviors could determine how long they live. A person's behavior is determined by how they live or function in their daily life and by what a person values and what they believe, such as use of seat belts.

There are behaviors known as consumption behaviors like smoking, excessive alcohol use, overuse of prescribed or illicit drugs, or poor nutritional decisions, any one of which could negatively impact a person's health.

Other classifications of the behavior determinant elements are physical behavior and safety behavior. Someone who is very sedentary every day and has limited physical activity could become less healthy. An example of a safety behavior is a parent who owns a gun and does not make sure the gun is locked away from their child's access.

These are just some of the behaviors that are elements in the behavior health determinant, which determine one's health status, whether they stay healthy, become healthy, develop a chronic health condition like diabetes, or die prematurely.

Some behaviors are influenced by the social health determinant elements because a person's culture or financial situation influences how they behave, what they eat, or purchasing decisions such as a bike helmet. Some behaviors are influenced by the biological health determinant elements (gender) because the person is a man and "macho men" do not wear seatbelts or do not wear a helmet on a bike. Another behavior may be avoiding any type of vaccinations, which is an element of the biological health determinant. The avoidance may be due to fear, or culture (the social determinant), or inability to find a healthcare provider (access determinant).

Application of Behavioral Health Determinants

"Tobacco smoking is one of the world's largest health problems today" (Ritchie & Roser, 2023). Both the Asian and European countries experience the highest number of deaths (globally) due to smoking tobacco (Ritchie & Roser, 2023). Smoking behavior has an impact on the biological health determinant as exhibited by increased cardiovascular diseases such as strokes and heart attacks and in lung diseases like congestive obstructive pulmonary disease (COPD) and lung cancer. According to research, approximately "8.7 million people (globally) die prematurely from tobacco use every year" (Ritchie & Roser, 2023). Smoking behavior in China is also associated with their culture of patriotism as the Chinese believe smoking benefits their economy (Xing et al., 2023). Both elements of culture and economy are examples of social health determinants that impact health. Therefore, a single health determinant, such as behavioral health, does not affect health alone.

SOCIAL DETERMINANTS

The many elements of the social determinants of health (SDOH) are: (a) family structure; (b) social networks; (c) social roles; (d) work setting; (e) income; (f) culture; (g) crime; (h) education; (i) housing; (j) values and beliefs; and (k) policies.

According to WHO, "social determinants (of health), are the conditions in which people are born, grow, live, work, and age that are shaped by the distribution of money, power, and resources at [the] global, national, and local levels" (Holtz, 2022). The SDOH, together with the physical environment determinants, can contribute to 20% of premature deaths.

Any one of the SDOH elements by itself can have a positive or negative effect on health, staying healthy, or trying to become healthier. Health begins with the SDOH, which are where one lives, studies, plays, and works—both the type of work and the safe environment of work. To understand the impact of the SDOH, one needs to adjust the preconception that health begins and ends in the healthcare system. Each of the SDOH elements influences how a country, a district, and a local government allocates their financial resources and are instrumental in achieving a nation's, a state's, a community's goals for health, education, and well-being. Being healthy begins with the social determinant elements in combination with the biological, behavioral, and environmental determinants.

Application of Social Determinants

People who have a quality education have a better chance to stay healthy and live longer (Tulane University, 2021). For example, Israel has a 98% literacy rate and a life expectancy of 82 years, versus India with a 71% literacy rate and life expectancy of 68 years. Such facts support the concept that a person who is better educated may live longer (Johnson et al., 2018).

ENVIRONMENTAL DETERMINANT

The environmental health determinants (EHD) relates to the physical conditions that surround the body, support the body, or impact the body such as: (a) housing stability; (b) air and water quality and water availability; (c) safety; (d) toxic substances including pesticides and electronic waste; (e) urban versus rural living, (f) design of vehicles and roadways; (g) sanitation; and (h) climate change.

"Threats to any one of the EHDs can have an adverse impact on health and well-being at the population level" (Pan American Health Organization & World Health Organization, n.d.). Some threats in the environment are naturally occurring; some occur because of social conditions and how a population lives.

Some dwellings are safe, others are affected by germ-carrying rodents and bug infestations. In some countries and in American cities with homeless populations, the dwellings are made of cardboard or are flimsy tents. The lack of cleanliness, security, and safety of a dwelling can provide a living environment that has a negative impact on the inhabitants' health.

In many communities and villages around the world, including even in developed countries, the air and water quality are below standard, and the access to any life-sustaining quantity of water is difficult. Some communities experience toxic fumes from industrial plants or industrial contaminants leaking into the air or underground water systems, negatively impacting the air and water environments. Other communities are located near toxic chemical or electronic waste dumps which can affect air, water, and safety quality.

For some rural areas, paved road construction is limited causing hazardous driving conditions. In other communities, the excess in the number of vehicles on the roadways increases the environmental safety for everyone.

Application of Environmental Health Determinants

Contaminated food, lack of proper sanitation, and/or poor quality of drinking water cause significant diarrheal diseases and many child deaths and illness globally, mostly in South Asia and sub-Saharan Africa (UNICEF, 2021). "In 2020, around one in four people lacked safely managed drinking water in their homes and nearly half the world's population lacked safely managed sanitation" (UNICEF, 2021). In developing, low-income countries, many children under the age of 3 years have multiple episodes of diarrhea every year (UNICEF, 2024) caused by bacteria, viruses, and parasites mostly from contaminated water. These data demonstrate a combination of the EHD, the biological health determinants, and the social health determinants affecting health status.

ACCESS DETERMINANT

The access to care health determinant elements are: (a) availability of hospitals, clinics, and health personnel; (b) affordability; (c) insurance; (d) technology; (e) spoken language; (f) location of services; (g) time of services; (h) treatments and screenings; and (i) prevention.

Various studies have demonstrated that "medical care played a relatively minor role in reducing early deaths, accounting for only 10% of premature deaths" (Committee on Population, 2015). Unlike the elements of the behavioral health determinant, which can contribute 40% to 50% of premature death, accessing healthcare services contributes the least to overall premature death rates.

The access-to-care health determinant is dependent on many other systems, such as the financial system, insurance system, higher education system, and government system, all of which influence how or where one receives healthcare services. The education system can determine how many people receive an education to practice in the healthcare system. The government system of policymaking can determine how much government funding supports services in the healthcare system.

The access determinant covers many aspects of receiving healthcare. Access to care is affected by the cost to deliver care. This cost is not the same as the charges to the patient; rather, it is the money that goes into providing care given by a hospital or a clinic. It includes the salaries of the healthcare providers; the cost of the equipment used in exams and in treatments (like x-ray and MRI machines); the upkeep on hospital and clinic buildings (maintenance); the electricity, cooling and heating of the building; the water; and general supplies, like needles and exam gloves. So, if cost is a limiting factor for a healthcare provider, then some types of healthcare services may not be made available to the patients.

Regardless of insurance coverage, ensuring that access to care is financially sustainable for the patient is essential to achieving equitable health outcomes. If someone has health insurance, then the insurance company pays for part of the charges incurred by the patient. If the patient does not have health insurance, then the patient must have money to pay for the healthcare services provided. If the patient does not have adequate income to pay for healthcare, then they may decide not to seek healthcare, which is also an access to care issue.

As well, access to healthcare is affected by the location of healthcare services. In some rural areas, healthcare services are limited or nonexistent. Such areas are referred to as medically underserved areas (MUA). There may be general family doctors in rural areas, but healthcare specialists, like a cardiologist or surgeon, may be only in the large metropolitan areas, which then limits access to care for the person living in a rural area.

Access to healthcare is influenced by culture and by spoken languages. Some cultures require a woman to be examined only by a woman healthcare provider. Some cultures believe in extraordinary providers who practice non-Western medicine. If that type of provider is not available, then access to care is not possible. If English is the only language spoken in a hospital or clinic, then someone who does not understand or cannot communicate in English may not be able to completely access healthcare services at that hospital or clinic. Thus, the SDOH elements can combine with the access-to-healthcare determinant which impact how a person receives healthcare services.

A social determinant that interacts with the access-to-care determinant is the level of education of the person needing healthcare services. If the person is unable to read, then they may not know how or when to access care, or what kind of care is provided at what hospital or clinic. It is also the person's perception of what "access" means. Is their perception that they are delayed care because they believe they are experiencing discrimination? Or is their perception that they are denied care because they desire something different in healthcare?

Other factors impacting access to healthcare and the ability to pay for healthcare, are a low-paying job, limited benefits in a health insurance policy, high deductible in the health insurance policy, or lack of health insurance through an employer. These are the SDOH linked to income and, thus, impact and influence the access to health care determinant.

Finally, other factors, such as access to transportation (an element of SDOH) for individuals with handicaps, and health literacy (another element of SDOH) all figure into what correlates with the access to healthcare determinant. Many physical environmental barriers, such as lack of sidewalks to navigate a wheelchair, play a role in how a person receives healthcare or is limited in the healthcare they seek.

Application of Access Determinant

As presented, access can be understood from many aspects. Access can be affected by how much a government spends of their gross domestic product (GDP) on healthcare. For example, in countries like Egypt, 6.4% of their GDP is devoted to healthcare (Holtz, 2022); the United States spends 18% of GDP on health, and Cuba spends 11% of GDP on healthcare (Birn et al., 2017). Also, the national policy on whether access is a right or privilege to care and the type of health insurance affect access. France, the United Kingdom, and Canada's national policies dictate access to healthcare services is a **right** and provide universal insurance to all citizens, versus the United States, which considers access to healthcare services as a **privilege**, does not offer universal insurance.

CONCLUSION

"Although the determinant categories are listed independently, they have substantial and complex interactions over the life course of an individual or group" (Knickman & Elbel, 2019). It is imperative for every country, community, village, and all policymakers to think in tandem regarding the health determinants. No determinant is any more important than the other—each element of each determinant can impact how an element in another determinant will respond or function. If a person cannot read (SDOH), then they may not be able to read the medicine label on the prescribed medication (biological determinant) even though they were able to receive care at a clinic (access determinant). All health determinants collectively determine the health, morbidity, and early mortality of a country's population and, thus, health and morbidity globally.

LEARNING ACTIVITIES

CourseConnect

To access self-assessment questions and interactive, competency-based learning activities for this chapter, visit www.springerpub.com/courseconnect. See inside front cover and tear-out for CourseConnect details.

REFERENCES

American Medical Association. (2024, July 9). *Trends in health care spending*. https://www.ama-assn.org/about/research/trends-health-care-spending

Birn, A. E., Pillay, Y., & Holtz, T. H. (2017). *Textbook of global health* (4th ed.). Oxford University Press

Committee on Population. (2015, February 24). *Measuring the risks and causes of premature death: Summary of workshops*. U.S. Department of Health and Human Services, National Institutes of Health. https://www.ncbi.nlm.nih.gov/books/NBK279974

Goliber, T. (2002, July). *The status of the HIV/AIDS epidemic in sub-Saharan Africa*. Population Reference Bureau. https://www.prb.org/resources/the-status-of-the-hiv-aids-epidemic-in-sub-saharan-africa/

Hartman, M., Martin, A., Whittle, L., & Catlin, A. (2023, December 13) National health care spending in 2022: Growth similar to prepandemic rates. *Health Affairs, 43*(1), 6–17. https://doi.org/10.1377/hlthaff.2023.01360

Holtz, C. (2022). *Global health care: Issues and policies* (4th ed.). Jones and Bartlett Learning.

Jacobsen, K. H. (2019). *Introduction to global health*. Jones and Bartlett Learning.

Johnson, J., Stoskopf, C., & Shi, L. (2018). *Comparative health systems: A global perspective* (2nd ed.). Jones and Bartlett Learning.

Knickman, J. R., & Elbel, B. (Eds.). (2019). *Jonas & Kovner's health care delivery in the United States* (12th ed.). Springer Publishing Company. https://doi.org/10.1891/9780826172730

Kyruus Health. (2022). *Biological and physical determinants of health: Why they matter to providers*. https://kyruushealth.com/biological-and-physical-determinants-of-health/

Merriam-Webster. (n.d.). Fitness; wholesomeness; wellness. *Merriam-Webster.com dictionary*. https://www.merriam-webster.com/dictionary/health

Mosby, C. V. (2009). *Mosby's medical dictionary* (8th ed.). Scientific Research. https://www.scirp.org/reference/referencespapers?referenceid=2519759

National Library of Medicine. (n.d.). *Measuring the risks and cause of premature death: Summary of workshops*. https://www.ncbi.nlm.nih.gov/books/NBK279971/

Pan American Health Organization & World Health Organization. (n.d.). *Environmental determinants of health*. https://www.paho.org/en/topics/environmental-determinants-health

Rakshit, S., McGough, M., & Amin, K. (2024, January 30). *How does U.S. life expectancy compare to other countries?* Health Systems Tracker Kaiser Family Foundation. https://www.healthsystemtracker.org/chart-collection/u-s-life-expectancy-compare-countries/#Life%20expectancy%20at%20birth,%20in%20years,%201980-2022

Rakshit, S., McGough, M., Amin, K., (2025, January 31). How does U.S. life expectancy compare to other countries? Health Systems Tracker Kaiser Family Foundation. https://www.healthsystemtracker.org/chart-collection/u-s-life-expectancy-compare-countries/#Life%20expectancy%20at%20birth,%20in%20years,%201980-2023

Ritchie, H., & Roser, M. (2023). *Smoking*. Our World in Data. https://ourworldindata.org/smoking

Sartorius, N. (2006, August). The meanings of health and its promotion. *The Croatian Medical Journal, 47*(4), 662–664. PMID: 16909464; PMCID: PMC2080455.

Tulane University. (2021, January). *Education as a social determinant of health*. https://publichealth.tulane.edu/blog/social-determinant-of-health-education-is-crucial/

UNICEF. (2021). *Billions of people will lack access to safe water, sanitation and hygiene in 2030 unless progress quadruples—warns WHO, UNICEF*. https://www.unicef.org/press-releases/billions-people-will-lack-access-safe-water-sanitation-and-hygiene-2030-unless

UNICEF Data. (2024, January). *Diarrhoea*. https://data.unicef.org/topic/child-health/diarrhoeal-disease

U.S. Department of Health and Human Services. (2018). *Healthy People 2020*. https://www.slu.edu/law/health/2020-symposium/-pdf/social-determinants-of-health-healthy-people-2020.pdf

World Factbook. (2022). *HIV/AIDS—Adult prevalence rate*. Central Intelligence Agency. https://www.cia.gov/the-world-factbook/about/archives/2022/field/hiv-aids-adult-prevalence-rate/country-comparison

World Health Organization. (1948–1986). *Constitution*. https://apps.who.int/gb/bd/PDF/bd47/EN/constitution-en.pdf?ua=1

World Health Organization. (2024, March). *Diarrhoeal disease*. https://www.who.int/news-room/fact-sheets/detail/diarrhoeal-disease#:~:text=In%20low%2Dincome%20countries%2C%20children,to%20fall%20ill%20from%20diarrhoea

Xing, E., Dai, Z., Madar, A., Welding, K., Clegg Smith, K., & Cohen, J. E. (2023). The problematic use of cultural symbols on Chinese cigarette packs. *Tobacco Induced Diseases, 21*(May), 65. https://doi.org/10.18332/tid/162301

PART II: Health and Healthcare in North America

CHAPTER 4

OVERVIEW OF NORTH AMERICA

Anna Foucek Tresidder

INTRODUCTION

Understanding the health systems of North America necessitates a multifaceted exploration of its geography, history, population demographics, socioeconomic factors, and health outcomes. Comprising the United States, Canada, Mexico, and various territories, North America exhibits diverse dynamics that influence health at the individual, community, and national levels. North America is home to two distinct healthcare systems: the predominantly private system in the United States and the predominantly publicly funded systems in Mexico and Canada. Despite differences in organization and financing, these countries face similar challenges, including rising healthcare costs, access disparities, and the need for quality improvement.

GEOGRAPHY

North America is the third largest continent, covering approximately 24.7 million square kilometers (Figure 4.1). It extends from the Arctic region in the north to the Isthmus of Panama in the south, bordered by the Atlantic Ocean to the east and the Pacific Ocean to the west. Diverse landscapes, including the Rocky Mountains, the Great Plains, and extensive coastal regions characterize the continent. Major rivers like the Mississippi, Yukon, Rio Grande, and Colorado Rivers provide vital water resources and transportation routes. The geography of North America significantly influences its climate, ecosystems, and population distribution. The northern regions experience a polar climate, while the southern areas enjoy a tropical climate. This variation affects agricultural productivity, economic activities, and health outcomes in different regions (U.S. Geological Survey, 2025).

HISTORY

The history of North America is complex, marked by Indigenous cultures, European colonization, and the emergence of modern nation–states. Indigenous peoples, including the Navajo, Sioux, and Inuit, have inhabited the continent for centuries, developing rich cultures and societies. European exploration began in the late 15th century, culminating in the colonization of vast territories by Spain, France, and England.

The United States emerged as an independent nation in 1776, followed by Canada in 1867 and Mexico in 1821. The historical context of colonization, including the forced displacement of Indigenous peoples and the transatlantic slave trade, has had long-lasting impacts on the demographic and socioeconomic landscape of North America (Hofstadter, 2008). The legacy of colonialism continues to shape contemporary health disparities and access to healthcare among different populations. North America's history is marked by Indigenous civilizations, colonialism, and waves of immigration, which have shaped its social, political, and economic landscapes. The impact of colonization has had enduring effects on Indigenous health and well-being, including loss of land, cultural disruptions, and disparities in healthcare access. Understanding this historical context is essential for comprehending contemporary health disparities and inequities within the region.

FIGURE 4.1 Map of North America.

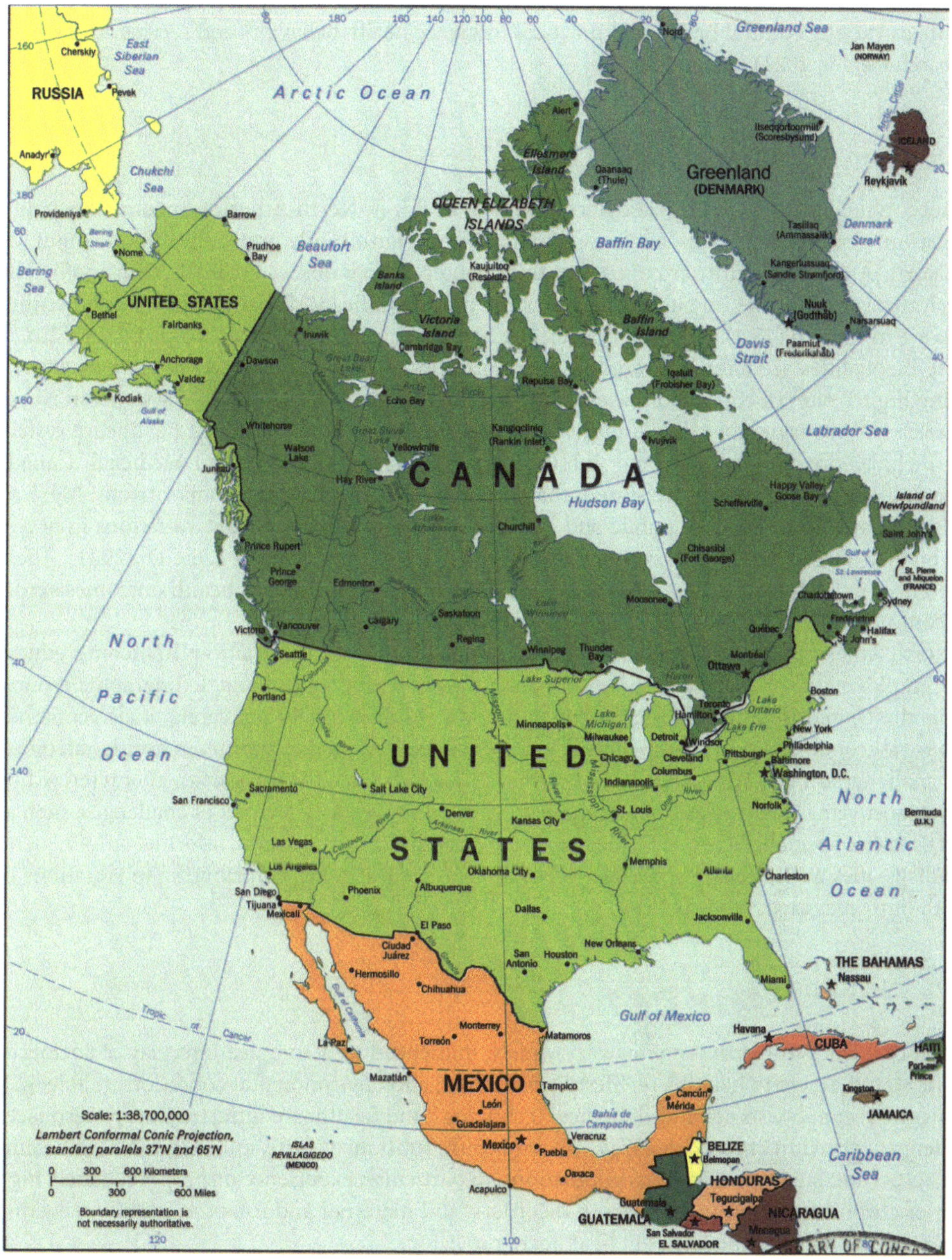

Source: U.S. Central Intelligence Agency. (1998). *North America*. https://www.loc.gov/item/99440663/

POPULATION

As of 2023, North America has an estimated population of over 579 million people, making it one of the most populous regions in the world (World Bank Group, 2023). The population is diverse, comprising a multitude of ethnicities, languages, and cultures. The United States is the most populous country, followed by Mexico and Canada. Population dynamics in North America are influenced by immigration, which plays a significant role in shaping cultural and demographic trends.

For instance, the United States and Canada have seen substantial immigration from Latin America, Asia, and Africa, contributing to multicultural societies. These demographic shifts affect public health, as varying cultural beliefs and practices influence health behaviors and service access (Pew Research Center, 2021).

SOCIOECONOMIC FACTORS

Socioeconomic factors are critical determinants of health in North America. Income inequality, education, employment status, and access to healthcare significantly impact health outcomes. Of the North American countries covered in this chapter we can observe that the Gini coefficient, which measures income inequality, indicates the most significant disparities in wealth distributions are in Mexico (45.4), the United States (41.5), and Canada (33.3; U.S. Census Bureau, 2022). These inequalities are often mirrored in health metrics, with marginalized populations experiencing higher rates of chronic diseases and lower life expectancies. Healthcare systems in North America vary considerably. The United States operates primarily on a mixed healthcare system that includes private insurance and public programs such as Medicare and Medicaid. Canada has a publicly funded healthcare system that provides universal coverage to its citizens. Mexico's healthcare system is a mix of public and private providers, with significant variations in access and quality (Organisation for Economic Co-operation and Development [OECD], 2021). These differences in healthcare access and financing contribute to disparities in health outcomes across the continent.

North America exhibits significant socioeconomic diversity, with variations in income, education, employment, and access to social services across different regions and demographic groups. While the United States boasts a high gross domestic product (GDP) per capita, it also contends with socioeconomic disparities, including income inequality, racial disparities in health outcomes, and challenges in accessing affordable healthcare. Canada's healthcare system, characterized by universal coverage, addresses some of these disparities but faces its own set of challenges, such as wait times for specialized services. Mexico grapples with issues of poverty, informal employment, and disparities in healthcare access between urban and rural areas, contributing to variations in health outcomes across the country.

HEALTH OUTCOMES

Health outcomes in North America vary widely, influenced by a complex interplay of socioeconomic status, access to healthcare, lifestyle behaviors, and environmental conditions (Table 4.1). While the region boasts advanced medical technology and healthcare infrastructure, it also faces challenges related to chronic diseases, mental health, substance abuse, and disparities in healthcare access and quality. Indigenous populations, in particular, experience disproportionately high rates of chronic diseases, mental health disorders, and maternal and infant mortality, reflecting historical and ongoing inequities in healthcare provision.

The United States has one of the highest rates of obesity globally, with approximately 36.2% of adults classified as obese (Centers for Disease Control and Prevention [CDC], 2024). This is linked to lifestyle factors, including diet and physical activity, which socioeconomic status influences. Mental health is another critical concern, exacerbated by social determinants such as poverty, unemployment, and social isolation. The prevalence of mental health disorders is rising, with only a fraction of those affected receiving adequate treatment (World Health Organization [WHO], 2022). Furthermore, Indigenous populations face unique health challenges, including higher rates of substance abuse and mental health disorders, often stemming from historical trauma and systemic inequities (Gameon & Skewes, 2021).

TABLE 4.1 HEALTH STATISTICS OF NORTH AMERICAN COUNTRIES

COUNTRY	LIFE EXPECTANCY AT BIRTH (YEARS)	INFANT MORTALITY RATE (PER 1,000 LIVE BIRTHS)	MATERNAL MORTALITY RATIO (PER 100,000 LIVE BIRTHS)	LEADING CAUSE OF MORTALITY
United States, Canada, and Mexico combined	76.4	11.5	47	Heart disease
United States	77.2	5.4	19	Heart disease
Canada	82.3	4.5	8	Cancer
Mexico	75.2	12.1	33	Diabetes

Sources: Centers for Disease Control and Prevention. (2023). *National vital statistics reports: Deaths, final data for 2022*. U.S. Department of Health and Human Services. https://www.cdc.gov/nchs/products/nvsr.htm; Government of Canada. (2023). *Life expectancy and mortality*. Statistics Canada. https://www.statcan.gc.ca/en/subjects-start/health/life_expectancy_and_deaths; Instituto Nacional de Estadística y Geografía. (2023). *Estadísticas de mortalidad en México* [Mortality statistics in Mexico]. https://www.inegi.org.mx/programas/mortalidad/; Pan American Health Organization. (2023). *Health in the Americas: Maternal and child health statistics*. https://www.paho.org/en/topics/child-health; United Nations Children's Fund. (2023). *State of the world's children 2023: Infant and maternal mortality statistics*. https://data.unicef.org/resources/sowc-2023/; World Health Organization. (2023). *Global health estimates: Leading causes of death*. https://www.who.int/data/gho/data/themes/mortality-and-global-health-estimates/ghe-leading-causes-of-death

CONCLUSION

North America presents geographic diversity, historical complexities, and a multifaceted population landscape that shapes the health and well-being of its inhabitants. Socioeconomic factors critically shape health outcomes, highlighting the need for targeted public health interventions that address inequalities. Understanding these dynamics is essential for developing effective health systems that promote equitable health for all populations in North America. North America's healthcare systems exhibit strengths and weaknesses, reflecting the region's diverse socioeconomic, political, and cultural contexts. While Canada's publicly funded system provides universal coverage and promotes equity in access to care, challenges such as wait times and resource constraints require ongoing attention. In the United States, efforts to expand access to healthcare coverage and improve quality of care have yielded mixed results, underscoring the need for comprehensive healthcare reform. In Mexico, while public healthcare initiatives aim to provide universal coverage through a mix of government programs, disparities in care quality, regional access, and significant out-of-pocket expenses highlight the need for continued investment in the healthcare infrastructure and equitable service delivery. In this section, our authors cover Canada, Mexico, and the United States.

LEARNING ACTIVITIES

CourseConnect

To access self-assessment questions and interactive, competency-based learning activities for this chapter, visit www.springerpub.com/courseconnect. See inside front cover and tear-out for CourseConnect details.

REFERENCES

Centers for Disease Control and Prevention. (2024). *Adult obesity facts*. https://www.cdc.gov/obesity/adult-obesity-facts/index.html

Gameon, J.A., & Skewes, M.C. (2021). Historical trauma and substance use among American Indian people with current substance use problems. *Psychology of Addictive Behaviors, 35*(3), 295–309. https://doi.org/10.1037/adb0000729

Hofstadter, R. (2008). *The American political tradition and the men who made it.* Vintage Books.

Organisation for Economic Co-operation and Development. (2021). *Health at a glance 2021: OECD indicators.* OECD Publishing.

Pew Research Center. (2021). *The future of world religions: Population growth projections, 2010–2050.* https://www.pewresearch.org/religion/2015/04/02/religious-projections-2010-2050/

U.S. Census Bureau. (2022). *Income and poverty in the United States: 2021.* https://www.census.gov/library/publications/2022/demo/p60-276.html

U.S. Geological Survey. (2025). *Geologic map of North America.* https://www.usgs.gov/media/images/geologic-map-north-america

World Bank Group. (2023). *Population, total - North America.* https://data.worldbank.org/country/north-america

World Health Organization. (2022). *Mental health, brain health and substance use.* https://www.who.int/teams/mental-health-and-substance-use

CHAPTER 5

THE UNITED STATES OF AMERICA

Thomas Foley, Sara Mar, Anna Foucek Tresidder, Kellan E. Baker, and Sharon Bryant

INTRODUCTION

The United States of America is a demographically and geographically diverse country known for both healthcare innovation and health inequities. Given the country's immense financial wealth and high quality of healthcare research, training, and services, the United States is viewed as having an underperforming healthcare system with glaring health disparities. As you read this chapter it is important to think about the following question: Why, given its wealth of resources and quality healthcare training and innovation, does the United States rank behind many other countries in key healthcare outcomes such as prevalence of preventable chronic diseases and life expectancy at birth?

GEOGRAPHIC AND DEMOGRAPHIC FEATURES

The United States of America is one of the largest countries in the world, with a total surface area of more than 9.83 million square kilometers (World Bank Group, 2024). It is a federal democratic republic that consists of 50 states, a federal district (District of Columbia), five territories (American Samoa, Guam, Northern Marina Island, Puerto Rico, and the U.S. Virgin Islands), over 500 federally recognized American Indian and Alaska Native entities, and more than 300 federally recognized Indian Reservations. The United States includes densely populated cities such as New York City, New York, with approximately 11,314 people per square kilometer, and sparsely populated rural areas such as Yukon-Koyukuk, Alaska, with approximately 0.02 people per square kilometer (USAGov, n.d.).

Just as the land area of the United States is large and diverse, so is its population. In 2023, more than 339 million people lived in the United States, ranking it behind India and China. The positive net migration in the United States during 2023 was nearly 1 million people, adding diversity to its large population and helping to offset the effects of population aging and declining fertility (UN Data Portal, n.d.). As the United States becomes more diverse, there is a greater need for person-centered and culturally and linguistically appropriate healthcare that promotes health equity and mitigates health disparities. Table 5.1 provides estimates of key U.S. demographic information.

BRIEF COUNTRY HISTORY

Millions of Indigenous people lived across North America in different tribes for thousands of years before the arrival of European colonizers during the 15th and 16th centuries. Early in the 17th century, the British established their first permanent colonies in what is now the United States. Colonization had near-genocidal impacts on the Indigenous population through massacres, spread of infectious diseases, and significant losses of land, natural resources, and culture. To this day, Indigenous populations are marginalized. The first British permanent settlements also led to the colonizers' involvement in the trade of Africans as slave labor to be used on tobacco and cotton plantations. Approximately 15 million Africans were kidnapped from their lands and forced into slavery in the Americas via the Middle Passage, including about 500,000 in the land that is now the United States. Slavery was not abolished in the United States until the ratification of the Thirteenth Amendment in December of 1865. After slavery was abolished, legalized racial segregation continued for another century. Prohibitions of racial discrimination in public

TABLE 5.1 ESTIMATES OF KEY U.S. DEMOGRAPHIC INFORMATION	
Median age, 2023	38.1 years
Percent of population by age, 2023	0–19 years: 24.3% 20–64 years: 58% 65+ years: 17.7%
Fertility rate, 2023	1.64 children per woman
Percent of population by ethnicity/race, 2022	Non-Latinx White: 59% Latinx: 19% Non-Latinx Black: 12% American Indian/Alaska Native: 7% Asian/Pacific Islander: 6% Note: People reporting mixed ethnicities/races was greater than 2%.
Languages, 2019	Total: There are more than 350 spoken and signed languages. English: 78% of the population aged 5 years and older speak only English at home. Spanish: 62% of people aged 5 years and older who speak a language other than English speak Spanish. Sign language: More than 6 million people use sign language. Others: Chinese, Tagalong, Vietnamese, and Arabic are other common languages.
Female-to-male ratio, 2023	1.02 females per 1.00 male
Intersex, 2024	1.7% of the population
Nonbinary, 2022	1% of the population
Transgender, 2022	0.6% of the population
Sexual orientation, 2022	7.2% of the population is bisexual, lesbian, gay, or another sexual minority.
Urban, 2022	82% of the population is urban.

Sources: Adapted from Mitchell, R.E., Young, T.A. Bachleda, B., & Karchmer, M.A. (2006). *How many people use ASL in the United States? Why estimates need updating*. Sign Language Studies. https://gallaudet.edu/wp-content/uploads/gcloud/gal-media/Documents/Research-Support-and-International-Affairs/ASL_Users.pdf; UN Data Portal. (n.d.). *OHCHR and the human rights of LGBTI people*. https://www.ohchr.org/en/sexual-orientation-and-gender-identity; U.S. Census Bureau. (n.d.). *Population*. https://www.census.gov/topics/population.html

accommodations and the allocation of federal funds were not signed into federal law until 1964 via the Civil Rights Act. Racially discriminatory housing practices, referred to as **redlining**, were not made illegal nationwide until the passage of the Fair Housing Act of 1968 (Mintz & McNeil, 2018).

Relatively speaking, the United States is a young nation, gaining its independence from Great Britain in 1776 with the Declaration of Independence. It rapidly developed during the Industrial Revolution, which began in the later part of the 17th century and lasted into the early 20th century. During this time, migration to the United States from countries worldwide resulted in a population boom and a large workforce. Work shifted from predominately agricultural to industrial because of manufacturing and technological advances. After the Industrial Revolution, the United States became a global economic and geopolitical leader. During this period, civil rights also progressed. In addition to the advancement in prohibiting racial discrimination, civil rights improved for women, people living with disabilities, and the bisexual, lesbian, and gay communities. In 1972, Title IX of the Education Amendments prohibited sex-based discrimination in schools. In 1990, the Americans with Disabilities Act (ADA) established the civil rights of people living with disabilities by prohibiting discrimination based on disability, and requiring the provision of reasonable accommodations to allow people with disabilities to participate in school, the workplace, and other areas of everyday life. In 2022, the Respect for Marriage Act was enacted, requiring all U.S. states and territories to recognize same-sex marriages. Even with these civil rights advances, social injustices persist today (Library of Congress, n.d.). Women continue to earn less money than men for similar work. People with disabilities have fewer educational and work opportunities, creating significant pay and wealth inequities. Communities of color continue to face barriers to quality healthcare due to segregation, racial bias, and exclusion from high-paying jobs that offer benefits like healthcare insurance. In 2023, more than 500 anti-LGBTQ+ bills were introduced in states across the country, seeking to marginalize LGBTQ+ people by limiting medical care for transgender people, banning educational curricula that mention LGBTQ+ populations and history, and banning expressions of LGBTQ+ culture (American Civil Liberties Union [ACLU], 2024).

HEALTH OUTCOMES

LIFE EXPECTANCY FROM BIRTH AND THE LEADING CAUSES OF MORTALITY

During the 20th century, the United States made significant gains in life expectancy. Life expectancy at birth increased from 47 years in 1900 to 77 years in 2000. Such gains, however, slowed during the 21st century In 2023, life expectancy at birth was 79.4 years, placing the United States behind more than 50 other countries (UN Data Portal, n.d.). There are also significant racial and ethnic disparities in life expectancy. In 2020, the life expectancy at birth was 67 years for AI/AN, 71.5 years for non-Latinx Blacks, 77.5 years for non-Latinx Whites, 78 years for Latinx, and 83.5 years for Asians (NCHS, 2024).

There are several reasons why gains in life expectancy stalled in the United States in the 21st century. One key reason is the high mortality rate of preventable chronic diseases. About 60% of all adults in the United States live with at least one chronic disease, and 40% live with two or more chronic diseases. Chronic diseases account for approximately seven out of 10 deaths. In 2021, heart disease was the leading cause of death in the United States, accounting for approximately one out of every five deaths. Cancer was the second leading cause of death, and lung cancer was the leading cause of cancer mortality. Cigarette smoking and exposure to secondhand smoke are estimated to cause 90% of lung cancer deaths. Other preventable chronic conditions such as stroke, Alzheimer disease, type 2 diabetes, chronic hepatic steatosis and cirrhosis, and chronic renal disease are also among the top causes of mortality in the United States (NCHS, 2024). Figure 5.1 displays the leading causes of U.S. mortality during 2020 and 2021 (NCHS, 2024).

While the United States has been a leader in preventing mortality from communicable diseases, there is concern that antivaccination movements and the high prevalence of chronic diseases are placing people in the United States at risk of harm from preventable infectious diseases. From 2020 to 2022, the COVID-19 death rate in the United States was among the top 20 in the world. Before the start of 2024, more than 100 million people in the United States had been infected with COVID-19, and more than 1.15 million died of COVID-19 (KFF, 2024). Influenza and pneumonia continue to be deadly infectious diseases in the United States as vaccination rates remain low and the prevalence of chronic diseases remains high. In 2022, less than 50% of all adults and children age 6 months to 17 years received an influenza vaccination, and less than 25% of adults had ever received a pneumococcal vaccination. The combination of influenza/pneumonia was the 13th-ranked cause of mortality in the United States in 2022 (NCHS, 2024).

INFANT AND MATERNAL MORTALITY

In 2021, the U.S. maternal mortality ratio was about 33 maternal deaths per 100,000 live births. Maternal mortality has been increasing over the past several years, and racial and ethnic disparities

FIGURE 5.1 Leading causes of mortality in the United States during 2020 and 2021.

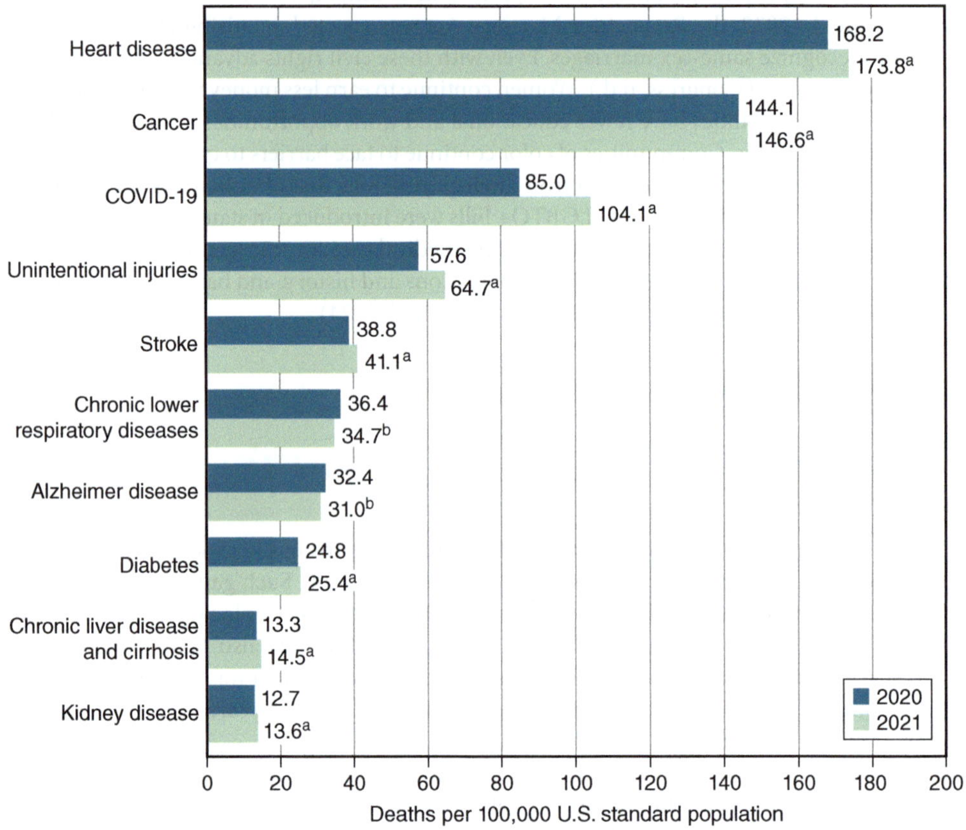

Note: A total of 3,464,231 resident deaths were registered in the United States in 2021. The 10 leading causes of death accounted for 74.5% of all U.S. deaths in 2021. Causes of death are ranked according to number of deaths. Rankings for 2020 data are not shown. Access data table including the number of deaths for leading causes and the percentage of total deaths at https://www.cdc.gov/nchs/data/databriefs/db456-tables.pdf#4.

[a] Statistically significant increase from 2020 to 2021 ($p < .05$).
[b] Statistically significant decrease from 2020 to 2021 ($p < .05$).

Source: National Center for Health Statistics. (2024). *Data collection systems*. https://www.cdc.gov/nchs/index.html

persist. Compared to non-Latina White and Latina women, maternal mortality is about 2.5 times greater for non-Latina Black women. Maternal mortality was 4.5 times greater for women age 40 and older when compared to women age 25 to 39 (National Center for Health Statistics [NCHS], 2024).

The infant mortality rate in the United States during 2023 was 4.9 infant deaths per 1,000 live births. In 1950, infant mortality was 31.7 deaths per 1,000 live births (UN Data Portal, n.d.). While infant mortality rates have improved, racial, ethnic, and age disparities exist. In 2021, non-Latinx Black (10.6), Native Hawaiian/Other Pacific Islanders (7.8), and American Indian/Alaska Native (AI/AN; 7.5) infant mortality rates were significantly higher when compared to Latinx (4.8), non-Latinx White (4.4) and Asian/Pacific Islander (3.7) infant mortality rates. Infant mortality was higher when maternal age was either less than 25 years or 40 years or more (NCHS, 2024).

MENTAL HEALTH

In 2021, nearly 60 million U.S. adults—more than one in five—experienced a mental health disorder, of which anxiety and major depressive disorder were the two most common. Despite the high prevalence, less than 50% of adults with a mental health disorder received treatment in 2021, and an estimated 164 million people in the United States lived in a mental health provider shortage area (MHPSA). In particular, rural populations receive mental health care less frequently, as more than 60% of rural Americans live in an MHPSA (National Alliance on Mental Illness [NAMI], 2023).

In 2021, suicide was the second leading cause of death among youths age 10 to 14 and the third leading cause of death among people age 15 to 24. Approximately 90% of people who died by suicide experienced symptoms of mental illness. Marginalized populations such as LGBTQ+ people are often more at risk for mental health concerns due to trauma, societal discrimination, and lack of access to culturally competent healthcare. Transgender people were almost nine times more likely to report attempting suicide and 66% of transgender young adults age 18 to 25 have reported suicidal ideation. Lesbian, gay, and bisexual youth were four times more likely to report attempting suicide when compared to heterosexual youths (NAMI, 2023). Expanding access to culturally competent care is an essential part of closing mental health disparities. For example, access to gender-affirming care for transgender and nonbinary people improves quality of life and mental health, and decreases depression, anxiety, and suicidal ideation. **Gender-affirming care** includes social, behavioral, medical, and/or physiologic services that focus on understanding and validating an individual's gender identity (ACLU, 2024).

DETERMINANTS OF HEALTH

HEALTH BEHAVIORS

In the United States, health behavior risk factors are drivers of preventable chronic-disease morbidity and mortality. To drastically lower the risk of developing a preventable chronic disease, the Centers for Disease Control and Prevention (CDC) recommends the following four health behaviors: do not smoke, eat healthy, be active, and limit drinking alcohol. While the use of tobacco cigarettes has decreased in the United States, there were still more than 30 million adult smokers in 2020. In 2019, approximately 6% of high school students smoked tobacco cigarettes, and more than 25% used e-cigarettes. People of all age groups in the United States fail to meet crucial dietary intake recommendations for whole grains, fruits, and vegetables. In addition, people are overconsuming refined grains, meat, added sugar, saturated fat, and sodium. As well, nearly 75% of adults in the United States fail to meet the national recommendations for physical activity and over 80% of young people failing to meet the national physical acivity recommendations for youths (National Center for Chronic Disease Prevention and Health Promotion [NCCDPHP], n.d.). In 2019, more than 14 million people age 12 and older had alcohol use disorder (AUD) and less than 10% of people with an AUD received treatment. The COVID-19 pandemic increased alcohol use and alcohol-related harm. In 2020, during the first year of the pandemic, more people used alcohol as a coping technique when compared to 2019. Nearly 100,000 people died from an alcohol-related cause in 2020, which was an increase of about 25% from 2019 (National Institute on Alcohol Abuse and Alcoholism [NIAAA], n.d.).

ENVIRONMENTAL FACTORS

The environments in which we live, work, and play significantly impact our health. Access to healthy environments in the United States, however, is not equal as communities of color and people who live with disabilities are more likely to experience environmental injustices. For example, Black people are 75% more likely than White people to live in **fenceline communities**, which are communities that are adjacent to industrial facilities. People who live in fenceline communities are at increased risk of being exposed to toxic waste and air and water pollution, developing several chronic conditions such as cancer and respiratory infections, experiencing mental health crises, and having lower life expectancy. Black and Latinx communities are more likely to be located in food swamps (National Research Development Corporation [NRDC], 2021). A **food swamp** is an environment with a high density of corner stores and fast-food restaurants offering unhealthy food options and a low density of grocery stores and farmers' markets offering nutritious food (Singleton et al., 2023). Communities of color and people with disabilities also lack equitable access to green spaces such as community parks. Green spaces improve air quality and mental and physical health and mitigate the impacts of extreme heat from climate change (Wong et al., 2022).

SOCIAL AND ECONOMIC FACTORS

The United States is the world's wealthiest country based on gross domestic product (GDP). In 2022, the United States accounted for nearly 25% of the world's GDP. Per-capita GDP in the United States during 2022 was approximately $76,330, which was well above the world average of $12,688 (World Bank Group, 2024). In addition, the United Nations recognizes the United States as a country with "very high" human development based on a combination of standards of living, health, and education. In 2022, the U.S. Human Development Index score was .927, which was 20th in the world (UN Human Development Programme, 2024).

Despite being a wealthy nation recognized for high human development, the United States has significant income and educational attainment inequities that impact health disparities. While poverty in the United States has been cut in half since 1950, the poverty rate has remained relatively constant during the 21st century. The poverty rate in 2021 was approximately 11.5%, similar to that in 2000. AI/ANs (25%), non-Latinx Blacks (17%), and Latinx (17%) are more likely to live in poverty when compared to Asians (8.5%) and non-Latinx Whites (8.5%). People with disabilities are three times more likely to live in poverty when compared to people without disabilities. In 2021, about 91% of people age 25 or older in the United States had at least a high school diploma. An undergraduate university degree was the highest level of education for nearly one quarter of the population and about 14% of the population had an advanced university degree such as a master's or doctorate. AI/ANs and Latinx were less likely to have a high school diploma and less likely to have a college degree when compared to other races and ethnicities. People living without disabilities are more than twice as likely to have at least an undergraduate degree (U.S. Census Bureau, 2023). Low educational attainment and poverty are associated with a greater risk of experiencing environmental injustices such as living in a food swamp, being predisposed to unhealthy behaviors such as poor diet, having lower life expectancy, and encountering barriers to healthcare (Raghupathi & Raghupathi, 2020).

HEALTHCARE SYSTEM

FINANCING AND INSURANCE

The United States is viewed as having an overly complex, expensive, and underperforming healthcare system with glaring inequity-driven health disparities. The U.S. healthcare system is a multipayer system without universal healthcare coverage. The system operates on a near-equal split between public and private insurance. The public system ensures that older adults, low-income adults, and children from low-income households can access healthcare. Public financing primarily comes from the government via taxes and subsidies. The public insurance system comprises the **Children's Health Insurance Program (CHIP)**, **Medicaid**, and **Medicare**. Medicare is public insurance for older adults and adults with severe disabilities. Medicaid is public insurance for adults with low income. CHIP is the public insurance system for children of low-income households. Individual states set income eligibility requirements for CHIP and Medicaid as a percentage of the federal poverty level (FPL). Private healthcare financing comes mostly from employer/employee contributions. Many employers offer healthcare for employees and their dependents as an employment benefit, and employees pay toward their healthcare coverage via a combination of premiums, deductibles, and copays or coinsurance (Commonwealth Fund, 2024). The private insurance system predominately relies on three types of managed care plans: **health maintenance organizations (HMOs)**, **preferred provider organizations (PPOs)**, and **high deductible health plans (HDHPs)**. HMOs are managed care plans that cost less if members stay within the HMO network of healthcare providers. PPOs are plans that offer an expanded network of providers; however, PPOs have more expensive monthly premiums. HDHPs typically provide an expanded network similar to PPOs while keeping monthly premiums low like an HMO; however, annual deductibles and out-of-pocket maximums are much higher in HDHPs. Many HDHP plans also offer the option to create an individual **health savings account** in which the employee and their employer can make pre-tax contributions to cover future medical expenses (KFF, 2024).

DELIVERY

Hospitals have become the backbone of outpatient and inpatient care in the United States. There are more than 6,100 hospitals in the United States and about 50% are **private, nonprofit hospitals** owned by nongovernmental entities such as philanthropic organizations and are intended to benefit local communities. About 20% are **private for-profit hospitals**, which are investor owned. Physician-owned specialty hospitals, such as orthopedic hospitals, are standard private for-profit hospitals. **Public hospitals** are owned by federal, state, or local government agencies and are not necessarily open to the public. For example, hospitals owned by the federal government benefit historically marginalized populations such as Indigenous populations and veterans. **Community hospitals** are nonfederal, short-stay hospitals whose services are open to the public. More than 80% of hospitals in the United States are considered to be community hospitals (American Hospital Association [AHA], 2024). **Community health centers (CHCs)** also play an essential role in outpatient healthcare delivery. CHCs are federally funded and offer essential primary and dental care services as a safety-net provider for underserved regions such as rural areas and for marginalized populations such as people experiencing homelessness. In 2021, CHCs served more than 30 million people in thousands of locations nationwide. Of the people served at CHCs in 2021, approximately 90% were low-income and 20% were uninsured (National Association of Community Health Centers [NACHC], 2024).

There are two main sectors of long-term care (LTC) facilities in the United States: community-based and institutionalized LTC facilities. Community-based LTC facilities include home healthcare, adult day and senior centers, and informal care. Institutionalized LTC facilities include assisted living facilities, nursing homes, and subacute and specialized care facilities. In 2018, approximately 69,000 paid, regulated LTC providers served more than 9.5 million people. Paid LTC comes from home health aides, certified nursing assistants, physicians, nurses, and therapists (NCHS, 2024). However, a significant portion of LTC is unpaid, **informal care** that friends, family, and neighbors deliver. In 2021, approximately 38 million informal caregivers in the United States provided unpaid care, estimated to be worth nearly $600 billion (Reinhard et al., 2023).

The U.S. healthcare system is a leading employer in the United States, accounting for more than 10% of employment. Healthcare employment is among the fastest-growing employment areas, including home healthcare aides and allied health professionals. Allied health professionals account for most of the healthcare workforce in the United States and are essential to addressing the chronic disease epidemic and healthcare provider shortages. The allied health field is diverse and includes healthcare professionals such as dentists and dental hygienists, dieticians and nutritionists, healthcare administrators, occupational and physical therapists, pharmacists, physician assistants, psychologists, social workers, and speech–language pathologists. While the continued growth of the allied health professions is essential to improving healthcare and health outcomes in the United States, the historical backbone of the U.S. healthcare system has been physicians and nurses. Physicians need to graduate from an accredited medical school that awards the degree of medical doctor (MD) or doctor of osteopathic medicine (DO). More than one million physicians are licensed to practice in the United States, translating to about three physicians per 1,000 people. Physician shortages exist in fields such as primary care and geriatrics, and extend to certain geographic regions such as rural areas. Nurses account for the most significant percentage of non-informal healthcare providers. **Registered nurses (RNs)** complete an associate degree program in nursing (ADN) or a bachelor of science degree in nursing (BSN) and provide basic nursing care. **Advanced practice registered nurses (APRNs)** have graduate degrees in specialty areas and clinical experience beyond that required of an RN (U.S. Bureau of Labor Statistics, 2024).

TRADITIONAL AND COMPLEMENTARY CARE

Traditional healthcare favors preventing and treating illnesses by using more natural practices such as diet, social cohesion, and respect for the environment and spirituality. For example, many AI/ANs view life and health as a connection among the individual, family, community, and world and a balance among emotional, mental, physical, and spiritual dimensions (Dapice, 2006). Native Hawaiians also view life and healthcare from a more ecological perspective. Native Hawaiians' concept of ***lokahi*** promotes harmony and balance among the person, the land, and spirituality. The mental and physical health of the person, family, community, environment, and spirits are linked together (Daniels et al., 2022). There are efforts to integrate traditional healthcare practices into the allopathic medical system as a form of complementary care. For example, **naturopathic doctors** receive training in allopathic medicine but primarily utilize individualized and noninvasive lifestyle treatments that focus on underlying causes such as diet and stress. Naturopathic doctors attend accredited schools and practice evidence-based healthcare in clinics, hospitals, and integrated medical centers alongside other allied health professionals, nurses, and physicians (Association of Accredited Naturopathic Medical Colleges [AANMC], 2023).

ACCESS, QUALITY, AND COST

Although the United States spends more on healthcare than any other country and has the world's highest per-capita healthcare spending, it lags far behind in critical health and healthcare outcomes. In 2022, healthcare expenditures in the United States were $4.4 trillion. Per-capita healthcare spending was $12,555 per person. Total out-of-pocket spending for healthcare was more than $470 billion. On a per-capita basis, out-of-pocket spending on healthcare in the United States was greater than every other country except Sweden (Peterson-Kaiser Family Foundation, 2024).

The U.S. healthcare system also ranks last in accessibility and affordability compared to other high-income countries (Commonwealth Fund, 2024). Of the millions of adults lacking healthcare coverage in the United States, 85% report that it is difficult to afford healthcare and more than 60% report delaying or skipping needed healthcare because of cost. AI/ANs, Latinx, and non-Latinx Blacks are uninsured at much higher rates when compared to non-Latinx Whites and Asians. The cost of insurance and not meeting restrictive coverage eligibility requirements are the top two reasons people lack healthcare insurance in the United States. The **Patient Protection**

FIGURE 5.2 Number of uninsured nonelderly people in the United States from 2010-2022.

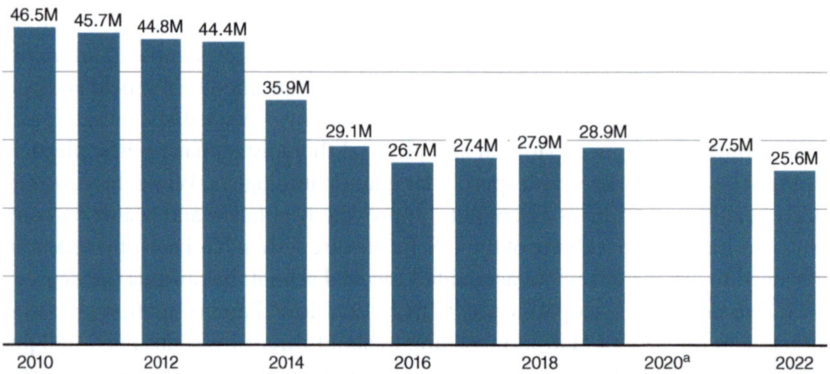

Note: Includes nonelderly individuals aged 0–64.

[a] Due to disruptions in data collection during the first year of the pandemic, the Census Bureau did not release American Community Survey 1-year estimates in 2020.

Source: KFF. (2024). *Key facts about the uninsured population*. https://www.kff.org/uninsured/issue-brief/key-facts-about-the-uninsured-population/

and Affordable Care Act of 2010 (ACA) was a significant step forward regarding healthcare access. The ACA expanded Medicaid coverage and provided subsidies to lower the cost of health insurance. Because of the ACA, the number of uninsured nonelderly Americans decreased from over 46.5 million in 2010 to nearly 25 million in 2022. Figure 5.2 shows the decrease in uninsured nonelderly adults in the United States from 2010 to 2022. The ACA also improved the quality of coverage by mandating that health insurance plans include essential benefits such as maternity and pediatric care and rehabilitative and preventive services (KFF, 2024).

CONCLUSION

While the United States has exceptional healthcare training and services, the U.S. healthcare system is expensive and underperforming (Peterson-KFF, 2024). Compared to other high-income countries, the United States has lower life expectancy and poor healthcare accessibility. Historically marginalized groups such as communities of color and the LGBTQ+ community disproportionately experience health disparities and challenges accessing quality healthcare and healthy environments. The United States is slowly addressing these challenges through expanding Medicaid eligibility, incentivizing preventive services, and designing person-centered approaches to care. As you reflect on this chapter, answer the following question: What can the United States do to make healthcare more accessible, mitigate healthcare disparities and social injustices, increase life expectancy, and decrease morbidity and mortality from preventable diseases?

LEARNING ACTIVITIES

CourseConnect

To access self-assessment questions and interactive, competency-based learning activities for this chapter, visit www.springerpub.com/courseconnect. See inside front cover and tear-out for CourseConnect details.

REFERENCES

American Civil Liberties Union. (2024). *Issues*. https://www.aclu.org/

American Hospital Association. (2024). *Fast facts on U.S. hospitals, 2024*. https://www.aha.org/statistics/fast-facts-us-hospitals

Association of Accredited Naturopathic Medical Colleges. (2023). *What is naturopathic medicine?* https://aanmc.org/naturopathic-medicine/

Commonwealth Fund. (2024). *Topics*. https://www.commonwealthfund.org/topics

Daniels, S. A. P., Kauahikaua, L., Kaio, C., Casson-Fisher, J. N., & Ku, T. (2022). Conceptualizing a new system of care in Hawai'i for native Hawaiians and substance use. *Hawaii Journal of Health & Social Welfare, 81*(12 Suppl 3), 43–51.

Dapice, A. N. (2006). The medicine wheel. *Journal of Transcultural Nursing, 17*(3), 251–260. http://doi.org/10.1177/1043659606288383

KFF. (2024). *Trending*. https://www.kff.org/

Library of Congress. (n.d.). *Legislation*. https://www.congress.gov/search

Mintz, S., & McNeil, S. (2018). *Digital history*. http://www.digitalhistory.uh.edu

National Alliance on Mental Illness. (2023). *Mental health by the numbers*. https://www.nami.org/about-mental-illness/mental-health-by-the-numbers/

National Association of Community Health Centers. (2024). *America's health centers: By the numbers*. https://www.nachc.org/resource/americas-health-centers-by-the-numbers/

National Center for Chronic Disease Prevention and Health Promotion. (n.d.). *Centers of Disease Control and Prevention*. https://www.cdc.gov/nccdphp/index.html

National Centre for Health Statistics. (2024). *Data collection systems*. Centers for Disease Control and Prevention. https://www.cdc.gov/nchs/index.htm

National Institute on Alcohol Abuse and Alcoholism. (n.d.). *Alcohol and its effects on health*. National Institutes of Health. https://www.niaaa.nih.gov/alcohols-effects-health

National Research Development Corporation. (2024). *Food apartheid: Racialized access to healthy affordable food.* https://www.nrdc.org/bio/nina-sevilla/food-apartheid-racialized-access-healthy-affordable-food

Peterson-Kaiser Family Foundation. (2024). *Health systems tracker.* https://www.healthsystemtracker.org/

Raghupathi, V., & Raghupathi, W. (2020). The Influence of education on health: An empirical assessment of OECD countries for the period of 1995-2015. *Archives of Public Health, 78*(20). https://doi.org/10.1186/s13690-020-00402-5

Reinhard, S. C., Caldera, S., Houser, A., & Choula, R. B. (2023). *Valuing the invaluable 2023 update: Strengthening supports for family caregivers.* AARP Public Policy Institute.

Singleton, C. R., Wright, L. A., McDonald, M., Archer, I. G., Bell, C. N., McLoughlin, G. M., Houghtaling, B., Stowers, K. C., & Steeves, E. A. (2023). Structural racism and Geographic access to food retailers in the United States: A scoping review. *Health & Place, 83.* 103089. https://doi.org/10.1016/j.healthplace.2023.103089

UN Data Portal. (n.d.). *UN population division data portal.* United Nations. https://population.un.org/dataportal/home/

UN Human Development Programme. (2024). *Human development reports.* https://hdr.undp.org/

USAGov. (n.d.). *The U.S. and its government.* U.S. General Services Administration. https://www.usa.gov/about-the-us

U.S. Bureau of Labor Statistics. (2024). *Occupational outlook handbook: Healthcare occupations.* https://www.bls.gov/ooh/healthcare/home.htm

U.S. Census Bureau. (2023). *Topics.* https://www.census.gov/topics.html

Wong, S., Rush, J., Bailey, F., & Just, A. C. (2022). Accessible green spaces? Spatial disparities in residential green space among people with disabilities in the Untied States. *Annals of the American Association of Geographers, 113*(2), 527–548. https://doi.org/10.1080/24694452.2022.2106177

World Bank Group. (2024). *The World Bank open data.* https://data.worldbank.org/

CHAPTER 6

CANADA

Serdar Atav

INTRODUCTION

Canada is a vast and prosperous nation in the northern part of the North American continent. Reflecting Canada's progressive and social democratic leanings, one of the defining features of its healthcare system is the universal single-payer model. This model aims to provide comprehensive healthcare coverage to all Canadian citizens, irrespective of their financial circumstances or ability to pay. This approach reflects Canada's commitment to ensuring no one is left behind when accessing essential medical care. For many Canadians, their healthcare system fosters a sense of national pride, making it a cornerstone of their national identity (Martin et al., 2018). However, while its universal **single-payer healthcare system** ensures equitable access to health services, the Canadian healthcare system also faces challenges that require ongoing attention and improvement to address funding, long wait times, primary care access, and regional differences.

GEOGRAPHY AND GOVERNANCE

Canada is the world's second-largest country, boasting a total area of 3,855,100 square miles. Its only mainland border, stretching an impressive 5,525 miles, is with the United States, making it the longest international border in the world. Of Canada's total population of 39.1 million, more than 90% live within 150 miles of the international border, and this underpins the close relationship and interconnectedness between these two neighboring countries. Canada's large landmass is divided into ten provinces and three territories. The provinces are in the southern part of the country, and the territories are in the northern regions (Figure 6.1).

Canada's political system is rooted in the Westminster parliamentary tradition, mirroring the democratic models prevalent in Western Europe. Like the United Kingdom and some other European parliamentary democracies, Canada is a constitutional monarchy with a bicameral legislature consisting of an elected House of Commons and an appointed Senate. As the head of government, the prime minister is drawn from the party holding the most seats in the Commons and serves as the nation's chief executive. Politically and administratively, the provinces in Canada are similar to the states in the United States. They possess a significant degree of autonomy and authority within their jurisdictions. On the other hand, the sparsely populated territories have more limited powers and authority as the federal government delegates their governance. This division between provinces and territories reflects Canada's massive geographical expanse and the diverse needs of its regions, allowing for a balanced distribution of power and self-governance across the nation.

As a member of the Group of Seven (G7) and the North Atlantic Treaty Organization (NATO), Canada is firmly entrenched among the world's most advanced democratic nations and a key player in promoting global security and economic cooperation.

FIGURE 6.1 Map of Canada.

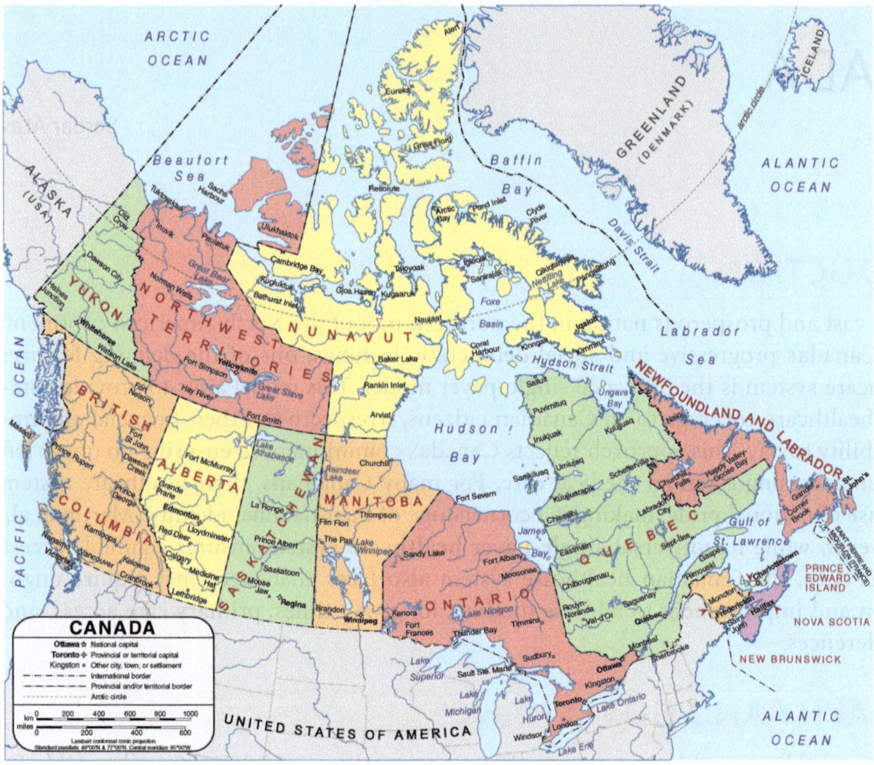

Source: Map Grid. (2020, November 15). *Political map of Canada with English labels.* https://commons.wikimedia.org/w/index.php?title=File:Canada_political_map_-_en.svg&oldid=951799837.

CANADA'S POPULATION DYNAMICS

Due to recent immigration patterns, Canada's population is 41,638,486 in 2025 and growing every day, up from 38.93 million in 2022 (Statistics Canada, 2025). Despite this growth, Canada maintains a relatively low population growth rate, 0.77% in 2021 and 0.85% in 2022. Statistics Canada (2024a) indicates that the primary characteristics of Canada's relatively small but growing population are:

- *Aging demographics*: In 2022, around 15.4% of Canadians were age 0 to 14, 65.7% were 15 to 64, and 18.9% were 65 years and over. Canada's median and average ages in 2023 were 40.6 and 41.6, respectively, reflecting an aging population.
- *High immigration rates*: Canada's net migration rate was 5.46 migrants per 1,000 population in 2022, driven mainly by economic policy and family reunification. Between 2011 and 2016, immigrants accounted for two thirds of Canada's population growth.
- *Urbanization*: In 2021, 81.7% of Canadians lived in urban areas, with an annual urbanization rate of 0.95%. Major cities with over 1 million population include Toronto, Montreal, Vancouver, Calgary, Edmonton, and Ottawa (the capital).
- *Ethnic and linguistic diversity*: According to the 2016 census, the largest ethnic group was White (69.8%). The racialized groups consisted of South Asians (7.1%), Indigenous Peoples (5%), Chinese (4.7%), Blacks (4.3%), Filipinos (2.6%) and Arabs (1.9%). English (55.97%) and French (20.61%) are the official languages, but many other languages are spoken, including Mandarin, Cantonese, Punjabi, and Spanish.

The population pyramid of Canada (Figure 6.2) confirms that the nation is in the demographic transition toward an aging population structure. This aligns with Canada's lower fertility rates and high life expectancies.

FERTILITY AND MORTALITY

In 2022, Canada's fertility rate hit an all-time low of 1.33 children born per woman. This number places Canada in the middle among the other selected high-income countries, ranging from 0.78 in South Korea to 1.80 in France. The infant mortality rate under 1 year was 4.7 deaths per 1,000 live births, while life expectancy at birth in 2022 was 83.8 years (81.52 years for males and 86.21 years for females; Statistics Canada, 2024b). Canada's population dynamics reflect a complex interplay of demographic factors, including aging, immigration, urbanization, and cultural diversity, shaping the nation's demographic landscape and future trajectory.

SEX AND SEXUAL ORIENTATION

Canada legalized same-sex marriage nationwide in 2005. Canada was the first country in the world to provide census data on transgender and nonbinary people. According to data from the 2021 census, out of the approximately 30.5 million individuals aged 15 and over residing in private households across Canada, 100,815 identified as transgender or nonbinary. This figure comprised 59,460 transgender individuals and 41,355 nonbinary individuals, collectively representing

FIGURE 6.2 Population pyramid: Men and women, 2021.

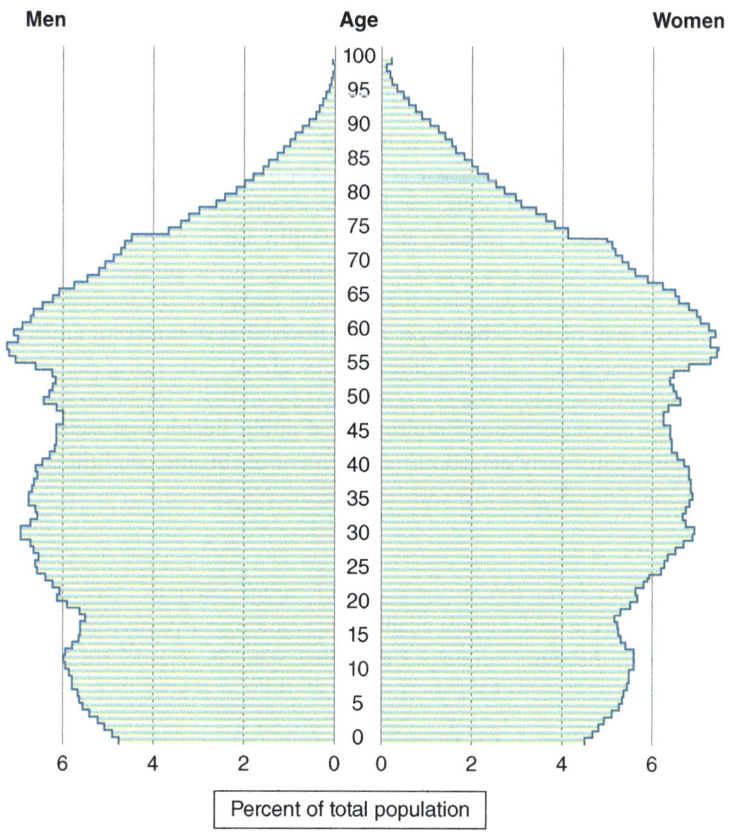

Source: Statistics Canada. (2021). *Comparison age and gender pyramid*. https://www12.statcan.gc.ca/census-recensement/2021/dp-pd/dv-vd/pyramid/index-eng.cfm

0.33% of the Canadian population within this age group. According to Statistics Canada, Canada is home to approximately 1 million people who are LGBTQ+, accounting for 4% of the total population aged 15 and older in 2018 (Statistics Canada, 2021).

HEALTH OUTCOMES

LEADING CAUSES OF MORTALITY

In line with other prosperous nations, the leading causes of mortality in Canada primarily reflect an epidemiologic transition toward noncommunicable diseases and conditions associated with aging populations. However, the COVID-19 pandemic has also left a significant impact. The top causes of death can be categorized as follows (Statistics Canada, 2023).

Noncommunicable diseases:

- Cancer (malignant neoplasms)
- Cardiovascular diseases (diseases of the heart, cerebrovascular diseases)
- Chronic respiratory diseases (chronic lower respiratory diseases)
- Diabetes mellitus

Communicable disease:

- COVID-19

Injuries:

- Unintentional injuries (accidents)

Other causes:

- Alzheimer disease and other dementias
- Chronic liver disease and cirrhosis

While noncommunicable diseases have traditionally dominated the leading causes, the COVID-19 pandemic emerged as a significant cause of mortality in Canada in 2022, ranking third overall. This highlights the substantial toll of the viral outbreak on the nation's public health landscape. Unhealthy lifestyle behaviors like tobacco use, unhealthy diets, physical inactivity, and alcohol consumption remain significant risk factors contributing to the prevalence of noncommunicable conditions like cancer, cardiovascular diseases, and diabetes. The leading causes of death in Canada highlight two major health challenges— the prevalence of noncommunicable diseases like cancer, heart conditions, and respiratory illnesses associated with aging populations, as well as the resurgence of communicable diseases exemplified by COVID-19. From a policy perspective, this epidemiologic profile necessitates a multipronged public health approach focusing on health promotion, preventive care, early detection/management of chronic conditions, preparedness for disease outbreaks, and providing quality care for an aging population across the continuum of care.

QUALITY OF LIFE

Canada consistently ranks at the top of various quality of life rankings. According to *U.S. News & World Report*, Canada has the third highest quality of life ranking, surpassed only by the much smaller Sweden and Norway. In the same rankings, the United States is placed 23rd (U.S. News & World Report, 2024).

CANADA'S HEALTHCARE SYSTEM

HISTORY OF THE CANADIAN HEALTHCARE SYSTEM

Canada's healthcare system, known as Medicare, evolved through incremental efforts at the provincial level since the late 1940s, culminating in a decentralized **universal coverage model**. The province of Saskatchewan pioneered the first universal hospital services plan in 1947, followed by similar schemes in British Columbia (1948) and Alberta (1950). In 1957, the federal government's Hospital Insurance and Diagnostic Services Act set conditions for provinces to receive cost-sharing funds for universal hospital coverage. By 1961, all provinces had agreed to this federal framework.

Building on this, Saskatchewan implemented universal coverage for physician services in 1962. The 1966 federal **Medical Care Act** encouraged other provinces to follow suit through conditional grants. By 1971, every province had established universal coverage for hospital care and medical services, forming the foundation of Medicare—a decentralized system administered provincially but adhering to federal standards and primarily funded through federal transfers (Marchildon et al., 2020).

KEY FEATURES

Universal Coverage

Canada's healthcare system is designed to provide universal access to essential medical services for all citizens, regardless of their employment status or ability to pay out-of-pocket fees.

The financing model is primarily single payer, with provincial and territorial governments acting as the primary insurers, funding healthcare through tax revenues collected at their respective levels. While the public system covers core hospital and physician services, private insurance plays a supplementary role in providing additional benefits such as vision and dental care.

Comprehensive Benefits

Besides hospital and physician care, provinces/territories provide supplementary benefits like prescription drug coverage and home care services, though specifics vary.

Emphasis on Primary Care

Family physicians serve as the main point of entry, focusing on preventive care, early intervention, and managing patients' overall health.

Public Administration

Healthcare is publicly administered, and facilities are predominantly nonprofit. Most physicians are paid through a blend of fee-for-service and alternative payment models.

Funding

Healthcare is funded primarily through federal transfers to provinces and territories and provincial and territorial tax revenues. Globally, the Canadian healthcare system ranks higher than other countries (Hutchison, 2017). However, within the high-income countries, it achieves only a middling performance, highlighting the mixture of its successes in specific dimensions, such as administrative efficiency and goal attainment, and failures in other areas, such as long waiting times, primary care access, and financial sustainability. Patients and providers often cite problems with primary care access and policy strategies for improvement (Philpott, 2024; Zang, 2024).

Canada's single-payer system is often cited as a model for its comprehensive benefits. Yet, it also ranks among the most expensive healthcare systems globally regarding per-capita expenditures (2021). According to the latest data from the World Economic Forum (2023), Canada's healthcare expenditure per capita stood at $5,905 in 2021 (Figure 6.3). While this ranks Canada as the fourth most expensive healthcare system globally, its spending levels are comparable to other Western European nations and advanced economies. The staggering costs of the U.S. healthcare system, which amounted to $12,318 per capita in the same year, underscore the substantial gap between the two neighboring nations. Canada's expenditures, while still significant, are less than half of those in the United States.

Canada's healthcare system only covers traditional medical care. Alternative or complementary therapies are not covered under the insurance scheme.

FIGURE 6.3 Per-capita health expenditures in selected countries in 2021.

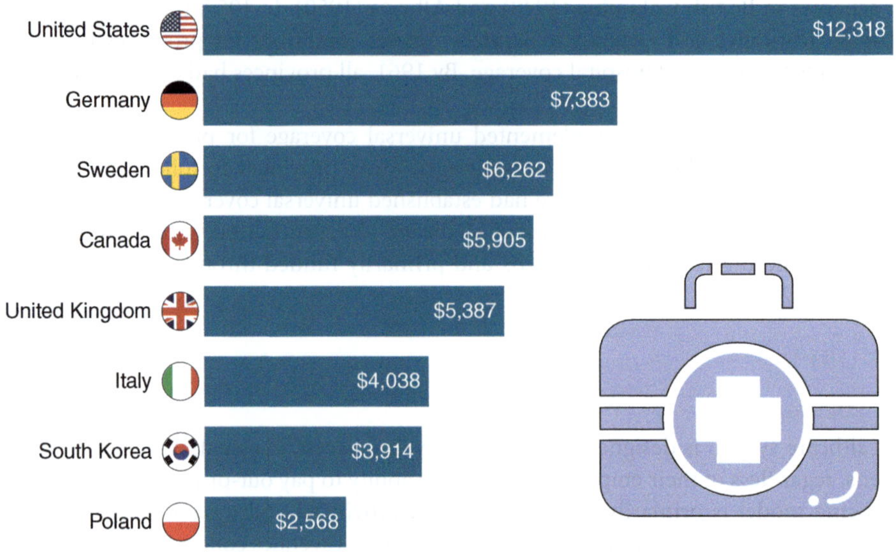

Note: Includes government and private/compulsory and voluntary spending.

Source: Statista. (n.d.). *The U.S. has the most expensive healthcare in the world.* https://www.statista.com/chart/8658/health-spending-per-capita/

Canada's health system boasts several world-class hospitals and healthcare facilities that rank among the best globally, including Toronto General Hospital, Princes Margaret Cancer Centre, McGill University Health Centre, and Vancouver General Hospital. These hospitals attract top medical talent, employ the latest medical technologies, and adhere to rigorous quality standards. Additionally, Canada has several internationally accredited academic health science centers that integrate multidisciplinary patient care, research, and medical education under one umbrella. The quality of Canada's healthcare facilities is further bolstered by robust accreditation programs through organizations like **Accreditation Canada**, which ensure healthcare organizations meet national safety and quality requirements. While challenges persist in waiting times, Canada's world-class hospitals and healthcare facilities are vital in delivering high-quality, specialized care to Canadians.

Canada's single-payer, universal healthcare systems have distinctive advantages for providers. For example, providers in Canada enjoy practicing without corporate and governmental restrictions. Their autonomy is far greater than that in the United States. Even though reimbursements are lower in Canada, the simplicity, predictability, and prompt payments through the single-payer system make the Canadian system attractive to some providers. Furthermore, malpractice insurance is much cheaper in Canada, and the risk of being sued is lower (Shaw, 2005).

DETERMINANTS OF HEALTH

SOCIOECONOMIC STATUS AND INEQUALITY

Canada has a high-functioning economy, with a projected gross domestic product (GDP) per capita of $60,495 in 2024, ranking 25th globally. However, this wealth is not equally distributed. Marginalized groups, particularly **Indigenous peoples** (First Nations, Inuit, and Métis), experience higher poverty rates due to the legacy of colonial practices, racist policies, and ongoing discrimination. While the national poverty rate stands at 7.4%, it nearly doubles to 13.9% among Indigenous populations (National Advisory Council on Poverty, 2023).

EDUCATION

Canada's education system, with strong public education traditions, follows the European model. Education is free and mandatory from ages 6 to 16. Major universities are public institutions with relatively low tuition fees regulated by provincial and territorial governments. Despite an official 99% literacy rate, concerns about functional literacy levels required for a knowledge-based economy persist.

EMPLOYMENT AND INCOME SUPPORT

As of 2024, Canada's unemployment rate was 6.1%, varying across provinces. The Employment Insurance (EI) program provides income support for up to 45 weeks, replacing 55% of an individual's income. While social safety nets related to food and nutrition security are generally robust, gaps remain, particularly for Indigenous and marginalized communities.

HEALTH BEHAVIORS

Like other Western nations, Canadians face challenges with health risk behaviors. According to the government, the most prevalent issues are physical inactivity, unhealthy eating, alcohol misuse, tobacco smoking, and substance use (Public Health Agency of Canada, 2016).

Human Rights and Social Justice

Canada positions itself as a progressive nation, supporting social justice and human rights domestically and internationally. The government focuses on inclusive governance, pluralism, respect for diversity, and promoting the rights of women, children, Indigenous Peoples, LGBTQ+ individuals, and refugees (Global Affairs Canada, 2023).

Environmental Issues

Canada's record on environmental issues is mixed. While strongly supporting United Nations' efforts on climate change, biodiversity loss, and curbing methane emissions, the country's significant mining and oil sectors have devastating environmental impacts globally, including forest loss, water contamination, community displacement, and greenhouse gas emissions.

In summary, Canada's determinants of health reflect a complex interplay of socioeconomic advantages and disparities, with marginalized groups facing more significant challenges in areas like poverty, education, and access to social support despite the nation's overall prosperity and progressive policies.

CONCLUSION

Canada's universal healthcare system performs comparably to other high-income nations, ranking higher globally than most countries. Financially, Canada's per-capita healthcare spending of $5,905 in 2021 was less than half of the exorbitant $12,318 spent in the United States for the same year. Yet, Canada achieves significantly better population health outcomes. However, the Canadian system faces several serious challenges that require attention. Access to primary care delivered by family physicians is frequently cited as a significant issue by patients, providers, and policymakers alike, nearing a crisis point that demands immediate reforms. Long wait times, especially for specialist consultations and surgical procedures, are often mentioned as a detriment impacting public satisfaction with the healthcare system. Additionally, dental and vision care are not covered under the core Medicare benefits, leaving approximately one third of Canadians without supplemental private insurance to access these services (Allin et al., 2020).

Furthermore, regional disparities in access to healthcare services persist across Canada's vast geography. This is unsurprising for a country of such immense size, but marginalized populations like Indigenous communities are disproportionately affected by these access inequities, mirroring other socioeconomic disadvantages they face. After 50 years since its inception, there is a consensus among patients, healthcare providers, and policymakers that Canada's Medicare system needs an overhaul to address these short-term access issues and ensure its long-term financial sustainability and continued delivery of high-quality care.

LEARNING ACTIVITIES

CourseConnect

To access self-assessment questions and interactive, competency-based learning activities for this chapter, visit www.springerpub.com/courseconnect. See inside front cover and tear-out for CourseConnect details.

REFERENCES

Allin, S., Marchildon, G., & Merkur, S. (2020). Canada's health system: Struggling to modernize a half-century old system. *European Journal of Public Health, 30*(Suppl_5). https://doi.org/10.1093/eurpub/ckaa165.1001

Global Affairs Canada. (2023, July 19). *Canada's efforts to address global issues*. https://www.international.gc.ca/world-monde/issues_development-enjeux_developpement/human_rights-droits_homme/advancing_rights-promouvoir_droits.aspx?lang=eng

Hutchison, B. (2017). Canadian health care: An overview. *PLoS Medicine, 14*(3), e1002268. https://doi.org/10.1371/journal.pmed.1002268

Marchildon, G. P., Allin, S., & Merkur, S. (2020). Canada: Health system review. *Health Systems in Transition, 22*(3), 1–194. PMID: 33527903.

Martin, D., Miller, A.P., Quesnel-Vallée, A., Caron, N.R., Vissandjée, B., Marchildon, G.P. (2018). Canada's universal health-care system: Achieving its potential. *Lancet, 391*(10131), 1718-1735. https://linkinghub.elsevier.com/retrieve/pii/S0140673618301818

National Advisory Council on Poverty. (2023). *Blueprint for transformation: The 2023 report of the National Advisory Council on Poverty*. https://www.canada.ca/content/dam/esdc-edsc/documents/programs/poverty-reduction/national-advisory-council/reports/2023-annual/NACP_2023-Report-EN%20Final.pdf

Philpott, J. (2024). *Health for all: A doctor's prescription for a healthier Canada*. Signal-Mcleland & Steward.

Public Health Agency of Canada. (2016). *How healthy are Canadians?: A trend analysis of the health of Canadians from a healthy living and chronic disease perspective*. http://publications.gc.ca/collections/collection_2017/aspc-phac/HP40-167-2016-eng.pdf

Shaw, J. (2005). Oh Canada: Comparing single-payer health care with practice in the United States. *The American Journal of Medicine, 118*(10), 1064–1066. https://doi.org/10.1016/j.amjmed.2005.07.007

Statistics Canada. (2021, June 15). *A statistical portrait of Canada's diverse LGBTQ2+ communities*. https://www150.statcan.gc.ca/n1/daily-quotidien/210615/dq210615a-eng.htm

Statistics Canada. (2023, November 27). *Leading causes of death, total population, by age group*. https://www150.statcan.gc.ca/n1/daily-quotidien/231127/t001b-eng.htm

Statistics Canada. (2024a, May 27). *Population and demography statistics*. https://www.statcan.gc.ca/en/subjects-start/population_and_demography

Statistics Canada. (2024b, June 7). *Life expectancy*. https://www150.statcan.gc.ca/n1/en/subjects/health/life_expectancy_and_deaths/life_expectancy

Statistics Canada. (2025, July 16). *Canada's population clock (real-time model)*. https://www150.statcan.gc.ca/n1/pub/71-607-x/71-607-x2018005-eng.htm

U.S. News & World Report. (2024). *Quality of life rankings*. https://www.usnews.com/news/best-countries/rankings/quality-of-life

World Economic Forum. (2023, February 23). *These countries spend the most on healthcare*. https://www.weforum.org/agenda/2023/02/charted-countries-most-expensive-healthcare-spending/

Zang, T. (2024). *The doctor dilemma: Improving primary care access in Canada (Commentary No. 660)*. C.D. Howe Institute.

CHAPTER 7

MEXICO

Itzel Eguiluz Cárdenas, Sarah Ratkovich González, and Irma Marcela González-Treviño

GEOGRAPHY, SIZE, AND DEMOGRAPHICS

IMPORTANT GEOGRAPHIC FEATURES AND DIVISIONS

The United Mexican States has a territorial extension of 1,964,375 square kilometers (1,220,606 square miles; Government of Mexico, 2014), which makes it one of the biggest countries in the world. It occupies the 13th place, and the capital, Mexico City, is the fifth most populated city in the world when counting its metropolitan area.

Mexico is divided into 32 federative entities, split into various municipalities along geographic and political lines (Instituto Nacional de Estadística y Geografía [INEGI], 2020). Each state has its own constitution and penal code.

POPULATION SIZE

According to 2020 data from the INEGI, the year of the last available national census, Mexico had a population of 126,014,024 inhabitants, composed of 64,540,634 women (51.2%) and 61,473,390 men (48.8%; INEGI, 2020).

AGE DISTRIBUTION

There is a greater concentration in the age range of 10 to 14 years, composed of 10,943,540 people, followed by the group 15 to 19 years old, consisting of 10,806,690 people. Mexico still has a young population, although this is changing rapidly (Figure 7.1).

MEDIAN AGE AND BIRTH RATES

Additionally, the median age of the country's population was 29 years (INEGI, 2020). The number of registered births for the year 2020 was 1,629,211, while for the year 2022, a total of 1,891,388 births were reported. Furthermore, women age 15 to 49 years have an average of 1.5 live births per 1,000 (INEGI, 2020). These numbers vary from state to state. For example, the fertility rate in Mexico City is less than 1.5 birth per 1,000 while in the southern state of Chiapas is 2.7 live births per 1,000

MIGRATION PATTERNS

Between 2015 and 2020, a total of 802,807 individuals emigrated to other countries, with the majority falling within the 18 to 29 age group (47%). The primary reasons for these residential changes were to reunite with family (36.5%), to seek employment (16.4%), and a job change or offer (12.4%; INEGI, 2020). According to 2020 data from the International Organization for Migration (2022), there was an unmodified population of approximately 11,186,000 immigrants in Mexico, less than 1% of the country's population. Most are nationals from the United States, Venezuela, Guatemala, Honduras, and Spain. Also, Mexico traditionally has been a country of emigration, but in the last 10 years, the number of people seeking refuge has risen.

FIGURE 7.1 Population by age and sex, Mexico 2023.

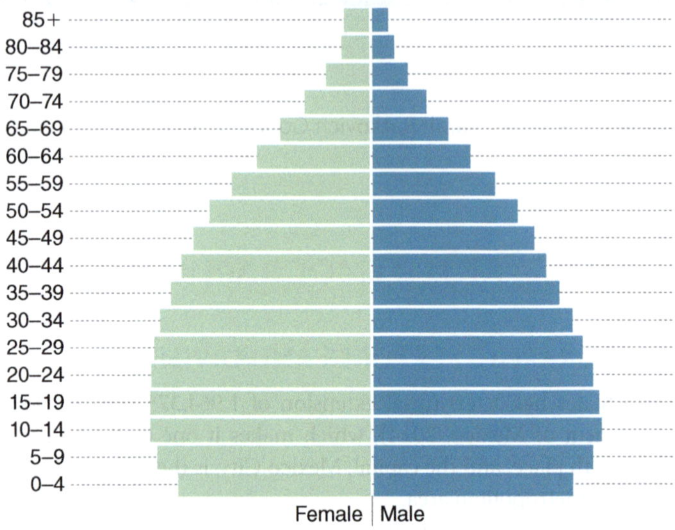

Source: World Health Organization. (2024). *Mexico, country overview*. https://data.who.int/countries/484

URBAN/RURAL: WHAT THIS MEANS TO MEXICO AND OTHER GEOGRAPHIC DISTRIBUTIONS

In Mexico, as elsewhere, population is the primary criterion for distinguishing between rural and urban distribution. A rural population is one in which fewer than 2,500 people reside, whereas an urban community is populated by a greater number. Considering these data, in 2020, 79% of the population lived in urban areas, while 21% resided in rural areas (INEGI, 2020).

MALE/FEMALE/LGBTTTIQ GROUPS

Considering data from the year 2021, there were approximately 5,000,000 people over the age of 15 years who identify as part of the LGBTTTIQ community, which accounts for 5.1% of the population in that age group. Of that number, 81.8% identify based on sexual orientation, 7.6% based on gender identity, and 10.6% based on both. Thus, 2,387,343 individuals identify as bisexual, 1,224,823 as homosexual, 489,835 as lesbian, and 518,811 indicate another type of sexual orientation. Additionally, 316,258 individuals are transgender, and 592,328 individuals have another gender identity (INEGI, 20221). Since 2021, in Mexico City trans identities have been legally identified, and starting in 2023, the National Electoral Institute approved nonbinary electoral cards for voting; also, with some flaws, same-sex marriage is recognized in all the Mexican states.

ETHNIC GROUPS: AFRO-MEXICAN POPULATION

Considering the country's ethnic groups, in 2020, 23.2 million people over 3 years old identified themselves as Indigenous. Of this population, 30.8% (7,364,645) spoke an Indigenous language, and 865,972 did not speak Spanish (INEGI, 2022). On the other hand, individuals who recognize themselves as Afro-descendants or Afro-Mexicans represent 2% of the population, equivalent to 2,576,213 people (INEGI, 2020).

CULTURAL BELIEFS

RELIGIONS

In Mexico, 97,864,218 people consider themselves Catholics, and 14,095,307 identify as Protestants or Evangelical Christians. Additionally, there are 58,876 practitioners of Judaism and 7,982 followers of Islam. Likewise, 29,985 people practice religions of Eastern origin, 33,372 engage in religious practices with various ethnic roots, 40,799 adhere to religions of African roots, and 36,764 consider themselves spiritualists. In contrast, other religions are comprised of 40,391 individuals. Finally, 10,211,052 people identify as nonreligious, 3,103,464 are without religious affiliation, and 491,814 are not specified (INEGI, 2020).

LANGUAGES

Mexico is considered a multilingual country due to the 68 Indigenous languages spoken. Among these languages, the most spoken are Nahuatl with 725,000 speakers, Maya with 859,000 speakers, Tzeltal with 556,000 speakers, Mixtec with 517,000 speakers, Tsotsil with 487,000, Zapotec with 479,000, Otomi with 307,000. Lastly, Totonac, Chol, and Mazatec each have more than 200,000 speakers (Ministry of Culture, 2019).

POLITICAL SYSTEM

Mexico has three primary government powers: the executive, which is the president with a 6 year term; the legislative, composed of the Congress of senators and deputies; and the judiciary, represented by the Supreme Court (Secretaría de Relaciones Exteriores, 2012). Although, some political positions in the country are open for reelection as majors.

HISTORICAL CONSIDERATIONS FOR CONTEXT AS COLONIALISM

Before the Spanish arrived in Mexico, there were reports of the region as being healthy by Fray Bartolome de las Casas, a Spanish priest and the denominated "protector of the Indigenous people." He had the opportunity to travel throughout the conquered territories and document his findings. He also stated that the local population decreased rapidly due to the physical abuse and the diseases the Spaniards brought with them such as smallpox and measles. It is also well known that the Mexican population lived under hygienic conditions—they washed their hands and food and cared for their teeth. The European conquerors had poor sanitation, and they ascribed the habit of bathing to the development of diseases, as well as "divine punishment" since they considered the rituals, which included drinking pulque, an alcoholic beverage called the "Gods drink," and the adoration of their deities as heresy who should be penalized by the Spanish god.

The Spanish began building hospitals and pharmacies to care for the conquered sick population. However, they still had poor housing conditions and no access to vaccination, which resulted in a continuum of ill health and an inability to work the land, leading to drought and more diseases. The local population, as well as the enslaved Black people, were nearly completely lost until the medical advances of the 18th century helped improve this situation and decreased the mortality rate (Mandujano, 2003).

HEALTH OUTCOMES

TOP 10 CAUSES OF DEATH AND MORTALITY RISK FACTORS

In the last 10 years (considering that the statistics come from 2022), Mexico has had a consistent death rate; however, since the COVID-19 pandemic, it has taken a giant leap and has not decreased to the previous rates.

Even if Mexico is unique, the leading causes of death are similar to the ones observed globally. According to INEGI, the first 10 causes of death (women and men combined) are shown in Table 7.1.

In the women/men distribution, the first three causes remain the same. However, stroke moves to number four in the case of women. Also, it is interesting to notice that cardiovascular diseases, which are the leading cause of death worldwide and the main cause in Mexico, account for more than twice as much as the second cause, which is diabetes mellitus (INEGI, 2022).

As we can see, the leading death causes are nontransmittable diseases; this is strictly related to the main risk factors associated with death in Mexico. According to the Institute of Health Metrics and Evaluation (IHME) in Mexico, the first risk factor associated with death is high blood sugar, which directly relates to the second cause of death, diabetes mellitus. Moreover, the other top five causes are high body mass index, dietary risks, kidney dysfunction, and high blood pressure. These risk factors are not mutually exclusive, and reveal a pattern of factors mostly related to metabolic diseases and mainly caused by behavioral risks, but not exclusively (IHME, 2021).

It is apparent that noncommunicable diseases are the leading cause of health burden in Mexico, especially when considering how they can relate to each other and how some risk factors are associated with more than one cause of death.

MENTAL HEALTH

Mental health care in Mexico faces significant challenges despite growing awareness and service demand. Although there is a high prevalence of mental health disorders, access to care is still limited, particularly in rural areas. Mental disorders have considerably increased since the only national mental health survey that used diagnostic criteria to evaluate their prevalence. It is important to invest in epidemiological studies, prevention, and care of mental disorders, which are among the leading causes of years lived with disability in the country (Medina-Mora et al. 2023).

Policies and programs in Mexico promote integrating mental health services into primary health care (PHC). However, these services remain largely unavailable in the country. Civil society organizations, including religious institutions, are the primary providers of migrant health care in Mexico. While there have been some government initiatives to improve mental health services, such as creating specialized clinics and training more mental health professionals, these efforts have been insufficient to address the growing need. There are also disparities in access to care based on socioeconomic status.

As a result of the pandemic, it is urgent to guarantee unconditional access to the national health system, including mental health care, for asylum seekers, refugees, and other vulnerable migrants, regardless of their documentation status (Hintermeier et al., 2024).

Efforts to improve mental health care in Mexico must focus on increasing funding, expanding services to underserved areas (rural), reducing stigma, and improving the quality of services. This requires a collaborative effort among government agencies, healthcare providers, and civil society organizations. Therefore, the 2023 to 2024 plan has three focus areas: Primary Health Care, Adequate Stewardship, and Intersectionality.

INFECTIOUS DISEASES

Data on infectious diseases in Mexico are quite comprehensive since the Health Secretary has a weekly epidemiologic report that condenses the overall incidence and prevalence of many infectious diseases—from vector-borne diseases to respiratory illnesses, and even a report for diseases preventable by vaccination.

Recalling the causes of death, we found COVID-19 unsurprisingly as the fifth cause, and other respiratory infections (influenza and pneumonia) in the ninth and tenth places. However, when discussing morbidity, we found that the first four diseases are infectious: acute respiratory, urinary, intestinal, and COVID-19, being the most prevalent (Single Information System for Epidemiological Surveillance [SUIVE], 2022).

TABLE 7.1 LEADING CAUSES OF DEATH AND NUMBER OF DEATHS, BY SEX (2022)

RANK	TOTAL	MEN	WOMEN
1	Heart diseases: 200,023 In 2021 there were 225,449	Heart diseases: 106,769 In 2021 there were 123,313	Heart diseases: 93,201 In 2021 there were 102,127
2	Diabetes mellitus: 115,025 In 2021 there were 140,729	Diabetes mellitus: 57,174 In 2021 there were 71,330	Diabetes mellitus: 57,837 In 2021 there were 69,396
3	Malignant tumors: 89,574 In 2021 there were 90,124	Malignant tumors: 42,889 In 2021 there were 45,503	Malignant tumors: 46,673 In 2021 there were 46,620
4	Liver diseases: 41,281 In 2021 there were 41,890	Liver diseases: 30,127 In 2021 there were 30,524	Cerebrovascular diseases: 17,919 In 2021 there were 18,090
5	COVID-19: 38,508 In 2021 there were 238,772	Accidents: 28,816 In 2021 there were 26,787	COVID-19: 15,255 In 2021 there were 93,652
6	Accidents: 37,450 In 2021 there were 36,613	Assaults (homicides): 28,816 In 2021 there were 31,263	Influenza and pneumonia: 14,131 In 2021 there were 21,492
7	Cerebrovascular diseases: 35,977 In 2021 there were 37,169	COVID-19: 23,250 In 2021 there were 145,115	Liver diseases: 11,147 In 2021 there were 11,362
8	Assaults (homicides): 33,287 In 2021 there were 35,700	Influenza and pneumonia: 18,905 In 2021 there were 33,101	Chronic obstructive pulmonary diseases: 8,772 In 2021 there were 8,579
9	Influenza and pneumonia: 33,049 In 2021 there were 54,601	Cerebrovascular diseases: 18,052 In 2021 there were 19,079	Accidents: 8,578 In 2021 there were 7,786
10	Chronic obstructive pulmonary diseases: 18,463 In 2021 there were 18,439	Chronic obstructive pulmonary diseases: 9,685 In 2021 there were 9,860	Renal insufficiency: 6,265 In 2021 there were 6,160

Note: Teal, dark green, and light green indicate communicable diseases; dark pink, light pink, grey, dark blue, and beige indicate noncommunicable diseases; light orange and dark orange indicate external causes.

Source: World Health Organization. (2024). *Mexico: Country overview*. https://data.who.int/countries/484

It is vital to note that, being a multidiverse country with many types of weather, including tropical weather which is a risk factor for vector-borne diseases, this has become of interest to the government. Dengue virus (DV) is a topic of concern in Mexico. Dengue has been a significant health issue for the last 10 years; it has been noted by the Epidemiological Vigilance System that every year from 2011 through 2024 (except for 2021), there have been more than 10,000 confirmed cases of dengue; 2013 and 2023 had higher confirmed cases (more than 60,000 and 50,000, respectively). It is of concern that out of the four subtypes of dengue, all of them have been reported in Mexico, changing the prevalence from DV-1 and 2 to DV-3 and 2. This is important because when people get a DV infection with one subtype, they have immunity for that one, but if they get infected by any of the other three, the risk for severe dengue increases (Secretaría de Salud, 2024).

Regarding HIV, the first case reported in Mexico was in 1983 (Centro Nacional para la Prevención y Control del VIH y el SIDA [CENSIDA], 2023). Subsequent reports indicated that approximately 370,000 people were living with HIV. According to the 95-90-86 UNAIDS goals for AIDS 2030, 95% of the population living with HIV will know their status, 90% of them will have antiretroviral treatment, and 86% of them will be in virological suppression. Mexico has 72-62-58, accounting for 230,000 people having access to treatment and 215,000 being in virological suppression (CENSIDA, 2023).

INFANT AND MATERNAL MORTALITY

In recent years, Mexico has seen significant improvements in infant and maternal mortality, yet challenges remain.

The good news about infant mortality is that it has decreased from 22.6 deaths per 1,000 live births in 2000 to 12.1 deaths per 1,000 live births in 2020, which represents a 46.2% decrease, according to the Pan American Health Organization (PAHO, 2022).

Of course, some challenges need to be addressed. Some of these are linked to disparities along regions and socioeconomic status, as social determinants of health where neonatal mortality (deaths within the first 28 days of life) remains a concern.

Concerning maternal mortality, its ratio has declined from an estimated 59.1 deaths per 100,000 live births in 2020, a 4.6% since 2000. Nonetheless, diverse challenges arose during the pandemic, and the maternal mortality ratio increased during the first 2 years, 2020 and 2021 (PAHO, 2022).

Some other impact factors related to social determinants of health are lack of access to prenatal and postnatal care, difficulties in accessing healthcare centers, and inadequate nutrition. Some initiatives address these factors, such as enhancing training and skills for healthcare providers, diverse infant nutrition programs, and increased breastfeeding.

LIFE EXPECTANCY

Life expectancy in Mexico has fluctuated in recent years. While there were significant improvements before 1990, life expectancy at birth in 2023 was 75.0 years, lower than in 2019 (Health in the Americas, 2022). Some of these changes may be related to the COVID-19 pandemic (World Health Organization [WHO], 2024).

In Mexico, as in most countries, women have a longer life expectancy than men, with a difference of more than 6 years. Some differences are higher for specific states or cities, as Nuevo León has a higher life expectancy than Guerrero or Chiapas, raising the need to address changes for social determinants of health.

QUALITY OF LIFE INDEXES

The UN Development Programme (UNDP, 2024) classified human index development as high, with a .781 for 2022. While it decreased during the COVID-19 pandemic, as with other indexes and indicators, it recovered to previous levels during the last year, situating Mexico in a lower range than the world average. The gender gap is a bit higher than the world average with .979, placing Mexico in the 33rd global position, being Mexico's most urgent topic among Participation and Economic Opportunities (UNDP, 2024).

HISTORICAL/THEORETICAL BACKGROUND OF HEALTHCARE

THE MEXICAN HEALTH SYSTEM

According to reports by WHO, the healthcare system in Mexico is divided into three main components: (a) social security based on employment, (b) public assistance services for nonbeneficiaries of social security, which is supported by a financial protection program, and (c) private sector comprised of service providers, insurance companies, and fabricants and distributors of pharmaceutical products and medical devices.

The evolution of the Mexican health system came as a consequence of the Industrial Revolution, where the workers needed insurance to cover accidents, as well as the 1917 Constitution (that came at the conclusion of the Mexican Revolution), followed by the establishment of the Social Security Mexican Institute (IMSS) during the first half of the 19th century. The driver to all of these was to improve the health quality of the rural and poor populations in the country as well as to protect the people from epidemics. The position of Health Secretary was created and articles were added to the Constitution regarding the professional practice of medicine and the protection of women and children as well as the workers' health as a fundamental right.

After the revolution, Mexico and the United States began a program to eradicate yellow fever, which, with joint efforts, was eliminated from Mexico in 1925; this collaboration also led to the forming of the School of Public Health of Mexico.

The National Institute of Social Security (INSS) was planned as a government-funded institution. The concept was first discussed in 1928 but later modified and rejected by the succeeding governments. Finally, the IMSS was established (changing the word "National" for "Mexican") in the middle of World War II in 1943. Initially, the IMSS only covered employees of a few private sector jobs and was not well received by workers and healthcare professionals. This eventually fell into place after the government made some adjustments to ensure more people would benefit from the IMSS and that healthcare workers got a small payment.

At the beginning of the 2000s and with a new government party in Mexico, Popular Insurance (Seguro Popular), was founded for the attention of the most economically **vulnerable populations** in the country, offering a high level of attention to its beneficiaries and covering costly diseases such as HIV/AIDS and a broad list of cancers; however, during the current administration it has had many administrative changes that are not homogeneous in every state (González Block, 2020). Then, these services were replaced with the INSABI (Instituto de Salud para el Bienestar [Institute of Health for Well-Being]); this change started just before the pandemic, and in 2024, the plan included moving these services to IMSS Bienestar, a branch of social security services.

HEALTHCARE TRAINING AND EDUCATION

The economically active population in Mexico in 2021 means that the professionals working actively in healthcare comprise 10% of the total professionals; 19% have technician training, 71% have a professional degree, and 9% have a postgraduate degree. Most healthcare professionals work in nursery and care, followed by medicine, odontology, therapy, and rehabilitation professionals. Most healthcare professionals (approximately 7%) work in diagnosis, pharmacy, public health, and multidisciplinary programs (INEGI, 2021).

More than two-thirds of Mexico's healthcare personnel are women. Nonetheless, there are significant gender gaps among physicians and nurses. These gaps also mean that while women make up most of the workforce in Mexico, their presence in leadership positions is still very scarce.

PREVENTIVE HEALTH

Preventive health and health promotion focus on preventing morbidity and mortality in a population by decreasing the risk factors and detecting diseases promptly. One of the main preventive activities in healthcare is vaccination. Mexico has a Universal Vaccination program, encompassing a manual of vaccines that includes the type of vaccination, age, and coverage; there is also a National Vaccination Card, specifically for children, women, men, and older adults. This vaccination program has 12 vaccines, many of which have multiple targets and are available for free in public healthcare centers (Centro Nacional para la Salud de la Infancia y Adolescencia [CeNSIA], 2015).

HEALTHCARE COST, QUALITY, AND ACCESS

In 2020, Mexico's public health expenditures were relatively low, accounting for only 3.3% of the gross domestic product (GDP) and 11.52% of total public expenditures. There is a significant reliance on out-of-pocket spending, representing 38.77% of total health expenditures. This financial burden on individuals and families can limit access to healthcare and lead to economic hardship, particularly for vulnerable populations. Increasing public health funding could alleviate this issue and improve healthcare outcomes for all Mexicans (World Bank Group, 2024).

One unique characteristic of the Mexican health system is the private clinics located in drug stores/pharmacies or even supermarkets. General practitioners offer primary medical care from these locations, such as contraceptive information, blood pressure measurements, and joint disease treatments, and treat conditions such as diarrhea or the flu. Some providers are now offering medical lab services in these pharmacy clinics. In the last national census (2020), 13.1% of the population and some immigrants reported using these clinics (INEGI, 2020) as they are widely available at reasonable costs. There have been criticisms of the services' quality, however, such as the high amount of antibiotics prescribed.

DETERMINANTS OF HEALTH

NATIONAL AND PER-CAPITA GROSS DOMESTIC PRODUCT AND POVERTY RATES

In 2023, the Mexican economy grew by 3.2% for the second year. Although slower than the post-pandemic rebound, this growth demonstrates a robust economy. Furthermore, there has been a significant poverty reduction, with the official multidimensional poverty rate dropping from 43.9% in 2020 to 36.3% in 2022 (World Bank Group, 2024). This positive shift has lifted an estimated 8.8 million Mexicans out of poverty, although progress in alleviating extreme poverty has been slower (World Bank Group, 2024). There is still a lot to do, especially for vulnerable populations affected by the lack of essential services in some states and rural areas.

EDUCATION, LITERACY, AND ECONOMIC RATES

Mexico has made significant strides in education in recent years. Between 2000 and 2020, the average number of years of schooling increased by 38.4%, reaching 9.2 years. Additionally, Mexico boasts a high literacy rate of 99.1%, with men at 99.2% and women at 99.0%.

The unemployment rate remained low in 2022 at 3.3%, with a negligible difference between men and women (3.3% and 3.4%, respectively). However, a significant number of people still work in nonformal economy employment. In 2024, the Congress approved an essential increase for the minimum number of annual vacation days, now 12 days, while previously it was 6 days.

In addition, 43.9% of the population was below the national poverty line in 2020, a decrease from 41.9% in 2018. In 2020, 3.1% of the population lived in poverty, defined as having an income of less than $1.90 per day, below the regional average of 3%.

FOOD AND NUTRITION

Mexico is characterized by its rich and varied cuisine, which includes essential ingredients such as corn, beans, chili, tomatoes, avocado, herbs, and spices. The cuisine varies from region to region, and traditional dishes and beverages encompass a wide range and are part of its culinary culture. However, there are concerns about the high consumption of processed foods rich in fats, sugars, and salt (INEGI, 2015).

Nutrition in Mexico encompasses various aspects of food, health, and social determinants, such as social, economic, and gender inequalities, access to healthcare and education, and health policies and programs (Hernández-Ávila et al., 2020).

In Mexico, food and celebrations are closely related, as food is considered a way to bring together family and friends, share experiences, and uphold the country's traditions. Another noteworthy aspect of Mexico's culinary diversity is its street food culture, including street vendors, markets, and culinary festivals (Martínez, 2018).

Considering the multidiversity of Mexico, related to its history of Indigenous populations and the colonial influence, there are many different traditions and celebrationss; According to the Cultural Information System, there are 1,256 celebrations in Mexico, many of them related to a religious entity, most of them of Catholic descent. Interestingly, one of the primary ways the events are celebrated in Mexico is through its gastronomy, declared in 2010 as the Cultural Patrimony of Humanity by UNESCO. Mexican festivities are always associated with certain foods; for example, the "pan de muerto," or bread of death, consumed on the Dia de Muertos, one of the most important in the country.

HEALTH BEHAVIORS

Health and dietary behaviors in Mexico are influenced by various factors such as cultural, socioeconomic, political, and environmental factors. The availability and access to food are the main factors determining an individual's eating pattern and behavior. However, this can be reversible with proper nutritional education. In Mexico, according to the National Health and Nutrition Survey (La Encuesta Nacional de Salud y Nutrición [ENSANUT], 2018), 75.2% of Mexican adults are overweight or obese, specifically 42.5% are overweight and 33.7% are obese. According to the same survey, 35.6% of preschool-age children (0 to 4 years old) are overweight or obese. In the age group of 5 to 11 years, the prevalence is 34.1%, which is genuinely concerning due to the onset of chronic degenerative diseases such as diabetes mellitus, high blood pressure, musculoskeletal disorders, certain types of cancer, to name a few. Nonetheless, there is also essential work to eliminate "fatphobia" from society and medical approaches.

SOCIAL JUSTICE, SUCH AS HUMAN RIGHTS ISSUES AND VULNERABLE AND UNDERSERVED POPULATIONS

Migrants and Refugee Health

There are challenges within the National Health System that are exacerbated when immigrant populations, especially those in irregular situations, try to access health services. The recent changes, by the transition from Seguro Popular to the centralized INSABI and now to IMSS-Bienestar, have further strained the country's capacity to respond effectively, especially during and in the aftermath of the COVID-19 pandemic. In Mexico, immigrant populations are theoretically covered by existing healthcare plans, but face significant barriers to accessing these services. The lack of clear guidelines for INSABI eligibility and the requirement for government-issued identification further marginalize this vulnerable group, leaving them at heightened risk.

Other Vulnerable Populations

Discrimination is an essential issue in many Mexican populations. This social rejection leads to difficulties when trying to access crucial services and human rights. In 2022 INEGI reported that the main interest groups for discrimination were people from the LGTB community (37.3%) and Afro-descendants (35.6%); of both groups, women were most targeted. Skin color was also a vital discrimination point; people who were discriminated against were mainly of a darker complexion with which more than a third of the population was identified.

These types of discrimination negate vulnerable individuals' rights, the most important being receiving economic social support, receiving medical attention, and receiving services in a government office. In the two former, women reported being the main subjects of discrimination; in the last, men were the majority.

Other important groups in this report were people with disabilities, older adults (60 and older), Indigenous people, and women who worked as housekeepers (INEGI, 2022).

ENVIRONMENTAL AND CLIMATE CHANGE ISSUES: VECTOR-BORNE DISEASES AND AIR POLLUTION

According to the IHME in 2021, out of the 10 main risk factors for death and disability in Mexico, the only one that is related to environmental risks is air pollution, which was in eighth place; in 2011 it was in seventh place, indicating a decrease; however, this could be due the COVID-19 pandemic. Air pollution is a significant risk factor for respiratory and cardiovascular diseases, as well as cancer development, which are among the top 10 death causes in Mexico (IHME, 2021).

HEALTH PRACTICES

TRADITIONAL AND COMPLEMENTARY

Midwives

Midwives play a crucial role in maternal and newborn health in Mexico, especially in some states with higher rural and Indigenous populations, such as Guerrero. In contrast, finding these practices in the northern states is more difficult. Midwives provide culturally relevant care, often combining nonacademic knowledge with clinical practices.

A midwife or *partera*'s main activities are prenatal care, labor and delivery support, and postnatal care. They also help and educate mothers in breastfeeding, newborn care, and family planning.

In Mexico, some parteras have learned their skills through apprenticeship and oral tradition, and they often incorporate local practices and remedies into their care. At the same time, others have received formal midwifery training and are usually employed by public hospitals or clinics. They combine their medical knowledge with cultural sensitivity to provide comprehensive care.

Although it has been demonstrated that partera offer safe practices, they still need recognition in clinical spaces. They have limited access to education and training, and often face stigma.

Organizations, including Compañeros en Salud (Partners in Health) and the International Confederation of Midwives (ICM), are working to support and strengthen midwifery in Mexico. By recognizing and supporting midwives' valuable contributions, Mexico can improve maternal and newborn health outcomes and women's health.

Traditional Medicine

When talking about **traditional medicine**, we tend to think only of ancestry, which, in the case of Mexico, is quite rich; however, conventional Mexican medicine is actually a cultural mix of current treatments and traditions. In 1552, a registry of medicinal plants in Mexico was documented in Nahuatl and Latin, and today, more than 80% of the country's population still use them in traditional medicine. It is estimated that more than 4,500 medicinal plants are inventoried in Mexico, most of which are reported by the Social Security Institute Herbarium. There is a significant effort to study both the scientific classification and the effects of these plants to have a more evidence-based use of the remedies.

Currently, in Mexico, in addition to medicinal plants, there are many traditional medicine practices in use by specialized therapists such as *hueseras* (people who work with bones), *sobadores* (people who massage or manipulate the body), and *curanderas* (people who use plants and rituals to cure the body). These practices were derived from the pre-Hispanic cultures and Catholic religious beliefs but also influenced the African costumes that came with the Spanish conquest (Bioversidad Mexicana, 2020).

CONCLUSION

Mexico is a multidiverse country with rich historical and cultural diversity, therefore generalizing the health of the Mexicans would be an oversight. With almost 2,000,000 square kilometers of land area a vast religious and ethnic variety, and different weather and geographic spaces, it is a unique space that encompasses many benefits and inequalities. The influence that the Spanish conquest had on Mexico'scultural baggage and beliefs is visible to this day, and shows in the racial discrimination and the sexism that is current in the country. The Mexican health system has changed during the last 20 years even though traditional medicine remains essential for a large population group. We will need to wait to see how the new government implements the current policies.

RECOMMENDATIONS TO IMPROVE HEALTH AND HEALTHCARE

Conducting surveys that include social determinants of health can help design programs and public policies based on the actual healthcare needs of all vulnerable populations, not just representative samples.

Another recommendation is the urgent need to improve access to care through expanding health service coverage in rural and vulnerable areas. Rethinking the need for identification or other documentation for migrant populations will be an asset to improving health access. Also, there is a need to improve mental health in primary care, training first-level personnel to deliver better care and aid prevention.

Many Mexicans do not know about the many resources available for the population, such as free vaccinations, the first level of healthcare without insurance or social security, and many programs of health benefits, including contraceptives. The government needs to connect more with the population, stressing the importance and availability of communication pathways to achieve more population coverage.

LEARNING ACTIVITIES

CourseConnect

To access self-assessment questions and interactive, competency-based learning activities for this chapter, visit www.springerpub.com/courseconnect. See inside front cover and tear-out for CourseConnect details.

REFERENCES

Bioversidad Mexicana. (2020). *Medicinal*. Comisión Nacional para el Conocimiento y Uso de la Biodiversidad. https://www.biodiversidad.gob.mx/diversidad/medicinal

Centro Nacional para la Prevención y Control del VIH y el SIDA. (2023). *Boletín de atención integral de personas con VIH: Centro nacional para la prevención y el control del VIH y el sida* [Comprehensive care bulletin for people living with HIV]. Gobierno de México. https://www.gob.mx/censida/documentos/boletin-de-atencion-integral-de-personas-con-vih

Centro Nacional para la Salud de la Infancia y Adolescencia. (2015). *Vacunación universal* [Universal vaccination]. Gobierno de Mexico. https://www.gob.mx/salud/censia/articulos/vacunacion-universal?state=published

González Block, M. A., Reyes Morales, H., Cahuana Hurtado, L., Balandran, A., & Mendez, E. (2020). *Mexico: Health system review*. World Health Organization. https://iris.who.int/bitstream/handle/10665/334334/HiT-22-2-2020-eng.pdf

Government of Mexico. (2014, February 13). *Datos básicos de México* [Basic facts about Mexico]. https://consulmex.sre.gob.mx/sanpedrosula/index.php/bienvenida-y-directorio/34

Hintermeier, M., Gottlieb, N., Rohleder, S., Oppenberg, J., Baroudi, M., Pernitez-Agan, S., Lopez, J., Flores, S., Mohsenpour, A., Wickramage, K., & Bozorgmehr, K. (2024). COVID-19 among migrants, refugees, and internally displaced persons: Systematic review, meta-analysis and qualitative synthesis of the global empirical literature. *EClinicalMedicine*, 74, 102698. https://doi.org/10.1016/j.eclinm.2024.102698

Instituto Nacional de Estadística y Geografía. (2015). *Encuesta intercensal 2015.* [2015 intercensal survey] https://www.inegi.org.mx/programas/intercensal/2015/

Instituto Nacional de Estadística y Geografía. (2020). *Panorama de las religiones en México* [Overview of religions in Mexico]. https://www.inegi.org.mx/contenidos/productos/prod_serv/contenidos/espanol/bvinegi/productos/nueva_estruc/889463910404.pdf

Instituto Nacional de Estadística y Geografía. (2021). *Encuesta nacional de ocupación y empleo* [National survey of occupation and employment]. https://www.inegi.org.mx/contenidos/programas/enoe/15ymas/doc/enoe_n_nota_tecnica_trim2_2021.pdf

Instituto Nacional de Estadística y Geografía. (2022). *Encuesta Nacional sobre Discriminacion* [National survey on discrimination]. https://www.inegi.org.mx/programas/enadis/2022/

Institute of Health Metrics and Evaluation. (2021). *Health research by location: Mexico.* https://www.healthdata.org/research-analysis/health-by-location/profiles/mexico#main-content

International Organization for Migrations. (2022). *Perfil migratorio de México, boletín anual 2022* [Mexico's migration profile, 2022 annual report]. En ONU Migración. https://mexico.iom.int/sites/g/files/tmzbdl1686/files/documents/2023-03/Perfil%20Migratorio-%20Boletin%20Anual%202022%20%283%29.pdf

Mandujano, A., Camarillo, L., & Mandujano, M. (2003). Historia de las epidemias en el México antiguo. Algunos aspectos biológicos y sociales History of epidemics in ancient Mexico: Some biological and social aspects. *Casa del Tiempo, [CE9]* 5, 9–21. https://www.uam.mx/difusion/revista/abr2003/mandujano.pdf.

Martínez, R. (2018). La relación entre la comida y las celebraciones en México: Un análisis antropológico [The relationship between food and celebrations in Mexico: An anthropological analysis]. *Revista Mexicana de Antropología, 22[CE10]* (1), 45–62.

Medina-Mora, M. E., Orozco, R., Rafful, C., Cordero, M., Bishai, J., Ferrari, A., Santomauro, D., Benjet, C., Borges, G., & Mantilla-Herrera, A. M. (2023). Mental disorders in Mexico 1990-2021. Results from the Global Burden of Disease 2021 study. *Gaceta medica de Mexico, 159*(6), 512–522. https://doi.org/10.24875/GMM.M24000828

Ministry of Culture. (2019). *México es uno de los países con mayor diversidad lingüística en el mundo* [Mexico is one of the countries with the greatest linguistic diversity in the world]. https://www.gob.mx/cultura/prensa/mexico-es-uno-de-los-paises-con-mayor-diversidad-linguistica-en-el-mundo#:~:text=Las%20lenguas%20que%20m%C3%A1s%20se,m%C3%A1s%20de%20200%20mil%20hablantes

Pan American Health Organization. (2022, September 24). *Mexico. Health in the Americas.* https://hia.paho.org/en/countries-22/mexico-country-profile

Sedas, A. C., Aguerrebere, M., Juarez, L. A. M., Alba, L. E. Z., Eguiluz, I., & Bhabha, J. (2020). *Situational brief: Migration in Mexico during the COVID-19 pandemic.* https://1bec58c3-8dcb-46b0-bb2a-fd4addf0b29a.filesusr.com/ugd/188e74_6f98530009f54edfa41096e8142b717b.pdf

Secretaría de Salud. (2024). *Análisis complementario de la situación epidemiológica de dengue en México* [Complementary analysis of the epidemiological situation of dengue in Mexico 2024]. https://www.gob.mx/salud/documentos/analisis-complementario-de-la-situacion-epidemiologica-de-dengue-en-mexico-2024

Single Information System for Epidemiological Surveillance. (2022). *Anuario de morbilidad 1984–2022, 20 Principales causas de enfermedad nacional* [Morbidity yearbook 1984–2022, 20 leading causes of disease in the nation]. Gobierno de Mexico. https://epidemiologia.salud.gob.mx/anuario/2022/principales/nacional/mes.pdf

UN Development Programme. (2024, March 13th). *Mexico. Specific country data.* https://hdr.undp.org/data-center/specific-country-data#/countries/MEX

World Bank Group. (2024, March 7). *World Bank in Mexico.* https://www.worldbank.org/en/country/mexico/overview

World Health Organization. (2024). *Mexico.* https://data.who.int/countries/484

PART III: Health and Healthcare in Central America

CHAPTER 8

OVERVIEW OF CENTRAL AMERICA

Leslie A. Bozeman and Luke Orgo

BRIEF HISTORY

Central America includes Belize, Costa Rica, El Salvador, Guatemala, Honduras, Nicaragua, and Panama (Figure 8.1). It lies between North America and South America, bordering Mexico and Colombia. Until 1821, when the region gained independence from Spain, five of the countries that make up modern day Central America (Costa Rica, El Salvador, Guatemala, Honduras, and Nicaragua) comprised what was then called the Kingdom of Guatemala. Belize, a former British colony known as British Honduras, gained independence from Britain in 1821 and then changed its name. It has experienced a longstanding border dispute with Guatemala (BBC News, 2023). Panama has a distinct relationship and history with the region. While it also became a part of Central America in 1821, it first aligned itself with Greater Colombia and then Colombia after Greater Colombia was dissolved. In 1903, Panama aligned with the United States to build the Panama Canal. The country, while part of the isthmus that connects North and South America, developed a distinct culture, population, and economy from the rest of the Central American countries (Wallace, 2017).

FIGURE 8.1 Map of Central America.

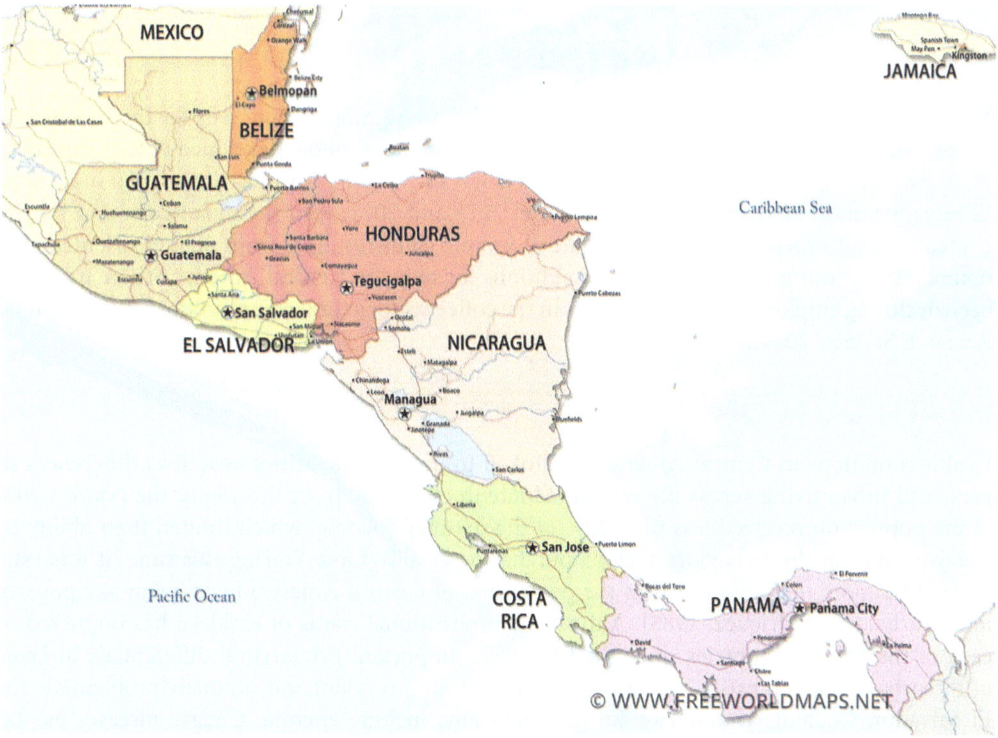

Source: FreeWorldMaps.net. (n.d.). *Central America*. https://www.freeworldmaps.net/centralamerica/

GEOGRAPHY

The region varies greatly with respect to landforms, climate, animals, soils, and vegetation (Carmack, 2017). It has four main natural areas: the highlands, northern lowlands, pacific lowlands, and southern isthmus. It is characterized by a tropical climate, mountains in the interior, several active volcanoes, and frequent earthquakes. Earthquakes and volcanic eruptions throughout the region's history caused the destruction of infrastructure and the relocation of cities (Perez-Brignoli, 1985). Along the coasts there are extensive lowlands and humid swamps. The climate is largely tropical, although cooler in higher elevations (Shally-Jensen, 2015).

POPULATION

The Indigenous groups of the region vary greatly by country. They include the Olmecs and the Pipils of El Salvador and the Maya in Belize, Guatemala, and parts of Honduras and El Salvador. The Monimbó, Subtiava, Matagalpa, the Miskito, Sumo, Rama and the Garifuna inhabited Nicaragua. The Bribrí, Cabécar, Boruca, Guatuso, and Térraba inhabited Costa Rica (Teaching Central America, 2025).

Modern day populations across the region consist of ***mestizos***—individuals of mixed ethnic heritage including Indigenous, European, and African descent. Approximately 40% of Central Americans live in rural areas (Huddleston, 2021). In 2023, the population of Central America was greater than 181 million. Guatemala, with a population of approximately 18.1 million, was the most populous Central American country in 2023, and Belize, with a population of approximately 411,000, was the least populated. The population density in Central America during 2023 was 74 people per square kilometer, which was above the global population density of 62 people per square kilometer. El Salvador's population density, 305 people per square kilometer, was exceptionally high. In contrast, Belize's population density, 18 people per square kilometer, was well below the global average (UN Data Portal, n.d.).

SOCIOECONOMIC FACTORS

Marginalization, discrimination, poverty, and health are significant concerns for the Indigenous peoples of Central America (Ramirez, 2020). According to a model developed at the University of Texas at Austin, an average of 407,000 people left the region's Northern Triangle (Guatemala, El Salvador, and Honduras) annually between 2018 and 2021, with the majority bound for the United States. Unfortunately, the moderate economic gains resulting from market-oriented economic reforms did not improve living conditions for many in Central America. There have also been declining employment opportunities in the coffee sector's rural communities (Congressional Research Service, 2024).

HEATH OUTCOMES

Health conditions in Central America are linked to income disparities as well as differences in rural and urban living across the region (Monteith et al., 2005). In the 1960s, the poorest 40% of the population received less than 10% of the national income, which limited their ability to engage in pro-health behaviors such as purchasing quality food. During this time, it was estimated that more than two thirds of the population of Central America lived below the poverty line (Garfield & Rodriguez, 1985). Although the nutritional status of children has improved in each of the region's countries since the late 1980s, important urban/rural differentials in favor of the urban area still exist. Health conditions that are prevalent and uniquely problematic for El Salvador, Guatemala, and Honduras, specifically, include anemia, Chagas disease, mental health issues, obesity, and soil-transmitted infections (Minnesota Department of Health, 2024).

From a global perspective, Central America has favorable health outcomes and Costa Rica is viewed as one of the world's healthiest countries. Population aging along with high incidences of noncommunicable diseases such as heart disease, stroke, diabetes mellitus, chronic obstructive pulmonary disease, and chronic kidney disease are of particular concern in Central America. In addition, Central America experienced significant mortality from the COVID-19 pandemic (Institute for Health Metrics and Evaluation [IHME], n.d.). Please refer to Table 8.1 for Central American health outcome data.

TABLE 8.1 HEALTH OUTCOMES OF CENTRAL AMERICA

REGION/ COUNTRY	LIFE EXPECTANCY AT BIRTH, 2023	INFANT MORTALITY, 2023	MATERNAL MORTALITY, 2020	LEADING CAUSE OF MORTALITY, 2021
Central America	74.96	11.5	64.5	—
Belize	73.57	8.7	129.8	COVID-19 and heart disease
Costa Rica	80.80	6.5	22	COVID-19 and heart disease
El Salvador	72.10	9.5	42.8	COVID-19 and heart disease
Guatemala	72.60	17.6	95.5	COVID-19 and heart disease
Honduras	72.88	13.0	71.8	COVID-19 and heart disease
Nicaragua	74.95	12.3	77.9	COVID-19 and heart disease
Panama	79.59	12.6	49.5	COVID-19 and heart disease

Sources: Institute for Health Metrics and Evaluation. (n.d.). *Health research by location: Country profiles*. https://www.healthdata.org/research-analysis/health-by-location/profiles; UN Data Portal. (n.d.). *UN population division data portal*. https://population.un.org/dataportal/home; UN Population Fund. (n.d.). *Maternal health*. https://www.unfpa.org/maternal-health

LEARNING ACTIVITIES

CourseConnect

To access self-assessment questions and interactive, competency-based learning activities for this chapter, visit www.springerpub.com/courseconnect. See inside front cover and tear-out for CourseConnect details.

REFERENCES

BBC News. (2023, April 10). *Belize country profile*. https://www.bbc.com/news/world-latin-america-18724590

Carmack, R. (2017). *The Indigenous peoples of Mesoamerica and Central America: Their societies, cultures, and histories*. Lexington Books.

Congressional Research Service. (2024). *Central American migration: Root causes and U.S. policy*. https://sgp.fas.org/crs/row/IF11151.pdf

Garfield, R., & Rodriguez, P. (1985). Health and health services in Central America. *Jounal of the American Medical Association, 254*(7), 936–943. https://jamanetwork.com/journals/jama/article-abstract/400091

Huddleston, E. (2021). *World studies: Central America*. Focus Readers.

Institute for Health Metrics and Evaluation. (n.d.). *Health research by location: Country profiles*. University of Washington. https://www.healthdata.org/research-analysis/health-by-location/profiles

Minnesota Department of Health. (2024). *Central American (Guatemalan, Honduran, Salvadoran) minors refugee health profile*. Center for Excellence in Newcomer Health. https://www.health.state.mn.us/communities/rih/coe/profiles/central.html#NaN

Monteith, S., Stupp, P., & McCraken, S. (2005). *Reproductive, maternal, and child health in Central America: Trends and challenges facing women and children: El Salvador, Guatemala, Honduras, Nicaragua*. U.S. DRH/CDC.

Perez-Brignoli, H. (1985). *A brief history of Central America*. University of California Press.

Ramirez, P. (2020). Indigenous Latino heritage: Destruction, invisibility, appropriation, revival, survivance. In V. Apaydin (Ed.), *Critical perspectives on cultural memory and heritage*. UCL Press. https://www.jstor.org/stable/j.ctv13xpsfp.15

Shally-Jensen, M. (2015). *Countries, people and cultures: Central and South America*. Grey House Publishing.

Teaching Central America. (2025). *History*. https://www.teachingcentralamerica.org/history

UN Data Portal. (n.d.). *UN population division data portal*. United Nations. https://population.un.org/dataportal/home/

Wallace, A. (2017, May 26). *¿Por qué muchos centroamericanos no piensan en Panamá cuando hablan de Centroamérica* (y viceversa)? https://www.bbc.com/mundo/noticias-america-latina-39655419

CHAPTER 9

COSTA RICA

Pablo Montero-Zamora and Jeancarlo Cordoba

DEDICATION

We dedicate this chapter to Dr. Pablo Ortiz-Roses, a cherished mentor and colleague of the authors, who passed away on June 14, 2024, during its development. His profound contributions to the Costa Rican healthcare system and Indigenous communities are immeasurable, leaving an indelible mark on both. Dr. Ortiz-Roses inspired hundreds of health preventionists and researchers worldwide, and his efforts were instrumental in shaping the healthcare system that Costa Rica enjoys today. His memory will forever endure as an example of dedication and compassion in public health.

INTRODUCTION

Costa Rica, known for its biodiversity and progressive environmental policies, pioneered universal healthcare and education. Since the abolishment of its army in 1942, the nation has channeled resources toward robust social services, including universal healthcare through the Costa Rican Social Security Fund (in Spanish *Caja Costarricense de Seguro Social* [CCSS]), and a strong emphasis on education. Despite these accomplishments, significant disparities persist among socioeconomic subgroups. Access to quality healthcare opportunities often varies based on income level, ethnicity, and geographic location. While Costa Rica continues to lead healthcare innovation, addressing these disparities remains a pressing challenge. Through comprehensive strategies prioritizing equity and inclusion, Costa Rica endeavors to create a society where all citizens have equal access to healthcare and prevention, reflecting its enduring commitment to peace, prosperity, and social justice.

GEOGRAPHY AND POPULATION

GEOGRAPHICAL FEATURES

Costa Rica, located in Central America, shares borders with Nicaragua to the north, the Caribbean Sea to the northeast, Panama to the southeast, and the Pacific Ocean to the southwest. Covering an area of 51,060 square kilometers, it supports a population of approximately 5 million people, predominantly concentrated in the densely populated Great Metropolitan Area, anchored by the capital city of San José. Costa Rica is organized into seven provinces (administrative divisions similar to states in the United States): San José, Alajuela, Heredia, Cartago, Guanacaste, Puntarenas, and Limón, and further divided into 83 cantons (administrative divisions similar to counties in the United States; García et al., 2023). Costa Rica's seven provinces contribute to the country's geographic diversity, encompassing various landscapes, including coastal areas, mountain ranges, and fertile plains. Costa Rica's diverse geography offers a multitude of experiences, ranging from bustling urban centers to remote rural communities, making it a popular and traditional tourism destination for many foreigners in the last decades (Echeverri et al., 2022).

Costa Rica's geography includes the following:

- *Mountain ranges*: Cordillera de Talamanca, Cordillera Central
- *Rivers*: Rio Grande de Tarcoles, Pacuare River
- *Valleys and lowlands*: Central Valley
- *Coastal areas*: Caribbean Sea, Pacific Ocean
- *Volcanic activity*: Arenal Volcano, Poas Volcano
- *Indigenous reserves*: Talamanca Reserve
- *Urban centers*: San Jose
- *Rural areas*: scattered across the country

DEMOGRAPHICS

According to the 2023 Population and Housing Census Estimate conducted by Costa Rica's National Institute of Statistics and Census (INEC), the country's population stands at approximately 5,262,237 individuals. These data signify an annual growth rate of roughly 1%, reflecting a stable trend in population expansion since the previous census. Among the population, there are 2,648,531 men and 2,613,705 women, resulting in a balanced gender distribution. Specifically, for every 100 women, there are 101 men in the country. These demographic figures underscore the consistent growth and gender composition within Costa Rica's population landscape (INDEC, 2023).

Age

Upon reviewing the population's age structure, it is evident that Costa Rica continues to undergo an aging process that mirrors those observed in developing countries. For instance, in 2022, 10.1% of the population was 65 years or older, compared to 5.6% in 2000. This implies that over a span of 22 years, the proportion of the older demographic nearly doubled. The reasons behind this shift include low fertility rates, stable mortality rates over an extended period, and consistently high life expectancy. This demographic trend has decreased the relative proportion of the population under 15 years of age over time. By 2022, it had declined to 20.8%, whereas in 2000, it stood at 31.9% (INDEC, 2023).

Sex

As already mentioned, in the demographic context, in 2023, the male population in Costa Rica amounted to 2,648,531 individuals, while the female population totaled 2,613,705 (INDEC, 2023). Fertility emerges as a pivotal factor, with a crude birth rate of 9.54 per 1,000 inhabitants and a total fertility rate of 1.22 per woman. Nevertheless, both the gross and net reproduction rates are recorded at 0.594 per woman. Mortality rates, notably among infants and children, manifest gender disparities, thus impacting the overall life expectancy at birth, which stands at approximately 77 years (Institute for Health Metrics and Evaluation [IHME], 2024a; INDEC, 2023). In comparison, neighboring Nicaragua reports a higher total fertility rate of 2.2 children per woman (IHME, 2025a), and Honduras has an even higher rate of 2.4 children per woman (IHME, 2025b), underscoring the demographic differences between Costa Rica and other countries in the region.

Ethnicity/Race

Race and ethnicity are integral components that shape the social dynamics and demographic composition of Costa Rica. Mestizos and Whites represent the predominant ethnic group, constituting 83.64% of the population. Additionally, the Mulatto, Indigenous, Black/Afro-Caribbean, Chinese, and other ethnic groups contribute to the cultural diversity of the nation. Despite the prominence of Mestizos and Whites, Costa Rica embraces a multicultural identity, with minority groups such as the Indigenous population comprising 2.42% and the Black/Afro-Caribbean community representing 1.05% of the populace. Costa Rica is home to eight Indigenous groups spread across 24 territories nationwide. The Black/Afro-Caribbean population, representing approximately 33% of Limón Province's population, primarily resides in small communities along the Caribbean coast.

The recent surge in asylum applications has further influenced Costa Rica's demographic landscape. The influx of migrants from Nicaragua, Venezuela, and Colombia underscores the country's role as a significant destination for individuals seeking refuge (INDEC, 2023). In response, the government has implemented changes to its asylum system to address the evolving sociopolitical dynamics in the region. Furthermore, the emigration of Costa Rican citizens to other countries of the Organisation for Economic Co-operation and Development (OECD) highlights global migration trends. The increasing number of individuals migrating to destinations such as the United States, Mexico, and Germany reflects both economic motivations and the pursuit of better opportunities abroad. As Costa Rica navigates the complexities of migration and asylum, embracing diversity and fostering inclusivity remain paramount (OECD, 2023b). These efforts are essential for building a cohesive and resilient society that celebrates its multicultural heritage.

Language

Costa Rica's linguistic diversity encompasses Indigenous languages like Maléku, Ngöbere, Cabécar, Bribri, Guaymí, and Buglere, alongside Spanish, spoken by approximately 98% of the population (Umaña, 2011). The Afro-Caribbean community in Limón Province primarily speaks English-based creole languages such as Mekatelyu or Patua (Cuneo et al., 2008).

BRIEF COUNTRY HISTORY

Costa Rica's evolution into a beacon of stability and social welfare is intricately intertwined with key historical events shaping its identity and trajectory. In 1821, amid the sweeping currents of change across Central America, Costa Rica boldly declared its independence from Spanish colonial rule. This pivotal moment observed the genesis of a new era, laying the groundwork for Costa Rica's emergence as an autonomous nation. However, it was not until 1838, after the dissolution of the United Provinces of Central America, that Costa Rica firmly established itself as an independent and sovereign state, cementing its commitment to democratic principles and civil freedom (Hall et al., 2000; Pesec, Ratcliffe, & Bitton, 2017).

Fast-forwarding to the mid-20th century, Costa Rica found itself at a critical juncture. In 1941, under the visionary stewardship of President Rafael Ángel Calderón Guardia, the CCSS was founded. This institution, colloquially referred to as "La Caja," represented a pioneering endeavor aimed at providing universal healthcare coverage to all Costa Ricans, regardless of socioeconomic status. The establishment of the CCSS epitomized a bold stride toward societal advancement, endeavoring to address the pressing healthcare needs of the populace and foster a more equitable society (Pesec, Ratcliffe, & Bitton, 2017; Pesec, Ratcliffe, Karlage, et al., 2017).

The 1940s were a period of global upheaval, and Costa Rica was not immune to the tide of revolution and reform sweeping across the world. In 1948, the nation became embroiled in a brief but intense civil conflict. This internal conflict, characterized by factions advocating for political and social change, culminated in a decisive victory for those espousing reform. Subsequently, President José Figueres Ferrer made an indelible mark on Costa Rican history by abolishing the country's military—a groundbreaking decision that underscored Costa Rica's unwavering commitment to peace and disarmament. Redirecting erstwhile military resources toward education, healthcare, and social programs, President Figueres Ferrer's action laid the cornerstone for a more inclusive and prosperous society (Pesec, Ratcliffe, & Bitton, 2017).

As the dust settled and Costa Rica embarked on a journey of postwar reconstruction, the CCSS emerged as a beacon of hope in a nation endeavoring to heal and rebuild. Funded through a blend of employer and employee contributions, supplemented by governmental support, the CCSS provided indispensable medical services to millions of Costa Ricans, ensuring access to primary care, hospitalization, and essential medications (Pesec, Ratcliffe, Karlage, et al., 2017; Sáenz et al.,

2011). Synonymous with Costa Rica's commitment to social justice and human dignity, the CCSS embodied the nation's values of inclusivity, equality, and solidarity.

Subsequent decades witnessed Costa Rica's steadfast evolution as a paradigm of stability and social progress within the region. Despite grappling with an array of challenges, including socioeconomic disparities and environmental pressures, Costa Rica remained resolute in its pursuit of a fairer and more equitable society (Braun et al., 2015). Costa Rica's abolition of the military and establishment of comprehensive social guarantees were foundational for its ongoing development.

POLITICAL SYSTEM

Costa Rica operates under a presidential republic, with elections held every 4 years. The president serves as both head of state and government. The political system embraces a multiparty structure, promoting diversity. In the Republic of Costa Rica, the government is divided into three branches: legislative, executive, and judicial. The legislative branch is responsible for creating laws and consists of the unicameral Legislative Assembly. The executive branch, led by the president, implements, and enforces rules. The judicial branch, headed by the Supreme Court, interprets laws and ensures their constitutionality. This separation of powers promotes checks and balances, preventing any one branch from exerting unchecked authority (Hybel, 2019). Costa Rica has made significant strides in healthcare policy. For example, the establishment of the CCSS provided universal healthcare, while the government continues to focus on addressing rising healthcare costs.

HEALTH OUTCOMES

In comparison to the average of OECD countries, the healthcare system in Costa Rica shows both strengths and weaknesses in key healthcare indicators. While it falls short on metrics such as maternal mortality ratio, obesity prevalence, and vaping, it excels in life expectancy, surpassing the OECD average. Preventable mortality in Costa Rica, at 148 per 100,000, aligns closely with the OECD average of 158, while treatable mortality, at 89 per 100,000, exceeds the OECD average of 79 years. Additionally, a lower percentage of Costa Ricans, at 3.4%, rate their health as bad or very bad compared to the OECD average of 7.9%. However, diabetes prevalence in Costa Rica exceeds the OECD average (OECD, 2023a).

LIFE EXPECTANCY FROM BIRTH

According to the global burden of disease (GBD) study, during the 21st century, Costa Rica witnessed significant slow improvements in life expectancy from birth. Over this period, life expectancy surged by 3.5 years, rising from 77 years in 1990 to 80.5 years in 2024 (IHME, 2024b). GBD estimations show that, by 2024, only Canada (83.1 years), Chile (81.7 years), and Colombia (80.8 years) boasted higher life expectancy rates than Costa Rica (IHME, 2024b). Notably, the Nicoya region of Costa Rica, known as a "Blue Zone," boasts an exceptionally long life expectancy attributed to lifestyle habits such as consuming unprocessed foods, prioritizing rest and friendships, and regular physical activity (Pes et al., 2022). Despite such achievements, there are notable disparities in life expectancy among different demographic groups within Costa Rica. In 2022, male life expectancy from birth was approximately 76.6 years, while female life expectancy was around 82.9 years (Vollset et al., 2024).

LEADING CAUSES OF MORTALITY

Several factors have contributed to recent life expectancy trends in Costa Rica. A significant issue is the high mortality rate associated with preventable chronic diseases, as reflected by changes in

disability-adjusted life years (DALYs) per 100,000 population between 2011 and 2021. DALYs are a health measure used to quantify the overall disease burden. One DALY represents the loss of 1 year of healthy life due to either premature death or time lived with disability. It combines both years of life lost (YLL) and years lived with disability (YLD) to provide a comprehensive view of health outcomes. Among the most critical changes is the dramatic increase in DALYs due to high body mass index, which escalated by 657.5%, reflecting widespread obesity. During the same period, DALYs associated with elevated fasting plasma glucose levels rose by 720%, indicating a growing diabetes crisis (IHME, 2024a). High blood pressure saw a 212.3% increase in DALYs, signaling greater cardiovascular risks (IHME, 2024a). Poor dietary habits led to a 275.2% rise in DALYs related to dietary risks, further exacerbating health issues. Kidney dysfunction, with an increase of 241.8% in DALYs, is closely linked to chronic conditions such as diabetes and hypertension (IHME, 2024a).

Despite the known risks, tobacco use resulted in a 68.8% increase in DALYs, contributing to respiratory and cardiovascular diseases. Alcohol consumption saw a 202.5% rise in DALYs, posing significant health threats, including liver disease. High low-density lipoprotein cholesterol, with a 38.0% increase in DALYs, highlights challenges in managing blood lipid levels. Conversely, improvements in malnutrition and air pollution have been observed, with decreases in DALYs of 277.3% and 93.3%, respectively, suggesting positive outcomes from public health interventions (IHME, 2024a). However, the overall trend underscores the urgent need for comprehensive strategies to combat these escalating health challenges in Costa Rica. Despite these challenges, Costa Rica remains committed to enhancing its public health infrastructure and implementing preventive measures to mitigate the impact of chronic diseases. Through continued efforts to promote health education and disease prevention, Costa Rica strives to improve overall life expectancy and health outcomes for its population.

NONCOMMUNICABLE DISEASES

In Costa Rica, noncommunicable diseases (NCDs) have emerged as the predominant causes of mortality, ranking second only behind COVID-19 in 2021. Ischemic heart disease retained its status as the primary contributor to NCD-related deaths, exhibiting a slight increase in mortality rates (+1.7%) between 2011 and 2021. Meanwhile, stroke, previously the second leading cause of NCD-related deaths in 2011, went to third place, with a notable escalation in mortality rates (+7.8%) over the same decade. Of notable concern is the escalation of chronic kidney disease, ascending from the third leading NCD in 2011 to the second by 2021, marked by a substantial increase in mortality rates (+10.2%). Moreover, other NCDs, such as Alzheimer disease and diabetes, showcased upward trajectories in mortality rates, underscoring the significant burden of these conditions on Costa Rica's populations (IHME, 2024a). In addition, concerning cancer, prostate cancer saw a staggering increase of 125% during the same period. In 2021, it emerged as the leading cause of cancer-related deaths, followed by breast cancer and colorectal cancer (IHME, 2024a). The evolving health landscape in Costa Rica, as delineated by these trends in NCDs, needs immediate scholarly inquiry and robust public health responses. It underscores the exigency for evidence-based interventions and comprehensive policy frameworks to mitigate the prevalence of NCDs and their consequential impact on population health and well-being.

COMMUNICABLE DISEASES

Through widespread vaccination campaigns, Costa Rica has been at the forefront of combating mortality from communicable diseases. However, mirroring trends seen in countries like the United States, there is growing concern over rising antivaccination sentiment and increasing vaccine hesitancy within Costa Rica (Faerron Guzmán et al., 2021). This stance, coupled with the high prevalence of chronic diseases, poses a significant risk to the population, leaving Costa Ricans vulnerable to preventable infectious diseases. Among the common infectious diseases in Costa Rica are genital herpes, tuberculosis, trichiniasis, chlamydia, and, notably, COVID-19 (IHME, 2024a).

COVID-19

From 2020 to 2022, COVID-19 posed a significant challenge to Costa Rica's health system, causing approximately 9,200 deaths as of March 2023 (Johns Hopkins Coronavirus Resource Center, 2023). By 2021, it became the leading cause of death in the country, with a mortality rate of 93.3 deaths per 100,000 inhabitants. This rate was comparable to that of developed countries like the United States, which recorded 83.12 deaths per 100,000 people during the same year. Notably, Costa Rica ranked as the Latin American country with the second lowest mortality rate, only behind Panama, which reported 75.5 deaths per 100,000 people. This achievement surpassed mortality rates observed in countries such as Mexico (289 per 100,000 people), Brazil (227.4 per 100,000 people), and Colombia (210.7 per 100,000 people; IHME, 2024a). Costa Rica's effective COVID-19 response, resulting in low mortality rates compared to its Latin American counterparts, was driven by proactive testing, contact tracing, strategic healthcare resource allocation, public awareness campaigns, and timely vaccinations led by the Ministry of Health (MoH). The CCSS also implemented structural changes, including a specialized COVID-19 center and optimized healthcare processes, ensuring continuity of essential services for non-COVID-19 patients. These efforts were supported by Costa Rica's integrated health system and robust healthcare infrastructure (Mora-García et al., 2024).

Lower Respiratory Infections

According to the Global Burden of Disease (GBD) study, lower respiratory infections (LRIs) such as pneumonia or bronchiolitis are significant causes of mortality and morbidity in Costa Rica. From 2009 to 2018, Costa Rica experienced a notable 75% increase in lower respiratory mortality. However, between 2018 and 2021, there was a considerable 28% decrease in mortality from LRIs. This decline might be attributed to the impact of COVID-19, which resulted in increased lockdown measures (IHME, 2024a), which reduced the risk of pneumonia or bronchiolitis in vulnerable youth populations within Costa Rica.

DETERMINANTS OF HEALTH

HEALTH BEHAVIORS

Tobacco Use

Similar to other countries, Costa Rica has presented very comprehensive legislation on tobacco control based on the World Health Organization Framework Convention on Tobacco Control (Burci, 2003) that allowed the country to achieve a reduced tobacco consumption rate of 8.7% in 2022 based on the Global Adult Tobacco Survey, with a marked difference between men (13.1%) and women (4.3%; Institute on Alcoholism and Drug Dependence [IAFA], 2022). Also, regarding cessation services in 2021, 15 Comprehensive Medication Care Centers, 34 Tobacco Cessation Clinics, and a virtual assistant (i.e., *mSalud* Commission) were established (Costa Rica Ministry of Health, 2022). A new legislation to control new tobacco products such as electronic cigarettes, vapes, and heat-not-burn tobacco products was put in place in 2021 (The Legislative Assembly of the Republic of Costa Rica, 2021), complying with international regulation on tobacco control. As a result of tobacco control measures put in place in the country, the average age of initiation of tobacco consumption increased from 16 to 18 when comparing 2015 and 2022 (IAFA, 2022).

Poor Dietary Intake

Regarding dietary intake, the most vulnerable populations are being threatened by food system crises, food taxes, and the consequences of the COVID-19 pandemic. For example, women who lead households have a higher degree of food insecurity than men in the same situation. In the first income quintile, 36% of households in Costa Rica were forced to reduce the quality or quantity of food they consumed. Additionally, 6% of households spent all day without eating due to the lack of money or other resources (González-Rivera et al., 2023).

According to González-Rivera et al. (2023), in 2020, 22% of households with children under 5 years of age had moderate to severe nutritional food insecurity, which demonstrates a lack of access to food. This leads to food deficiency and inability for a healthy and active lifestyle in vulnerable populations of the quintiles with the highest poverty levels in households primarily led by women, and households that have small children.

Conversely, obesity is exhibited at a high frequency in all age groups; the greatest prevalence is between 40 and 64 years old, according to the period from 2018 to 2021 (González-Rivera et al., 2023). The mortality rates from events related to malnourishment or obesity are low, but the impact of inadequate nutrition is significant in Costa Rica. The mortality rates from nutritional events must be considered alongside associated events, as between the ages of 55 and 79, the probability of dying from causes associated with malnutrition, obesity, or overweight increases significantly (González-Rivera et al., 2023).

Physical Inactivity

In 2016, a study indicated that Costa Rica was the sixth most sedentary country in the world, where 46.1% of adults (38% of men and 54% of women) did not do enough physical activity to maintain good health (Pan American Health Organization/World Health Organization [in Spanish, *Organización Panamericana de la Salud/Organización Mundial de la Salud*], 2016). Similarly, another study in 2023 showed similar data when found that on average, it was observed that, in Costa Rica, 37.4% of the study population does not perform the minimum recommended physical activity; this percentage is even higher among women (Gómez et al., 2023). These data demonstrate that physical inactivity is a threat to the population´s health, especially when combined with poor diet and some other unhealthy behaviors such as tobacco and alcohol consumption, leading to a challenge to the healthcare system. Likewise in 2018, a National Survey of Physical Activity and Nutritional Surveillance among high school students showed that of those students who are active once or twice a week, 38% of them are obese, demonstrating the need for better options in physical activity (Caravaca Rodriguez, 2020).

Alcohol Abuse

Based on the 2022 VII National Survey on the Consumption of Psychoactive Substances in the population aged 12 to 70 in households, alcoholic beverages remain the main psychoactive consumer product in Costa Rica. The largest number of alcoholic beverage consumers are in the 20 to 29 age group, with 31% of people in that age group (Lopez, 2023). In Costa Rica, data from 2019 show that the total alcohol consumption per capita (liters of pure alcohol, ages 15 and older) is 3.5, a bit lower than other countries in the region such as Nicaragua (4.2), Panama (6.6), Colombia (4.9), Mexico (5.7; World Bank Group, 2024).

SOCIAL AND ECONOMIC FACTORS

Costa Rica is notable for its success in development. It is considered a middle-income country with consistent economic growth over the past 25 years. This increase in growth was derived from an outward-oriented strategy, which was based on the practice of openness to foreign investment and the gradual liberation of trade. The per capita GDP in Costa Rica in 2024 is $18,030 locating the country as the 84th of the major economies in the world (International Monetary Fund, 2024).

Educational Attainment

In 2019, only one third of young adults in Costa Rica had completed tertiary education, the majority being bachelors degrees. However, people with a tertiary degree (i.e., refers to bachelor's, master's, or doctoral degree) earn at least twice the income of those with a lower secondary degree (OECD, 2025). Tertiary-educated women who work full time in Costa Rica have almost the same income as men. Their wages are 97% of the income of men with the same education; however, they only have 75% of the average income for tertiary-educated individuals across OECD countries (OECD, 2025). Women with a third degree who work full time in Costa Rica have almost the same income as men. Their wages are 97% of the income of men with the same education; however, they only have 75% of the income of OECD countries. More than half of the 25- to 34-year-olds had not completed high school in Costa Rica in 2018. Despite increases in educational achievement, some problems associated with providing a high-quality secondary education still exist. Preprimary education initiatives have increased the number of enrolled students, but the services provided to children under 3 years are still lacking (OECD, 2025).

Poverty

By February 2024, the poverty rate was 20.61%, reflecting a continuous, steady decrease from 23.02% in February 2023—a reduction of 2.4 percentage points. Also, there is a decrease in extreme poverty, although this is less apparent than the general decrease. In this context, stability has been apparent since the last month of 2015, and by February 2024, represents 5.93% of the population. Every year, the average is 1.2% lower (Cordoba et al., 2023). Regarding the right to employment, by 2021, 42.3% of households in poverty **had noncompliant labor laws** (i.e., labor regulations in the country that do not fully align with national legal standards or international conventions, such as those set by the International Labour Organization); 34.1% of families participated in informal employment and 24.9% did not follow the minimum wage. Additionally, 11.5% of the population was unemployed at that date. It is crucial to recognize that these percentages have changed very little since the mid-1990s (Cordoba et al., 2023). However, something important to highlight about the population economy in Costa Rica is inequalities. The distribution of income in Costa Rica is unequal, which may explain the deterioration of the country's average social inequality index. Specifically, the Gini coefficient for 1990 placed the country above the regional average, with a value of 0.374. In 2021, however, the same measurement showed a value of 0.524, making Costa Rica the most unequal country in the world (Cordoba et al., 2023).

HEALTHCARE SYSTEM

OVERVIEW

The financing and governance of healthcare in Costa Rica is declared by the Constitution Act of the country, which mandates that Social Security should be implemented for manual and intellectual workers. This is done through a system of mandatory contributions from the state, employers, and workers (**tripartite system model**) that aim to shield them from the risk of illness, disability, childbirth, death, and other conditions as determined by the law. The Constitution Act also stipulates that the Social Security system will be operated and governed by the CCSS indicating as well that Social Security funds and reserves cannot be moved or utilized for other than their intended purposes (Gobierno de Costa Rica, 1949). The way the CCSS is structured to protect Social Security is one of the main keys to achieving universal health coverage in Costa Rica (Pesec, Ratcliffe, & Bitton, 2017).

FINANCING AND INSURANCE

The CCSS and its tripartite system model offer the following three Social Security regimes under its administration:

- Seguro de Enfermedad y Maternidad (SEM) regime (Illness and Maternity Insurance)
- Invalidez, Vejez y Muerte (IVM) regime (Disability, Old Age, and Death)
- Noncontributive regime

The mandatory contributory regime applies to all employees in the formal sector and is financed by a 15% payroll tax. This tax is funded by contributions from employers, employees, and government at rates of 9.25%, 5.5%, and 0.25%, respectively, as stipulated under the legal framework, which also dictates that premiums paid by workers should never exceed those paid by employers (Pesec, Ratcliffe, & Bitton, 2017; Sáenz et al., 2011). In addition to this system, retired persons contribute with a rate of 14% on their retirement pension income toward social health insurance. There also exists a Voluntary Health Insurance Regime financed by individuals at a 10.25% rate of reported income for independent workers; however, once enrolled contributions become mandatory as the individual cannot withdraw from enrollment in social health insurance. In the end, the CCSS represents a large risk pool, collecting contributions from all subcomponents of the population and pooling risks across the system, thereby allowing lower-income and higher-risk groups to access health services (Slon, 2017).

DELIVERY

The population's health demand is marked by its diversity and range of issues. Similarly, the response to technological innovation and service provision (offering) has also diversified, overspecialized, and increased in complexity and cost. For cost–benefit reasons and technical rationality, it is necessary to define the health priorities to be attended to and to stagger the offer into two or more levels of care according to the installed health capacity and the country's economic possibilities (Salas Chaves, 2010).

In that sense, Costa Rica´s healthcare delivery, through the CCSS, is divided into three levels of care. The first level of care is the building block of the system, presenting a basic offer of services, including a home-visit program for the entire community, outpatient care, community activities with local stakeholders, and strong connections with educational institutions of the region. The first level of care is organized through a Basic Comprehensive Health Care Team (abbreviated as EBAIS in Spanish). The team comprises a general practitioner, nursing assistant, technical assistant in primary care (abbreviated as ATAP in Spanish), and medical data clerk in charge of administrative procedures, but also includes a pharmacy health technician, depending on the geographic location (Cuccia et al., 2019). The EBAIS is vital to the system's foundation due to the closeness to the community. Based on regulations, each EBAIS oversees approximately 5 thousand people, and every household in the catchment area is visited at least once a year, offering a perspective of the health status of the population with a real primary health focus.

The second level of care includes outpatient and inpatient care of some major medical specialties, such as internal medicine, psychiatry, pediatrics, obstetrics and gynecology, and general medicine. The third level of care, composed of the major hospitals in the country, offers all the medical subspecialty services in outpatient and inpatient care (Salas Chaves, 2010). In addition, Costa Rica has six specialized hospitals to treat specific populations, such as children, older people, women, people with mental health issues, and people in need of physical rehabilitation (García-González, 2004). Something unique about the organization of Costa Rica´s healthcare system is the role of the Ministry of Health, which, in fact, oversees and regulates the healthcare industry instead of being a provider as happens in some other countries globally. The Costa Rica Ministry of Health, as the governing body of the health sector, has an organizational and functional structure designed to promote institutional, interinstitutional, and intersectoral coordination. Another function of the Ministry of Health in Costa Rica is to implement policies, programs, and projects focused on individuals and communities, with the aim of expanding equitable access to healthcare (García-González, 2004).

Providers

The CCSS is the backbone of Costa Rica's universal healthcare system, providing coverage to over 95% of the country's population. Despite this, the private market is largely unregulated. Since 2000, the number of private medical practices that provide primary care has increased, and the percentage of primary care that occurs in private practices has also increased. A growing number of people rely on private primary care providers over the course of a year, and private secondary care providers are also increasing in number. Private primary care is typically funded out-of-pocket by Costa Ricans, and some individuals supplement their CCSS insurance with additional private health insurance that covers the out-of-pocket costs of their private sector expenditures. Particularly in San José, patients who have money to pay for private healthcare choose this form of care over other options (Pesec, Ratcliffe, & Bitton, 2017). As of 2024, Costa Rica has 15 public hospitals administered by the CCSS and four major private hospitals: CIMA, Hospital Clínica Bíblica, Hospital Metropolitano, and La Católica. Both the public and private healthcare sectors are planning to expand their infrastructure in the coming years to meet the increasing demand for healthcare services (International Trade Administration & U.S. Department of Commerce, 2024)

CHALLENGES

Regarding challenges for the health system, Costa Rica has some potential for improvement in different areas that can position the country among the best healthcare systems in the world due to its conditions. According to the Pan American Health Organization (2022), some of those challenges are

1. achieving universal healthcare with a focus on interculturality, ensuring that healthcare services are accessible and relevant to all cultural groups within the population;
2. improving accessibility, quality, and equity in healthcare by developing systems to identify and address persistent barriers to healthcare access;
3. strengthening the Ministry of Health's leadership by creating mechanisms for continuous monitoring and evaluation of the healthcare system, aligned with the national framework for universal access;
4. recognizing the importance of primary healthcare in the overall healthcare delivery system, ensuring its role is central to achieving better health outcomes;
5. enhancing resource efficiency and financial sustainability by exploring alternative funding sources for healthcare and implementing methods to evaluate the financial protection of current health spending;
6. conducting studies on the fundamental functions of public health to ensure the system remains responsive to evolving health needs; and
7. addressing the growing prevalence of noncommunicable diseases by implementing preventive measures and improving care for chronic conditions.

CONCLUSION

Costa Rica's healthcare system, renowned for its emphasis on equitable universal health coverage and bolstered by a robust primary healthcare framework established during the 1990s reforms, faces both longstanding successes and emerging challenges. The system excels in life expectancy and maintains a strong foundation for comprehensive healthcare delivery. However, it confronts issues such as an aging population contributing to a rise in NCDs and connectivity problems to secondary and tertiary care, compounded by lengthy wait times for specialized services.

Furthermore, the incomplete implementation of the EBAIS (i.e., Basic Comprehensive Health Care Team) model in urban areas adds complexity. Despite these challenges, Costa Rica's healthcare system is poised to address these issues through ongoing reforms, strategic infrastructure investments, and a continued focus on preventive care and health promotion.

LEARNING ACTIVITIES

CourseConnect >

To access self-assessment questions and interactive, competency-based learning activities for this chapter, visit www.springerpub.com/courseconnect. See inside front cover and tear-out for CourseConnect details.

REFERENCES

Braun, Y. A., Dreiling, M. C., Eddy, M. P., & Dominguez, D. M. (2015). Up against the wall: Ecotourism, development, and social justice in Costa Rica. *Journal of Global Ethics, 11*(3), 351–365. https://doi.org/10.1080/17449626.2015.1100653

Burci, G. L. (2003). World Health Organization (WHO): Framework convention on tobacco control. *International Legal Materials, 42*(3), 515–539.

Caravaca Rodríguez, I. (2020). *Encuesta colegial de vigilancia nutricional y actividad física: Costa Rica 2018* [School-based nutritional surveillance and physical activity survey: Costa Rica 2018]. Ministerio de Salud de Costa Rica. https://www.ministeriodesalud.go.cr/index.php/biblioteca-de-archivos-left/documentos-ministerio-de-salud/vigilancia-de-la-salud/normas-protocolos-guias-y-lineamientos/vigilancia-nutricional/censos-y-encuestas/encuesta-colegial-de-vigilancia-nutricional-y-actividad-fisica-2018-vigilancia-de-la-salud/5296-informe-de-resultados-encuesta-colegial-2018/file

Cordoba, D., Oviedo, L., & Robalino, J. (2023). *Análisis del mercado laboral, pobreza y desigualdad en Costa Rica al II trimestre 2023* [Analysis of the labor market, poverty, and inequality in Costa Rica in the second quarter of 2023]. https://iice.ucr.ac.cr/2023/07/27/analisis-del-mercado-laboral-pobreza-y-desgigualdad-en-costa-rica/

Costa Rica Ministry of Health. (2022). *Global adult tobacco survey. Comparative data sheet.* https://www.ministeriodesalud.go.cr/index.php/biblioteca-de-archivos-left/documentos-ministerio-de-salud/ministerio-de-salud/control-de-tabaco-e-informacion-relacionada/encuesta-de-consumo-de-tabaco-en-adultos/7264-datos-comparativos-gats-2015-2022/file

Cuccia, L., Chadwick, J., Hassan, A., Kim, A., Sivarajan, R., & Wang, V. (2019). Costa Rica's health care reform: Impact and success of the EBAIS model. *McGill Journal of Global Health, 8*(1), 24–35.

Cuneo, C. N., McCabe, A., & Melzi, G. (2008). Mestizaje: Afro-Caribbean and Indigenous Costa Rican children's narratives and links with other traditions. In A. McCabe, A. L. Bailey, & G. Melzi (Eds.), *Spanish-language narration and literacy: Culture, cognition, and emotion* (pp. 237–270). Cambridge University Press.

Echeverri, A., Smith, J. R., MacArthur-Waltz, D., Lauck, K. S., Anderson, C. B., Monge Vargas, R., Alvarado Quesada, I., Wood, S. A., Chaplin-Kramer, R., & Daily, G. C. (2022). Biodiversity and infrastructure interact to drive tourism to and within Costa Rica. *Proceedings of the National Academy of Sciences of the United States of America, 119*(11), e2107662119. https://doi.org/10.1073/pnas.2107662119

Faerron Guzmán, C. A., Montero-Zamora, P., Bolaños-Palmieri, C., Araya-Amador, J., Benavides-Rawson, J., & Ávila-Agüero, M. L. (2021). Willingness to get a COVID-19 vaccine and its potential predictors in Costa Rica: A cross-sectional study. *Cureus, 13*(10), e18798. https://doi.org/10.7759/cureus.18798

García-González, R. (2004). *El Sistema Nacional de Salud en Costa Rica: Generalidades* [The national health system in Costa Rica: Overview]. http://www. cendeisss. sa. cr/cursos https://www.binasss.sa.cr/opac-ms/media/digitales/El%20Sistema%20nacional%20de%20salud%20en%20Costa%20Rica.%20Generalidades.pdf

García, Y. E., Chou-Chen, S. W., Barboza, L. A., Daza–Torres, M. L., Montesinos-López, J. C., Vásquez, P., Calvo, J. G., Nuño, M., & Sanchez, F. (2023). Common patterns between dengue cases, climate, and local environmental variables in Costa Rica: A wavelet approach. *PLOS Global Public Health, 3*(10), e0002417. https://doi.org/10.1371/journal.pgph.0002417

Gobierno de Costa Rica. (1949). *Constitución política de Costa Rica* [Political constitution of Costa Rica]. https://www.tse.go.cr/pdf/normativa/constitucion.pdf

Gómez, G., Hidalgo, E. S., Oreamuno, A. S., & Ferrari, G. (2023). *Physical activity in Costa Rican urban population and its relationship to socio-demographic and anthropometric patterns*. https://www.scielo.sa.cr/scielo.php?script=sci_abstract&pid=S1659-44362023000100003&lng=en&nrm=iso

González-Rivera, C., Caravaca-Rodríguez, I., & Bolaños-Cruz, A. (2023). *Análisis del panorama de la situación del sobrepeso y la obesidad en niños, niñas y adolescentes en Costa Rica* [Analysis of the landscape of overweight and obesity among children and adolescents in Costa Rica]. https://www.unicef.org/lac/media/42591/file/Reporte-obesidad-intantil-Costa-Rica.pdf

Hall, C. A. S., Hall, M., & Aguilar, B. (2000). Chapter 2—A brief historical and visual introduction to Costa Rrica. In C. A. S. Hall, C. L. Perez, & G. Leclerc (Eds.), *Quantifying sustainable development* (pp. 19–42). Academic Press. https://doi.org/10.1016/B978-012318860-1/50005-8

Hybel, A. R. (2019). *The challenges of creating democracies in the Americas: The United States, Mexico, Colombia, Venezuela, Costa Rica, and Guatemala*. Springer.

Institute for Health Metrics and Evaluation. (2024a). *Costa Rica*. https://www.healthdata.org/research-analysis/health-by-location/profiles/costa-rica

Institute for Health Metrics and Evaluation. (2024b). *GBD foresight visualization*. Institute for Health Metrics and Evaluation. https://vizhub.healthdata.org/gbd-foresight

Institute for Health Metrics and Evaluation. (2025a). *Honduras*. https://www.healthdata.org/research-analysis/health-by-location/profiles/honduras

Institute for Health Metrics and Evaluation. (2025b). *Nicaragua*. https://www.healthdata.org/research-analysis/health-by-location/profiles/nicaragua

Institute on Alcoholism and Drug Dependence. (2022). *Executive summary*. Global Adult Tobacco Survey 2022. https://iafa.go.cr/wp-content/uploads/2023/11/iafa-gats-costa-rica-2022-resumen-ejecutivo.pdf

Instituto Nacional de Estadísticas y Censos. (2023). *Encuesta nacional de hogares* [National household survey]. INEC. https://inec.cr/estadisticas-fuentes/encuestas/encuesta-nacional-hogares

International Monetary Fund. (2024). *Costa Rica*. DataMapper. https://www.imf.org/external/datamapper/profile

International Trade Administration & U.S. Department of Commerce. (2024, February 3). *Costa Rica—Healthcare sector*. https://www.trade.gov/country-commercial-guides/costa-rica-healthcare-sector

Johns Hopkins Coronavirus Resource Center. (2023). *Costa Rica. COVID-19 overview*. Johns Hopkins Coronavirus Resource Center. https://coronavirus.jhu.edu/region/costa-rica

Lopez, P. (2023, October 24). *IAFA presenta Encuesta Nacional: Alcohol y cannabis con más consumidores en grupo de 20 a 29 años* [IAFA presents national survey: Alcohol and cannabis are the most common users in the 20-29 age group]. IAFA—Instituto sobre Alcoholismo y Farmacodependencia. https://iafa.go.cr/comunicado/iafa-presenta-encuesta-nacional-alcohol-y-cannabis-con-mas-consumidores-en-grupo-de-20-a-29-anos/

Mora-García, C. A., Pearson, A. A., & Prado, A. M. (2024). Maintaining essential health services during a pandemic: Lessons from Costa Rica's COVID-19 response. *BMJ Global Health, 8*(Suppl 6), e014143. https://doi.org/10.1136/bmjgh-2023-014143

Organisation for Economic Co-operation and Development. (2023a). *Health at a glance 2023*. https://doi.org/10.1787/7a7afb35-en

Organisation for Economic Co-operation and Development. (2023b). *International migration outlook 2023: Costa Rica*. OECD iLibrary. https://doi.org/10.1787/b0f40584-en

Organisation for Economic Co-operation and Development. (2025). *Costa Rica*. https://doi.org/10.1787/048cf07b-en

Pan American Health Organization. (2022, September 13). *Costa Rica—Country profile*. Health in the Americas. https://hia.paho.org/en/countries-22/costa-rica-country-profile

Pan American Health Organization/World Health Organization. (2016). *Factores de riesgo de las enfermedades no transmisibles en la región de las Américas: Consideraciones para fortalecer la capacidad regulatoria* [Risk factors for noncommunicable diseases in the Americas: Considerations for strengthening regulatory capacity]. https://iris.paho.org/handle/10665.2/28227?locale-attribute=es

Pes, G. M., Dore, M. P., Tsofliou, F., & Poulain, M. (2022). Diet and longevity in the Blue Zones: A set-and-forget issue? *Maturitas, 164*, 31–37. https://doi.org/10.1016/j.maturitas.2022.06.004

Pesec, M., Ratcliffe, H., & Bitton, A. (2017). *Building a thriving primary health care system: The story of Costa Rica* [Case Study]. Ariadne Labs. https://www.ariadnelabs.org/wp-content/uploads/2017/12/CostaRica-Report-12-19-2017.pdf

Pesec, M., Ratcliffe, H. L., Karlage, A., Hirschhorn, L. R., Gawande, A., & Bitton, A. (2017). Primary health care that works: The Costa Rican experience. *Health Affairs, 36*(3), 531–538. https://doi.org/10.1377/hlthaff.2016.1319

Sáenz, M. del R., Acosta, M., Muiser, J., & Bermúdez, J. L. (2011). The health system of Costa Rica. *Salud Pública de México, 53*, s156–s167. http://www.scielo.org.mx/scielo.php?script=sci_arttext&pid=S0036-36342011000800011&lng=en&tlng=es

Salas Chaves, Á. (2010). Organización de la oferta de los servicios de salud en Costa Rica [Organization of the provision of health services in Costa Rica]. In I. Vargas & W. Vargas (Eds.), *La salud pública en Costa Rica: Retos y perspectivas* [Public health in Costa Rica: Challenges and perspectives] (pp. 169–193). Universidad de Costa Rica, Facultad de Medicina, Escuela de Medicina, Departamento en Salud Pública.

Slon, P. (2017). Universal health coverage assessment: Costa Rica. *Global Network for Health Equity (GNHE)*. http://gnhe.org/blog/wp-content/uploads/2015/05/GNHE-UHC-assessment_CostaRica.pdf

The Legislative Assembly of the Republic of Costa Rica. (2021). *Law number 10066: Regulation of electronic nicotine delivery systems (SEAN), similar systems without nicotine (SSSN), and electronic devices that use heated tobacco and similar technologies*. https://pgrweb.go.cr/scij/Busqueda/Normativa/normas/nrm_texto_completo.aspx?param2=1&nValor1=1&nValor2=96116&nValor3=128587&nValor4=NO&strTipM=TC

Umaña, A. C. (2011). La diversidad lingüística de Costa Rica: Las lenguas indígenas [The linguistic diversity of Costa Rica: The indigenous languages]. *Revista de Filología y Lingüística de la Universidad de Costa Rica, 37*(2), 93–106. https://doi.org/10.15517/rfl.v37i2.6424

Vollset, S. E., Ababneh, H. S., Abate, Y. H., Abbafati, C., Abbasgholizadeh, R., Abbasian, M., Abbastabar, H., Magied, A. H. A. A. A., ElHafeez, S. A., Abdelkader, A., Abdelmasseh, M., Abd-Elsalam, S., Abdi, P., Abdollahi, M., Abdoun, M., Abdullahi, A., Abebe, M., Abiodun, O., Aboagye, R. G., . . . Murray, C. J. L. (2024). Burden of disease scenarios for 204 countries and territories, 2022–2050: A forecasting analysis for the Global Burden of Disease Study 2021. *The Lancet, 403*(10440), 2204–2256. https://doi.org/10.1016/S0140-6736(24)00685-8

World Bank Group. (2024). *Total alcohol consumption per capita (liters of pure alcohol, projected estimates, 15+ years of age)*. World Bank Open Data. https://genderdata.worldbank.org/en/indicator/sh-alc-pcap-li

CHAPTER 10

EL SALVADOR

L. Esther Aranda and Wolfgang Munar

OVERVIEW

Since ending its civil war in 1992, El Salvador has improved its people's health and well-being. By 2022, life expectancy had increased by 6 years, and infant and maternal mortality had declined by 76% and 65%, respectively (World Bank Group, 2024a; World Health Organization [WHO], 2024a). The country also had the second-lowest income inequality in Latin America (World Bank Group, 2024b).

In 2009, healthcare reforms based on universal **primary healthcare** (PHC) were introduced. These reforms prioritized access and coverage for the poorest in the country (Ministerio de Salud [MINSAL] Publica y Asistencia Social, 2009). A central element of these reforms was implementing a new community-based family healthcare delivery model, which centered on multiprofessional PHC teams providing services in health facilities and the community (MINSAL, 2017). The 2009 **health reforms** resulted in improved healthcare delivery, access, utilization, and quality, particularly benefiting the poorest rural populations and contributing to enhanced health indicators related to maternal and child health (Aranda et al., 2023; Báscolo et al., 2019; Bernal & Martinez, 2020; MINSAL, 2019b; World Bank Group, 2018). However, despite these improvements, there is still room for further progress. Ongoing **health disparities** suggest the need for additional reforms addressing the systemic root of persistent health disparities.

DEMOGRAPHICS

El Salvador, the smallest and most densely populated country in Central America, had a population of 6.4 million in 2023, the majority (76%) living in urban areas (Pan American Health Organization [PAHO], 2024a). In the most recent census conducted in 2007, 86.3% of the population identified as *mestizo* (or "mixed," a blend of mostly Spanish and Indigenous heritages), followed by 12.7% White, 0.2% Indigenous, 0.1% Black, and 0.6% other (Gobierno de El Salvador, Oficina Nacional de Estadistica y Censos, 2008). The life expectancy at birth in 2022 was 71.5 years, and the median age was 27.6 years (PAHO, 2024a). The fertility ratio and birth rate were 1.8 per woman and 16 per 1,000 people, respectively (World Bank Group, 2024a). However, El Salvador has a high adolescent fertility rate (54.6 per 1,000 women age 15–19 years in 2022; PAHO, 2024a). About 75% of the population falls between the ages of 15 and 64, 18% are under 15, and 7.5% are over 64, indicating a predominantly youthful population (WHO, 2024a). However, the country is undergoing a demographic transition characterized by slower population growth, a decrease in the youth population, and a gradual shift toward an aging population.

INCOME AND POVERTY

In 2023, per capita income was $5,344, and gross domestic product (GDP) growth was 3.5% (World Bank Group, 2024a). In 2022, remittances from Salvadorans living abroad were equivalent to nearly one quarter (24%) of GDP (World Bank Group, 2024b). Most (73%) of the economically active population works in the informal sector, and most informal sector workers (94%) live in poverty (Lopez & Ruiz-Arranz, 2020). The poverty rate declined nearly by half, from 52% in 2000 to 28% in 2022 and is higher in rural areas than in urban areas (World Bank Group, 2024b). A 4.1% increase in the poverty rate from 2019 to 2021 was primarily attributed to the COVID-19 pandemic (Organisation for Economic Co-operation and Development [OECD], 2023).

GEOGRAPHY AND CLIMATE

El Salvador, located along the Central American volcanic axis, borders the Pacific Ocean, Honduras, and Guatemala. Its geographic location and climate make it vulnerable to volcanic eruptions, earthquakes, tsunamis, landslides, hurricanes, floods, droughts, and extreme weather events, leading to annual losses of 2.5% of GDP (World Bank Group, 2021). El Salvador experiences two distinct seasons: a rainy wet season from May to October and a dry season from November to April (World Bank Group, 2024a). The country is divided administratively into 14 departments and 262 municipalities.

HEALTH OUTCOMES

As noted earlier, health and well-being have improved since the end of the civil conflict, leading to increased life expectancy and better maternal and child health. However, noncommunicable diseases (NCDs) currently account for the majority (65%) of the disease burden (WHO, 2024a). The remaining burden is due to interpersonal violence and injuries (19%) and infectious diseases (16%; WHO, 2024a). Ischemic heart disease was the top cause of death between 2009 and 2019, but in 2020, COVID-19 became the leading cause of death (WHO, 2024b). Table 10.1 lists the top 10 causes of death for 2009, 2019, and 2020.

Interpersonal violence is a significant health concern in El Salvador; however, these deaths have decreased by 69% between 2010 (64.7 per 100,000) and 2023 (20.3 per 100,000; OECD, 2023). The high levels of violence in El Salvador have physical and mental health implications. Violence, particularly gang related, hinders delivery and access to healthcare services in both rural and urban areas (Lopez & Ruiz-Arranz, 2020). Intergenerational violence affects the mental health of men, women, and children, contributing to suicides (OECD, 2023).

SOCIAL AND ENVIRONMENTAL DETERMINANTS OF HEALTH

Despite economic growth and policies implemented between 2009 and 2019 to reduce inequalities, educational disparities persist. Males average 7.6 years of schooling and females 6.8 years (PAHO, 2024a). Moreover, urban attendance for upper secondary education is higher (74%) than

TABLE 10.1 TOP 10 CAUSES OF DEATH (BY RANK) 2009, 2019, AND 2020 IN EL SALVADOR

CAUSE OF DEATH	2009	2019	2020
COVID-19	—	—	1
Ischemic heart disease	1	1	2
Interpersonal violence	2	2	3
Kidney disease	3	3	4
Diabetes mellitus	5	4	5
Stroke	6	5	6
Lower respiratory infections	4	6	7
Cirrhosis of the liver	8	8	8
Alzheimer disease and other dementias	10	9	9
Chronic obstructive pulmonary disease	9	10	10
Road Injury	7	7	—

Source: Adapted from World Health Organization. (n.d.). *Global health estimates: Leading causes of death*. https://www.who.int/data/gho/data/themes/mortality-and-global-health-estimates/ghe-leading-causes-of-death

in rural areas (51%; OECD, 2023). This difference underscores the challenges in ensuring equitable opportunities across different regions, likely contributing to socioeconomic disparities.

Environmental factors such as water quality, poor sanitation, and air pollution also influence health outcomes in El Salvador. Climate change exacerbates the effects of such factors on population health (World Bank Group, 2021). Furthermore, El Salvador's vulnerability to natural disasters exacerbates food insecurity, especially in rural areas where high poverty levels persist (World Food Programme, 2024).

HEALTHCARE IN EL SALVADOR

El Salvador's health sector provides a mix of public and private services. While most Salvadorans depend on public coverage, some may opt for private sector services, leading to high out-of-pocket expenses (MINSAL, 2019a). In 2022, out-of-pocket expenses amounted to 27% of current health expenditures (PAHO, 2024a).

The **public health system** is decentralized and is characterized by segmentation and fragmentation, with four distinct entities providing services to different population segments without effective care coordination or pooling of financial resources. MINSAL is the largest provider of healthcare services, primarily serving the rural poor and populations in marginalized urban areas. The Salvadoran Institute for Social Security (known as ISSS), the second largest provider, caters to formal sector workers and their families. The other two entities are the Military Health Command (COSAM) and the Institute for Teacher Welfare (ISBM), which cater to the military and educators, respectively. In 2018, per-capita spending by these entities was inversely correlated with population coverage: $616 by ISBM, $491 by COSAM, $292 by ISSS, and $135 by MINSAL (2019a).

The private healthcare sector consists of for-profit and nonprofit organizations. For-profit providers operate hospitals and clinics primarily in urban areas (OECD, 2023). Nonprofit providers include nongovernment organizations (NGOs), church groups, and others who render services mainly in rural areas (OECD, 2023).

2009 HEALTHCARE REFORMS

MINSAL offers universal access to PHC services as part of its 2009 health reforms. PHC is the entry point to MINSAL's integrated network of healthcare facilities (2013, 2019b). Before 2009, the public health system suffered from underfunding and limited access to care in rural areas (MINSAL, 2019b). In 2007, a law was passed to create a unified health system. Still, it was not until 2009 that a national healthcare plan, titled "Building Hope: Strategies and Recommendations for Health," outlined the implementation of **universal health coverage** based on comprehensive PHC (MINSAL Publica y Asistencia Social, 2009).

The latter plan was grounded on four fundamental principles: health as a human right, equity, intersectoral collaboration, and social participation. It aimed to strengthen MINSAL's regulatory and steering role over the public and private health sectors while improving coverage, access, and healthcare service quality. It also proposed strengthening healthcare infrastructure and human resources, reorganizing MINSAL's facilities into an integrated network, building a unified health information system, improving intersectoral collaboration, and providing platforms for civic and professional organizations to continue to engage in health reform decisions. The plan introduced a new **community and family care model**, prioritizing its initial deployment to the poorest rural communities (MINSAL, 2019b).

REORGANIZATION OF THE MINISTRY OF HEALTH

To support the implementation of the health reform agenda, MINSAL established a new directorate specifically focused on PHC. The directorate's responsibilities included supervising, monitoring, and evaluating PHC services within its integrated care network. It further delegated oversight to five regions and supervision to 17 departmental offices. Guidance from PAHO and WHO on implementing integrated healthcare networks influenced the organization of the health network

(MINSAL, 2013). MINSAL also integrated multiple information systems into a unified platform to enhance monitoring and analysis, facilitating informed decision-making based on epidemiologic and operational data (MINSAL, 2019b).

NEW COMMUNITY AND FAMILY CARE MODEL

The reform introduced a novel community-based family care model to provide services at PHC facilities and within the community. To achieve this, multidisciplinary PHC teams (known as Equipos Comunitarios de Salud Familiar [ECOS-F]) were formed, consisting of a doctor, two nurses, and up to three health promoters. Specialized PHC teams (known as ECOS-E or Especializados) were also created. These teams included pediatricians, obstetricians/gynecologists, nutritionists, and dentists. PHC teams were deployed in the 100 poorest municipalities (MINSAL, 2017, 2019a). In addition to offering clinical services at healthcare facilities, PHC teams engage in community outreach, health promotion activities, and home visits to provide preventive care.

Each PHC team serves up to 300 families in rural areas, up to 1,800 families in urban areas, up to 6,000 families in rural areas, and up to 9,000 in urban areas (MINSAL, 2017). MINSAL (2019b) reported 529 teams operating in vulnerable areas.

FINANCING THE 2009 HEALTH REFORMS

During the early stages of the health reform, fee-for-service payments were eliminated from public sector facilities. Such out-of-pocket expenditures had been identified as barriers to accessing healthcare services (MINSAL, 2019b). The resulting revenue loss was more than replaced by domestic funds from taxes. Figure 10.1 shows a steady increase in the PHC budget from 2008 to 2019, resulting in an 81% rise in real spending (Gobierno de El Salvador, 2024). By 2019, the PHC budget accounted for 33% of domestic health spending, marking it the highest percentage over 10 years. During this period, the country's health spending increased from 4.1% of GDP in 2008 to 4.7% in 2019, a 13% increase (PAHO, 2024a).

The government also obtained loans from the Inter-American Development Bank (IADB) and the World Bank that helped cover a portion of the capital costs generated by the health reform

FIGURE 10.1 Primary healthcare budget ($2,022) in El Salvador.

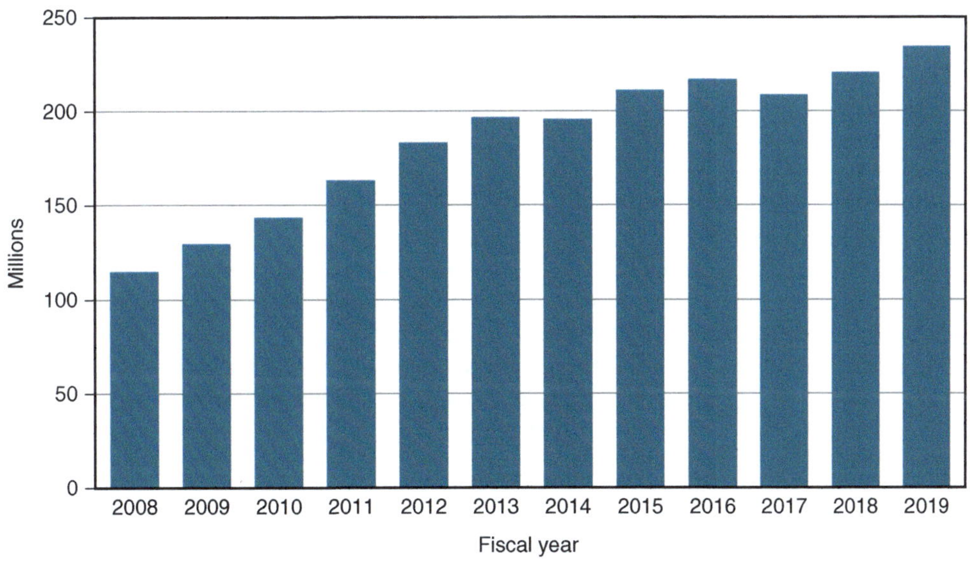

Source: Data from Ministerio de Salud. (n.d.). *Budget reports 2008 to 2019.* https://w3.salud.gob.sv/download/informe-de-labores-2018-2019/

(IADB, 2010; World Bank Group, 2018). In 2010, the IADB provided a $100 million loan to build PHC infrastructure, strengthen the country's health information system, and provide technical assistance, among other key funded activities (IADB, 2010). In 2011, the World Bank extended an $80 million loan to expand healthcare services coverage, quality, and equity and to strengthen MINSAL's stewardship capacity (World Bank Group, 2018).

MINSAL also received aid from various bilateral and multilateral organizations to support the implementation of health reform priorities (MINSAL, 2019a). For instance, the IADB provided results-based aid through a public/private partnership called the **Salud Mesoamerica Initiative** (SMI), which aimed to improve maternal and child health in Central America (IADB, 2024). Furthermore, between 2011 and 2019, SMI, hosted by the IADB, provided nonreimbursable financing to support the government's priorities in PHC. A brief case study of SMI in El Salvador is presented in Box 10.1, illustrating some of the innovations the initiative introduced in the country.

HEALTH REFORM IMPACTS ON HEALTH AND THE HEALTH SYSTEM

Evaluations of the 2009 healthcare reforms and SMI projects supporting the reform have found significant improvements in health system performance in maternal and child health, service utilization, coverage, and quality care, particularly in rural poor areas between 2009 and 2019. For example, an evaluation of an SMI in-kind incentive intervention between 2015 and 2017 found these incentives contributed to increasing antenatal checkups, family planning, and institutional deliveries (Bernal & Martinez, 2020). Furthermore, explanatory case study research conducted between 2011 and 2017 reported gains in PHC system performance (Aranda et al., 2023; Munar et al., 2018).

Looking at the broader effects, in 2019, PAHO assessed the progress of the health reforms using its PHC evaluation framework (Báscolo et al., 2019). The results, not yet published, found that the community and family model of care, which emphasizes prevention and health promotion, contributed to reducing costs, improving health outcomes for women and children, and building trust in the public health system (Báscolo et al., 2019). Additionally, it found that the most significant gains in health improvements for women and children occurred in targeted rural areas, closing the equity gap between rural and urban areas (Báscolo et al., 2019).

BOX 10.1 Case Study of the Salud Mesoamerica Initiative in El Salvador: Healthcare Service Delivery Innovations

Salud Mesoamerica Initiative (SMI) is a public-private partnership in the Central American region where donors and governments share the program's cost (Inter-American Development Bank [IADB], 2024). It is a results-based aid model in which governments agree to performance targets for maternal and child health service delivery outputs and quality care. If governments achieve at least 80% of those targets (as verified by an external evaluator), SMI reimburses them for half of their investment in the program. Those monies can then be used in any area of health.

Between 2011 and 2023, SMI funded 75 primary healthcare (PHC) teams in 14 of El Salvador's 100 poorest communities. SMI was implemented in three phases, with targets set in areas such as reproductive health, maternal health, child health, and nutrition. Phase one focused on service delivery readiness, ensuring that facilities had the essential equipment, supplies, and medicines to deliver PHC services. Phase two introduced team-based, in-kind incentives, offering PHC teams material goods for use in the facility or community. Finally, phase three focused more on meeting performance targets related to health outcomes and quality.

SMI introduced innovative implementation approaches and interventions to improve service delivery and quality, such as policy dialogues between SMI and Ministry of Health (Ministerio de Salud [MINSAL]) officials to set performance targets and evaluate novel service intervention options, learning events to exchange knowledge among PHC teams, micronutrient distribution to reduce anemia, and team in-kind incentives to improve performance (Aranda et al., 2023; Bernal et al., 2020; Bernal & Martinez, 2020).

REMAINING CHALLENGES

NCDs present a considerable challenge to the country's healthcare system. The increasing demand for health services, coupled with inadequate resources and infrastructure, hinders the effective treatment and prevention of NCDs such as cardiovascular disease, diabetes, and cancer. These challenges are exacerbated by sedentary lifestyles, smoking, and poor dietary habits, requiring an intersectoral approach (PAHO, 2024b).

Another challenge is sustaining the progress made before the COVID-19 pandemic and expanding the strategies outlined in the Building Hope Plan. As of 2019, only one third of the planned PHC teams were operational, barely reaching 22% of the population (Báscolo et al., 2019). Continuous investments are also needed to ensure facilities have essential supplies, equipment, and medicines to deliver PHC services.

The long-term goal of establishing an integrated public health system remains a challenge. Progress will depend on political will and sustained engagement of the civil society in enhancing the healthcare system, as evidenced over the past decade (Clark, 2015; MINSAL, 2019b). Political leadership is essential in further supporting the pending reforms to streamline financing, reduce segmentation, and improve coordinated quality care.

CONCLUSION

El Salvador implemented a rights-based health reform prioritizing care for the country's poorest communities, reducing geographic and socioeconomic health disparities. However, the progress of the health reform was disrupted by the COVID-19 pandemic in 2020, which coincided with a change in the central government. The impact of these two events on the progress made by the health reform in improving the country's healthcare system and overall health is still unclear.

ACKNOWLEDGMENT

The authors wish to acknowledge the support provided by Lari Hernandez-Perez, Graduate Research Assistant at the Gill Lebovic Center for Community Health in the Caribbean and Latin America.

LEARNING ACTIVITIES

CourseConnect

To access self-assessment questions and interactive, competency-based learning activities for this chapter, visit www.springerpub.com/courseconnect. See inside front cover and tear-out for CourseConnect details.

REFERENCES

Aranda, L. E., Arif, Z., Innocenti, C., Wahid, S. S., Frehywot, S., & Munar, W. (2023). Characterizing the implementation of performance management interventions in a primary health care system: A case study of the Salud Mesoamerica Initiative in El Salvador. *Health Policy and Planning, 38*(5), 579–592. https://doi.org/https://doi.org/10.1093/heapol/czad020

Báscolo, E., Cid, C., Houghton, N., & Luque, H. (2019). *En el camino a la salud universal. Diez años de reforma del Sistema de Salud en El Salvador* [On the road to universal health. Ten years of health system reform in El Salvador]. Pan American Health Organization.

Bernal, P., Ajzenman, N., Kettle, S., Boo, F. L., & Iriarte, E. (2020). *Designing behaviorally informed health interventions: Adherence to micronutrient treatment in El Salvador*. https://publications.iadb.org/en/designing-behaviorally-informed-health-interventions-adherence-to-micronutrient-treatment-in-el-salvador

Bernal, P., & Martinez, S. (2020). In-kind incentives and health worker performance: Experimental evidence from El Salvador. *Journal of Health Economics, 70*, 102267. https://doi.org/10.1016/j.jhealeco.2019.102267

Clark, M. A. (2015). The new left and health care reform in El Salvador. *Latin American politics and society, 57*(4), 97–118. https://doi.org/10.1111/j.1548-2456.2015.00291.x

Gobierno de El Salvador. (2024). *Portal de transparencia* [Transparency portal]. https://www.transparencia.gob.sv/institutions/minsal/documents/presupuesto-actual

Gobierno de El Salvador, Oficina Nacional de Estadistica y Censos. (2008). *Censo de población y vivienda 2007, El Salvador* [Population and housing census 2007, El Salvador]. https://onec.bcr.gob.sv/servers/redatam/htdocs/CPV2007S/index.html

Inter-American Development Bank. (2010). *El Salvador integrated health program loan proposal.* https://www.iadb.org/en/project/ES-L1027

Inter-American Development Bank. (2024). *Salud Mesoamerica initiative.* Inter-American Development Bank. https://www.saludmesoamerica.org/en/mesoamerica

Lopez, A., & Ruiz-Arranz, M. (2020). *Inequality and social discontent: How to address them through public policy: Economic report on Central America, the Dominican Republic, Haiti, Mexico, and Panama.* https://www.iadb.org/en/news/idb-addresses-how-use-public-policy-mitigate-social-risk-brought-pandemic

Ministerio de Salud. (2013). *Manual de organización y funciones de las RISS* [Manual of organization and functions of the RISS]. https://asp.salud.gob.sv/regulacion/pdf/manual/Manual_de_Organizacion_y_Funciones_de_las_RIISS.pdf

Ministerio de Salud. (2017). *Lineamientos técnicos para los ecos familiares y ecos especializados* [Technical guidelines for family ecos and specialized ecos]. San Salvador, El Salvador: Ministerio de Salud. https://asp.salud.gob.sv/regulacion/pdf/lineamientos/lineamientos_tecnicos_para_los_Ecos_Familiares_y_Ecos_Especializados.pdf

Ministerio de Salud. (2019a). *Informe de labores 2018–2019* [Work report 2018-2019]. https://w3.salud.gob.sv/download/informe-de-labores-2018-2019/

Ministerio de Salud. (2019b). *Transformación de la salud en El Salvador. Diez años de reforma hacia la salud universal* [Health transformation in El Salvador: Ten years of reform towards universal health]. Ministerio de Salud de El Salvador. https://w3.salud.gob.sv/download/libro-transformacion-de-la-salud-en-el-salvador-10-anos-de-reforma-hacia-la-salud-universal/

Ministerio de Salud Publica y Asistencia Social. (2009). *Construyendo la esperanza. Estrategias y recomendaciones en salud* [Building hope: Strategies and recommendations in health]. Editorial del Ministerio de Salud. https://w5.salud.gob.sv/archivos/pdf/PoliticaNacSalud2009-2014/Pol%C3%ADtica+de+Salud+-+Construyendo+la+Esperanza.pdf

Munar, W., Wahid, S. S., Mookherji, S., Innocenti, C., & Curry, L. (2018). Team- and individual-level motivation in complex primary care system change: A realist evaluation of the Salud Mesoamerica Initiative in El Salvador. *Gates Open Research, 2*, 55. https://doi.org/10.12688/gatesopenres.12878.1

Organisation for Economic Co-operation and Development. (2023). *Multi-dimensional review of El Salvador.* https://www.oecd-ilibrary.org/content/publication/2f3d5e1f-en

Pan American Health Organization. (2024a). *Core indicators portal.* Region of the Americas. https://opendata.paho.org/en/core-indicators

Pan American Health Organization. (2024b). *ENLACE: Data portal on noncommunicable diseases, mental health, and external causes.* https://www.paho.org/en/enlace

World Bank Group. (2018). *Implementation completion and results report. IBRD-80760 on a loan in the amount of US$80 million to the Republic of El Salvador for an strengthening public health care system (P117157).* https://documents1.worldbank.org/curated/en/766911544812115606/pdf/approved-icr-el-salvador-p117157-from-portal-november-29-11292018-636803354311107418.pdf

World Bank Group. (2021). *El Salvador.* Climate Change Knowledge Portal. https://climateknowledgeportal.worldbank.org/country/el-salvador/climate-data-historical

World Bank Group. (2024a). *Data.* El Salvador. https://data.worldbank.org/country/el-salvador

World Bank Group. (2024b). *Poverty and inequality platform. Country profile, El Salvador.* https://pip.worldbank.org/country-profiles/SLV

World Food Programme. (2024). *El Salvador.* https://www.wfp.org/countries/el-salvador

World Health Organization. (2024a). *Data: El Salvador.* https://data.who.int/countries/222

World Health Organization. (2024b). *The global health observatory. Global health estimates: Leading causes of death.* https://www.who.int/data/gho/data/themes/mortality-and-global-health-estimates/ghe-leading-causes-of-death

CHAPTER 11

GUATEMALA

Victor Puac-Polanco, Aida Barrera, Alejandra Paniagua-Avila, and Dorian Ramirez-Flores

GEOGRAPHY, SIZE, AND DEMOGRAPHICS

Guatemala is located in Central America and shares borders with Mexico, Honduras, El Salvador, and Belize. It is bordered to the south by the Pacific Ocean and to the northeast by the Gulf of Honduras. With an area of 180,928 square kilometers (112,423 square miles), Guatemala is divided into four regions: the central-western highlands; the low northern plateau; the southern volcanic belt, which is dominated by 27 volcanoes that extend about 186 miles; and the tropical coastal lowlands. The country has political and administrative divisions comprising 22 departments and 340 municipalities. As of 2023, Guatemala's population is estimated to be around 17.6 million, representing a 42% increase over the last 20 years (Instituto Nacional de Estadistica, 2019a). The population is expected to increase by 2.7% between 2023 and 2025. The crude birth rate decreased from 39% in 1990 to 21% in 2023. Guatemala's net migration rate has declined by 1.9 per 1,000 inhabitants between 2023 and 2024. Individuals aged 0 to 14 account for 31.4% of the population, ages 15 to 64 make up 62.9%, and adults older than 65 make up 5.7%. The median age in Guatemala has increased from 21.6 years in 1990 to 27.8 years in 2023. Approximately 50.8% of the population is female, while 49.2% are male. No official estimations exist regarding LGBTQI+ populations as individuals cannot self-identify gender in official documents. Moreover, the country's law does not prohibit discrimination based on sexual orientation, gender expression, or sex characteristics nor does it recognize LGBTQI+ individuals, couples, or their families (U.S. Embassy in Guatemala, 2024). Guatemala, a country with a diverse and rich culture, is home to around 24 ethnic groups, each with unique traditions and customs. These include the Maya (41.7%), Ladino (56%), Garifuna (0.1%), Xinka (1.8%), and Afro-Descendants/Creole/Afro-Mestizo (0.2%). At the beginning of 2024, around 53.3% of Guatemala's population lived in urbanized areas, whereas 46.7% lived in rural areas.

CULTURAL BELIEFS

RELIGIONS

Guatemala's constitution guarantees religious freedom. According to a 2016 survey, 45% of the population was Catholic, 42% Protestant, 11% did not profess any religious affiliation, and 2% of the population professed various beliefs identifying as Buddhists, Hindus, Muslims, Jews, and adherents of the Mayan, Xinca, and Garifuna (Office of International Religious Freedom, 2021). Catholics and Protestants are constant in all ethnic groups and regions of the country. Clergy and leaders of Maya spirituality organizations indicate that many Indigenous Catholics and some Protestants practice some form of religious **syncretism**, defined as the union of different practices from Christian and Maya religious beliefs and practices. This religious syncretism is more evident in the south and northeast of the country, while Maya spirituality is more common in the west.

Although Catholicism was predominantly practiced in Guatemala due to religious imposition from the Spanish conquest, the number of Protestants multiplied by seven between 1960 and 1985, with the fastest religious conversion rate in all of Latin America (Samandu et al., 1988). In Guatemala, healthcare is a fragmented system comprising various public, private, and semiprivate providers and facilities. The diverse range of health providers includes many associated with religious institutions, and their faith-based approach is evident in how they address challenges and care for the people they serve. Guatemala's vibrant religious landscape features numerous Catholic healthcare facilities and programs, as the Catholic Church is the largest and longest-established religious institution in the country. Additionally, there are various decentralized Protestant church initiatives. Traditional Mayan spiritual practices, beliefs, and healers are also interwoven throughout the healthcare landscape. Medical missions are generally short-term visits sponsored by religious-affiliated institutions outside the country that provide healthcare, but that rarely translate into establishing long-term health systems (Marshall, 2016).

LANGUAGES

The official language of Guatemala is Spanish. According to data from the latest national population survey of 2018, 70% of the Guatemalan population over 5 years old communicated in Spanish. The remaining 30% speak one of the 23 Mayan languages preserved since before the arrival of the Spaniards on the continent. The main Mayan languages spoken in the country are Q'eqchi', K'iche', Mam, Kacqchikel, and Q'anjob'al (25%; INE, 2019b). Many speakers of Mayan languages also speak Spanish. A small percentage (0.02%) speak Xinca and Garífuna languages. Unfortunately, the multilinguistic context is often not accounted for in health decision-making. For example, most healthcare services are provided in Spanish. While this is not a challenge in urban areas, it does add an access barrier to rural populations, especially Indigenous women who are more likely to experience discrimination. The lack of culturally appropriate and respectful care ultimately decreases the use of healthcare facilities by marginalized populations. Read the interview with Ingrid Sub Cuc in Box 11.1.

POLITICAL SYSTEM

According to its Constitution, Guatemala is a free, independent, and sovereign state. Its system of government is democratic and representative, organized into three branches: the executive, the legislative, and the judicial, which operate independently. The executive, led by the president (head

BOX 11.1 Perspectives on Indigenous Maya Health

Interview with Ingrid Sub Cuc, MSC in Public Health, third-year PhD student in Native American Studies at the University of California, Davis. She is a Kaqchikel and Q'eqchi' woman, originally from Sololá, Guatemala.

Indigenous health systems continue to be used because they relate to language, worldview, and belonging; moreover, trust in healers allows them to provide therapeutic support to people with *nervios* (anxiety or depression) and other problems. Trust is a very important and valued issue in Indigenous communities. Indigenous traditional medicine is mainly based on the use of medicinal plants, the *temascal* or *tuj*, prayers, and offerings, with language as a cohesive element because language shapes the way of understanding life, the world, health, and disease. That is why it is so difficult to integrate Indigenous therapy into the official health system because it becomes decontextualized, and the vital importance of the native language is not considered.

Other reasons for the failure of the attempts to integrate the public health system with Indigenous medicine are that it is about extracting "what is good" in the Indigenous health system and implementing it in the Western public system, but it is not integrated. The background is discrimination and racism, not only toward health knowledge but also toward Indigenous languages and philosophical conceptions. Indigenous users feel discriminated against by Indigenous health workers themselves, who do not know how to accept their identity and prefer to speak in Spanish rather than to be known as Indigenous among their colleagues. Education and sensitization are needed to overcome these historical challenges that divide us as a country. Decolonization is necessary.

of state), fulfills the state's executive functions, along with the vice president, ministers, and other officials. The president is elected for 4 years and serves as the commander-in-chief of the national armed forces. The legislative branch formulates and reviews laws for approval, modification, or repeal. It also represents their electors. Legislators have the authority to oversee public officials, and individuals engaged in public affairs. Lastly, the judicial branch administers justice guided by the Constitution and all the laws. Judges deliver justice through the court system (Dabroy, 2022).

IMPORTANT TRADITIONS, PRACTICES, EVENTS, OR LEISURE PURSUITS

In Guatemala, religious events are celebrated in every town, often accompanied by annual fairs. Football soccer is a sport that mobilizes the population, with people of all ages participating in it. Television serves as a significant source of entertainment for the population. The country's traditions are a fusion of ancestral Indigenous traditions and customs brought by the Spanish, mostly linked to Catholic religious celebrations. For example, during Holy Week, colorful flower and sawdust carpets are made for religious parades, and on All Saints' Day, traditional foods are enjoyed, while giant kites are flown in some towns of the central highlands (Stansifer et al., 2024).

HISTORICAL CONSIDERATIONS FOR CONTEXT

The territory of modern Guatemala was the heart of the Maya civilization, conquered by the Spanish in the 16th century. Guatemala gained independence in 1821 and was part of the Federal Republic of Central America from 1823 to 1841. The country endured instability and civil strife in the latter half of the 19th century and was governed by a series of U.S.-backed dictators in the early 20th century. A military coup in 1944 sparked a decade-long revolution and led to significant social and economic reforms. A U.S.-backed military coup in 1954 ended the revolution and established a dictatorship. From 1960 to 1996, Guatemala experienced a brutal civil war between the U.S.-backed government and leftist rebels, which included genocidal massacres of the Maya population. The United Nations mediated a peace accord, resulting in economic growth and successive democratic elections (Stansifer et al., 2024).

HEALTH OUTCOMES

TOP 10 CAUSES OF DEATH

Guatemala is experiencing a demographic and epidemiologic transition in which the population is aging, and the leading causes of mortality are transitioning from communicable and maternal/neonatal diseases to noncommunicable diseases and injuries. Gains in life expectancy during the 20th and 21st centuries can be attributed to improvements in preventing communicable diseases and maternal and neonatal mortality. During most of the 20th century, the leading causes of mortality were from communicable diseases. In the 21st century, the percentage of deaths due to communicable and maternal/neonatal deaths decreased from 55.72% to 21.36% in 2019. In contrast, the percentage of deaths attributed to noncommunicable diseases increased from 31.39 in 1990 to 64.17% in 2019. In 1990, the leading causes of death were attributed to lower respiratory infections, enteric infections, and maternal/neonatal diseases. In 2019, the leading causes of death were lower respiratory infections, ischemic heart disease, diabetes, and chronic kidney disease. In 2020 and 2021, COVID-19 was the leading cause of death, followed by ischemic heart disease, lower respiratory infections other than COVID-19, and diabetes (Institute for Health Metrics and Evaluation [IHME], 2024a).

MENTAL HEALTH

According to the only National Mental Health Survey in Guatemala, conducted in 2009, 27.8% of the surveyed population reported mental health conditions. The most prevalent conditions were anxiety/somatoform and mood conditions at 20.2% and 8.0%, respectively (Cobar Herrera et al., 2009). Similar to other noncommunicable diseases, the public health system has not been able to keep up with the increasing prevalence of mental health conditions among the Guatemalan population. As an example, the mental health treatment gap in Guatemala is 84.9% among the population in need of any mental health services (Kohn et al., 2018).

INFECTIOUS DISEASES

Communicable and maternal/neonatal diseases still contribute to an important portion of deaths and disability in Guatemala.

COVID-19

According to PAHO, Guatemala ranked 22nd in the number of deaths from COVID-19 in the Americas region in 2021, with a cumulative 914.7 deaths per million population over 2 years. Guatemala registered 4,813 deaths directly caused by COVID-19 in 2020 and 11,293 in 2021 (PAHO, 2024). However, limited COVID-19 testing led to underestimating the actual number of cases and deaths attributed to COVID-19. For instance, a study estimated a peak of 73% excess mortality in July 2020 compared to previous years, and a total number of 8,036 deaths in 2020, which was 46% higher than the official COVID-19 mortality count (Martinez-Folgar et al., 2021). As of 2023, less than 50% of the Guatemalan population had received at least one COVID-19 vaccine dose. COVID-19 vaccination coverage has been low due to limited supply, limited access, and vaccine hesitation among the population.

Respiratory Infections

In 2019, respiratory infections contributed to 11.31% of deaths in Guatemala with lower respiratory infections, including pneumonia, as the cause of most of these deaths (IHME, 2024a). Deaths attributed to tuberculosis have decreased from 2.7 fatalities per 100,000 inhabitants in 2005 to 1.2 fatalities per 100,000 inhabitants in 2021 (Instituto Nacional de Estadistica, n.d.).

Enteric Infections

Enteric diarrheal infections contributed 13.55% in 2019 to the overall country's disease burden. Diarrhea, together with chronic and acute undernutrition, are among the main contributors to mortality among children under 5 years. Diarrheal infections are caused in part by limited water and poor sanitation systems, particularly among the rural Indigenous populations (IHME, 2024a).

NONCOMMUNICABLE DISEASES

The deaths and disability attributed to noncommunicable diseases in Guatemala have been increasing for the past decades. A public health system, which has traditionally prioritized communicable and maternal/neonatal diseases, has been unable to respond to the increasing prevalence of cardiovascular diseases among the Guatemalan population.

Cardiovascular Diseases

In 2021, close to one in five deaths in Guatemala were attributed to cardiovascular diseases, including ischemic heart disease, hypertension, stroke, and other less common heart diseases (e.g., atrial fibrillation, cardiomyopathy; IHME, 2024a). The increasing percentage of cardiovascular deaths in the Guatemalan population has been attributed to lifestyle changes among the population. While data are limited, studies suggest that both males and females are presenting behavioral risk factors for cardiovascular diseases at a young age. According to the Pan-American Health Organization (PAHO) indicators, 55.9% of people 15 years or older were overweight or obese in 2016. Among the same group, the prevalence of tobacco use was 10.4%. Also, 74.2% of the population reported insufficient physical activity or exercise (PAHO, 2024).

Diabetes Mellitus

Data about diabetes in Guatemala are limited. The most robust survey in Guatemala, conducted in 2006 among an urban and ethnically mixed population, showed an adjusted prevalence of adult diabetes of 9.6%, which was similar to the prevalence in countries like the Unite—d States at that time (Barcelo et al., 2012). According to PAHO, the prevalence of diabetes mellitus among urban populations has increased from 7.4% in 2000 to 9.7% in 2014 (PAHO, 2024). Less robust studies conducted within health facilities suggest that the prevalence of diabetes among the rural, Indigenous populations is also high.

LIFE EXPECTANCY FROM BIRTH

Guatemala made significant gains in life expectancy from birth during the second half of the 20th century and the first two decades of the 21st century. Life expectancy increased by more than 25 years from 46 years in 1960 to 73 years in 2019. During the civil war, life expectancy decreased from 55 years in 1975 to 50 years in 1982. More recently, during and after the COVID-19 pandemic, life expectancy decreased to 72 years in 2020 and 69 years in 2021. In 2022, Guatemala's life expectancy at 69 years was the third lowest in Latin America and the lowest in the Central American region (World Bank Group, 2024a).

DETERMINANTS OF HEALTH

NATIONAL AND PER-CAPITA GROSS DOMESTIC PRODUCT AND POVERTY RATES

Guatemala is classified as an upper middle-income economy (PAHO, 2024). In 2022, Guatemala´s national gross domestic product (GDP) amounted to $95 billion, with a per capita GDP of $5,473.2 and an interannual growth rate of 4.1% (World Bank Group, 2024b). In 2000, 56.2% of the population lived in poverty and 15.7% in extreme poverty, whereas by 2014, the overall poverty rose to 59.3% and extreme poverty to 23.4% (Instituto Nacional de Estadistica, 2023a). In 2023, the country's poverty rate was 55.1%, especially among Indigenous populations (World Bank Group, 2024b). Additionally, in 2014, 76.3% of the Guatemalan population had a low income, 22.7% had a middle income, and 1% had a high income (Velasquez, 2022).

EDUCATION AND LITERACY RATES

In 2018, the illiteracy rate of the population aged 7 years or older was 18.5%, with a higher prevalence among women (21.7%) compared to men (15%; Instituto Nacional de Estadistica, 2019b). In 2021, the enrollment rate was 60.8% in preschool, 90.2% in primary school, 48.3% in middle school, and 25.3% in high school (UN Development Programme, 2022). In 2010, the higher education enrollment rate was 10.4% of the population between 20 and 34 years of age (Tobar Piril, 2011).

UNEMPLOYMENT RATES

Guatemala's overall unemployment rate increased from 2% in 2019 to 2.2% in 2021 and 3% in 2022. This trend was more noticeable in rural areas and among women. In 2022, Guatemala City had an unemployment rate of 0.4% for men and 0.7% for women. Other urban areas had rates of 0.3% for men and 0.4% for women, and the rural regions reported rates of 0.6% for men and 0.7% for women. The informal economy accounted for 71.1% of employment, complemented by 28.9% of the formal sector. Besides, the rate of visible underemployment—individuals aged 15 years or older who unwillingly work less than 8 hours a day but wish to work more hours and are available to do so—was 11.3%. The most affected by underemployment were men, Ladinos, Mayans, individuals older than 24 years, and those working in commerce, agriculture, and services (Instituto Nacional de Estadistica, 2023b).

FOOD AND NUTRITION

During the period from 2020 to 2023, on average, Guatemala had 2.3 million undernourished people (13.3%) and 10.5 million people affected by moderate or severe food insecurity (59.8%; 4.1 million female adults and 3 million male adults). Regarding food availability, the average **dietary energy supply adequacy** was 124%. The prevalence of anemia among women of reproductive age (15 to 49 years) dropped from 22.4% in 2000 to 7.4% in 2019, and the prevalence of obesity in the adult population (18 years and older) rose from 12.9% in 2000 to 21.2% in 2016 (Food and Agriculture Organization, 2024). In children under the age of 5 years, chronic undernutrition prevalence was 46.5% in 2015, affecting more in rural areas (53%), the northwest (68.2%), southwest (51.9%), and the north of the country (50%), as well as Indigenous children (58%), those with less educated mothers (67%), and those from economically disadvantaged households (65.9%).

HEALTH-RELATED BEHAVIORS

In 2015, the prevalence of tobacco use among Guatemalans age 13 to 15 years old was 17.1% (males, 19.5%; females, 14.4%), whereas the prevalence among adults was 22.2% for men and 1.6% for women (PAHO, 2024). There is little information about physical activity in Guatemala. One study reported a 9.7% prevalence of physical inactivity among Guatemalan adults. However, this could be an underestimation, given that other countries from the Americas reported prevalences greater than 80% (Oldridge, 2008). In 2016, the alcohol consumption per capita among people aged 15 years and older was 11.2 liters of pure alcohol for males and 4.2 for females. In the same age group, the prevalence of heavy episodic drinking (defined as consuming at least 60 grams of pure alcohol on at least one occasion within the past 30 days) was 17.2% for males and 2.5% for females, whereas among people with an alcohol use disorder, the prevalence was 44.6% for men and 14.9% for women (Poznyak & Rekve, 2017).

TOP 10 MORTALITY RISK FACTORS

The 10 leading risk factors for death and disability in 2021 were malnutrition; high fasting plasma glucose; high body mass index; air pollution; high alcohol abuse; kidney dysfunction; high blood pressure; dietary risks; water, sanitation, and hygiene; and occupational risks (IHME, 2024b).

SOCIAL JUSTICE SUCH AS HUMAN RIGHTS ISSUES AND VULNERABLE AND UNDERSERVED POPULATIONS

The Guatemala 2022 Human Rights Report informed the killings of social activists and the involvement of police officers and agents in organized crime. Legal proceedings against two former presidents and several military officers for alleged genocide against Indigenous communities during the internal armed conflict (1960–1996) faced significant, yet not justifiable, delays. Due to political persecution, a former general attorney, along with various judges, prosecutors, and justice officials, have been forced to leave the country in recent years. Other human rights issues included in the report are inhumane prison conditions, arbitrary arrest, and detention, repression, independence of the judiciary system problems, restrictions on free expression and media, gender-based violence, violence against Indigenous groups as well as LGBTQ+ persons, individuals with disabilities, and restrictions on workers' freedom of association (U.S. Embassy in Guatemala, 2024).

ENVIRONMENTAL AND CLIMATE CHANGE ISSUES

In 2023, Guatemala's concentration of particulate matter, a measure of air pollution, is four times higher than the threshold recommended by the World Health Organization (WHO; Guatemala = 21 mcg/m^3 vs. recommendation = 5 mcg/m^3 annual mean). Such air pollution accounted for 37% of deaths from stroke and ischemic heart disease. Despite these high levels of air pollution, Guatemala does not have a policy establishing limits for particulate matter. Moreover, 44% of the population lives without safe drinking water, while 58% of deaths are due to diarrhea caused by unsafe drinking water, poor sanitation, and inadequate personal hygiene. Although the country had a national health and climate change plan or strategy by 2023, there were insufficient data to assess the extent of the problem of climate change and its impact on health (WHO, 2023).

HISTORICAL/THEORETICAL BACKGROUND OF HEALTHCARE

The current healthcare system was developed during the Civil War. While the system has been modified with some reforms, it still faces significant problems. It is mainly divided into three: the public sector, the private for-profit sector, and the private nonprofit sector. The public sector, managed by the Ministry of Public Health and Social Assistance (MSPAS), provides services to 70% of the population; the private nonprofit sector (IGSS) provides coverage to 17.4%.; and the private for-profit sector provides coverage to approximately 12% to 18% of the population (Becerril-Montekio & Lopez-Dávila, 2011). The funding for the MSPAS comes from state tax revenues, external aid, loans, and international donations. However, the public health system is severely underfunded, and in most years, resources are insufficient to cover the population's needs. In addition, the public sector focuses on treating diseases rather than implementing public health prevention programs, creating a basic primary care system where most of the scarce financial resources are spent on tertiary-level hospitals. Wide gaps exist between the quality of services provided in Guatemala City's public hospitals versus those offered to the population in other cities' healthcare facilities, especially in rural areas.

HEALTHCARE TRAINING AND EDUCATION

Healthcare training is delivered by one public university and 13 private universities. All 14 universities provide diverse training programs in the healthcare sector, covering undergraduate, graduate, master's, and doctoral degrees. Healthcare professionals include physicians, nurses, dentists, psychologists, nutritionists, pharmacists, medical specialists, and many more. In 2020, the number of physicians per 1,000 population was 1.3 and nurses 2.3 (World Bank Group, 2024b).

HEALTHCARE COST, QUALITY, AND ACCESS

As per the Constitution, every citizen has the right to universal healthcare. The reality is that few citizens have access to comprehensive healthcare, with rural areas experiencing vast access inequities. In this context, the private health insurance market has witnessed significant growth during the last decade. In 2024, gross written premiums for health insurance reached $390 million, a 5.45% increase compared to 2023. This growth rate is projected to continue at a steady 4.56% annual rate. The average spending per capita on health insurance is estimated to be $19.01 in 2024. While the health insurance market in Guatemala is experiencing a surge in demand, the costs of healthcare services are expected to increase with time due to the aging demographic and the subsequent surge in chronic diseases. In 2021, household out-of-pocket health expenditure was $3.66 billion. This is the highest value ever recorded and shows an overall increasing trend that in 2010 amounted to approximately $1.5 billion, which represented 6.4% of the Guatemalan GDP (Mendoza, 2024). The quality and accessibility of healthcare services have been negatively impacted by factors like the constant shift of health authorities and personnel responsible for ensuring quality standards. Quality assurance has not been fully integrated as a nationwide core component of the health system. Notably, the unit for the quality assurance had been dismantled in 2012 and again in 2014 (Ávila et al., 2015).

GAPS IN CARE OR HEALTHCARE SHORTAGE AREAS

Significant disparities exist in accessibility to healthcare services and medications across different segments of society, with accompanying inequalities in health outcomes, especially among the economically disadvantaged, Indigenous People, individuals with low education levels, and those who live in rural areas (Ávila et al., 2015).

HEALTHCARE PRACTICES

ALLOPATHIC MEDICINE

Also known as conventional medicine, allopathic medicine is the predominant form of healthcare in Guatemala. The country has both public and private healthcare providers that offer allopathic medical services. The public sector, overseen by the MSPAS, delivers care through a network of hospitals and health centers, especially in urban areas. However, access to these services can be limited in rural regions, where traditional medicine practices are more prevalent.

Private healthcare facilities, such as hospitals and clinics, are available in Guatemala, especially in larger cities. These facilities often provide a broader range of specialized services and may have shorter waiting times compared to public institutions. However, private healthcare can be more expensive and may not be accessible to everyone. The use of medicinal plants and spiritual healing, especially among Indigenous populations, is often integrated with allopathic medicine to provide holistic healthcare.

TRADITIONAL MEDICINE

To understand traditional Maya medicine, one must consider that it originates from the Maya worldview of the constant search for the meaning of life, including spirituality and the sciences that meticulously explain cosmology. It comprises sacred rituals, codices, stone inscriptions, ideograms, technology, art, weaving, music, oral tradition, organization, rules of coexistence, and the personal, family, and social interactions practiced by millennial-old traditions of the Maya. Maya traditional medicine is based on the use of natural inputs such as medicinal plants (herbal medicine), minerals, animal oils, and the restoration of mechanical (sunken fontanelle), emotional ("fright"; nerves or sadness), energetic ("evil eye"), and hot-cold balance in the body (facial paralysis). The therapy used depends on the origin of the disease. In Maya medicine, there are specialists; for example, *Lyom*/midwife, *Ajq'ayis*/healer with herbs, *Ajb'aq*/masseur or bone setter, *Ajtuj*/healer with sauna, *Ajchay*/healer with obsidian, *Ajeyaj*/dentist, and *Ajch'ut*/healer with snake teeth or thorns (Barrios Escobar, 2016).

Although non-Indigenous populations use some practices of Maya traditional medicine, their use is more widespread among the Indigenous population of the country's western highlands and northeastern regions. These populations have less access to allopathic medicine due to language barriers, travel distances to care services, discrimination, and lack of trust in healthcare providers and settings. Although efforts have been made since the peace agreements to implement cultural education to respect and accept the traditional healthcare system, challenges still exist toward true integration of allopathic–traditional systems (Avila et al., 2015).

COMPLEMENTARY MEDICINE

According to the Guatemalan Ministry of Health, complementary or alternative medicine encompasses practices and products that are not part of conventional medical care. This includes acupuncture, acupressure, reflexology, naturopathy, herbal medicine, chiropractic, iridology, and homeopathy, which must be practiced by a licensed technician with valid registration, and the complementary medicine center must be accredited by the Ministry of Health (Muñoz, 2023).

CONCLUSION

The Guatemalan healthcare system and its universal coverage approach continue to be expensive for the state and inequitable for the population. Moreover, out-of-pocket healthcare expenses increase every year, posing a considerable financial strain on the population. In the past 10 years, private health insurance has become a popular alternative for healthcare services. While the entrance of the health insurance market will benefit a growing portion of the population, it is critical for stakeholders and policymakers to set up regulations and norms that will prevent an inequitable distribution of health benefits, expand the coverage to low-income groups, incentivize primary care prevention, and allow investment into interventions that seek integration of the large Maya traditional and allopathic medical systems.

LEARNING ACTIVITIES

CourseConnect

To access self-assessment questions and interactive, competency-based learning activities for this chapter, visit www.springerpub.com/courseconnect. See inside front cover and tear-out for CourseConnect details.

REFERENCES

Avila, C., Bright, R. Gutierrez, J., Hoadley, K., Coite, M., Romero, N., & Rodriguez, M.P. (2019). *Guatemala health system assessment, August 2015*. Health Finance & Governance Project, Abt Associates Inc. https://internationalmedicalrelief.org/wp-content/uploads/2019/07/Guatemala-HSA-_ENG-FULL-REPORT-FINAL-APRIL-2016.pdf

Barcelo, A., Gregg, E. W., Gerzoff, R. B., Wong, R., Perez Flores, E., Ramirez-Zea, M., Cafiero, E., Altamirano, L., Ascencio Rivera, M., de Cosio, G., de Maza, M. D, del Aguila, R., Emanuel, E., Gil, E., Gough, E., Jenkins, V., Orellana, P., Palma, R., Palomo, R . . . CAMDI Collaborative Study Group. (2012). Prevalence of diabetes and intermediate hyperglycemia among adults from the first multinational study of noncommunicable diseases in six Central American countries: The Central America Diabetes Initiative (CAMDI). *Diabetes Care, 35*(4), 738–740. https://doi.org/10.2337/dc11-1614

Barrios Escobar, L. E. (2016). *El rostro y el ser de los cuatro pueblos de Guatemala. Elementos para la interculturalidad* [The face and being of the four peoples of Guatemala: Elements for interculturality] (2nd ed.). Ministerio de Cultura y Deporte. https://mcd.gob.gt/wp-content/uploads/2017/02/El-Rostro-y-el-Ser-de-los-Cuatro-Pueblos.pdf

Becerril-Montekio, V., & Lopez-Dávila, L. (2011). Sistema de salud de Guatemala. *Salud Publica Mex, 53*, S197.

Cobar Herrera, M. I., De la Roca Ordaz, M. W., Dávila Valenzuela, K. D., Dalila, K., Cutz, C., Ismael, M., Pappa, D., Gómez Gómez, C.E., Bautista Fuentes, N.E., González Rivera, B.A., Campos Correa, V.R., Vaides Guillermo, A.O., Donald, H....et al. (2009). *Encuesta nacional de salud mental: Descripción epidemiológica de trastornos de salud en hombres y mujeres de 18 a 65 años de edad realizada en la República de Guatemala mayo-julio 2009* [National mental health survey: Epidemiological description of health disorders in men and women aged 18 to 65 years, conducted in the Republic of Guatemala May-July 2009]. Publication Number MFN:008255, Graduate, Universidad de San Carlos de Guatemala. https://biblioteca.medicina.usac.edu.gt/tesis/pre/2009/015.pdf

Dabroy, J. (2022). *Elementos fundamentales del sistema político guatemalteco: Institucionalidad pública* [Fundamental elements of the Guatemalan political system: Public institutions]. https://asies.org.gt/wp-content/uploads/pdfs/elementos_fundamentales_del_sistema_politico_guatemalteco_institucionalidad_publica.pdf

Food and Agriculture Organization. (2024). *FAOSTAT: Guatemala*. https://www.fao.org/faostat/en/#country/89

Institute for Health Metrics and Evaluation. (2024a). *Global health data exchange*. https://ghdx.healthdata.org/

Institute for Health Metrics and Evaluation. (2024b). *Guatemala*. https://www.healthdata.org/research-analysis/health-by-location/profiles/guatemala

Instituto Nacional de Estadistica. (n.d.). *Tema/indicadores: Series historicas con la tasa de mortalidad por tuberculosis desagregada por departamento* [Topic/indicators: Historical series with the tuberculosis mortality rate disaggregated by department]. https://www.ine.gob.gt/vitales/

Instituto Nacional de Estadistica. (2019a). *Estimaciones y proyecciones de poblacion a largo plazo 1950–2050* [Long-term population estimates and projections 1950–2050]. https://www.ine.gob.gt/proyecciones/

Instituto Nacional de Estadistica. (2019b). *XII censo nacional de poblacion y VII de vivienda* [XII national population census and VII housing census]. https://censo2018.ine.gob.gt/explorador%20%0d7

Instituto Nacional de Estadistica. (2023a). *Encuesta nacional de condiciones de Vida - ENCOVI- 2023* [National survey of living conditions - ENCOVI - 2023]. https://www.ine.gob.gt/sistema/uploads/2024/08/22/20240822115045oP9hz3bt6r44qxs2amGK6YQqIpGhNdg0.pdf

Instituto Nacional de Estadistica. (2023b). *Principales resultados de la encuesta nacional de empleo e ingresos 2022 (ENEI)* [Main results of the 2022 national survey of employment and income (ENEI)]. https://www.ine.gob.gt/sistema/uploads/2023/03/23/20230323142069Odm3oxU9mTY58hkborwzylm7MJop05q.pdf

Kohn, R., Ali, A. A., Puac-Polanco, Figueroa, C., López-Soto, V., Morgan, K., Saldivia, S., & Vicente, B. (2018). Mental health in the Americas: An overview of the treatment gap. *Revista Panamericana de Salud Pública, 42*, e165. https://doi.org/10.26633/RPSP.2018.165

Marshall, K. (2016). *Faces of health, poverty, and faith in Guatemala*. Georgetown University. https://berkleycenter.georgetown.edu/posts/faces-of-health-poverty-and-faith-in-guatemala

Martinez-Folgar, K., Alburez-Gutierrez, D., Paniagua-Avila, A., Ramirez-Zea, M., & Bilal, U. (2021). Excess mortality during the COVID-19 pandemic in Guatemala. *American Journal of Public Health, 111*(10), 1839–1846. https://doi.org/10.2105/AJPH.2021.306452

Mendoza, J. (2024). *Household out-of-pocket health spending in Guatemala 2010–2021*. https://www.statista.com/statistics/1285558/out-of-pocket-health-expenditure-guatemala/

Muñoz, C. (2023). *¿Qué es un centro de medicina alternativa?* [What is an alternative medicine center?]. MSPAC. https://www.facebook.com/MinisteriodeSaludPublicayAsistenciaSocial/videos/646152601012910/?_rdr

Office of International Religious Freedom. (2021). *Informe internacional sobre la libertad de religion: Guatemala* [International report on religious freedom: Guatemala]. https://uploads.mwp.mprod.getusinfo.com/uploads/sites/40/2022/06/SPANISH-GUATEMALA-2021-INTERNATIONAL-RELIGIOUS-FREEDOM-REPORT-final-CHECKED.pdf

Oldridge, N. B. (2008). Economic burden of physical inactivity: Healthcare costs associated with cardiovascular disease. *European Journal of Cardiovascular Prevention and Rehabilitation, 15*(2), 130–139. https://doi.org/10.1097/HJR.0b013e3282f19d42

Pan American Health Organization. (2024). *Health in the Americas: Guatemala*. https://hia.paho.org/en/countries-22/guatemala-country-profile

Poznyak, V., & Rekve, D. (2017). *Global status report on alcohol and health 2018*. https://www.who.int/publications/i/item/9789241565639

Samandu, L., Dary, C., & Similox Salazar, V. (1988). *El protestantismo en Guatemala* [Protestantism in Guatemala]. http://biblioteca.usac.edu.gt/folleto/USAC/digi/USAC_F_0338.pdf

Stansifer, C. L., Anderson, T. P., Horst, O. H., Anderson, T.P., & The Editors of Encyclopaedia Britannica. (2024). *Guatemala*. https://www.britannica.com/place/Guatemala

Tobar Piril, L. A. (2011). La educación superior en Guatemala en la primera década del siglo XXI. *Innovación Educativa, 11*(57), 69–80. https://www.redalyc.org/articulo.oa?id=179422350009

UN Development Programme. (2022). *Informe nacional de desarrollo humano. Desafíos y oportunidades para Guatemala: Hacia una agenda de futuro La celeridad del cambio, una mirada territorial del desarrollo humano 2002 - 2019* [National report of human development. Challenges and opportunities for Guatemala: Towards a future agenda, the speed of change, a territorial look at human development 2002-2019]. https://www.undp.org/es/guatemala/publicaciones/informe-nacional-de-desarrollo-humano-desafios-y-oportunidades-para-guatemala-hacia-una-agenda-de-futuro-la-celeridad-del

U.S. Embassy in Guatemala. (2024). *2023 Human rights report: Guatemala*. https://www.state.gov/reports/2023-country-reports-on-human-rights-practices/guatemala/

Velasquez, A. M. (2022). *La desigualdad social en Guatemala: Evolución y respuesta institucional* [Social inequality in Guatemala: Evolution and institutional response]. https://www.cepal.org/es/publicaciones/47938-la-desigualdad-social-guatemala-evolucion-respuesta-institucional

World Bank Group. (2024a). *Life expectancy at birth, total (years)*. https://data.worldbank.org/indicator/SP.DYN.LE00.IN

World Bank Group. (2024b). *Guatemala*. https://data.worldbank.org/country/guatemala?view=chart

World Health Organization. (2023). *Environmental health: Guatemala 2023 country profile*. https://www.who.int/publications/m/item/environmental-health-gtm-2023-country-profile

PART IV: Health and Healthcare in South America

CHAPTER 12

OVERVIEW OF SOUTH AMERICA

Leslie A. Bozeman and Luke Orgo

INTRODUCTION

South America is the fourth largest continent behind Asia, Africa, and North America. It includes Argentina, Bolivia, Brazil, Chile, Colombia, Ecuador, French Guiana, the Falkland Islands, Guyana, Paraguay, Peru, Suriname, Uruguay, and Venezuela (Figure 12.1). It was first and primarily colonized by Spain and Portugal. The two countries split the region, according to the Treaty of Tordesillas of 1494. The Treaty, signed by Spain's monarchs, King Ferdinand II of Aragon and Queen Isabella I of Castile, and Portugal's King John II, established a line of demarcation between the two crowns (UNESCO, n.d.). France, the Netherlands, and the United Kingdom established smaller colonies (Finlayson, 2025).

GEOGRAPHY

South America can be divided into three physical regions: mountains and highlands, river basins, and coastal plains and is home to dry deserts; dense, tropical rain forests; and grasslands. It boasts a rich biodiversity of plant and animal species. The Andes, the continent's primary mountain system, covers 5,500 miles. The region also has high plateaus, low plateaus, and glaciers. Its three most important river basins are the Amazon, the Orinoco, and the Paraguay/Paraná (National Geographic, 2025). The continent has been connected to Central and North America by the land bridge of the Panamanian Isthmus for approximately 3.5 million years and is bounded on the east by the Pacific Ocean, on the north by the Caribbean Sea, and on the west by the Atlantic Ocean (Cardenas, 2013).

CULTURE

South America is home to a variety of cultural groups including Indigenous tribes, enslaved people, and colonizers. Indigenous cultures of South America include Incas, Aymara, Amazonian tribes, Guarani, and Mapuche. The Inca Empire is the most well-known Indigenous culture of the region and was established in 1438 in Cuzco, Peru, and then expanded to Bolivia, Ecuador, Chile, and Colombia (National Geographic, 2025). The Incas were the architects of an expansive network of roads along which they built essential facilities that enabled them to rule widely. Beginning in the 16th century, African slaves were imported to South America, primarily to Brazil but also to present-day Venezuela, Colombia, coastal Ecuador and Peru, and northwestern Argentina (Britannica, n.d.). Their cultural practices were integrated with the beliefs of the region's Indigenous peoples as well as rituals brought by Europeans. Gauchos (cowboys) live in the Pampas of Argentina, Brazil, and Uruguay and are known for hunting and trading (National Geographic, 2025). The region's contemporary population comprises American Indians, Iberians, Africans, and immigrants from Italy, Germany, Lebanon, South Asia, and Japan (Britannica, n.d.). It is noteworthy that Brazil has the largest population of Japanese people outside of Japan (Connect Brazil, 2025).

FIGURE 12.1 Map of South America.

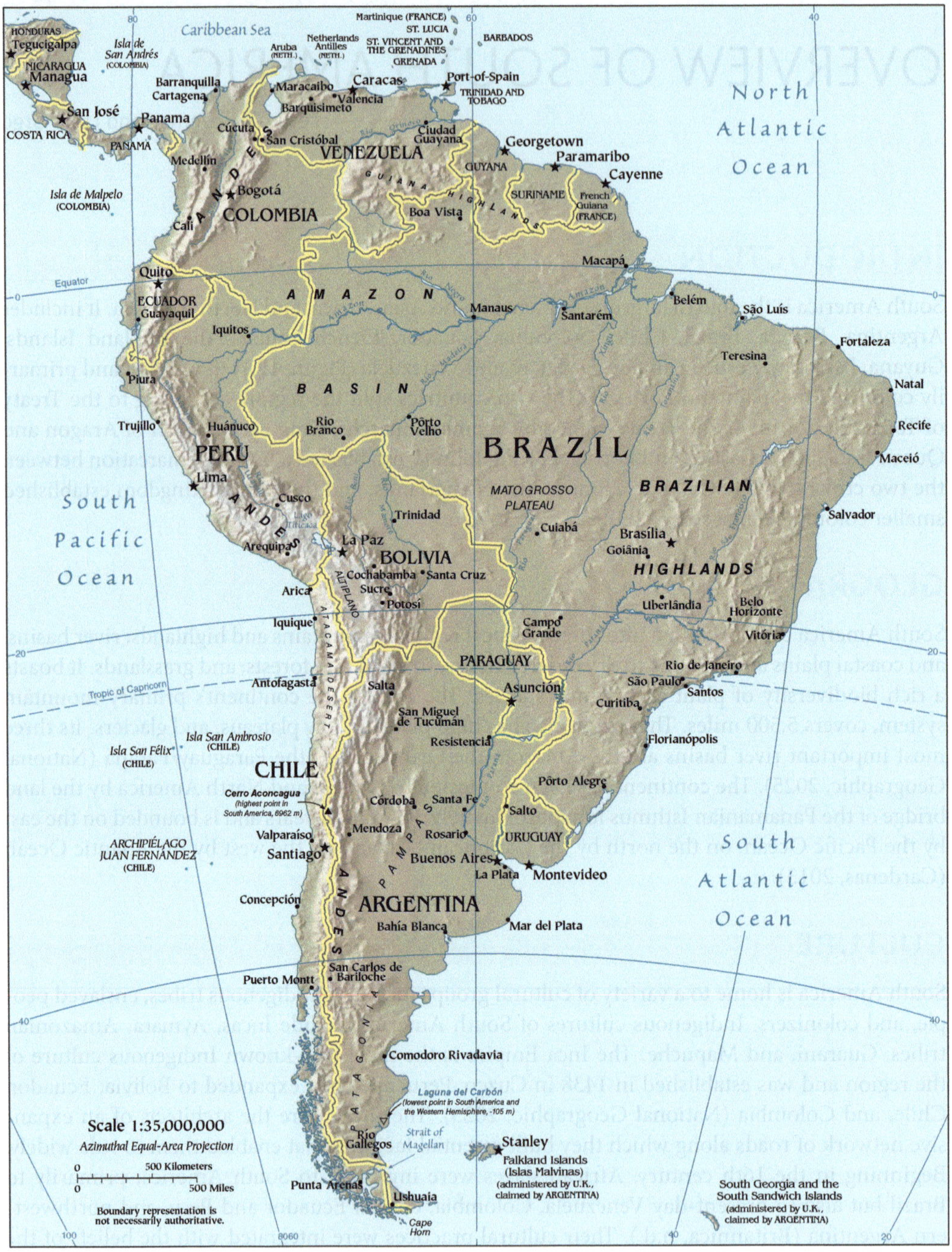

Source: Flores, P. (2006). *Map of South America*. https://en.wikipedia.org/wiki/File:Map_of_South_America.jpg

The majority of South Americans speak Portuguese and Spanish due to a long history of colonization; however, South America has more language families and languages than either North or Central America. Data show that there are 448 languages in South America, compared to 220 in North America and 273 in Central America. The most widely spoken native language of South America is Quechua, followed by Guarani (Tomedes, 2025). Quechua is spoken in Peru, Ecuador, and Bolivia, extending north into Colombia and extending south into northern Chile and northwestern Argentina (Blake, 2006).

There are more than 433 million people living in South America, and Brazil is one of the most populous countries in the world. In 2023, the population of Brazil was approximately 211.14 million people, accounting for nearly 50% of the South American population. To put this in perspective, Guyana, Suriname, French Guiana, and the Falkland Islands accounted for less than 1% of South America's population in 2023. There were fewer than 4,000 people living on the Falkland Islands during 2023 (UN Data Portal, n.d.).

SOCIOECONOMIC FACTORS

Poverty is a significant challenge across South America, where 86% of the population lives in urban areas. While rural poverty rates are higher, the number of urban poor is increasing at a faster rate (UN Development Programme, 2024). Accordingly, social inequality plagues the region, exacerbated by the COVID-19 pandemic. The disparity between rich and poor grew significantly between 2019 and 2022. Brazil, for example, the continent's largest country, "ranks among the 10 most unequal countries in the world: the richest 10% of its population earn more than 10 times the minimum wage and concentrate 59% of the total national income, while more than half of the population collectively earn about 10% of total national income." This inequality is often reflected in health services access disparities (Faria et al., 2023).

HEATH OUTCOMES

Life expectancy at birth continues to improve in South America, driven by the steady reduction in mortality at all ages, particularly reductions in infant and child mortality. Life expectancy at birth in South America was 76.21 years in 2023, which was greater than global life expectancy (73.17 years). The South American infant mortality rate in 2023, which was 12.3 infant deaths per 1,000 live births, was substantially lower than the global infant mortality rate, which was 27.3 infant deaths per 1,000 live births (UN Data Portal, n.d.). The South American maternal mortality ratio in 2020, which was 86.5 maternal deaths per 100,000 live births, was also substantially lower than the global ratio, which was 223.5 maternal deaths per 100,000 live births (UN Population Fund, n.d.). Interregion health disparities exist, however. Chile had the highest life expectancy at birth (81.17 years) and lowest infant mortality rate (4.1 infant deaths per 1,000 live births) in South America during 2023. Bolivia, on the other hand, had the lowest life expectancy at birth (65.58 years) and highest infant mortality rate (31.8 infant deaths per 1,000 live births) in South America during 2023 (UN Data Portal, n.d.).

Noncommunicable diseases cause the most mortality in South America, in particular, cardiovascular diseases, such as ischemic heart disease and stroke, which are the leading causes of mortality. While noncommunicable diseases are the primary leading causes of mortality in South America, it is important to note the deadly impact of the COVID-19 pandemic on South American countries. In 2021, COVID-19 was the leading cause of death in every South American country (Institute for Health Metrics and Evaluation [IHME], n.d.). In addition, youth and the older population across South America are suffer consequences from frequent and intense heatwaves. For example, heat-related deaths of people over the age of 65 have increased since the start of the 21st century (Hartinger et al., 2023). Refer to Table 12.1 for key South American health outcome data.

TABLE 12.1 HEALTH OUTCOMES IN SOUTH AMERICA

REGION/ COUNTRY	LIFE EXPECTANCY AT BIRTH (2023)	INFANT MORTALITY (2023)	MATERNAL MORTALITY (2020)	LEADING CAUSES OF MORTALITY (2021)
South America	76.21	12.3	86.5	COVID-19 and heart disease
Argentina	77.39	9.0	44.9	COVID-19 and heart disease
Bolivia	68.58	31.8	160.9	COVID-19 and heart disease
Brazil	75.85	12.1	72.1	COVID-19 and heart disease
Chile	81.17	4.1	15.0	COVID-19 and heart disease
Colombia	77.72	9.8	74.8	COVID-19 and heart disease
Ecuador	77.39	9.6	65.7	COVID-19 and heart disease
Falkland Islands	79.21	9.2	n/a	n/a
French Guiana	76.98	8.9	n/a	n/a
Guyana	70.18	21.3	111.1	COVID-19 and heart disease
Paraguay	7.84	14.0	71.1	COVID-19 and heart disease
Peru	77.74	11.7	68.5	COVID-19 and heart disease
Suriname	73.63	14.1	96.5	COVID-19 and heart disease
Uruguay	78.14	5.6	18.6	COVID-19 and heart disease
Venezuela	72.51	15.7	259.2	COVID-19 and heart disease

Sources: Institute for Health Metrics and Evaluation. (n.d). *Health research by location*. https://www.healthdata.org/research-analysis/health-by-location/profiles; UN Data Portal. (n.d). *UN population division data portal*. https://population.un.org/dataportal/home; UN Population Fund. (n.d.). *Data portal*. https://www.unfpa.org/data

LEARNING ACTIVITIES

CourseConnect

To access self-assessment questions and interactive, competency-based learning activities for this chapter, visit www.springerpub.com/courseconnect. See inside front cover and tear-out for CourseConnect details.

REFERENCES

Blake, J. (2006). Classification of languages. In K. Brown (Ed.), *Encyclopedia of languages and linguistics* (2nd ed.). Elsevier, Ltd.

Britannica. (n.d.). *South America.* https://www.britannica.com/place/South-America

Cardenas, L. (2013). Ecosystems of South America. In S. Levin (Ed.), *Encyclopedia of biodiversity* (2nd ed.). Academic Press.

Connect Brazil. (2025). *The history of Japanese in Brazil.* https://www.connectbrazil.com/the-history-of-japanese-in-brazil/

Faria, L., Alvarez, R., & Santos, L. (2023). *Socioeconomic inequality in Latin America and the Caribbean: The post-pandemic future for the training of health professionals.* História Ciências Saúde: Manguinhos. https://doi.org/10.1590/S0104-59702023000100029

Finlayson, C. (2025). *The South American colonial landscape.* LibreTexts. https://socialsci.libretexts.org/Bookshelves/Geography_(Human)/World_Regional_Geography_(Finlayson)/05%3A_Middle_and_South_America/5.03%3A_The_South_American_Colonial_Landscape

Hartinger, S., Yglesias-González, M., Blanco-Villafuerte, L., Palmeiro-Silva, Y., Lescano, A., Stewart-Ibarra, A., Rojas-Rueda, D., Melo, O., Takahashi, B., Buss, D., Callaghan, M., Chesini, F., Flores, E., Posse, C., Gouveia, N., Jankin, S., Miranda-Chacon, Z., Mohajeri, N., Helo, J., . . . Romanello, M. (2023). The 2022 South America report of The *Lancet* Countdown on health and climate change: trust the science. Now that we know, we must act. *The Lancet, 20*, 1–35, https://www.thelancet.com/action/showPdf?pii=S2667-193X%2823%2900044-3

Institute for Health Metrics and Evaluation. (n.d.). *Health research by location.* https://www.healthdata.org/research-analysis/health-by-location/profiles

National Geographic. (2025). *South America: Physical geography.* https://education.nationalgeographic.org/resource/south-america-physical-geography

Tomedes. (2025). *Languages of South America: The most spoken and Indigenous South American languages.* https://www.tomedes.com/translator-hub/languages-south-america

UN Data Portal. (n.d.). *UN population divisions data portal.* https://population.un.org/dataportal/home/

UN Development Programme. (2024). *The changing faces of poverty in Latin America and the Caribbean.* https://www.undp.org/latin-america/blog/changing-faces-poverty-latin-america-and-caribbean

UNESCO. (n.d.). *Treaty of Tordesilla.* https://www.unesco.org/en/memory-world/treaty-tordesillas

UN Population Fund. (n.d.). *Data portal.* https://www.unfpa.org/data

CHAPTER 13

ARGENTINA

Pablo Rodríguez del Pozo and Jorge Colina

INTRODUCTION

Argentina's vast extension, diverse climate, and varied orography pose a complex, heterogeneous epidemiologic landscape. While epidemiologic heterogeneity complicates healthcare and treatment, it is not Argentina's most problematic source of health determinants or healthcare troubles. Argentina's multiple healthcare systems constitute an overlapping and ultimately inefficient coverage that encompasses everything from provincial and federal free-for-all public hospitals to mandatory health plans owned by single-union workers guilds, private health plans, or a national healthcare institute for the retired. Such disorder has cultivated inefficiency and a lack of effectiveness, leading to a complete dilution of responsibility amongsystems and their administrators. All of this has left the Argentine population, particularly the poor, underserved and defenseless.

GEOGRAPHY AND POPULATION

GEOGRAPHICAL FEATURES

Spanning 2.8 million square kilometers (1.1 million square miles; World Bank Group, 2023a), Argentina is the eighth largest country in the world, extending from above the Tropic of Capricorn in the north to the Tierra del Fuego in the south, and from the Andes Mountains in the west to the Atlantic Ocean in the east. The territory, federally organized into 24 provinces, hosts nearly all climates and ecosystems: from tropical to frigid, from desertic to bountiful, from the tallest mountain in the Western hemisphere, to extensive flatlands (the pampas) and everglades. It houses the sultry jungles of its own Mesopotamia, and large portion of the bone-dry Atacama Desert. The Argentinean Sea consists of approximately 1.1 million square kilometers (684,000 square miles) of Atlantic Ocean, and a number of inhospitable former whale-hunting South Atlantic islands as well as the Malvinas/Falkland Island group, which are still disputed by the United Kingdom.

DEMOGRAPHIC FEATURES

Distribution

Although Argentina is roughly the size of India, its population of 46.7 million people represents just a 30th of the Asian giant's, placing Argentina among the 30 least densely populated countries in the world. With a scant 17 inhabitants per square kilometer, its population density is significantly lower than that of its neighbors, Chile (26 inhabitants per square kilometer), and Uruguay (20 inhabitants per square kilometer).

However, these aggregate data of the country's population density conceal a unique feature of Argentinian demographics: 90% of the population is concentrated in urban areas, mostly in the metropolitan area of Buenos Aires (AMBA [*Área Metropolitana de Buenos Aires*]), which houses roughly 32% of the population. The next largest urban conglomerates, Córdoba and Rosario, represent 3% of the country's population each. Outside of these massive urban centers other disparities arise; for example, Patagonia, in the country's southern region, has a density of two inhabitants per square kilometer, while that of the country's northern region is nine inhabitants per square kilometer (0.6 square miles). Those living in small towns with less than 2,000 inhabitants or in rural areas represent a mere 10% of the country's demographic statistics.

Thus, Argentina has large, nearly empty swatches of land as well as many isolated populations. These populations are too small for healthcare facilities and expensive, advanced medical technologies which require large population pools to be economically viable. This population distribution gives way to enormous disparities in terms of access to healthcare, while forcing rising costs and tremendous inefficiencies.

Racial and Ethnic Groups

Whether the Argentinian melting pot is a 19th century narrative—which arose as a much-needed shared history for a young nation of European immigrants whose population was booming (experiencing a tenfold increase; del Pozo, 2002), or myth manufactured by the dominant elites aimed at imposing social discipline over the *criollo* population (those of European descent born in the Americas; Golay, 2013)—it is undeniable that Argentina has a considerably mixed and diverse population.

Racial and ethnic tensions seem to be nonsystemic, but rather dispersed in microtensions and microdiscriminations, mostly toward new immigrants from neighboring Bolivia and Paraguay. We hypothesize that the melting pot notion may play a normative role in the way Argentinians conduct their social relationships and understand their courtship or marital prospects.

The Black population of African descent is proportionally small as integration likely began in 1813, after the abolition of at-birth slavery (called freedom of wombs) which was then expanded to complete abolition by the Constitution of 1853 (Candioti, 2016).

Such relatively narrow racial diversity (though diverse socioculturally, most Argentinians identify as of European descent) may explain the absence of screening programs aimed at ethnicity-specific epidemiology. Nearly all the population is Spanish speaking, with some areas adjacent to Paraguay also speaking the Guaraní language, mostly at home. There are no co-official languages.

Age

Argentina is no exception to the world's demographic transition (Institute for Health Metrics and Evaluation, 2024). Fertility rates have gone from 3.4 in 1977 to 1.9 in 2021 (World Bank Group, 2023b), while life expectancy has increased from 68 to 77 years over the same period. However, there are considerable regional disparities likely linked to the median income level of the different jurisdictions. The province of Misiones with a per-capita gross domestic product (GDP) of $4,000, has a natality rate of 16 deaths per thousand, while the wealthy City of Buenos Aires, with a per-capita GDP of $26,000, has a natality rate of just above nine deaths per thousand. These kinds of income-related regional inequalities are highlighted throughout in this chapter.

Moreover, the Argentine population is aging, with median age increasing from 26 years in 1977, to above 32 years in 2022 (Instituto Nacional de Estadística y Censos [INDEC], 2023). The 2022 population pyramids (Figure 13.1) represent Argentina's demographic transition: from moderate growth to stability with signs of regression. The male/female ratio is the statistical standard. Since 2012, the law allows the choice of gender on one's obligatory national identity document (DNI). Those who have opted for a gender not assigned at birth number 26 per 100,000 people (0.03% of the population; Registro Nacional de las Personas, 2022).

Argentina is a demographically uneven country. While some regions reflect an aging society, such as the City of Buenos Aires and other urban conglomerates, other regions show profiles closer to relatively young societies. The comparison between urban and rural areas can be seen in the differences between the demographic statistics of Buenos Aires, Tierra del Fuego, and Misiones. In Buenos Aires, those age between 0 and 14 years represent 15% of the population, while those over 65 represent 18%. In the wealthy southern region of Tierra del Fuego, those age 0 to 14 represent 23% of the population and those 65 and older a mere 7%. In the poor Misiones province, the figures are 27% and 8%, respectively (Argentina, Secretaría de Niñez, Adolescencia y Familia, 2021). These heterogeneous demographics are yet another cause of health disparities (INDEC, 2023).

FIGURE 13.1 Argentina's population pyramids.

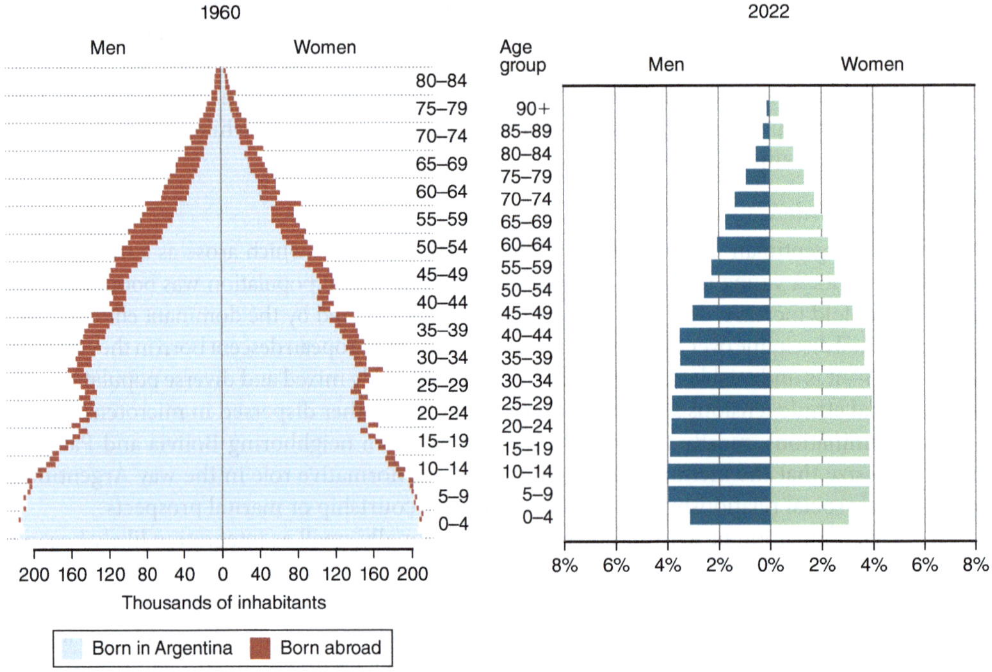

Source: National Institute of Statistics and Censuses. (n.d.). *National census 1960 and 2022*. https://www.indec.gob.ar/indec/web/Nivel3-Tema-2-41

Migrations

Internal rural-to-urban migrations have generally been the norm in Argentina, particularly in the first half of the 20th century. Most of these migrations were absorbed by the AMBA, contributing to the country's tremendously unbalanced population distribution. However, such migratory movements seem to have shifted in the last decades, with the bulk of internal movements being among urban areas. For example, the southern provinces of Patagonia and Tierra del Fuego are absorbing the exodus that is leaving the AMBA at a steady pace (Basso, 2023). At the same time Argentina is still attracting immigrants, mostly from neighboring impoverished populations in the Southern Cone, while decades of poor public policies are leading Argentinians to emigrate in large numbers. The immigration flux was 2,281,728 in 2020, a considerable number compared to 1,649,919 in 1990. Meanwhile, emigration was 1,076,148 in 2020, a populational bloodletting compared to the meager 430,155 emigrants in 1990 (United Nations, 2024). The National Census carried out in 2022 estimated that 4% of the population was born in a foreign country, a sharp contrast to the same figure in 1914 (30%) and 1947 (15%), showing that Argentina has stopped being a migrant-fed population.

HISTORY AND CULTURE

HISTORICAL CONSIDERATIONS

Being far from the main centers of Indigenous culture (Mexico, Central America, and Peru), Spanish colonization arrived comparatively late to Argentina (Ribeiro, 1972). Between the 16th and 18th centuries a strong Spanish colonizing population coexisted with a *mestizo* (mixed) population that would come to characterize the Argentine population. At the beginning of the 19th century, a desire for independence sparked the Argentine War of Independence with Spain (Donghi, 1972). Argentine victory ended the Spanish colonial period in 1820 but immediately triggered a fratricidal civil war between local *caudillos* (political or military leaders) in the provinces, which would eventually consolidate into the Argentine Republic in 1862 (Bethel, 1993).

Between 1862 and 1930, the new Argentine Republic entered the booming world economy of the second part of the 19th century and the beginning of the 20th century. During this time period, Argentina received substantial investments in its infrastructure from Great Britain, primarily for exploitation of its beef production and fertile plains (the humid pampas). From 1880 onward, Argentina began to receive a massive wave of immigration from Europe, which meant that by the beginning of the 20th century Argentina had a much more Europeanized racial demographic than the rest of Latin America (Bethel, 1993).

Between 1930 and 1943, the country underwent an abrupt and profound change. The Great Crisis of 1930 brought world trade to a halt, forcing the country to promote its incipient import substitution industrialization and replacing imports of consumer goods with domestic production (Prebish, 1948). At the political level, an influential number of military officers, explicit sympathizers of Italian and German fascism, banded together to oppose the traditional British influence in the military (Potash, 1971). This was thus a decade of a weakened democracy under pressure from two distinct factions of the armed forces—the pro-British and the pro-Germanicin constant tension and confrontation (Potash, 1971). At the same time, European immigration stopped. The fall of international commerce based on rural goods drove a massive internal immigration from the countryside to the city. This, combined with the attractiveness of internal urban industrialization, provoked a great concentration of the population in the metropolitan region.

In 1943, a coup d'état took place, giving way to the political emergence of Juan Domingo Perón, who, as the Secretary of Labor, began an active policy of labor regulations and rights to meet the needs of the massive concentration of workers that resulted from the collapse of international trade and the new industrialization (Page, 1998). In 1945 Perón was elected president; while the world returned to an intense international trade during the postwar period, Perón adamantly imposed a closed economic model. Perón organized a corporatist political model of greater industrial development focused on the domestic market and based on a heavy military industry (Mallon & Sourrouille, 1973), all with the aim of furthering Argentine development.

Between 1945 and 1983, Argentina was plunged into a chaos of political proscriptions. Coups d'états, political violence, and urban civil war marked the country until the recovery of a solid democracy in 1983, which it has maintained since then. However, it has not been able to dismantle the corporatist political model in place since 1943, which still coexists in conflict with the democratic institutions created in 1983. This may be one of the reasons why democracy could not translate into economic and social progress, leaving the country economically stagnant with increasing social deterioration and growing poverty.

RELIGIONS

According to a household survey held in 2019, 63% of the Argentine population identify as Catholic, 20% as atheist, 15% as Evangelist, and 2% as other religions. More women tended to be believers (15% stated they had no religion) while fewer men were (23% stated no religion). The tendency is toward more nonbelievers, since among those under 30 years old only half identified themselves as Catholic, and one quarter as nonbelievers (Conicet, 2020).

POLITICAL SYSTEM

Originally a loose league of autonomous provinces that had assigned the common defense to the province of Buenos Aires, Argentina became a federal republic in 1861. Modeled on U.S.

presidentialism, the republic is a classic liberal democracy in which the provinces retain every competence that has not been explicitly entrusted to the federal government. The provinces refer the sanction of the civil, commercial, and criminal codes to the federal government, as well as labor, mining, oil, and gas legislation. Health, primary education, and direct taxes, belong to the provinces by the Constitution of the Argentine Republic. However, a number of postconstitutional federal initiatives, together with agreements between the federal government and the provinces, have transitorily reverted some of those responsibilities onto the federal level, the main example being the federal collection of direct taxes, such as individual and company income tax. The federal government, besides exercising coordination among provinces on public health matters, has erected and funded numerous focused, disease-specific programs in each province. The tax system incentivizes the provincial jurisdictions to spend liberally, without being perceived as the tax collectors. This is because the national government (we use federal and national government as nearly interchangeable terms) imposed high value-added tax (VAT) and other indirect taxes, such as on fuel and energy, Social Security and other payroll taxes, sumptuary goods, or the high tax on personal and business income.

In healthcare matters, ambiguities in delimiting competencies between national and provincial jurisdictions, combined with the inadequate incentives stemming from the taxation model, result in numerous duplications of provincial and federal efforts, overlapping responsibilities, contradictions, and generalized inefficiency. This lack of clear jurisdictional accountability—whether federal or provincial—further exacerbates issues (Colina et al., 2004).

HEALTH OUTCOMES

Argentina has the health standards that can be expected for a mid- to low-income country. Virtually every health indicator is riddled with inequalities directly linked to the income levels of the population, often independent of the health insurance status of the individuals.

INFANT AND MATERNAL MORTALITY

A maternal mortality ratio of four to five per 10,000 live births has been quite stable in Argentina the last 20 years. Regrettably, this number is quite far from U.S. figures, which are consistently in the vicinity of two per 10,000 in the same period. The dispersion is quite significative among jurisdictions, though. San Luis, a mid-income province, showed 1.7 per 10,000 in 2020, while poor Northern Chaco had 9.2, and the wealthy City of Buenos Aires 4.3. We speculate, however, that some of the differences among provinces might be due to inconsistent registration methods. Statistics on mortality due to abortion are unreliable and still in their early stages in Argentina, where abortion was only legalized toward the end of 2020. Until then, underreporting was probably the norm.

The infant mortality rate is eight per 1,000 with a declining trend. However, in the northern provinces of the country, where low-income populations prevail, infant mortality rates are still in the double digits.

LIFE EXPECTANCY AND CAUSES OF DEATH

As mentioned, life expectancy at birth has increased in Argentina from 68 to 77 years between 1977 and 2021, predictably being 80 years for women and 74 years for men. These numbers vary from jurisdiction to jurisdiction, depending on income and demographic profiles. In the poor provinces of Chaco and Formosa in the north, life expectancy at birth is between 73 and 74 years, while in the wealthy City of Buenos Aires, or the oil-and-gas-rich provinces of Neuquén and Tierra del Fuego, it is above 77 years (Ministry of Health [MoH], 2023). The main causes of death in Argentina per 100,000 are cardiovascular disease (233 persons), tumors (136.1 persons), infections (110.5 persons), and accidents, homicides, and suicides (37.5 persons).

The distribution of these causes of death appears to follow a predictable provincial pattern, seemingly linked to income and climate. In the wealthier and cold southern provinces, such as Santa Cruz, Neuquén, and Tierra del Fuego, infectious diseases are the least prevalent. Meanwhile they prevail in the tropical, poorer provinces of Jujuy, Chaco, Formosa, and the great urban conglomerates, where cardiovascular disease is also the dominant cause of death. The distribution of tumoral disease as the cause of death seems to correlate with urban areas with comparatively aged population, such as the City of Buenos Aires, which tops the list (MoH, 2023).

Noncommunicable diseases account for 77% of mortality in Argentina, a number which leaves significant room for improvement as it demonstrates that communicable disease and accidents take a high proportion of Argentinean lives. Neighboring Chile and Uruguay's figures are a more hopeful 85% and 86% respectively, though still far from developed Germany and Spain's at 91% each (World Health Organization, 2022). It is worth noting that between 1997 and 2019, noncommunicable diseases have seen a slight but constant decline as cause of death. According to the Argentinean MoH, the reduction has been 3 percentage points, never surpassing the 1997 figure (MoH, 2023). These findings may indicate a concerning regression in Argentina's mortality profile toward that of less developed countries.

The number of deaths from cancer should also raise concerns. Lung cancer takes the most lives, representing 14.6% of all forms of mortal cancer. Colon cancer is a narrow second at 12.4%, followed by prostate cancer at 12.0%, breast cancer at 9.9%, and cervical cancer at 7.3%. It is unfortunate that these types of cancer, which are either curbed by reducing cigarette smoking (lung) or controllable by systematic screening (colon), top the list of mortal tumors. Argentina has significant room for a simple and cost-effective improvement in this matter (Instituto Nacional del Cáncer [Cancer National Institute], 2021).

MENTAL HEALTH

Anxiety and/or depression is reported by 18.4% of the population. This percentage rises to 22.3% among those in the lowest income quintile and drops to 15.7% among those in the highest income quintile. This trend is confirmed if education level is considered: Adults with less than secondary education are more likely to suffer from anxiety and/or depression (20.5% of cases) while the same figure drops to 16.9 in adults with secondary education or higher (INDEC, 2018).

The main causes of death are noncommunicable diseases, with lower respiratory infection being the only communicable disease among the 10 most prevalent causes, as shown in Table 13.1.

DETERMINANTS OF HEALTH

SOCIAL AND ECONOMIC FACTORS

Argentina's human development index (HDI) peaked during most of the 20th century, during which it was second only to the United States and Canada. In 1992 the United States had an HDI of 0.875 and Canada of 0.861, while Argentina stood at 0.724, closely followed by Chile and Uruguay in the region. However, while most developing countries have kept improving quite steadily, Argentina has stagnated at an HDI of 0.842 since 2012, eventually being overtaken by Chile in 2016 (UN Development Programme, 2022). We feel this reflects quite accurately the history of Argentina in the last four or five decades: The GDP per capita, which reached $10,000 in 2010, for example, has remained basically unchanged since 2021 (World Bank Group, 2023c). In the last few decades, the country has stalled economically in a never-ending downhill path of

TABLE 13.1 TOP 10 CAUSES OF DEATH IN ARGENTINA, 2019

2019 RANK	CAUSE	TYPE OF DISEASE
1	Ischemic heart disease	Noncommunicable
2	Lower respiratory infection	Communicable, maternal, neaonatal, and nutritional
3	Stroke	Noncommunicable
4	Chronic obstructive pulmonary disease (COPD)	Noncommunicable
5	Chronic kidney disease	Noncommunicable
6	Lung cancer	Noncommunicable
7	Colorectal cancer	Noncommunicable
8	Alzheimer disease	Noncommunicable
9	Diabetes	Noncommunicable
10	Cirrhosis of the liver	Noncommunicable

stagflation (Colina, 2021). Poverty rates, which were just 5% in 1974, have grown to 40% in 2023, reaching peaks of 47% in 1989 because of hyperinflation and 54% in 2002 because of hyperrecession. The total GDP has grown a mere 1% yearly between 2010 and 2021. Recurrent if not continuous crises seem to be the only stable feature of Argentina's economy.

This meager economic state translates into stagnant if not declining rates of basic and higher secondary education (UN Educational, Scientific, and Cultural Organization [UNESCO], 2024). Argentina middles the global table on the 2022 results of the Programme for International Student Assessment (PISA) tests. However, a closer look reveals a grim picture: Of all Argentine students, 77% score at a low level in math, with 55% and 54% scoring low in reading and science, respectively. These figures are significantly worse than the global averages of 31% in math, 26% in reading, and 24% in science (Organisation for Economic Co-operation and Development, 2022). The Argentinean unemployment rate seems quite stable, at approximately 7% of the economically active population. However, actual unemployment is masked by the fact that public employment acts as de facto, permanent unemployment insurance, rife informal employment.

HEALTH BEHAVIORS

Tobacco smoking in Argentina is lower than in the United States and most European countries. Only 22.2% of Argentinians smoke, against 24.3% of Americans in the former and around 30% of Europeans. There is not much difference between genders when it comes to smoking rates, similarly to Europe. Intriguingly the wealthiest districts, save the City of Buenos Aires, host the heaviest smokers: Tierra del Fuego with 24.9%, Santa Cruz with 27%, and oil-rich Neuquén and Chubut with 22% and 23%, respectively. The world trend is known to be the opposite. Cigarettes seem to be widely available in Argentina: almost half of the adult population, independent of their socio-economic level, has been to a store where tobacco is available (INDEC, 2018; United Nations, 2024). Alcohol consumption is lower than the average for industrialized countries. Heavy episodic drinking in the previous 30 days is 13.3% among the 18+, which is cause for concern.

The country is not exempt from the worldwide overweight, obesity and metabolic syndrome triad epidemics. Thirty-six percent of Argentinians self-reported being overweight, with a 25.5% total obesity rate. Predictably, while self-reported obesity affected 21.6% of those who completed secondary school and above, it climbed to 33.4% among those without full primary studies (INDEC, 2018). These are high prevalence figures. More worrisome, though, is that when obesity is determined by objective anthropometric measurements, the rate skyrockets to 45.9% among those with no primary studies. The rates of hyperglycemia follow these trends, with a total prevalence of 12.7% among the total population, but with 22.9% among those with no primary schooling, and a much healthier 10.3% within those who have secondary studies and above.

ARGENTINA'S HEALTHCARE MODEL

Argentina's healthcare model is one of redundancy, duplications, and overspending. Made with little forethought, this model arises as a natural consequence of the superposition of various independently developed provincial and federal efforts, and not the need for private services that address the desperation of patients and families. While some inefficiencies are an inevitable consequence of the country's territorial or populational challenges, the majority of these inefficiencies come from the absence of an individual-centered, consistent, synergic, country-wide model.

FINANCING

Argentina allocates approximately 10% of the country's GDP to fund their different healthcare systems. Resources come principally from three sources. The first is the provincial states, which fund 2% of national GDP with their general revenue budgets. The federal government contributes through several small programs that help provincial health systems, consisting of small subsidies, amounting to only 0.24% of the national GDP.

Payroll taxes are the second source of funding. Federal employees and those employed in private companies contribute 14% of their salaries to the national social security system. Provincial government employees, in turn, pay a similar percentage to their respective provincial social security systems. Lower-income, self-employed, and domestic workers make a smaller contribution to the national system. Pensioners contribute 6% of their retirement to finance their respective federal or provincial social security. Social security for healthcare represents 4% of the GDP.

The third source of healthcare funding in Argentina comes from underserved individuals who resort to out-of-pocket spending in private health insurance and direct payments to healthcare providers. Direct payment refers to copayments and often, fine print clauses. This source contributes yet another estimated 4% of the GDP, of which only 0.6% goes to private insurance while the remaining 3.4% are direct payments for healthcare products and services.

COVERAGE

Being a federal country, the bulk of Argentina's public healthcare system is in the hands of the provincial states. The provincial public systems are universal and have free access and very limited copayments. These systems are not organized as insurances but rather consist of an infrastructure of public hospitals and outpatient healthcare centers. These centers should provide services for 100% of the population in each jurisdiction, similar to a Beveridge funding model of the healthcare system in which healthcare facilities are owned and financed by the provincial governments. In a way, the provincial model has parallels to the public systems of Canada and Spain.

Social security at large covers 30 million inhabitants, of which 23 million are covered by the national system and 7 million are covered by the various provincial social security systems. Within the national social security system, roughly half of those covered are private or public salaried workers and their families. Three million are low-income, self-employed, or domestic workers, and 6 million are pensioners. Argentine social security healthcare systems resemble the Bismark's Krankenkassen model, which in broad strokes is a mandatory enrollment in an assigned state or union-run health insurer which is in turn financed by payroll taxes on companies and workers.

Private health insurance covers some 2 million people who pay out-of-pocket, while another 4 million are high salaried workers who are allowed to redirect their payroll tax to selected private health insurers, thus totaling 6 million lives on private health insurance.

As for the provision of services, provincial public healthcare systems and social security are not obligated to disclose their comprehensive healthcare package. However, it is generally understood that services should be as expansive as the available resources allow. The national social security system and private health insurance providers, in contrast, must provide an extensive medical program determined by law and regulations. This program includes services such as acute and chronic care; social benefits for disability, addictions; and mental health; in vitro fertilization; unlimited psychoanalysis sessions; and more with few limitations. Too often this prodigal spectrum of coverage exceeds the available resources and any actuarial calculation, not to mention any evaluation on medical need or effectiveness.

INSURANCE

The national social security systems operate through insurance entities (called *obras sociales*), akin to workers' mutual aid funds. They are like traditional German sickness funds and are owned by law by the trade unions. In Argentina each trade is represented by one single union, which bargains on behalf of all workers in each given trade, profession, or occupation. Collective bargaining is therefore highly concentrated. This model was established by Perón in the 1950s who was inspired by the Italian–Germanic system and remains in place today. Membership in the single union is compulsory, as well as a worker's affiliation to an obra social, which by default is the one owned by their single union. In theory however, the individual worker has the right to change to an obra social run by a different union, though collusion often prevents this. Salary discrepancies among different unions depending on their trades, leads to a great deal of financial inequality among obras sociales. Obras sociales owned by high-paying trades can afford generous packages that are out of reach for low-income trades, as they all depend on a flat 14% of their workers' salaries.

Provincial social security and national pensioner programs are state run and not managed by the unions. Private health insurance entities, known as *prepagas* (prepaid health plans), are comparable to the American health maintenance organizations (HMOs). Prepagas are privately run insurers that offer a variety of managed-care health plans, in which price and coverage are freely agreed upon by companies and users.

PROVIDERS

There are an estimated 200,000 practicing physicians in the country, which represents 4.3 physicians per 1,000 inhabitants. The number of nurses is similar, which reflects a severe lack of nursing personnel. Both physicians and nurses can work in the provincial public sector, social security, and private providers simultaneously. In fact, multiemployment in the health sector is one of the highest in the labor market.

Public systems have small outpatient centers of very low medical complexity. Outpatient and inpatient care is mainly provided by public hospitals (Sistema Integrado de Información Sanitaria Argentino [SISA], 2023).

There are 1,500 public hospitals with 80,000 beds, meaning there are 53 beds per hospital. This provider atomization is indicative of a dispersed population, in which each hospital tends to a small number of people on average. Social security has no more than 30 inpatient hospitals of its own. It therefore contracts services from private hospitals, clinics, or doctors. These private providers consist of 17,000 outpatient diagnostic and treatment centers and 3,800 private hospitals with 80,000 beds, with an average size of only 20 beds per hospital (SISA, 2023). Although the average available beds are low, there are 100 private hospitals with more than 100 beds; as in the public sector, this represents unavoidable inefficiencies due to

Argentina's populational dispersion. Practically all private hospitals are for-profit (ADECRA, 2005).

FUNCTIONING

The Argentinian healthcare system has tremendous dysfunctionalities which result in an inefficient, overlapping mosaic of heterogeneous entities combining Beveridge-type public systems, Bismarck-type social security entities, and American HMO-style prepagas. Every single Argentinian is covered by the provincial public healthcare system; if they work for a private company, they are also covered by social security (a dual coverage experienced by 30 million people), while still being entitled to the public services in their province. Finally, if unattended by their other two coverages, they opt for (if they can afford) a private insurance—as is the case for 2 million people—they end up with triple coverage, as they retain their right to both the public and social security systems. These overlaps create unique and wasteful inefficiencies in Argentina's healthcare provision.

For the national social security and private insurance entities, coverage is profligately defined by laws of the Congress, who provide no funding. As national social security legally entitles those covered to such extensive benefit packages that both low income *obras sociales* and privately contracting families often struggle to afford the mandatory package or the policies to buy it. There is no effective mechanism in place to balance financial availability between high and low-income *obras sociales*, nor for high- and low-income families. Consequently, many families are restricted bureaucratically or financially from healthcare services and must consequently shop around public hospitals in search of treatments. Despite being one of the countries that spends the most on medicine in terms of GDP, Argentina is the country in South America with the highest incidence of deaths due to side effects of medical treatment (Healthcare Access and Quality Collaborators, 2017; Reddy, 2016).

CONCLUSION

Argentina's healthcare model is expensive, inefficient and fragmented. Despite having hotspots of exceptional medical treatment, wastefulness plagues the country's healthcare spending. A significant overhaul or restructuring of the model has long been needed. Argentinian geography and population dispersion would present a challenge to any healthcare system, however, deeper issues of mismanagement and a departure from an individual-centered design are the true culprits of the system failure. As is always the case in pervasive inefficiencies, some stand to benefit from disorganization. Healthcare in Argentina is a free-for-all battleground in which no stakeholder is willing to renounce their slice of the inefficiency, while at the same time wants the popularity that comes with healthcare promises, leaving a landscape of half-measures in which nobody wins, and taxpayers lose the most.

LEARNING ACTIVITIES

CourseConnect

To access self-assessment questions and interactive, competency-based learning activities for this chapter, visit www.springerpub.com/courseconnect. See inside front cover and tear-out for CourseConnect details.

REFERENCES

ADECRA. (2005). La crisis de los prestadores institucionales de salud: un aporte a su solución. https://biblioteca.adecra.org.ar/la-crisis-los-prestadores-institucionales-salud-aporte-solucion-abril-2005/

Argentina, Secretaría de Niñez, Adolescencia y Familia. (2021). *Indicadores de niñez y adolescencia.* Aspectos demográficos. Buenos Aires.

Basso, M. (2023). Análisis de las migraciones internas en Argentina en el período 2005-2010. Astrolabio, Córdoba 2023. https://doi.org/10.55441/1668.7515.n30.35108

Bethel, L. (1993). *Argentina since independence.* Cambridge University Press.

Candioti, M. (2016). Abolición gradual y libertades vigiladas en el Río de la Plata. La política de control de libertos de 1813 [Gradual abolition and supervised freedoms in the Río de la Plata. The 1813 policy of control over freedmen]. *Corpus, 6*(1). https://doi.org/10.4000/corpusarchivos.1567

Colina, J., Giordano, O., & Rodríguez del Pozo, P. (2004). *El sistema de salud en la Argentina: Diagnósticos y propuestas* [The healthcare system in Argentina: diagnoses and proposals]. Fundación Arcor, Buenos Aires.

Colina, J. (2021). *Informe N°: 03/11/2021. Idesa, Buenos Aires, 2021.* https://idesa.org/mas-que-andar-conversando-con-el-fmi-hay-que-disenar-un-ordenamiento-integral-del-estado/

Conicet. (2020). *Encuesta nacional sobre creencias y actitudes religiosas en Argentina* [National survey on religious beliefs and attitudes in Argentina]. https://www.conicet.gov.ar/wp-content/uploads/Infografi%CC%81a-Encuesta-Religi%C3%B3n-1.pdf

del Pozo, J. (2002). *Historia de América Latina y del Caribe (1825–2001)* [History of Latin America and the Caribbean (1825-2001)]. Lom Ediciones.

Donghi, T. H. (1972). *Revolución y guerra: formación de una élite dirigente en la Argentina criolla* [Revolution and war: Formation of a ruling elite in Creole Argentina]. Editorial Siglo XXI.

Golay, I. (2013). *Argentina 'crisol de razas': Ficción y realidad* [Argentina, melting pot of races: Fiction and reality]. VII Jornadas de Jóvenes. https://www.aacademica.org/000-076/5

Healthcare Access and Quality Collaborators. (2017). Healthcare access and auality index based on mortality from causes amenable to personal health care in 195 countries and territories, 1990–2015. *Lancet, 390,* 231–266. http://doi.org/10.1016/S0140-6736(17)30818-8

Institute for Health Metrics and Evaluation. (2024). *Health research by location: Argentina.* https://www.healthdata.org/research-analysis/health-by-location/profiles

Instituto Nacional de Estadísticas y Censos. (2018). *National survey of risks factors.* https://www.indec.gob.ar/indec/web/Nivel4-Tema-4-32-68

Instituto Nacional de Estadísticas y Censos. (2023). *National census, 2022.* https://www.indec.gob.ar/ftp/cuadros/poblacion/censo2022_indicadores_demograficos.pdf

Instituto Nacional del Cáncer. (2021). *Estadísticas - mortalidad* [Statistics - mortality]. https://www.argentina.gob.ar/salud/instituto-nacional-del-cancer/estadisticas/mortalidad

Mallon, R., & Sourrouille, J. (1973). *La política económica en una sociedad sonflictiva* [Economic policy in a conflictive society: The Argentine case]. El Caso Argentino. Amorrortu Editores.

Ministry of Health. (2023). *Indicadores Básicos* [Basic indicators]. https://www.argentina.gob.ar/sites/default/files/indicadores-basicos_2023-web.pdf

Organisation for Economic Co-operation and Development. (2022). *Results: Factsheets - Argentina.* https://www.oecd.org/content/dam/oecd/en/publications/reports/2023/11/pisa-2022-results-volume-i-and-ii-country-notes_2fca04b9/argentina_3054c45c/09c7d993-en.pdf

Page, J. (1998). *Perón.* Editorial Javier Vergara.

Potash, R. (1971). *Ejercito y política en Argentina* [Army and politics in Argentina]. Editorial Hyspamérica.

Prebish, R. (1948). *Obras 1919–1948.* Fundación Raúl Prebish.

Reddy, K. S. (2016). Global burden of disease study 2015 provides GPS for global health 2023. *The Lancet, 388*(10053), 1448–1449. https://www.thelancet.com/journals/lancet/article/PIIS0140-6736(16)31743-3/fulltext

Registro Nacional de las Personas. (2022). *Caracterización sociodemográfica de las personas que rectificaron sus datos identificatorios de acuerdo a la Ley de Identidad de Género* [The sociodemographic characterization of people who have legally changed their identifying information under the Gender Identity Law]. Argentina, Dirección Nacional de Población. https://www.argentina.gob.ar/sites/default/files/2022/05/estudio_estadistico_cambio_de_identidad_de_genero_0.pdf (http://bit.ly/3MYpgm8)

Ribeiro, D. (1972). *Las Américas y la civilización* [The Americas and civilization]. Centro Editor de América Latina.

Sistema Integrado de Información Sanitaria Argentino. (2023). *National directorate of health information systems.* https://www.argentina.gob.ar/salud/digital

UN Development Programme. (2022). *Human development index (HDI)*. https://hdr.undp.org/data-center/human-development-index#/indicies/HDI

United Nations. (2024). *Population division.* https://population.un.org/wpp/

UN Educational, Scientific and Cultural Organization. (2024). *Education and literacy rates, Argentina.* http://sdg4-data.uis.unesco.org/

World Bank Group. (2023a). *Argentina overview.* https://www.worldbank.org/en/country/argentina/overview

World Bank Group. (2023b). *Fertility rate, total (births per woman): Argentina.* https://data.worldbank.org/indicator/SP.DYN.TFRT.IN?locations=AR

World Bank Group. (2023c). *GDP per capita (current US$) – Argentina.* https://data.worldbank.org/indicator/NY.GDP.PCAP.CD?end=2022&locations=AR&start=1983&view=chart

World Health Organization. (2022). *Noncommunicable diseases progress monitor 2022.* https://www.who.int/publications/i/item/9789240047761

CHAPTER 14

COLOMBIA

Ramon Abel Castano, Victoria Eugenia Soto, and Irieleth Gallo

GEOGRAPHY, SIZE, AND DEMOGRAPHICS

Colombia is in the tropical zone at the northwestern tip of South America, with coasts on the Atlantic and the Pacific Oceans. It is divided into 32 departments and the capital district of Bogotá. Its population as of 2024 is 52.7 million, which grew from 39.14 million in 2000, for an annual compound average growth rate of 1.2%.

The population shows a typical aging process, with an increase in life expectancy and a narrowing of the base of the pyramid. Life expectancy increased from 69.6 years for women and 63.3 years for men in 1985 to 78.9 and 72.1, respectively, in 2020. Regarding the pyramid base, as of 2000, the population percentage from age 0 to 14 was 32% and for people over age 60 it was 8.1%. For 2024, these figures were 21.9% and 15%, respectively. In addition, the aging index (the ratio between these older and younger age groups) was 25% in 2000 and 68% in 2024. The median age is 37, and birth rates are constantly decreasing, from 27 per 1,000 in 1990 to 14 per 1,000 in 2022.

Regarding the population distribution between rural and urban areas, the country has experienced a continued migration from rural to urban settings during the last decades. As of 1990, the urban and rural population share was 68% and 32%, respectively. By 2023, these figures were 76% and 24%, respectively.

The male:female ratio for 2023 was 0.953. The racial distribution is dominated by people who do not identify themselves as a specific race (76.82%), followed by those who identify themselves as Indigenous (14.3%), Afro-Descendants (7.54%), and other minorities (1.32%). The large share of the first group is explained by Latin American countries exhibiting a large mix of Caucasians, Indigenous People, and Afro-Descendants.

When asked about their religion in 2021, 78% of people reported themselves as Roman Catholics; the second most common category was no religion but belief in a superior being (7.5%), while the rest were composed of other Christian and non-Christian religions.

The official language is Spanish, and most people speak it, while most people from ethnic minorities preserve their native language along with Spanish.

The political system is a presidential republic with a bicameral Congress. Presidential elections take place every 4 years, and reelection is forbidden. The legislative branch consists of a 102-seat Senate and a 166-seat Chamber of Representatives, both elected to 4-year terms. The judiciary is independent and includes the Supreme Court, the Council of State, and the Constitutional Court. The 1991 Constitution established a decentralized unitary state, granting certain autonomy to territorial entities. The president serves as both head of state and head of government, leading the executive branch.

The primary sport is soccer, which mobilizes massive audiences for local and international games and championships. Soccer serves as a powerful social force, providing opportunities for youth development and community cohesion, while also historically linked to both moments of joy and challenges related to violence and politics in the country.

Colombia shares a legacy from colonization by Spaniards with most Latin American countries (except Brazil and other small Caribbean countries) dating to the arrival of Christopher Columbus in 1492. It means a common language (Spanish) and a dominant religion (Roman

Catholic), the influence of which lingered after the early 19th century period when most countries declared their independence from Spain.

One distinctive characteristic of Colombia, unlike most countries in Latin America, is the persistence of an armed conflict that has been ongoing since the mid-1960s, the oldest in the region. Although the government signed a peace agreement with the main rebel group in 2016, which led to their switching to civil life, dissident groups and new rebel groups have emerged, and the conflict is still active, although more concentrated in rural areas and certain areas of the country.

Besides armed conflict, the country also faces a persistent crime problem. Latin America in general has higher homicide rates and organized crime than the rest of the world; in 2022, Colombia was among the top 10 countries in the region for crime (UN Office on Drugs and Crime, 2023). Organized crime largely revolves around illicit drugs and illegal mining, and the armed conflict is also linked to these illegal activities, as they fuel money for their activities. The presence of armed conflict and illicit drugs is interdependent, and they coexist in most areas of the country that are affected by either of these two problems.

DETERMINANTS OF HEALTH

The national per-capita gross domestic product (GDP), expressed in purchasing-power parities, was $5,084 in 1990 and grew to $21,548 in 2023 (World Bank Group, 2024). Regarding poverty rates, the population living with less than $2.15 per day decreased from 17.5% in 2000 to 6% in 2022. Using a cutoff point of living on $6.85 per day, these percentages are 59.5% and 34.8%, respectively. Poverty rates are higher in rural areas and small villages in areas distant from large urban centers. The Human Development Index for 2021 was 0.752. Although it shows a constant growing trend from 0.61 in 1990 to 0.768 in 2019, the pandemic caused a fall in 2020 and 2021.

Literacy rates among people aged 15 or more grew from 92.8% in 2002 to 95.64% in 2020. When analyzed for the age subgroup between 15 and 24 years, literacy rates are higher and grew from 97.44% in 2002 to 98.91% in 2022. Interestingly, there is a slight advantage of approximately 1% favoring women.

Regarding employment, the working-age population increased from 68.52% in 2001 to 77.73% in 2024, reflecting the underlying change in the population pyramid. However, unemployment rates are still high, between 14.98% in 2001 and 10.17% in 2023. The lowest unemployment rate for this period was 9.2% in 2015. In addition, informal employment is a persistent problem, ranging between 54.5% of employed persons in 2001 and 55.8% in 2023. During this period, the lowest informality rate was 45.8% in 2017 and 2019; the highest rate was 59.3% in 2021 due to the effect of the pandemic in 2020.

Obesity is a growing problem in Colombia. In 2010, the prevalence of obesity among people between ages 18 and 64 was 16.5%, increasing to 18.7% in 2015 (Ministry of Health [MoH], 2023). Height stunting has improved from 26.1% of children under age 5 in 1990 to 10.8% in 2015.

According to the household surveys Encuesta de Calidad de Vida (DANE, n.d.) and Encuesta Nacional de Consumo de Sustancias Psicoactivas (DANE, 2020), adult tobacco consumption is decreasing, from 8.3% in 2016 to 6.1% in 2023.

HEALTH OUTCOMES

There were 265,047 total deaths in the year 2023: 31.5% were caused by cardiovascular diseases (17.2% by ischemic heart disease, 6.4% by cerebrovascular disease, 3.6% by hypertensive disease, and 4.2% by other cardiovascular diseases); 19.4% were caused by cancer (stomach 2%, lung/trachea/bronchi 1.8%, breast 1.4%, colorectal 1.3%, prostate 1.3%, hematopoietic 1%, cervical/uterine 0.7%, and the remaining 10% corresponds to other types of cancer); 12.7% were caused by external causes (5.3% by homicides, 3.2% by traffic accidents, 1.2% by suicide, and the remaining 3% correspond to other external causes). Communicable diseases accounted for 6.9% of total deaths. The remaining 30% of total deaths were caused by other diseases.

Colombia has shown a decreasing trend in potentially avoidable premature mortality during the last 20 years, which looks favorable compared to the average of the 20 largest countries in Latin America. As of 2000, Colombia had a rate of 340.9 potentially avoidable premature deaths per 100,000 people, while the average of the 20 countries was 312.76. By 2019, all countries in the region improved this indicator but Colombia's rate was below the 20 largest-country average, with 183.7 premature deaths per 100,000 people, while the 20 largest-country average was 252.73 (authors' estimations based on the Pan American Health Organization [PAHO] database; available at https://hia.paho.org/es/mortalidad-evitable).

Communicable diseases have reduced their share of total deaths from 7.5% in 2004 to 6.9% in 2023. HIV shows a growing incidence from 5,275 cases reported in 2012 to 12,919 in 2022, while prevalent cases grew from 37,325 to 141,787 in the same period, a growth in prevalence from 0.83 per 1,000 to 2.74 per 1,000.

As a tropical country, Colombia has a persistent problem with mosquito-borne diseases, particularly malaria and dengue. However, malaria has shown a descending pattern from 171,960 cases reported in 2000 to 50,301 in 2017 (MoH, 2024). This region of the Americas had a peak incidence of dengue in 2019, and the most recent outbreak in Colombia was reported in 2022 (MoH, 2023).

Regarding mortality due to noncommunicable diseases, between 2004 and 2023 cardiovascular diseases increased their rate from 29.5% to 31.5%, and cancer increased from 16.7% to 19.4%. External causes of death declined from 18.3% to 12.7% in the same period, which is largely explained by the deescalation of the armed conflict.

Mental health has been an explicit concern for public health policy, and a legal framework was passed in Congress in 2013. However, it has not been fully implemented, and the general approach to mental health is still too focused on curative rather than preventive interventions. Suicide rates have grown from 5.2 deaths per 100,000 inhabitants in 2005 to 6.1 in 2023. A survey of 49,756 respondents between ages 12 and 65 years showed that 84% report having ingested alcohol sometime in their lives, 54.5% during the last year and 30.1% in the previous month. Regarding marijuana use, the figures were 8.3%, 2.68, and 1.78 respectively, and for cocaine use, the figures were 2.07%, 0.57%, and 0.31%, respectively.

According to the PAHO (2024) country profile, Colombia had a maternal mortality ratio of 74.8 deaths per 100,000 live births in 2020. This figure reflects the impact of the COVID-19 pandemic and the immigration of Venezuelan pregnant women, as it was 65.4 in 2019. However, Colombia shows a stagnant pattern for this indicator, oscillating between 70 and 73 live births per 100,000 between 2008 and 2017.

The same PAHO (2024) source shows improvement regarding the infant mortality indicator, from 30 deaths per 1,000 live births in 1995 to 10.9 in 2021. However, stagnation was also evident between 2013 and 2021, as the indicators oscillated between 11.5 and 10.1.

HISTORICAL/THEORETICAL BACKGROUND OF HEALTHCARE

Colombia's current healthcare system started implementation after a significant healthcare reform in 1993. It is based on the principles of managed competition and has a competitive health insurance market. The government regulates the insurance premium and the benefits package.

The overall system is funded via general taxes plus payroll taxes. Collected taxes are pooled in a large country-level equalization fund, which sets a per-capita payment for each social health insurance system enrollee. Individuals can freely choose among 27 competing insurance funds, and the equalization fund transfers the per-capita payment to the insurer selected by each enrollee.

The social health insurance system is organized into two enrolment schemes: the contributory and the subsidized. The contributory scheme is aimed at workers in the formal sector (both private and public, salaried, or self-employed) and pensioners. In this scheme, the worker pays 4%

of their salary base and the employer pays an 8.5% tax on the salary base of employees earning above 10 times the statutory minimum wage. The subsidized scheme is aimed at informal and unemployed workers, meaning enrollees do not pay for their enrollment. Still, it is financed with part of the payroll taxes collected in the contributory scheme and general taxes.

As of June 2024, the enrollment figures were 23.3 million people in the contributory scheme and 26.5 million in the subsidized scheme. These figures add to 49.8 million Colombians covered by the social health insurance system, representing 94.5% of the population. The remaining 2.6 million individuals are distributed among special insurance schemes (the armed forces, the teachers' union, and the oil company), which enroll 2.2 million people; the rest are uninsured. This means Colombia has insurance coverage covering close to 99% of its population. By the start of the current system in 1993, social health insurance covered around 17% of the population, while the rest attended a supply-side subsidized network of public hospitals. Figure 14.1 shows the evolution of social health insurance enrolment.

All individuals in both insurance schemes are entitled to the same benefits package, which includes all necessary services and health technologies available in the country. Until 2015, the benefits package was defined as a positive list, namely, only those services explicitly included on the list were paid by the insurers. However, suppose a necessary service for a patient was not included in the positive list. In that case, the individual files a ***tutela***, a legal action to protect fundamental rights individually.

FIGURE 14.1 Evolution of out-of-pocket expenses as a percentage of Colombia's total health expenditure, 2011 to 2020.

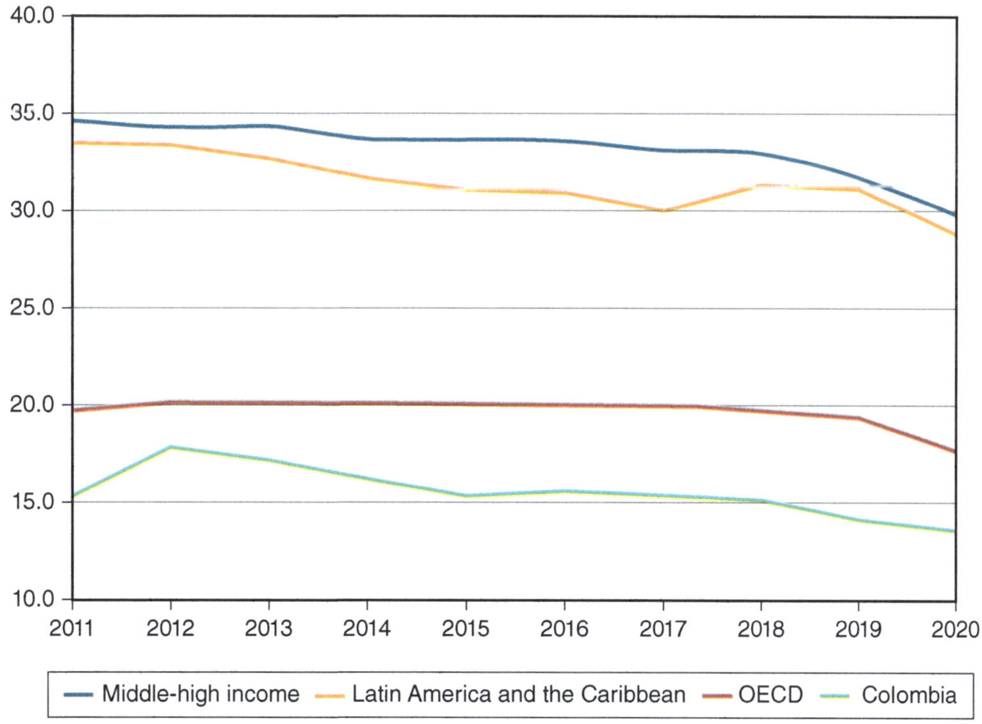

OECD, Organisation for Economic Co-operation and Development.

Source: Melo, L., Arango, L., Avila, O., Ayala-García, J., Bonilla-Mejía, L., Botero-García, J.A., Crispin-Fory, C., Cardona, M., Gallo, D., Granger-Castaño, C., Guzmán-Finol, K.K., Iregui-Bohórquez, A.M., Pinilla-Alarcón, D.E., Posso-Suárez, C.M., Ramírez-Giraldo, M.T., Ramos-Forero, J.E., Ramos-Veloza, M.A., Restrepo-Tobón, D.A., Restrepo-Zea, J.H., ... Vásquez-Escobar, D. (2023). *Aspectos financieros y fiscales del sistema de salud en Colombia* [Financial and fiscal aspects of the healthcare system in Colombia]. Ensayos Sobre Política Económica. No. 106. Banco de la República.

This led to new technologies being accessed via tutela (on a patient-by-patient basis) until they were added to the benefits package. These technologies accessed via tutela were paid directly by the central equalization fund on a fee-for-service basis. After 2015, a law was passed that changed the positive-list approach to a negative-list approach, which means that the government does not pay for services and technologies that are part of the explicitly excluded categories. These categories are

- experimental technologies;
- services and technologies without evidence of efficacy, safety, and effectiveness;
- technologies unavailable within the country;
- technologies with cosmetic purposes; and
- technologies that the regulatory agency does not authorize.

However, under this negative-list approach, new technologies are still approved via tutela on a patient-by-patient basis. Even new drugs that the national regulatory agency has not approved can be accessed via tutela or via an exceptional mechanism called *vital not-available*. This mechanism implies that the drug is imported only for one given patient.

Insurers are responsible for the purchasing function and all the benefits included in the benefits package. They can selectively contract with healthcare providers to set up their provider networks, using a range of contracting mechanisms from **fee-for-service** to prospective modalities such as **capitation**, **episode-of-care**, or **chronic-care capitation**. Fee-for-service is the most common payment mechanism for medium- and high-complexity services, but insurers are increasingly using some types of prospective payments. Capitation is the typical payment mechanism for primary care services.

Private providers dominate the healthcare delivery side. As of 2022, only 30% of the total hospital beds and 19% of the operating rooms were in the public sector (Jurado & Santos, 2022). The total beds per 1,000 people was 1.81 in 2019 (author's estimations, based on Integrated System of Information on Social Protection [Sistema Integrado de Información de la Protección Social in Spanish, or SISPRO] and the Chamber of Representatives [Cámara de Representantes, or REPS]). Although the MoH does not directly control public hospitals, they are organized as autonomous public entities with a board of directors that includes the local authorities and other interest groups. Most of the community low-complexity public hospitals are located in small municipalities and the poor areas of larger urban centers, representing 85.3% of the total facilities of the public sector. Medium- and high-complexity public hospitals are located in large urban centers, representing 11.8% and 2.8% of the total public facilities, respectively (MoH, 2022).

The larger share of private healthcare providers as a share of the total provider supply was achieved after a sustained growth during the last 30 years, since the start of the current healthcare system. This growth was partly fueled by healthcare professionals and private investors, and partly by private insurers in the social health insurance system, as they built vertically integrated networks or gave preference to other private providers. It caused public hospitals to lag in terms of state-of-the-art technologies and services, as well as a slower growth of hospital-bed supply. For example, as of 2017, 87.9% of cancer providers were in the private sector (Murcia et al., 2018).

Except for emergency care, the healthcare delivery system is organized by each insurer through closed networks. Health insurers operate in a similar way to health maintenance organizations in the United States, namely, they set up closed networks with primary care gatekeeping, control referrals to specialty care, and apply a wide range of managed care tools and strategies (such as authorizations, medical audits, payment denials, etc.) to keep costs under control. Although insurers can have vertically integrated providers, they cannot spend more than 30% of healthcare expenses in their providers.

Colombia´s healthcare system exhibits a high level of financial protection, as out-of-pocket expenses as a share of total health expenditures have been around 15% for the last decade.

This figure is lower than the average for middle- and high-income countries (33.2%), for Organisation for Economic Co-operation and Development (OECD) countries (19.8%; Melo et al., 2023), and for Latin America and the Caribbean (30%; PAHO, 2023). While there were plenty of media reports in other countries in the region about households that faced catastrophic expenditures forcing them to sell assets or acquire debt to pay for hospital bills, this was not reported in Colombia (Restrepo, 2021). From a longitudinal perspective, the percentage of households that incurred catastrophic expenses decreased from 10.62% in 1997 to 1.77% in 2023, and the percentage of households that faced zero expenditures for healthcare increased from 25% to 64% in the same period (authors' estimations based on household surveys).

Regarding access to primary care services, the Colombian system shows barriers to access, which are higher for people experiencing poverty and residents of rural areas. However, this problem has been partially reduced during the last 30 years. For example, in 1990 the percentage of pregnant women who had zero antenatal visits was 33.8% in the poorest wealth quintile and 2.9% in the richest wealth quintile, these figures went down to 6.7% and near zero, respectively, in 2015 (Castaño & Soto, 2022).

The managed competition model has created tensions among insurers, healthcare providers, and professionals because of the cost controls exerted by insurers. Although it is recognized that resources are finite and cost controls are necessary, some of the managed care tools and strategies used by insurers are considered too restrictive. Other insurers have been pointed out as appealing to abusive contracting practices and payment delays.

A deep financial sustainability crisis has been accumulating during the last 10 years, because the per-capita payment has been insufficient to cover the growing demand for healthcare and the increasingly costly medical technologies that enter the Colombian market (Espinosa et al., 2023). In addition, the generous interpretation of the right to healthcare that the Constitutional Court has advanced as the access to high-cost curative technologies increases has created a problem of runaway growth of health expenditures. This has caused some insurers to accumulate accounts payable, while others exit the market, leading to a large amount of unpayable debt to providers and suppliers.

The new president, who took office in August 2022, is the first left wing president in Colombia's history. His government team has advanced a healthcare reform introducing radical changes in the system's structure. The first radical change is to eliminate the managed competition model and shift toward a Beveridge-type model, where resources are allocated on a territorial basis. The delivery of services is organized through integrated delivery networks with a catchment area assigned based on geography.

The purchasing function is eliminated, and the national equalization fund is expected to pay directly to each healthcare provider for the services delivered to patients. A position similar to a third-party administrator (TPA) has been proposed, which is supposed to exert managed care tools and strategies. However, these TPAs have no incentive to optimize the financial resources because they will not receive a per-capita payment for each enrollee, as current insurers do, but will only accept a fee for administrative expenses.

A second radical change introduced by the government reform proposal is adopting a comprehensive scope of primary care; that is, not only first-contact healthcare facilities, but deployment of community-based healthcare teams that visit households periodically to identify people at risk and to intervene in those risks as much as possible at the community level. Although the implementation of primary care had been attempted previously, the insurance-based model, with its individual choice of insurer, led to the coexistence of population silos at a given territory, which undermined the implementation of community-wide interventions on health promotion and primary prevention (Castaño, 2023).

Congress rejected the government's healthcare reform bill in May 2024, and the government aims to submit a new bill that will be discussed during 2025. In addition to the government bill, other bills have been announced for this new legislative period, and at the time of writing of this chapter, it is impossible to predict the final design of the healthcare reform. It is clear, however, that the system will change radically and that the managed competition model will be profoundly modified.

CONCLUSION

As an upper middle-income country, Colombia exhibits characteristics similar to other countries in the same income level. Two distinctive characteristics stand out: the high crime rates and organized crime, and the persistence of an armed conflict. Its healthcare system is based on a managed competition model, with a competitive health insurance system but with premiums and benefits package regulated by the government. Private providers dominate healthcare delivery. The benefits packages are defined on a negative basis, and tutela is a very effective means to access high-cost technologies and treatments that are not included in the benefits package. However, the system is underfinanced and in deep financial crisis, making radical reform inevitable. Several reform bills have been discussed in Congress, and although it is difficult to predict the resulting system, the current system will be radically changed.

Our recommendations to improve health and healthcare start with a clear definition of the boundaries of the right to healthcare through an explicit priority-setting exercise to make the system sustainable. Under the current conditions of no explicit prioritization, no reform will be able to solve the sustainability crisis. In addition, strengthening primary care is an urgent policy that should be implemented soon to improve aggregate levels of health and reduce persistent equity gaps. Regarding the delivery of healthcare services, it is necessary to evolve toward more efficient network models and contracting strategies to make a more efficient use of available services.

LEARNING ACTIVITIES

CourseConnect

To access self-assessment questions and interactive, competency-based learning activities for this chapter, visit www.springerpub.com/courseconnect. See inside front cover and tear-out for CourseConnect details.

REFERENCES

Castaño, R. A. (2023). *Reforma a la salud ¿Sí o no?* [Health care reform, yes or no?] (pp. 98–104). Hipertexto.

Castaño, R. A., & Soto, V. E. (2022). *Aseguramiento versus acceso con equidad: ¿Qué muestran las encuestas ENDS?* [Insurance versus equitable access: What do the ENDS surveys show?]. PROESA. https://www.icesi.edu.co/proesa/politicas-en-breve-09

DANE. (n.d.). *Encuesta nacional de calidad de vida* [National quality of life survey]. https://www.dane.gov.co/index.php/estadisticas-por-tema/pobreza-y-condiciones-de-vida/calidad-de-vida-ecv

DANE. (2020). *Encuesta nacional de consumo de sustancias psicoactivas* [National survey on psychoactive substance use]. https://www.dane.gov.co/index.php/estadisticas-por-tema/salud/encuesta-nacional-de-consumo-de-sustancias-psicoactivas-encspa

Espinosa, O., Rodríguez, J., Urdinola, B., Do Nascimento Silva, P. L., Sánchez, A., Arias, M. L., Valdez, E. A., Cheng, T., & Fisher, S. E. (2023). Loss ratio of the capitation payment unit of the health-promoting entities in Colombia between 2017 and 2021: A financial–actuarial approach. *Cost Effectiveness and Resource Allocation, 21*(1), 73. https://doi.org/10.1186/s12962-023-00481-5

Jurado, C. E., & Santos, J. F. (2022, June 22). *Hospitales y clínicas: Eje articulador del sector salud* [Hospitals and clinics: The articulating axis of the health sector]. Revista A de la ANDI, Edición Especial. https://bit.ly/3PaJU3L

Melo, L., Arango, L., Avila, O., Ayala-Garcia, J., Bonilla-Mejia, L., Botero-Garcia, J. A., Cardona-Badillo, M., Crispin-Fory, C., Gallo-Monatano, D. P., Granger-Castano, C. J., Guzman-Finol, K., Iregui, A. M., Ospina, J., Pinilla-Alarcon, D., Posso-Suarez, C., Ramirez, M. T., Ramos-Foreo, J, E., Ramos-Veloza., M., Restrepo-Tobon, D. A., . . . Vasquez-Escobar. (2023). Aspectos financieros y fiscales del sistema de salud en Colombia [Financial and fiscal aspects of the health system in Colombia]. *Ensayos sobre Política Económica,* (106). Banco de la República. https://investiga.banrep.gov.co/es/espe/espe106

Ministry of Health. (2022). *Propuesta de redefinición de las características de operación de los hospitales públicos* [Proposal to redefine the operating characteristics of public hospitals]. chrome-extension://efaidnbmnnnibpcajpcglclefindmkaj/https://www.minsalud.gov.co/sites/rid/Lists/BibliotecaDigital/RIDE/VS/PSA/estudio-oferta-servicios-primarios-hospitales-publicos.pdf

Ministry of Health. (2023). *Análisis de situación de salud 2023* [Health situation analysis 2023]. https://www.minsalud.gov.co/sites/rid/Lists/BibliotecaDigital/RIDE/VS/ED/PSP/asis-colombia-2023.pdf

Ministry of Health. (2024). *Cifras de afiliación en salud* [Health affiliation figures]. https://minsalud.gov.co/proteccionsocial/Paginas/cifras-aseguramiento-salud.aspx

Murcia, E., Aguilera, J., Wiesner, C., & Pardo, C. (2018). Servicios oncológicos en Colombia [Oncology services in Colombia]. *Colombia Médica, 49*(1), 89–96.

Pan American Health Organization. (2023). *Gasto de bolsillo: Cifras confiables para el monitoreo de la salud universal* [Out-of-pocket expenditure: Reliable data to monitor universal health]. https://iris.paho.org/bitstream/handle/10665.2/59295/OPSHSSHS230009_spa.pdf?sequence=1

Pan American Health Organization. (2024). *Colombia country profile.* https://hia.paho.org/en/countries-2022/colombia-country-profile

Restrepo, J. (2021). Protección financiera en salud: ¿Qué ha pasado en América Latina en medio de la pandemia de COVID-19? [What has happened in Latin America amidst the COVID-19 pandemic?]. *Seguridad Social Latinoamericana–CLACSO, 6*, 22–30.

UN Office on Drugs and Crime. (2023). *Global study on homicide 2023.* https://www.unodc.org/documents/data-and-analysis/gsh/2023/Global_study_on_homicide_2023_web.pdf

World Bank Group. (2024). *PIB per cápita, PPA ($ a precios internacionales actuales) - Colombia* [GDP per capita, PPP (current international $) – Colombia]. https://datos.bancomundial.org/indicador/NY.GDP.PCAP.PP.CD?view=chart&locations=CO

CHAPTER 15

ECUADOR

Irene Torres, Mariana Pinto-Alvarez, Daniel Romero-Alvarez, and Daniel F. López-Cevallos

INTRODUCTION

Ecuador, located in northern South America, is a relatively small but demographically and geographically diverse country. While Ecuador is classified as a middle-income country (according to World Bank rankings), there are wide social, economic, and health inequalities that the country's health and social systems struggle to address. While reading this chapter, it is important to think about the following question: Why does Ecuador, despite its wealth of social, economic, and natural resources, rank behind many other peer countries in key health and healthcare outcomes such as infectious and noncommunicable diseases?

GEOGRAPHY AND POPULATION

GEOGRAPHICAL AND CLIMATE FEATURES

Located in northwestern South America, Ecuador is bordered by Colombia to the north, Peru to the south and east, and the Pacific Ocean to the west. It is the smallest of the Andean countries, with an area of about 252,000 square kilometers (156,585 square miles). The Andes Mountain range runs from north to south, reaching altitudes of over 5,000 meters (16,404 feet; Varela & Ron, 2018). Ecuador is divided into three main regions: the Coast (Costa), the Andes (Sierra), and the Amazon (Eastern). In addition, Ecuador has an archipelago located approximately 1,000 km (600 miles) off the coast, the Galápagos Islands. Ecuador experiences relatively minor weather variations throughout the year, with only two distinct seasons: wet or winter, and dry or summer. Altitude significantly influences Ecuador's climate, with annual temperatures ranging from approximately 0°C to 26°C (32°F–79°F; Varela & Ron, 2018).

POPULATION SIZE AND MAIN CHARACTERISTICS

According to the 2022 national census (Figure 15.1), Ecuador has 16,938,986 inhabitants, with Pichincha and Guayas being the most densely populated provinces. The country has a growth rate of 1.3%; there is a ratio of 95 men to 100 women, and the median age is 29 years. The 10 to 14 year and 15 to 19 year age categories constitute the largest groups. Starting with the third most common age category (20 to 24 years), the female population is consistently larger. The country is in a phase III of demographic transition; that is, there is decrease in both mortality and birth rates which indicates the population growth is slowing down. Furthermore, 63.1% of the population live in urban areas, 77.5% identify themselves as *mestizos* (mixed European and Indigenous ancestry), followed by Indigenous (7.7%) and Afro-Ecuadorian (4.8%; National Institute of Statistics and Census [INEC], 2022a).

Birth Rates

The birth rate in 2022 was 13.9 live births per 1,000 inhabitants. The percentage of live births with low birth weight in the same year was 9.3%. There were 2.3 live births per 1,000 females age 10 to 14 years in 2022, and 47.3 live births per 1,000 adolescents age 15 to 19 in the same year. However, 50.6% of pregnancies occurred in women age 20 to 29, followed by the 30 to 34 (18.9%) and 15

FIGURE 15.1 Age distribution of the Ecuadorian population.

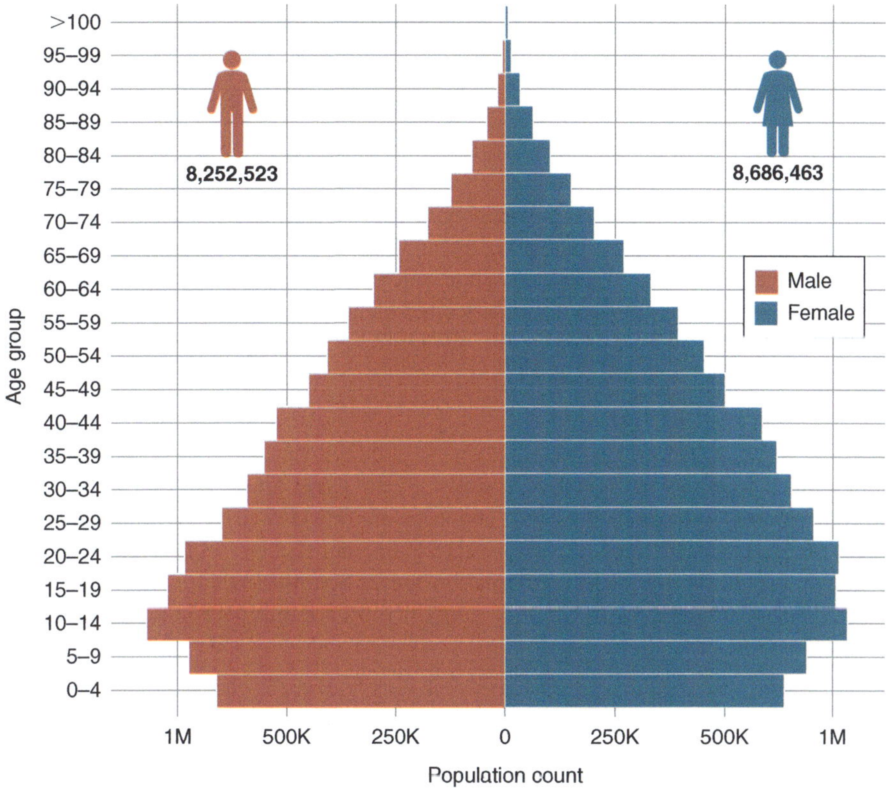

Source: National Institute of Statistics and Census. (2022a). *Censo Ecuador, resultados nacionales principales* [Ecuador census, main national results]. Instituto Nacional de Estadistica y Censos. https://www.censoecuador.gob.ec/

to 19 age groups (15.2%). The government also reported that in 2022, 96.7% of deliveries were attended by medical personnel, and in the private sector, 87.7% of births were by cesarean section, while in the public sector it was 36.9% (INEC, 2022b, 2023).

Migrant Populations

According to the 2022 census, Ecuador is home to 425,045 foreigners, with Venezuelans (54.5%), Colombians (23%), Spaniards (4.8%), and Peruvians (3.5%) being the most prominent. Half of the migrants are between 15 and 19 years old, and three out of four (78%) live in urban areas. The main reasons why foreigners choose to migrate to Ecuador are economic, such as dollarization and globalization, as well as access to quality healthcare and education, and the search for better living conditions. Since 2020, there has been an increase in the wave of migration, with a net migration balance above zero from 2010 to 2020 (INEC, 2022a).

Sex and Marital Status

Between 2010 and 2022, the ratio of men to women in urban and rural areas of the country declined similarly to the national level. That is, while in 2010 there were 102 men for every 100 women, in 2022 there were 98 men for every 100 women. Among the youngest age groups, the relationship is reversed compared to what was observed at the national level. That is, in the age group 0 to 19 years, the male population is in the majority (INEC Censos, 2024). Meanwhile, in the older age groups, the relationship remains the same as at the national level (more females than males), which could be explained by higher mortality or migration rates in the case of males. The marriage rate has decreased from 32.1 in 2021 to 30.8 in 2022 (compared to an increase in divorce rates from 12.7 to 13.7 during the same period), and the average age of marriage was 32 years for women and 35 years for men in 2022. In 2022, there were 260 registered same-sex marriages, with 127 male couples and 133 female couples, and 15 divorces among same-sex couples (INEC, 2022c).

CULTURAL BELIEFS

RELIGION AND SPIRITUALITY

The Constitution guarantees the right to choose, practice, and change one's religion and prohibits discrimination based on religion. Approximately 84% of Ecuadorians have a religious affiliation, with 65% identifying as Catholic and 19% as Evangelical, while 13% have no religious affiliation (Latinobarómetro, 2024). Indigenous communities often blend traditional beliefs with Christian practices, which are recognized by the country's Constitution (Constituent Assembly of Ecuador [Asamblea Constituyente del Ecuador], 2008).

LANGUAGES

Spanish is the official language of Ecuador; however, Kichwa and Shuar are official languages for intercultural relations and other ancestral languages are officially used by Indigenous peoples (Ministerio de Relaciones Exteriores y Movilidad Humana [Ministry of Foreign Affairs and Migration of Ecuador], 2021). Most of the population speaks Spanish (98.6%), followed by 3.9% speaking an Indigenous language (with Kichwa being the most common at 85.6%; INEC, 2024).

TRADITIONS AND MAJOR CELEBRATIONS

Ecuador boasts a rich tapestry of community traditions, practices, events, and leisure activities that reflect its diverse cultural heritage. One of the most important celebrations is the Inti Raymi, a sun festival inherited from Indigenous Andean cultures that honors the sun god, Inti. This event, marked by colorful costumes, music, and dance, underscores the deep connection between people and nature. Emphasizing harmony with nature can encourage sustainable lifestyles and environmental stewardship, which contribute to long-term health. Ecuadorians also take pride in their culinary heritage, with dishes like *ceviche* and *llapingachos* showcasing the fusion of Indigenous and Spanish cuisines (González, 2017). Ecuadorian cultural traditions strengthen community and social connections, which can greatly benefit public health. *Minga*, an Indigenous-origin communal work practice where people collaborate to achieve shared goals, extends to health-related efforts such as improving school, healthcare, or potable water treatment facilities. Additionally, traditional celebrations and rituals that bring people together may provide spaces for disseminating health promotion practices. Lastly, the emphasis on intergenerational family ties in Ecuadorian culture increases physical and mental health supports for vulnerable populations, such as the older population and children.

POLITICAL SYSTEM

Ecuador is a constitutional state, organized as a republic, with an emphasis on rights, justice, and democracy. Sovereignty rests with the people and is exercised through public power and direct participation, as defined in the 2008 Constitution (Constituent Assembly of Ecuador, 2008).

BRIEF COUNTRY HISTORY

Ecuador has been inhabited by Indigenous Peoples as early as the 10th century BCE. The Incas conquered what is now Ecuador at the end of the 15th century CE. Soon thereafter, the Spanish invasion of the Inca Empire capitalized on internal crises, facilitating their conquest, colonization, and subsequent exploitation (Ayala Mora, 2008). Between 1808 and 1812, the Revolution of Quito was sparked by Napoleon's intervention in the Iberian Peninsula, which prompted

American *criollos* (those of Spanish descent) to form juntas (military rulers) to govern in the name of the legitimate monarch. Despite initial setbacks, a sovereign junta seized power in Quito on August 10, 1809, but its reign was short-lived due to insufficient popular support and defeat at the hands of Spanish armed forces. However, the independence movement, led by Simon Bolívar, was reborn in Guayaquil in 1820, spread to Cuenca, and culminated in the Battle of Pichincha in 1822, which solidified Ecuador's independence. After their victory, key figures in Quito and Cuenca favored annexation to Colombia, with Venezuela and New Granada forming Gran Colombia in 1819. Although Bolívar held the title of president, he had centralist tendencies that clashed with the liberal policies of vice-president Santander. Bolívar's efforts to establish a dictatorship faltered, resulting in the dissolution of Gran Colombia in 1830, with the southern district of Ecuador subsequently gaining independence (Ayala Mora, 2008).

HEALTH OUTCOMES

MORBIDITY AND MORTALITY

Life expectancy in Ecuador is 74.5 years for men and 80 years for women (Ministerio de Salud Pública del Ecuador [MSP], 2022). Ecuador has an overall mortality rate of 5.0 per 1,000 inhabitants. In 2022, the leading cause of death in Ecuador was ischemic heart disease (Figure 15.2), accounting for 15% of total deaths, followed by diabetes mellitus and cerebrovascular disease. Homicide also accounted for a significant proportion of deaths at 5%. Among men, heart disease and homicide were the leading causes of death, while among women, heart disease and diabetes mellitus were more prominent. It is important to note that cancer is not a leading cause of death in Ecuador (INEC, 2022d).

Infant mortality rate is 8.6 per 1,000 live births and the under-five mortality rate is 10.6 per 1,000 live births. In addition, the neonatal mortality rate was recorded at 5.4 per 1,000 live births. Maternal mortality ratio is 33.9 deaths per 100,000 live births. In 2002, among 2,855 child deaths, certain prenatal conditions account for 56%, followed by congenital malformations at 22% (INEC, 2022d). There were 155 maternal deaths in 2021, with 18.1% attributed to direct obstetric causes. Of these, gestational hypertension with significant proteinuria accounts for 17.4%, followed by postpartum hemorrhage at 6.5% (INEC, 2022d).

In 2021 and 2022, Ecuador experienced a variety of causes of morbidity, with notable shifts in the prevalence of certain conditions. The COVID-19 virus, both identified and unidentified,

FIGURE 15.2 Leading causes of death in Ecuador (2022).

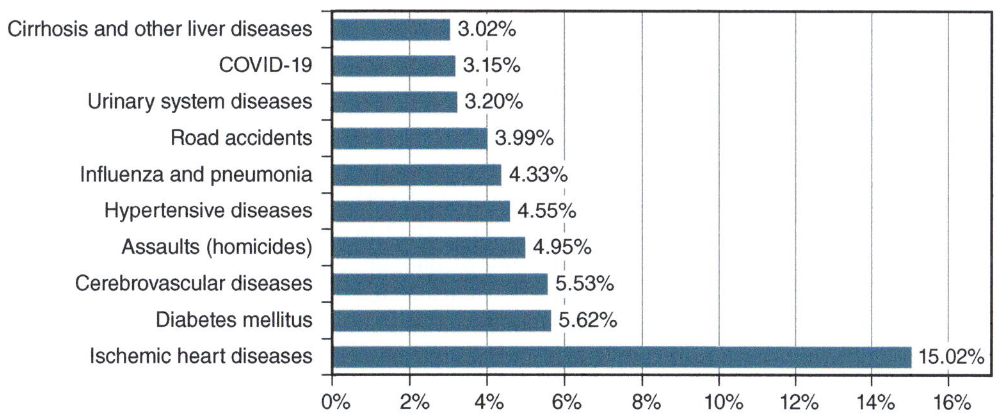

Source: Ecuador National Institute of Statistics and Census. (2022). *Defunciones generales* [General deaths]. https://www.ecuadorencifras.gob.ec/documentos/web-inec/Poblacion_y_Demografia/Defunciones_Generales_2022/Principales_resultados_EDG_2022.pdf

remained a significant health concern, with reported cases decreasing from 64,491 in 2021 to 14,552 in 2022. Similarly, from 2021 to 2022, conditions such as cholelithiasis (i.e., gallstones) decreased from 41,367 to 49,223 cases and acute appendicitis from 30,014 to 29,662 cases continued to affect a significant number of people (INEC, 2022d).

MENTAL HEALTH

Ecuador has experienced a steady increase in mental health problems, such as depression and anxiety disorders. The prevalence rate of mental disorders is estimated at 14.8% of the population, with a notable increase in incidence among children and adolescents due to increasing violence and socioeconomic stressors (World Health Organization [WHO], 2020). In 2020, mood disorders (depression, dysthymia, bipolar disorder) were the leading morbidity profile, followed by anxiety disorders (anxiety, severe stress reaction, panic), paranoid schizophrenia, cognitive impairment, and substance use disorders. Emergency or hospitalization cases often involved physical or pharmacologic restraints, mainly for severe depression, schizophrenia, mental, cognitive impairment, and personality disorders (MSP, 2022).

INFECTIOUS DISEASES

As in much of the rest of the world, the COVID-19 pandemic became the most important cause of infectious disease mortality. In 2020, Ecuador had 64% more deaths than expected, with COVID accounting for 21% of total (signaling a lack of diagnostic capacity; Cuéllar et al., 2021). Other than COVID-19, lower respiratory infections compromise 3.65% of the population. Tuberculosis and HIV/AIDS represent Ecuadorian mortality at 0.37% and 0.86%, respectively (Pan American Health Organization [PAHO], 2022).

DETERMINANTS OF HEALTH

FOOD AND NUTRITION

Food insecurity in Ecuador has increased significantly in recent years, disproportionately affecting different regions and vulnerable groups. Food insecurity rates are 37.9% in the Coast, 33.9% in the Amazon, and 19.4% in the Andes. In addition, malnutrition rates in Ecuador are alarming, with 27% of children under the age of 2 years suffering from chronic malnutrition, which rises to 39% among Indigenous children. The *Food Security Report* also found that one in four people surveyed had only one meal a day (UN Office for the Coordination of Humanitarian Affairs [OCHA], 2021). Ecuador faces a double burden of malnutrition, where one in four children under 5 years of age suffers from chronic malnutrition, and at the same time more than half of the adult population is overweight or obese (INEC, 2018).

TOBACCO AND ALCOHOL CONSUMPTION

The prevalence of smoking in Ecuador is relatively low compared to global and regional estimates. In 2020, approximately 11.3% of the population smoked, with a significant gender gap: 18.4% of men and 4.2% of women. Among the population aged 12 to 18 years, 2.5% consume alcoholic beverages. In addition, 41.8% of people consume alcohol on a weekly basis, and 79.2% of them drink beer. In 2021, high alcohol consumption was associated with 670.04 disability-adjusted life sear (DALYs) per 100,000 inhabitants and tobacco consumption with 644.16 DALYs per 100,000 inhabitants (Institute for Health Metrics and Evaluation [IHME], 2024).

NONCOMMUNICABLE DISEASES

In Ecuador, approximately 65% of the population aged 19 and above are overweight or obese, a major contributing factor to noncommunicable diseases (NCDs; Fernández & Martínez, 2017).

NCDs are estimated to account for 72% of deaths. The primary causes of death from NCDs are cardiovascular conditions; ischemic heart disease and stroke account for 9.21% and 5.01% of all deaths attributed to NCDs, respectively. The third is chronic kidney disease (5.24% of all NCD deaths), with 567 patients per million population using renal replacement therapy (Torres et al., 2022) and surpassing diabetes, which is the fourth NCD-related cause of death (3.62%). Still, these statistics are an underestimation as Ecuador has limited diagnostic capacity. In fifth place, cirrhosis of the liver, which has been linked to alcohol consumption, accounts for 2.1% of all deaths attributed to NCDs.

SOCIAL DETERMINANTS OF HEALTH

Socioeconomic Conditions

Ecuador, classified as a middle-income country, has experienced fluctuations in its economic indicators. According to the Central Bank of Ecuador (BCE), gross domestic product (GDP) per capita rose from $3,178 in 1995 to $4,374 in 2014; it then fell to $4,163 in 2019 and further to $3,785 in 2020 due to the COVID-19 pandemic. There was a slight recovery to $3,892 in 2021. This economic instability is reflected in social aspects, particularly in poverty rates. While the poverty incidence decreased from 58.3% in 2001 to 21.5% in 2017, it increased to 33% in 2020 before leveling off at 27.7% in 2021. Fiscal austerity policies implemented since 2018 in the context of negotiations with the International Monetary Fund (IMF) led to a reduction in government spending, particularly on social services (Johnston & Vasic-Lalovic, 2023).

In 2024, Ecuador's unemployment rate was approximately 3.8%, a significant decline from the peak of 13.3% recorded in the second quarter of 2020 during the COVID-19 pandemic. This decline reflects a broader trend of recovery in the labor market. Historically, Ecuador's unemployment rate has averaged around 4.7% over the past decade, which is relatively low compared to the regional average for Latin America. The employment landscape in Ecuador continues to be influenced by factors such as economic growth, labor force participation, and the prevalence of informal employment, which remains a notable feature of the country's labor market (The Global Economy, 2024).

HEALTHCARE SYSTEM

Ecuador's National Health System is based on constitutional principles that recognize healthcare as a fundamental human right. Healthcare is provided according to principles of equity, quality, and accessibility, and involves an integrated public network of government facilities, social security institutions, and other providers. Service delivery is mixed, involving government, private, autonomous, and community entities. Citizen participation in monitoring and improving the quality of healthcare is encouraged through mechanisms such as Citizens' Oversight Committees (Romero-Alvarez et al., 2024).

The biomedical health system in Ecuador (Figure 15.3) faces multiple challenges that affect the overall health and well-being of the population. The dominance of the medical–industrial complex, while strengthening tertiary care, neglects critical public health needs such as access to potable water and sanitation, particularly in rural areas, contributing to the persistence of infectious diseases and growth stunting. In addition, the prevalence of obesity is exacerbated by the growing influence of the loosely regulated processed food industry, perpetuating health inequities. A narrow focus on healthcare delivery hinders the multisectoral collaboration needed to address broader public health issues (Torres & López-Cevallos, 2017, 2018).

HEALTH INSURANCE AND HEALTHCARE DELIVERY

Ecuador's MSP leads the national health system, formulating policies and overseeing sector entities. Working with stakeholders through the National Health Council (Consejo Nacional de Salud

FIGURE 15.3 Ecuador's biomedical healthcare system.

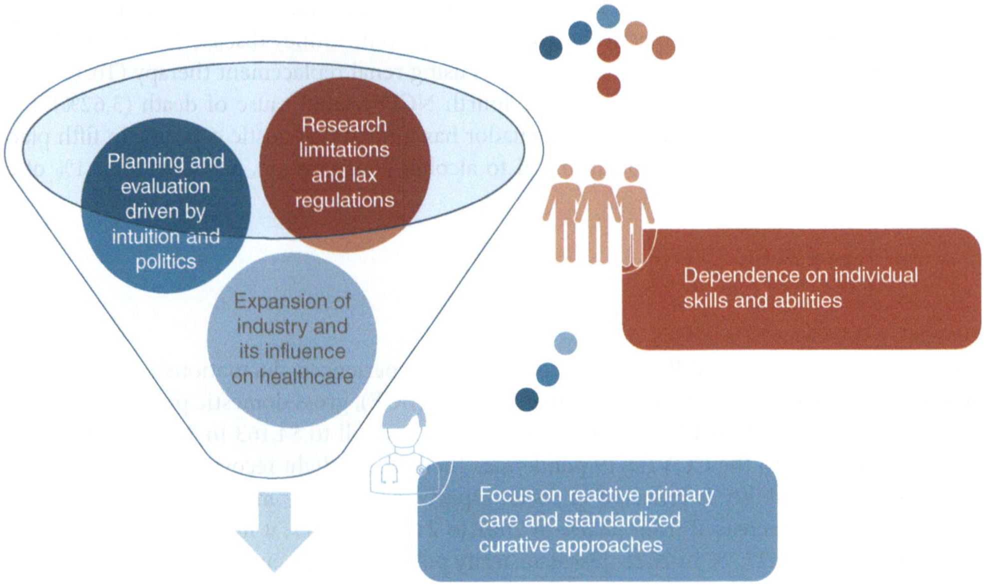

Source: Adapted from Torres, I., & López-Cevallos, D. F. (2018). Institutional challenges to achieving health equity in Ecuador. *The Lancet Global Health*, 6(8), E832–E833. https://doi.org/10.1016/S2214-109X(18)30245-6

[CONASA]), the MSP promotes consensus on sector policies. The Organic Health Law mandates that CONASA ensures the efficient use of financial resources for universal health coverage. The MSP, along with the Ministry of Economic and Social Inclusion and municipal health services, provide healthcare to the uninsured. Social security institutions cover the employed populations (PAHO, 2022; Romero-Alvarez et al., 2023).

HEALTHCARE COSTS AND ACCESS

National health expenditures represented 6.4% of Ecuador's GDP (public expenditures were $5,626 million; private expenditures were $1,747 million in 2022). In addition, out-of-pocket household spending was 32.6%. The production of hospital activities was $2,425 million in the public sector and $1,231 million in the private sector (INEC, 2022e). In 2022, there were a total of 632 registered health facilities nationwide, including 180 in the public sector, 412 in the for-profit private sector, and 40 in the nonprofit private sector. In terms of available hospital beds, there were 14,017 in the public sector and 9,378 in the private sector, for a ratio of 1.3 hospital beds per 1,000 inhabitants. In addition, a total of 1,843 intensive care unit (ICU) beds were reported in both public and private health facilities in the same year (INEC, 2022f). In 2020, the rate of doctors was 23.2 per 10,000 inhabitants, with a total of 40,587 doctors. For dentists, the rate was 3.0 per 10,000 population, accounting for 5,203 practitioners. Nurses had a rate of 15.4 per 10,000 population, comprising 27,017 individuals (INEC, 2020).

TRADITIONAL AND COMPLEMENTARY CARE

Traditional medicine in Ecuador is deeply rooted in the country's multicultural and multiethnic context. From regional associations formed by Indigenous groups to state-led initiatives, traditional healing practices coexist with formal biomedical health systems. However, the integration of traditional medicine faces challenges stemming from differences in treatment, diagnosis, and health beliefs between traditional healers and biomedical health workers. Ecuador's legal framework, including the Health Code of 1971 and subsequent constitutional reforms in 1998 and 2008, recognize traditional medicine as an integral part of the national health system. The 2006 Organic Health Law further promotes the implementation and monitoring of traditional medicine practices and aims to bridge the gap between traditional healers and formal healthcare providers. Despite these efforts, barriers such as a lack of recognition, dialogue, and clearly defined roles persist, hindering effective collaboration within primary care teams (Bautista-Valarezo et al., 2021; Garrido, 2021).

CONCLUSION

Although there is increased recognition of the broader social, economic, and political power structures in causing health inequities, the Ecuadorian healthcare system is based on a biomedical curative system approach. While recent reforms have strengthened tertiary (hospital) care, public health demands outside of the healthcare system (e.g., lack of potable water and sanitation leading to the persistence of vector-borne diseases) remain unsolved. To address persistent systemic inequities, Ecuador's efforts should consider building a community-based system aimed at fostering communication for health promotion and prevention initiatives that tackle, rather than reinforce, systemic inequities. Policy and programmatic efforts should involve community voices in decision-making, particularly underserved, marginalized, and politically disempowered groups such as low-income, rural, and Indigenous communities, and be accompanied by independent scientific research and evaluation.

LEARNING ACTIVITIES

CourseConnect

To access self-assessment questions and interactive, competency-based learning activities for this chapter, visit www.springerpub.com/courseconnect. See inside front cover and tear-out for CourseConnect details.

REFERENCES

Asamblea Constituyente del Ecuador. (2008). *Constitución de la República del Ecuador* [Constitution of the Republic of Ecuador]. Tribunal Constitucional del Ecuador. Registro oficial No 449 (2008): 79–93. https://www.oas.org/juridico/pdfs/mesicic4_ecu_const.pdf

Ayala Mora, E. (2008). *Resumen de historia del Ecuador* [Summary of the history of Ecuador] (3rd updated ed.). Corporación Editora Nacional. https://repositorio.uasb.edu.ec/bitstream/10644/836/1/AYALAE-CON0001-RESUMEN.pdf

Bautista-Valarezo, E., Duque, V., Verhoeven, V., Mejia Chicaiza, J., Hendrickx, K., Maldonado-Rengel, R., & Michels, N. R. M. (2021). Perceptions of Ecuadorian Indigenous healers on their relationship with the formal health care system: Barriers and opportunities. *BMC Complementary Medicine and Therapies, 21*(65). https://doi.org/10.1186/s12906-021-03234-0

Cuéllar, L., Torres, I., Romero-Severson, E., Mahesh, R., Ortega, N., & Pungitore, S. (2021). Excess deaths reveal unequal impact of COVID-19 in Ecuador. *BMJ Global Health, 6*(9), e006446. https://doi.org/10.1136/bmjgh-2021-006446

Fernández, A., & Martínez, R. (2017). *The cost of the double burden of malnutrition: Social and economic impact. Summary of the pilot study in Chile, Ecuador and Mexico.* UN Economic Commission for Latin America and the Caribbean (ECLAC). https://reliefweb.int/report/world/cost-double-burden-malnutrition-social-and-economic-impact-summary-pilot-study-chile

Garrido, V. V. (2021). *Perceptions of traditional medicine in Ecuador* [Master's thesis, Center for International Studies, Ohio University]. https://etd.ohiolink.edu/acprod/odb_etd/ws/send_file/send?accession=ohiou1618062150942875&disposition=inline

González, J. (2017). *Ecuadorian traditions*. https://www.ecuador.com/culture/

Institute for Health Metrics and Evaluation. (2024). *Global burden of disease 2021: Findings from the GBD 2021 study*. Institute for Health Metrics and Evaluation.

Johnston, J., & Vasic-Lalovic, I. (2023). *Ecuador: A decade of progress, undone*. Center for Economic and Policy Research. https://cepr.net/wp-content/uploads/2023/08/Ecuador-Brief-Final-PDF-8.15.2023.pdf

Latinobarómetro. (2024). *Informe Latinobarómetro 2024: La Democracia Resiliente* [Latinobarómetro report 2024: Resilient democracy]. https://www.latinobarometro.org/lat.jsp

Ministerio de Relaciones Exteriores y Movilidad Humana. (2021). *Ecuador*. https://www.cancilleria.gob.ec/bolivia/wp-content/uploads/sites/22/2021/07/ECUADOR.pdf

Ministerio de Salud Pública del Ecuador. (2022). *Informe de Evaluación del Plan de Salud Mental 2014-2017* [Evaluation report of the mental health plan 2014–2017]. https://www.salud.gob.ec/salud-mental/

National Institute of Statistics and Census. (2018). *Encuesta nacional de salud y nutrición* [National health and nutrition survey]. Instituto Nacional de Estadística y Censos. https://www.ecuadorencifras.gob.ec/ensanut-ajustada-2018/

National Institute of Statistics and Census. (2020). *Principales resultados. Recursos y actividades de salud (RAS) 2020* [Main results. Health resources and activities (RAS) 2020]. Instituto Nacional de Estadística y Censos. https://www.ecuadorencifras.gob.ec/documentos/web-inec/Estadisticas_Sociales/Recursos_Actividades_de_Salud/RAS%1F_2020/Principales_resultado_RAS_2020.pdf

National Institute of Statistics and Census. (2022a). *Censo Ecuador, resultados nacionales principales* [Ecuador census, main national results]. Instituto Nacional de Estadística y Censos. https://www.censoecuador.gob.ec/wp-content/uploads/2023/09/InfoNacionalDatos.pdf

National Institute of Statistics and Census. (2022b). *Presentación de estadísticas vitales: Nacidos vivos y defunciones fetales 2022* [Presentation of vital statistics: Live births and fetal deaths 2022]. Instituto Nacional de Estadística y Censos. https://www.ecuadorencifras.gob.ec/documentos/web-inec/Poblacion_y_Demografia/Nacimientos_Defunciones/Nacidos_vivos_y_def_fetales_2022/Presentacion_ENV_y_EDF_2022.pdf

National Institute of Statistics and Census. (2022c). *Principales resultados: Matrimonios y divorcios 2022* [Main results of marriages and divorces 2022]. Instituto Nacional de Estadística y Censos. https://www.ecuadorencifras.gob.ec/documentos/web-inec/Poblacion_y_Demografia/Matrimonios_Divorcios/2022/Principales_resultados_MYD_2022.pdf

National Institute of Statistics and Census. (2022d). *Principales resultados: Defunciones generales 2022* [Main results of general deaths 2022]. Instituto Nacional de Estadística y Censos. https://www.ecuadorencifras.gob.ec/documentos/web-inec/Poblacion_y_Demografia/Defunciones_Generales_2022/Principales_resultados_EDG_2022.pdf

National Institute of Statistics and Census. (2022e). *Cuentas satélite de salud* [Health satellite accounts]. Instituto Nacional de Estadística y Censos. https://www.ecuadorencifras.gob.ec/cuentas-satelite-de-salud/

National Institute of Statistics and Census. (2022f). *Presentación de estadísticas de camas y egresos hospitalarios 2022* [Presentation of hospital beds and discharges statistics 2022]. Instituto Nacional de Estadística y Censos. https://www.ecuadorencifras.gob.ec/documentos/web-inec/Estadisticas_Sociales/Camas_Egresos_Hospitalarios/Cam_Egre_Hos_2022/Presentacion_ECEH_2022.pdf

National Institute of Statistics and Census. (2023). *Proyecciones de población y omisión censal* [Population projections and census omissions]. Instituto Nacional de Estadística y Censos. https://www.ecuadorencifras.gob.ec/documentos/web-inec/Poblacion_y_Demografia/Proyecciones_Poblacionales/censo_2022/2024-02-18_Proyeccciones_presenta_VF.pdf

National Institute of Statistics and Census. (2024). *Boletín de segunda entrega – Marzo 2024* [Bulletin of second delivery – March 2024]. Instituto Nacional de Estadística y Censos. https://www.ecuadorencifras.gob.ec/documentos/web-inec/Inflacion/2024/Marzo/Boletin_tecnico_03-2024-IPC.pdfl

Pan American Health Organization. (2022). *Perfil de País: Ecuador* [Country profile: Ecuador]. Organización Panamericana de la Salud. https://hia.paho.org/es/paises-2022/perfil-ecuador

Romero-Alvarez, D., Borbor-Córdova, M., Cañizares Fuentes, W. R., Ortiz-Prado, E., & Torres, I. (2024, November 12). *Implications of the limited availability and usefulness of publicly shared health data in Ecuador*. Preprint. https://doi.org/10.21203/rs.3.rs-5356211/v1

Romero-Alvarez, D., López-Cevallos, D. F., & Torres, I. (2023). Doctors for the people? The problematic distribution of rural service doctors in Ecuador. *Health Policy and Planning, 38*(7), 851–861. https://doi.org/10.1093/heapol/czad040

The Global Economy. (2024). *Ecuador: Unemployment rate (monthly)*. https://www.theglobaleconomy.com/Ecuador/unemployment_rate_monthly/

Torres, I., & López-Cevallos, D. (2017). ¿Reforma de salud en Ecuador como modelo de éxito? Crítica al número especial de la Revista Panamericana de Salud Pública [Ecuadorian health reform as a success model? A critique of the special issue of the Pan American Journal of Public Health]. *Revista Panamericana de Salud Pública, 41*, e148. https://doi.org/10.26633/RPSP.2017.148

Torres, I., & López-Cevallos, D. F. (2018). Institutional challenges to achieving health equity in Ecuador. *Lancet Global Health, 6*(8), E832–E833. https://doi.org/10.1016/S2214-109X(18)30245-6

Torres, I., Sippy, R., Bardosh, K. L., Bhargava, R., Lotto-Batista, M., et al. (2022). Chronic kidney disease in Ecuador: An epidemiological and health system analysis of an emerging public health crisis. *PLoS One, 17*(3), e0265395. https://doi.org/10.1371/journal.pone.0265395

UN Office for the Coordination of Humanitarian Affairs. (2021). *Informe de seguridad alimentaria: Evaluación remota – Ecuador* [Food security report: Remote assessment – Ecuador]. Oficina de las Naciones Unidas para la Coordinación de Asuntos Humanitarios. https://ecuador.un.org/es/161834-informe-de-seguridad-alimentaria-evaluacion-remota-ecuador

Varela, L. A., & Ron, S. R. (2018). *Geografía y clima del Ecuador* [Geography and climate of Ecuador]. BioWeb. Pontificia Universidad Católica del Ecuador. https://bioweb.bio/geografiaClima.html

World Health Orgnization. (2020). *Mental health atlas, Ecuador 2020: Country profile*. https://www.who.int/publications/m/item/mental-health-atlas-ecu-2020-country-profile

PART V: Health and Healthcare in the Caribbean

CHAPTER 16

OVERVIEW OF THE CARIBBEAN

Thomas Foley

GEOGRAPHY

The Caribbean is a region within the Americas that is known for its rich culture and geographic beauty. It is predominately compromised of hundreds of island nations within the Caribbean Sea and its surrounding borders and can be broken into the following broad regional categories: Greater Antilles, Lesser Antilles, Lucayan Archipelago (Brereton & Clarke, 2023), and areas of mainland Central and South America that include Belize, Guyana, Suriname, and French Guiana (Heuman, 2018). The **Greater Antilles** consists of six major island nations in the northern region of the Caribbean Sea: Cuba, Cayman Islands, Jamaica, Haiti, Dominican Republic, and Puerto Rico. The **Lesser Antilles** consists of an arc of islands along the eastern boundary of the Caribbean Sea and southern islands that are located north off of mainland Venezuela. The Lesser Antilles can be divided into three main regions: Leeward Islands, Windward Islands, and Leeward Antilles.

- The *Leeward Islands* consist of the northeastern islands of the Lesser Antilles, and include the Spanish Virgin Islands, U.S. Virgin Islands, British Virgin Islands, Anguilla, Saint Martin/Sint Maarten, Saint Barthelemy, Saba, Sint Eustatius, Saint Kitts and Nevis, Antigua and Barbuda, Montserrat, and Guadeloupe. Figure 16.1 shows Trunk Bay in the U.S. Virgin Islands.

FIGURE 16.1 Trunk Bay in the U.S. Virgin Islands.

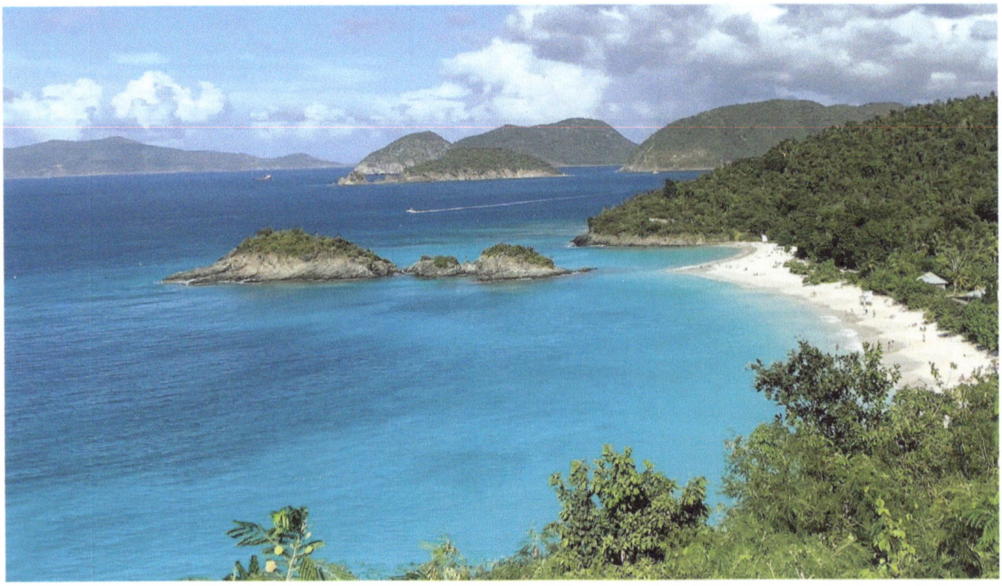

Source: National Park Service. (n.d.). *Trunk Bay*. U.S. Department of the Interior. https://www.nps.gov/places/trunk-bay.htm

- The *Winward Islands* consist of the southeastern islands of the Lesser Antilles. The Winward Islands include Dominica, Martinique, Saint Lucia, Barbados, Saint Vincent and the Grenadines, Grenada, and Trinidad and Tobago.
- The *Leeward Antilles* consist of the southwestern islands of the Lesser Antilles, which are located just north of mainland Venezuela. The Leeward Islands include the islands of the State of Nueva Esparta, the islands of the Federal Dependencies of Venezuela, Aruba, Bonaire, and Curacao.

The **Lucayan Archipelago** is neither located in the Caribbean Sea nor on its border; however, is commonly considered to be part of the Caribbean. The Lucayan Archipelago is located in the western area of the Northern Atlantic Ocean, north of Cuba and southeast of Florida. It includes the Bahamas and Turks and Caicos. Figure 16.2 shows a map of the Caribbean.

POPULATION

In 2023, there were more than 44.6 million people living in the Caribbean. About 90% of the Caribbean population lives in the most populous nations of the Greater Antilles: Haiti (11.7 million), Dominican Republic (11.3 million), and Cuba (11.1 million). Montserrat (4,400) and Saint Barthelemy (11,000) in the Lesser Antilles are the least populous (UN Data Portal, n.d.). The Caribbean is a relatively young region with approximately 31% of the population under the age of 20 years and only approximately 10.75% of the population over the age of 65 and older. However, age-based demographics in the Caribbean are significantly influenced by Haiti. Haiti's under-20 population accounted for more than 40% of Haiti's total population in 2023 while the older adult population accounted for less than 5%. There are several less populated Caribbean nations that are experiencing population aging. In Guadeloupe, for example, the older population accounted for more than 20% of the population during 2023 (UN Data Portal, n.d.).

FIGURE 16.2 Map of the Caribbean

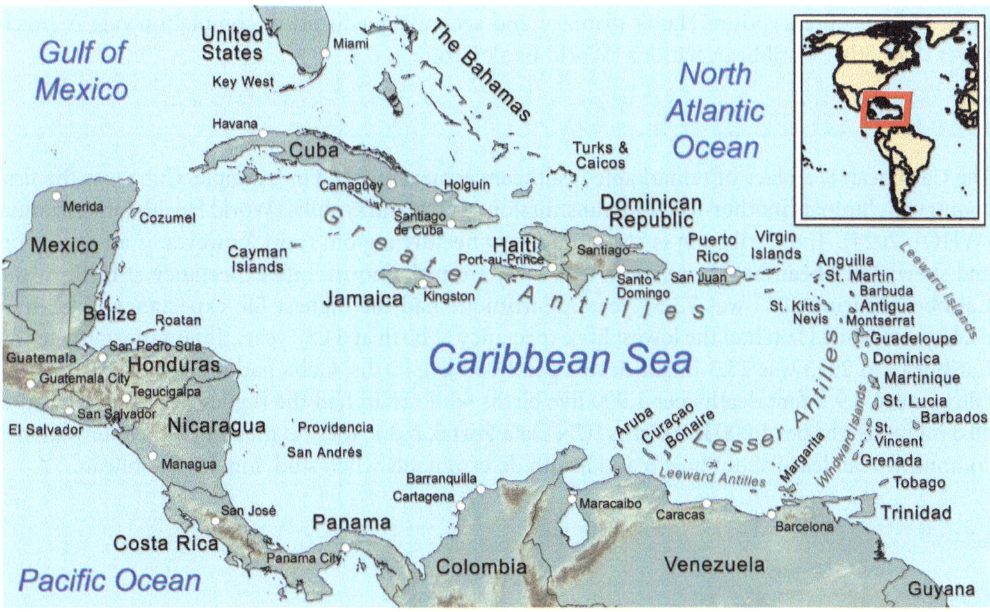

Source: Kmusser. (n.d.). *General map of the Caribbean*. https://commons.wikimedia.org/wiki/File:Caribbean_general_map.png

BRIEF HISTORY

The original settlement of the Americas spread into the Caribbean Islands from Central and South America several thousand years ago. The native populations of the Caribbean Islands such as the Taino in the Greater Antilles and the Igneri in the Lesser Antilles thrived for a few thousand years prior to the arrival of European colonizers who brought disease, death, and exploitation of the land and native people (Estevez, 2019). The European colonizers also transported enslaved people from Africa to work in the fields and mines of the Caribbean Islands. Early in the 1700s, nearly 80% of the Caribbean population was from Africa (National Museums Liverpool, 2024). After the abolishment of slavery, the colonizers exploited hundreds of thousands of people from South Asian countries, such as India, to work in the Caribbean under the slavelike practice of indentured servitude during the mid-19th to early-20th centuries (Roopnarine, 2022).

Self-liberated enslaved Haitians established the independent nation of Haiti in 1804 by defeating Napoleon's French Army during the Haitian Revolution, making Haiti the first independent nation of the Caribbean (Roy & Labrador, 2024). The latest Caribbean country to establish independence was St. Kitts and Nevis, which declared independence from the British in 1983 (Nicolas et al., 2012). Because of its history, the Caribbean is a culturally diverse country drawing from the Afro-Caribbean, Asian-Caribbean (predominately Indo-Caribbean), European-Caribbean, Hispanic-Caribbean, and Caribbean Native populations (Caribbean Community Secretariat, 2025). There are more than 70 languages used in the Caribbean. Spanish is the most common in the Greater Antilles and English is the most common in the Lesser Antilles (The Department of Modern Languages and Linguistics, n.d.).

SOCIOECONOMIC FACTORS

The Caribbean has notable socioeconomic disparities. The Cayman Islands is one of the wealthiest places in the world with a per-capita gross domestic product (GDP) of about $100,000. Haiti is one of the poorest countries in the world with a per-capita GDP of less than $2,000. With the exception of Haiti, the nations of the Caribbean are either near or above the world average per capita GDP. While the completion rate of primary and secondary education in the Caribbean is high, Haiti is an exception. Haiti's primary and secondary education completion rate is much lower than other Caribbean nations (World Bank Group, n.d.).

HEALTH OUTCOMES

The Caribbean is a place of remarkable healthcare achievements. For example, Cuba was the first country to eliminate mother-to-child transmission of HIV and syphilis (World Health Organization [WHO], 2024). The Caribbean is also a relatively healthy region. Haiti, however, is an exception and skews Caribbean health outcome data away from the norm. Life expectancy at birth in the Caribbean during 2023 was 73.33 years. Martinique had the highest life expectancy at birth at 84.45 years while Haiti had the lowest life expectancy at birth at 64.57 years. Infant mortality in the Caribbean in 2023 was 25.3 infant deaths per 1,000 live births. Cuba had the lowest infant mortality rate at 3.9 infant deaths per 1,000 live births while Haiti had the highest infant mortality at 40.8 infant deaths per 1,000 live births (UN Data Portal, n.d.). There is much that the international community can learn about health and health determinants when studying the Caribbean.

LEARNING ACTIVITIES

CourseConnect

To access self-assessment questions and interactive, competency-based learning activities for this chapter, visit www.springerpub.com/courseconnect. See inside front cover and tear-out for CourseConnect details.

REFERENCES

Brereton, B. M., & Clarke, C. G (2023). *West Indies*. Britannica. https://www.britannica.com/place/West-Indies-island-group-Atlantic-Ocean/Decolonization

Caribbean Community Secretariat. (2025). *Our people*. CARICOM. https://caricom.org/our-community/who-we-are/our-people/

The Department of Modern Languages and Linguistics. (n.d.). *Languages of the Caribbean*. The University of the West Indies, St. Augustine. https://sta.uwi.edu/fhe/dmll/languages-caribbean

Estevez, J. B. (2019). *Meet the survivors of a "Paper Genocide."* National Geographic. https://www.nationalgeographic.com/history/article/meet-survivors-taino-tribe-paper-genocide

Heuman, G. (2018). *The Caribbean: A brief history* (3rd ed.). Bloomsbury Atlantic.

National Museums Liverpool. (2024). *Slavery in the Caribbean*. https://www.liverpoolmuseums.org.uk/archaeologyofslavery/slavery-caribbean

Nicolas, G., Jean-Jacques, R., & Wheatley, A. (2012). Mental health counseling in Haiti: Historical overview, current status, and plans for the future. *Journal of Black Psychology, 38*(4), 509–519. https://psycnet.apa.org/doi/10.1177/0095798412443162

Roopnarine, L. (2022). *Latin American history: South Asian diaspora in the Caribbean*. Oxford University Press.

Roy, D., & Labrador, R. C. (2024). *Haiti's troubled path to development*. Council on Foreign Relations. https://www.cfr.org/backgrounder/haitis-troubled-path-development.

UN Data Portal. (n.d.). *UN population division data portal: Interactive access to global demographic indicators*. United Nations. https://population.un.org/dataportal/home

World Bank Group. (n.d.). *The World Bank open data*. The World Bank Group. https://data.worldbank.org/

World Health Organization. (2024). *WHO validates elimination of mother-to-child transmission of HIV and syphilis in Cuba*. https://www.who.int/news/item/30-06-2015-who-validates-elimination-of-mother-to-child-transmission-of-hiv-and-syphilis-in-cuba

CHAPTER 17

TRINIDAD AND TOBAGO

Kimberly D. Harry

INTRODUCTION

The **Republic of Trinidad and Tobago (T&T)** is a twin-island country in the Caribbean region with a unique societal structure, traditions, history, and religious backgrounds that influence health and healthcare practices. Although T&T is proactively advancing its healthcare service and delivery, worthwhile opportunities remain to ameliorate healthcare administration, implement healthcare innovation, and institute healthcare reforms and policies that benefit all its citizens and residents.

GEOGRAPHY

The twin-island Republic of T&T lies south of Grenada and approximately 6 to 7 miles northeast of mainland Venezuela. T&T is the most southerly country of the Caribbean archipelago and covers a total land area of 5,131 square kilometers (3,188 miles; Central Intelligence Agency [CIA], 2024). The country is subdivided into 15 primary geographical regions shown on the map in Figure 17.1, and operates three main port cities of Port-of-Spain, San Fernando, and Scarborough.

FIGURE 17.1 Map showing Trinidad and Tobago's geolocation and country subdivisions.

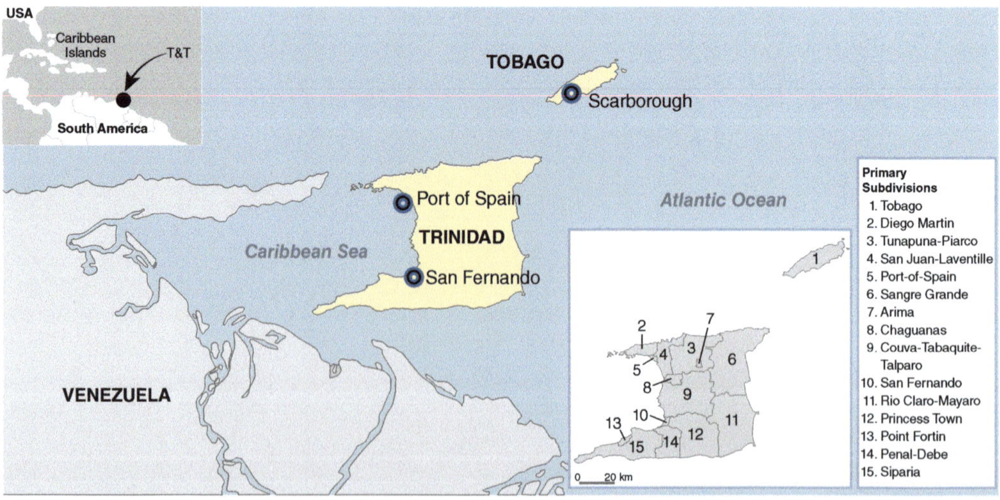

DEMOGRAPHIC FEATURES

OVERVIEW

T&T's population in 2023 was approximately 1.5 million people (UN Data Portal, n.d.), with just an estimated 4% of its total population living on the much smaller island of Tobago. The majority of the country's population consists of people of African and East Indian descent living in close proximity to or within urban centers. There are also sparsely populated rural communities distributed across both islands. Diversity within the nation's growing population and its various communities spans the demographic and cultural dimensions of age, race, ethnicity, and language (Central Statistical Office [CSo], 2023).

AGE

T&T has a rapidly aging population. The 2021 **aging index,** given by T&T's CSO, is 43.5. This aging index represents the number of older individuals (65+) per 100 persons younger than 15 years old within the population (CSO, 2023). T&T's median age in 2023 was 36.7 years, well above the world average of 30.4, and an increase of slightly more than 10 years when compared to the start of the 21st century. In 2023, approximately 75% of the population was 20 years old or older. Adults age 65 or older accounted for nearly 12% of the total population. At the turn of the century, less than 5% of the total population in T&T was 65 years or older. In addition, the birth rate has been declining in T&T from 14.9 births per 1,000 people to 10.7 per 1,000 in 2023 (UN Data Portal, n.d.).

ETHNICITY/RACE AND IMMIGRATION/EMIGRATION

T&T is a cosmopolitan mix of two major ethnicities, Afro-Trinidadians and Indo-Trinidadians, together with smaller ethnic groups consisting of Whites, Chinese, Latinx, Filipino/a, Middle Eastern people (predominantly Syrian/Lebanese), and people of mixed heritage (CSO, 2023). Data provided by Warner et al. (2018) indicate population distributions of 31.76% Afro-Trinidadians, 37.01% Indo-Trinidadians, 23.52% mixed heritage, and less than 1.0% non-Afro/Indo-Trinidadian/Mixed Heritage. An influx of migrants to T&T has started to reshape the racial/ethnic profile of the population, mainly through the growth of the Latinx and mixed heritage groups. According to a UN High Commissioner for Refugees (UNHCR) estimate, immigration of over 40,000 Venezuelan migrants occurred, largely due to the geopolitical and economic crisis surrounding Venezuela in recent years (Centers for Disease Control and Prevention [CDC], 2025).

Since 2010, T&T has also experienced high emigration rates of mostly high-skilled workers to Organisation for Economic Co-operation and Development (OECD) destinations, including the United States (Pekkala-Kerr et al., 2017). Furthermore, Pekkala-Kerr et al. (2017) note that many origin countries have limited educational capacities and fiscal resources to train workers or to replace those that have emigrated. Nunes and Stevenson's (2009) research highlights the challenges T&T faces in attracting and retaining primary care doctors, a key issue impacting the country's healthcare delivery system's effectiveness. Their study underscores the importance of primary care in the healthcare system, particularly in managing the shift from infectious to chronic noncommunicable diseases (namely, ischemic heart disease and diabetes mellitus), a trend prevalent in T&T. The migration dilemma, physician retention, and the future need as it relates to primary care are crucial in understanding the broader context of healthcare provision and the need for strategic planning in medical education and healthcare workforce development (Nunes & Stevenson, 2009).

LANGUAGE

English is the accepted official language of T&T, although **Bhojpuri** (a Hindi dialect) and **French patois** (Creole) are popular **colloquial languages** (informal/conversational and common) appearing in speech and music, mostly in the rural areas of T&T. Communication between healthcare providers and recipients of medical care in T&T is viewed as an area of concern related to the issue of migration (Modeste-James & Huggins, 2022). Modeste-James and Huggins (2022) explored the language barrier faced by Spanish-speaking Venezuelan migrants in accessing healthcare in T&T. Their study reveals that language barriers could potentially hinder optimal care coordination, suggesting a gap that could inhibit the ability of the nation's healthcare system to adequately respond to the needs of a linguistically diverse population. Further, their research points to the necessity for developing inclusive healthcare policies that ensure equitable access to healthcare services for all of the country's residents, including migrant populations (Modeste-James & Huggins, 2022).

HEALTH OUTCOMES

LIFE EXPECTANCY AT BIRTH

Life expectancy at birth in T&T during 2023 was approximately 73.5 years—a gain of nearly 5 years when compared to the start of the 21st century when life expectancy at birth in T&T was approximately 68.6 years. In addition, T&T's life expectancy at birth in 2023 was slightly above the world average of 73.17 and the Caribbean regional average of 73.13 years (UN Data Portal, n.d.).

NEONATAL, INFANT, AND MATERNAL MORTALITY

The recorded maternal mortality ratio in T&T during 2020 was 26.6 maternal deaths per 100,000 live births—well below the 2020 global maternal mortality ratio, which was 223.5 maternal deaths per 100,000 live births (UN Population Fund, 2024). The infant mortality rate for T&T in 2023 was 13.5 deaths per 1,000 live births (UN Data Portal, n.d.). While the infant mortality rate in T&T was below the Caribbean regional average, some Caribbean countries had more favorable infant mortality rates, including Cuba (4.4 deaths per 1,000 live births), Antigua and Barbuda (7.5), and Barbados (9.4). While the infant mortality rate represents the number of deaths per 1,000 live births associated with the age range of 0 to 12 months, **neonatal mortality** represents the newborn mortality period during the first 28 days of life for a given year (UNICEF, 2023). The neonatal mortality rate for T&T in 2021 was recorded as 10.3 deaths per 1,000 live births (UN Population Fund, 2024) and is expected to drop to 10 deaths per 1,000 live births in 2024, a target set below the United Nations goal of 12 deaths per 1,000 live births (UNICEF, 2023).

LEADING CAUSES OF MORTALITY AND LEADING MORBIDITY AND MORTALITY RISK FACTORS

In 2021, the leading causes of mortality in T&T were COVID-19, cardiovascular disease (CVD), diabetes mellitus, stroke, chronic kidney disease (CKD), prostate cancer, interpersonal violence, Alzheimer disease, and colorectal cancer (Institute for Health Metrics and Evaluation [IHME], n.d.). Refer to Figure 17.2 (IHME, n.d.) for a comparison of the leading causes of mortality in T&T during 2011 and 2021.

The leading morbidity and mortality risk factors in T&T represent a country that is rapidly aging and experiencing significant mortality from noncommunicable conditions such as CVD, diabetes, and CKD. In 2021, T&T's leading risk factors were high fasting-plasma glucose, high body mass index, hypertension, poor diet, air pollution, kidney dysfunction, tobacco use, high low density lipoprotein cholesterol, and alcohol abuse (IHME, n.d.).

NONCOMMUNICABLE AND COMMUNICABLE DISEASES

T&T has undergone an epidemiologic transition over time characterized by a decline in deaths from communicable diseases and an increase in morbidity and mortality from noncommunicable

FIGURE 17.2 Leading causes of mortality in Trinidad and Tobago during 2011 and 2021.

Cause	2011 rank	2021 rank	Change in deaths per 100k, 2011–2021
COVID-19	–	1	↑ +235.0
Ischemic heart disease	1	2	↑ +26.9
Diabetes	2	3	↑ +34.1
Stroke	3	4	↑ +22.7
Chronic kidney disease	4	5	↑ +16.4
Prostate cancer	6	6	↑ +7.9
Interpersonal violence	5	7	↓ −1.6
Hypertensive heart disease	7	8	↑ +4.7
Alzheimer disease	10	9	↑ +5.1
Colorectal cancer	12	10	↑ +5.4

Communicable, maternal, neonatal, and nutritional diseases; Noncommunicable diseases; Injuries

Source: Institute for Health Metrics and Evaluation. (n.d.). *Trinidad and Tobago*. https://www.healthdata.org/research-analysis/health-by-location/profiles/trinidad-and-tobago

diseases (NCDs). Diether Beuermann et al. (2018) indicate that NCDs account for 78% of mortality in T&T and the six common NCDs (diabetes, cancer, chronic respiratory illness, heart disease, hypertension, and cerebrovascular disease) account for 60% of mortality. While chronic respiratory illnesses continue to cause significant mortality in T&T, there has been a drastic reduction in the percentage of deaths caused by bronchitis and emphysema (i.e., COPD) and asthma over the past several decades.

In the 1980s and 1990s, HIV/AIDS was a major problem in T&T. Infection and death rates were high and steadily increasing. The country received assistance from the United States to combat HIV/AIDS via the President's Emergency Plan for AIDS Relief (PEPFAR), which included the provision for expanding access to treatment for HIV-infected individuals. HIV/AIDS morbidity and mortality in T&T have vastly improved as a result; however, there is concern about rising HIV incidences in younger populations between the ages of 15 and 25 years (CDC, 2025).

MENTAL ILLNESS, SERVICE DELIVERY, AND FACILITIES

Psychosis and schizophrenia are two common mental health disorders prevalent in T&T. Primary mental health concerns in T&T stem from substance abuse (primarily from alcohol and cannabis use) and suicidal ideation (Hutchinson, 2023). Limited resources supporting mental health services pose challenges to T&T's ability to address mental health concerns. Increasing awareness in mental health, improving access to mental health services, and integrating mental health into primary healthcare are viewed as some of the necessary steps in addressing mental health issues such as psychosis, schizophrenia, suicide ideation, and substance abuse disorders. Furthermore, Hutchinson (2023) points to the vulnerability of young men living in urban areas to psychosis risk factors such as cannabis use and a family history of mental health disorders (Hutchinson, 2023).

Mental health services are administered at a major public hospital in the capital city, **Port of Spain.** Additionally, there are about 14 mental health clinics spread throughout T&T to facilitate mental health service delivery in keeping with the nation's mental health policy and plan. Psychiatric units are also available at a large general hospital in the south of Trinidad and one of the district hospitals in Tobago (Berkeley, 2019).

DETERMINANTS OF HEALTH

HEALTH BEHAVIORS

Health behavior is a function of a number of sociodemographic variables, including different ethnicities, socialization, social class, geographic zones, and culturalization (Bourne, 2009). Modifiable lifestyle risk factors for CVD, a known preventable NCD, include unhealthy diet, inadequate exercise, unhealthy weight, smoking/tobacco misuse, excessive alcohol use, stress, birth control, and hormone replacement therapy, and are related to these sociodemographic variables (Baer et al., 2011). In T&T, these lifestyle risk factors are key influencers of morbidity and mortality associated with CVD and other preventable NCDs such as diabetes and CKD (Maharaj et al., 2017).

SOCIAL AND ECONOMIC FACTORS

The gross domestic product (GDP) of T&T in 2023 was $28.14 billion. The per-capita GDP was $18,333, an outcome considered as high human development (HHD). In addition, T&T has low unemployment (4.2% in 2023), as the economy has been steadily improving (World Bank Group, n.d.).

T&T is generally regarded as a country with a high literacy rate (UN Population Fund, 2024) and a country continuously aligning with the 21st-century knowledge economy. However, Shah et al. (2020, p. 229) provide insights into the effect that heads of household lacking primary school-level education (PSE) could have on the resiliency of households within the rural communities of agriculture-based counties such as Caroni and Nariva (see subregions 3, 8, 9 [Caroni] and 6, 11 [Nariva] in Figure 17.1). Shah et al. (2020) note that in the Caroni County region, one in five persons possess PSE, while in the Nariva County region, one in three persons possess PSE. Further, Shah et al. (2020) demonstrate empirically that resiliency is linked to household food security. The findings emphasize the need for increasing literacy rates in at-risk geographic zones to ensure food-secure communities.

The **Human Development Index (HDI)** is a metric developed by the United Nations that considers the performance of a country in three main achievement areas: life expectancy at birth, knowledge/literacy rate, and standard of living quality (GDP per capita). Based on its HDI of 0.81, T&T is classified as a developing nation with very high human development and a low level of poverty (UN Development Programme, 2025). T&T continues to progress in the area of social justice as a country willing to protect human rights. The country generally allows domestic and international human rights groups to investigate and publish their findings on human rights issues and violations. The government of T&T, working together with the UNHCR office and other humanitarian organizations, continues to seek and provide protection and assistance needed by refugee and asylum-seeking migrants, as well as other vulnerable groups. A 2020 policy draft seeking the provision of public healthcare services for nonnationals is noted as an important step toward promoting equity for these vulnerable populations (Lyons & Bhagwandeen, 2023).

RELIGIOUS ASPECTS

T&T has a diversity of religious beliefs and practices. The religious makeup of the twin island republic includes Roman Catholics (21.6%), Protestants (12.9%), Hinduists (18.2%), Muslims (5%), Anglicans (5.7%), Baptists (6.9%), Adventists (4.1%), Presbyterians (2.5%), Jehovah Witnesses (1.5%), nondenominational (2.2%), and other religions (19.4%; CIA, 2024). The diversity of religious beliefs and practices affects health and healthcare in T&T. Research involving prostate cancer among men in T&T identified various religious and cultural factors that prevent individuals from seeking conventional (allopathic) medical treatment (King-Okoye et al., 2019; Teye-Kwadjo et al., 2023). Bourne advises on the usefulness of understanding people's health-care-seeking behaviors that are influenced by religion, as it is a critical component in the planning of health policy (Bourne, 2009). To address conditions of ill health, some people may resort to seeking out religious leaders or spiritual advisors for faith-based healing, prayer, and spiritual therapy and may even refuse to seek the services of conventional healthcare practitioners (Teye-Kwadjo et al., 2023). King-Okoye et al.'s (2019) work highlights how religious beliefs and perceptions among male adults (including some of African descent) with prostate illness influence their health behaviors. Teye-Kwadjo et al. (2023) commented on research conducted at an oncology clinic in T&T, which indicated that medicinal herbs and spiritual therapy interventions offered perceived benefits and satisfaction to individuals. Moreover, Afro-Trinbagonian women, who are descendants of Africans brought to the Caribbean (including T&T) during the Atlantic slave trade, often practice forms of traditional healthcare with religious influences.

HEALTHCARE SYSTEM

HEALTHCARE SYSTEM STRUCTURE

T&T operates its healthcare system using the universal healthcare model (Bahall, 2018). The country has a dual public/private healthcare system consisting of government-run public hospitals and health centers and privately owned medical facilities. Under the universal healthcare model, the public has access to a wide range of healthcare services at zero cost to beneficiaries. However, if the private healthcare system is accessed, financial payments are needed for the services provided. In some instances, and in urgent cases, long waiting times for medical treatments through the public health system may require accessing the private healthcare system. Members of the public may also perceive that a higher quality of care is available from certain sections of the private care system.

The **T&T Ministry of Health** (MoH) is the leading authority with responsibility for supervising the country's entire health system. The central role of the T&T MoH is to protect the population's health and to ensure that all organizations and institutions providing healthcare services and products are compliant with local and international safety standards. Autonomy for the actual delivery of public healthcare services to the population resides with **regional health authorities (RHAs).** RHAs own and operate health facilities within their various sectors, providing a suite of services that include accident and emergency services; surgical, laboratory, pharmacy, medical imaging, and dental health services; clinics for treating chronic and/or lifestyle diseases; antenatal, postnatal, family planning, and child health clinics; and health promotion fitness programs. Examples of RHAs include the Eastern Regional Health Authority, the North Central Regional Health Authority, the Northwest Regional Health Authority, the Southwest Regional Health Authority, and the Tobago Regional Health Authority (Berkeley, 2019).

HEALTHCARE DELIVERY, FINANCE, INSURANCE, AND PAYMENT

Citizens are entitled to healthcare services at existing public facilities without making payments. No health insurance is required, and medicines are free at public healthcare facilities. Funding for public medical services is made via the government's fiscal contributions to its various RHAs. The delivery of primary-level public healthcare services occurs within more than 90 health centers and nine district health facilities. Secondary-level public healthcare is delivered at the country's nine regional public hospitals under the management and direction of the T&T MoH. The public health system provides a variety of services, including basic and specialized examinations, treatments for chronic diseases, kidney dialysis treatment, renal transplants, angioplasty, laparoscopic and open-heart surgery, lithotripsy, and other specialized treatments (Bahall, 2018).

The private healthcare sector in T&T is relatively small, mainly comprised of individual physicians, about 10 medical facilities with the capacity for handling up to 39,000 patients, and private pharmacies. Private medical facilities are located mainly in urban districts and private healthcare is delivered on a fee-for-service basis and financed by private health insurance or out-of-pocket expenses. Although the government does not finance private medical institutions, authority may be granted for the public health sector to subcontract private healthcare services (Diether Beuermann et al., 2018).

HEALTHCARE TRAINING AND EDUCATION

Colwill et al. (2008) forecasted that world population growth and aging would increase physician's workload by 29% between 2005 and 2025 (Colwill et al., 2008). Further, they predicted that only a 7% increase in the number of physicians would be occurring simultaneously, thereby creating a shortfall of physicians needed to provide medical services. Nunes and Stevenson (2009) describe the extreme need for T&T to provide and retain an adequate number of primary care physicians. Caribbean medical schools must ensure an adequate flow of doctors into primary healthcare services. In T&T, the shortage of nurses has also been a major issue regarding the delivery of healthcare. Factors such as migration, retirement, and change of career collectively contribute to the nursing shortages. Prioritizing incentives is needed to retain nurses within the healthcare system (Onuoha et al., 2015). Educational advancements at T&T institutions such as the University of the West Indies (UWI) School of Nursing at St. Augustine, together with motivational elements aligned with career service, will play an integral role in the future of the nursing profession in T&T. Barton (2008) discusses the role of UWI in the evolution of healthcare in the Caribbean, including T&T. UWI's contribution to medical education and research over the past 60 years has been instrumental in shaping healthcare policies and practices in the region. The development of medical education and research capabilities has influenced policy decisions, particularly in areas such as maternal health, infectious disease control, and chronic disease management. This evolution underscores the importance of academic institutions in driving policy changes and innovations in healthcare (Barton, 2008).

HEALTHCARE PRACTICES

TRADITIONAL MEDICINE

Traditional medicine or "**bush medicine**" (i.e., plant/herbal medicine) is a cultural practice in T&T and other Caribbean countries. The practice of bush medicine among T&T's population comes from the cultural fusion of practices inherited from the Indigenous People and ethnic migrant groups that lived in the country. In traditional healthcare, plants with medicinal properties, found in cultivated gardens or uncultivated lands, are used to treat various medical conditions. Naturopathic doctors and herbal practitioners usually prescribe bush medicines. Clement et al. (2015) underscore the medicinal value of various herbs, fruits, and vegetables used to prevent and cure ailments in T&T and other nations in the Caribbean.

ALTERNATIVE MEDICINE

Alternative medicine is a widely used and popular form of healthcare in T&T (Clement et al., 2015). Segments of the population hold the view that alternative practices offer a more holistic approach to healthcare. Alternative practices include the use of herbal medicine (for treating a variety of health conditions), acupuncture (for promoting healing and stimulating energy flow), massage therapy (for reducing stress, relieving muscle tension, and promoting relaxation), energy healing (utilizing energy fields to which the body is exposed), and aromatherapy (for removing stress and anxiety, improving sleep, and boosting energy).

CONCLUSION

Modern healthcare systems are shifting toward the adoption of a more patient-centered approach in the delivery of healthcare services. This is a global trend that T&T must progressively embrace in order to promote health equity and high quality of life outcomes. In addition, the country must continue to embrace and utilize best practices for the provision of quality primary care and maternal and newborn/infant healthcare to safeguard human capital. Furthermore, the shift in the disease pattern in T&T (Diether Beuermann et al., 2018) emphasizes the need for sharpening the focus on NCDs by pursuing developments and continuous improvement in NCD policy and action plans and for Caribbean medical schools and institutions to maintain efficient and effective capabilities and capacities for ensuring adequate training, development, and supply of doctors and nurses for primary care. More emphasis should be placed on strategic planning in medical education and healthcare workforce development (Nunes & Stevenson, 2009). Lastly, there is a need for policy reforms that accommodate the healthcare needs of migrants and provide equitable access to healthcare (Modeste-James & Huggins, 2022).

LEARNING ACTIVITIES

CourseConnect

To access self-assessment questions and interactive, competency-based learning activities for this chapter, visit www.springerpub.com/courseconnect. See inside front cover and tear-out for CourseConnect details.

REFERENCES

Baer, H. J., Glynn, R. J., Hu, F. B., Hankinson, S. E., Willett, W. C., Colditz, G. A., Stampfer, M., & Rosner, B. (2011). Risk factors for mortality in the nurses' health study: A competing risks analysis. *American Journal of Epidemiology, 173*(3), 319–329. doi:10.1093/aje/kwq368

Bahall, M. (2018). Health equity and access to health care in Trinidad and Tobago. *World Journal of Public Health, 3*(3), 83. doi:10.11648/j.wjph.20180303.13

Barton, E. N. (2008). Sixtieth anniversary of the University of the West Indies. *PubMed, 57*(6), 523–524.

Berkeley, B. (2019). An analysis of the problems users experience in public health care facilities in Trinidad and Tobago. *OALib, 6*(7), 1–13. https://doi.org/10.4236/oalib.1105364

Bourne, P. A. (2009). Health status and medical care-seeking behaviour of the poorest 20% in Jamaica. *International Journal of Collaborative Research on Internal Medicine and Public Health, 1*(6), 167–185.

Centers for Disease Control and Prevention. (2025). *HIV and TB overview: Trinidad and Tobago.* https://www.cdc.gov/global-hiv-tb/php/where-we-work/trinidadtobago.html

Central Intelligence Agency. (2024). *Country profiles: Trinidad and Tobago.* https://www.cia.gov/the world-factbook/countries/trinidad-and-tobago/

Central Statistical Office. (2023). *Population statistic.* https://cso.gov.tt/subjects/population-and-vital-statistics/population/

Clement, Y. N., Baksh-Comeau, Y. S., & Seaforth, C. E. (2015). An ethnobotanical survey of medicinal plants in Trinidad. *Journal of Ethnobiology and Ethnomedicine, 11*(1), 1–28. https://doi.org/10.1186/s13002-015-0052-0

Colwill, J. M., Cultice, J. M., & Kruse, R. L. (2008). Will generalist physician supply meet demands of an increasing and aging population? *Health affairs (Project Hope), 27*(3), w232–w241. https://doi.org/10.1377/hlthaff.27.3.w232

Diether Beuermann, Schwartz, M., Juan Pedro Schmid, Dippel, C., Jeetendra Khadan, Fajgenbaum, J., Loser, C., Wright, A., Waithe, K., Bollers, E., Bonnett, K., Mejia, C., Mooney, H., & Smets, L. (2018). *Nurturing institutions for a resilient Caribbean.* Inter-American Development Bank.

Hutchinson, G. (2023). Trinidad and Tobago. In C. Morgan, A. Cohen, & T. Roberts (Eds.), *Psychosis: Global perspectives* (pp. 265–278). Oxford University Press EBooks. https://doi.org/10.1093/med/9780198735588.003.0011

Institute for Health Metrics and Evaluation. (n.d.). *Health research by location: Country profiles.* University of Washington. https://www.healthdata.org/research-analysis/health-by-location/profiles

King-Okoye, M., Arber, A., & Faithfull, S. (2019). Beliefs that contribute to delays in diagnosis of prostate cancer among Afro-Caribbean men in Trinidad and Tobago. *Psycho-oncology, 28*(6), 1321–1327. https://doi.org/10.1002/pon.5085

Lyons, N., & Bhagwandeen, B. (2023). Examining healthcare needs and decisions to seek health services among Venezuelan migrants living in Trinidad and Tobago using Andersen's behavioral model. *Frontiers in Public Health, 11*, 1212825. https://doi.org/10.3389/fpubh.2023.1212825

Maharaj, R. G., Motilal, M. S., Babwah, T., Nunes, P., Brathwaite, R., Legall, G., Reid, S. D., Canavan, M. E., & Bradley, E. H. (2017). National alcohol survey of households in Trinidad and Tobago (NASHTT):

Alcohol use in households. *BMC Public Health, 17*(1), 347. https://doi.org/10.1186/s12889-017-4266-z

Modeste-James, A., & Huggins, C. (2022). Barriers to healthcare for Venezuelan migrants: Physicians' perspective. *International Journal of Health Governance, 27*(3), 329–341. https://doi.org/10.1108/ijhg-08-2021-0078

Nunes, P., & Stevenson, K. (2009). Providing quality primary care in the Caribbean. *Quality in Primary Care, 17*(6), 381–383.

Onuoha, P. C., Ramcharan, M., London, N., Ramlal, I., Sheen-Daniel, L. A., & Ezenwaka, C. E. (2015). Motivational factors and techniques at the workplace: Perspective of nurses in two major hospitals in Trinidad. *Asian Journal of Science and Technology, 6*(5), 1388–1392.

Pekkala-Kerr S., Kerr, W.,Ozden, C., Parsons, C. R. (2017). High-skilled migration and agglomeration. *Annual Review of Economics, 9*(1), 201–234.

Shah, K. U., Dulal, H. B., & Awojobi, M. T. (2020). Food security and livelihood vulnerability to climate change in Trinidad and Tobago. In J. Connell & K. Lowitt (Eds.), *Food security in small island states.* Springer. https://doi.org/10.1007/978-981-13-8256-7_12

Teye-Kwadjo, E., Goka, A. S., & Ussher, Y. A. A. (2023). Complementary and alternative medicine use by Ghanaian patients with breast cancer. *Trends in Psychology,* 1–21. https://doi.org/10.1007/s43076-023-00327-2

UNICEF. (2023, January). *Neonatal mortality—UNICEF data.* https://data.unicef.org/topic/child-survival/neonatal-mortality/

UN Data Portal. (n.d.). *UN population division data portal.* United Nations. https://population.un.org/dataportal/home/

UN Development Programme. (2025). *Human development index.* https://hdr.undp.org/data-center/human-development-index#/indicies/HDI

UN Population Fund. (2024). *Data portal.* United Nations. https://www.unfpa.org/data

Warner, W. A., Lee, T. Y., Badal, K., Williams, T. M., Bajracharya, S., Sundaram, V., Bascombe, N. A., Maharaj, R., Lamont-Greene, M., Roach, A., Bondy, M., Ellis, M. J., Rebbeck, T. R., Slovacek, S., Luo, J., Toriola, A. T., & Llanos, A. A. M. (2018). Cancer incidence and mortality rates and trends in Trinidad and Tobago. *BMC Cancer, 18*(1), 712. https://doi.org/10.1186/s12885-018-4625-x

World Bank Group. (n.d.). *The World Bank open data.* https://data.worldbank.org/

CHAPTER 18

BARBADOS

Heather Harewood and Roger Sealy

GEOGRAPHIC AND DEMOGRAPHIC FEATURES

Barbados, a **small island developing state (SIDS;** Box 18.1), spanning 430 square kilometers (267 square miles), is the easternmost island in the Caribbean (Central Intelligence Agency [CIA], 2024). The name Barbados derives from the Portuguese **Los Barbados** (the bearded ones), due to the bearded fig trees observed on the island's shores. Barbados is flat with a unique limestone composition in contrast to other volcanic Caribbean islands. The highest point, Mt. Hillaby (336 meters or 1,100 feet above sea level), is in the north central Scotland District with clay soil prone to land slippage (Commonwealth Network, 2013).

Barbados is one of the most populous Caribbean Island nations located in the Lesser Antilles. In 2023, the population of Barbados was 282,336 (UN Data Portal, n.d.). Barbados is also one of the most densely populated countries in the world with approximately 668 inhabitants per square kilometer (or within .5 square miles) and approximately 89% of the population residing in the urban corridor. It is divided into 11 parishes. The capital, **Bridgetown**, is in the most populous parish, which is St. Michael (**Ministry of Health and Wellness [MHW] of Barbados**, n.d.). The ethnic landscape of Barbados is predominantly of African descent (92.4%), followed by mixed (3.1%), White (2.7%), East Indian (1.3%), other (0.2%), and unspecified (0.2%; Ministry of Industry, Innovation, Science and Technology [MIST], 2024; Population and Housing Census, 2010, 2013). Net migration in Barbados peaked at 526 in 2008. It fell to –80 in 2023 (UN Data Portal, n.d.).

Barbados' highly dense population is experiencing population aging. The median age in Barbados during 2023 was 38.9 years and adults 65 years and older accounted for approximately 16% of the population. In 2023, Barbados' rate of natural population change was 0.6, well below the global average of 8.7, further reflecting the demographic shift occurring in Barbados. The birth rate in Barbados during 2023 was 11.2 births per 1,000 people, while the crude death rate was 10.6 deaths per 1,000 people. By 2050, adults 65 years and older are estimated to account for one quarter of the entire Barbadian population (UN Data Portal, n.d.). Decreasing birth rates and increased life expectancy in Barbados signify more economically dependent individuals as evidenced by an increasing dependency ratio rising from 47% in 2015 to 50% in 2022 (World Bank Group, n.d.). Population aging also presages more chronic noncommunicable disease (NCD) comorbidities and an attendant increase in healthcare expenditure (MHS-Barbados, n.d.). Table 18.1 includes key Barbados demographic statistics from 2011, 2017, and 2023.

BOX 18.1 Definition of Small Island Developing State

Small island developing states (SIDS) are a group of small island countries noted for shared sustainable development challenges that include geographic isolation, frequency of natural disasters, limited resources, and growing populations.

Source: Adapted from United Nations. (n.d.). *Office of the High Representative of the Least Developed Countries, Landlocked Developing Countries and Small Island Developing States: Small developing island states.* https://www.un.org/ohrlls/content/about-small-island-developing-states

TABLE 18.1 BARBADOS DEMOGRAPHIC INFORMATION

	2010	2017	2023
Total population	275,244	280,171	282,336
0–4 years	6.64%	5.82%	5.59%
5–14 years	13.52%	12.84%	11.89%
15–24 years	13.61%	13.20%	13.09%
25–64 years	54.41%	54.63%	53.33%
65 years and over	11.82%	13.52%	16.09%
Women 15–49 years (reproductive years)	71,023	67,740	65,572
Live births	3,514	3,258	3,155
Birth rate (per 1,000 population)	12.8	11.6	11.2
Deaths occurring during each year	2,553	2,641	2,996
Crude death rate (per 1,000 population)	9.2	9.4	10.6

Source: UN Data Portal. (n.d.). *UN population division data portal: Interactive access to global demographic indicators.* United Nations. https://population.un.org/dataportal/home

BRIEF OVERVIEW OF HISTORY AND CULTURE

From about 350 CE, Barbados was populated by various Indigenous groups arriving from South America, including the **Taino Arawaks** in 800 CE and the **Kalinago Caribs** in the mid-1200s. The English first claimed the island in 1625, and it became a hub for the transshipment of enslaved Africans to labor in the sugar industry until the abolition of slavery in 1838. Politically, Barbados became an independent member of the British Commonwealth on November 30, 1966 and a republic on November 30, 2021. Barbados is the world's third oldest **parliamentary democracy**, in which the government is led by the Prime Minister and the President is the head of state. English is the official language (Commonwealth Network, 2013).

The ethnic mix of Barbados reflects the milieu of the early European colonizers; enslaved, indentured, and imprisoned British people; enslaved West and Central Africans; other Europeans arriving in the mid-19th century; and East Indians, Syrio-Lebanese, and Asians arriving in the 20th century. Reflecting the island's heritage, the religious profile of Barbados is a complex mix of Eurocentric, Pan-African, and Asian beliefs. Approximately 75% of Barbadians who identify as religious are Christians. The main forms of Christianity are Anglicanism and Evangelical Protestantism. Other religious groups include Hindus, Muslims, and Rastafarians. One out of every four Barbadians do not identify as religious (Commonwealth Network, 2013).

HEALTH OUTCOMES

LIFE EXPECTANCY AND LEADING CAUSES OF MORTALITY

Barbados has shown steady gains in average life expectancy at birth in the postindependence era—increasing by approximately 9 years for both men and women in between 1966 and 2023. In 2023, life expectancy at birth was 78.61 years for Bajan women and 73.63 years for Bajan men (UN Data Portal, n.d.). The age-adjusted mortality rate for premature deaths decreased by 29.5% from 281.5 per 100,000 in 2000 to 198.5 per 100,000 in 2019. The major causes of death in Barbados are attributable to NCDs. In 2019, the age-adjusted mortality rate was 82.7 deaths per 100,000 people for communicable diseases and 477 deaths per 100,000 people for NCDs (Pan American Health Organization [PAHO], n.d.). Figure 18.1 lists the leading causes of death in Barbados during 2011 and 2021 (Institute for Health Metrics and Evaluation [IHME], n.d.).

NONCOMMUNICABLE DISEASES

Barbados has a significant burden of disease attributable to NCDs. Approximately one out of every four Barbadian has at least one NCD, and approximately 80% of all deaths in Barbados are caused by NCDs. The top three causes of mortality are stroke, ischemic heart disease, and diabetes mellitus. The total number of acute myocardial infarction (heart attacks) cases increased from 439 in 2016 to 537 in 2019. The 2019 myocardial infarction case fatality rate of 25% ranked higher than the 3% to 12% average for developed countries. Approximately 20% of Bajan adults have type 2 diabetes. There were 563 strokes in 2010 compared to 758 in 2019 (MHW-Barbados, n.d.).

In Barbados, there is also substantial morbidity and mortality attributed to cancer. The most frequent forms of cancer are prostate, breast, colon, rectal, uterine, stomach, lung, multiple myeloma, non-Hodgkin lymphoma, and pancreatic. The **National Cancer Plan** was formulated to address factors such as patient education, risk factor reduction, screening, and a clinical pathway review for the cancers of epidemiological concern. Cancer, hypertension, diabetes, asthma, epilepsy, and glaucoma accounted for at least 50% of the prescription volume and 72% of healthcare expenditures in 2019 to 2020. NCDs are a policy priority in the National Strategic Plan for Health (MHW-Barbados, n.d.).

INFECTIOUS DISEASES

Barbados has a strong history of preventing morbidity and mortality from common vaccine-preventable diseases via its **Expanded Programme on Immunisation (EPI)**, which has a primary

FIGURE 18.1 Leading causes of mortality in Barbados, 2011 and 2023.

Cause	2011 rank	2021 rank	Change in deaths per 100K, 2011–2021
Stroke	1	1	↑ +15.3
Ischemic heart disease	3	2	↑ +22.9
Diabetes	2	3	↑ +12.0
COVID-19	–	4	↑ +96.1
Chronic kidney disease	5	5	↑ +10.5
Lower respiratory infections	4	6	↓ −7.6
Colorectal cancer	6	7	↑ +5.1
Prostate cancer	8	8	↑ +8.7
Breast cancer	7	9	↑ +0.3
Hypertensive heart disease	9	10	↑ +4.4

● Communicable, maternal, neonatal, and nutritional diseases

● Noncommunicable diseases

Source: Institute for Health Metrics and Evaluation. (n.d.). *Barbados*. https://www.healthdata.org/research-analysis/health-by-location/profiles/barbados

vaccine coverage target of 95%. There were no confirmed measles, mumps, rubella, polio, tetanus, or pertussis cases between 2019 and 2020. A decline in primary vaccine coverage occurred during the COVID-19 pandemic with coverage falling to 85% to 89%, compared to 90% to 100% in 2019 (MHW-Barbados, n.d).

The **Integrated Mosquito Vector Management** program employs a multisectoral strategy to prevent and control arboviral diseases including the endemic dengue fever transmitted by *the Aedes aegypti* mosquito. All four dengue serotypes are present in Barbados, increasing the risk of hemorrhagic disease. There were major outbreaks in 2016, 2020, and in 2023 to 2024. However, the outbreaks resulted in only a small number of deaths. Vector control measures using Geographical Information Systems data guides targeted interventions at all phases of the mosquito life cycle (MHS, Barbados, n.d.; Vision Nova Inc., n.d.)

During 2019, approximately 1.5% of Barbados' population lived with HIV. Risky sexual behaviors are the primary means of HIV transmission in Barbados. The subpopulation with the highest prevalence is female sex workers. Priority interventions include maintaining **vertical transmission** (mother-to-child) below 2%, testing, pre- and postexposure prophylaxis, and treatment for high-risk groups including men who have sex with men, sex workers, and transgender individuals. As of 2019, 87% of persons living with HIV knew their status, 59% of diagnosed people were receiving treatment, and, of these, 77% were virally suppressed (MHW-Barbados, n.d).

The first two COVID-19 cases in Barbados were recorded on March 17th, 2020. The first COVID-19 death was reported on April 5th, 2020. Up to March 2024, there were 110,692 cases (49,933 male and 60,759 female) and 648 deaths. Approximately 57% of the population had been fully vaccinated (Barbados Government Information Service, 2024). The government prioritized COVID-19 management by providing designated quarantine areas and a bespoke isolation facility, Harrison Point, for management of cases to protect the lone public hospital. During the pandemic, the government partnered with the PAHO, the Global Vaccine Alliance, and various governments to procure adequate supplies of COVID-19 vaccines (MHW-Barbados, n.d.).

INFANT AND MATERNAL MORTALITY

Barbados has experienced favorable trends in maternal and child health. The infant mortality rate in Barbados has fallen steadily postindependence from 50.6 infant deaths per 1,000 live births in 1966 to 9.4 infant deaths per 1,000 live births in 2023 (UN Data Portal, n.d.). The maternal mortality ratio in Barbados during 2020 was 39.1 maternal deaths per 100,000 live births, which was far below the global ratio of 223.5 maternal deaths per 100,000 live births (UN Population Fund, n.d.).

MENTAL HEALTH

Mental health services are jointly delivered via a combination of public residential hospital-based care and primary care community-based ambulatory services and by private specialist providers. In 2020, there were 983 admissions to the psychiatric hospital—a sharp decline from 2019 when 1,209 people were admitted. In 2020, the top three discharge diagnoses were schizophrenia, substance abuse, and psychotic disorder. Males accounted for 63% of the first admissions to the psychiatric hospital. Among females, the most common discharge diagnosis was schizophrenia, whereas substance abuse was most common among men. The substance most abused is marijuana, followed by alcohol and cocaine. In 2019, **parasuicide** (an act of self-harm that mimics suicide; however, the aim is not to kill oneself) cases comprised 23 men and 55 women. Although the suicide rate is below global levels, concern about health and societal implications of suicide and self-harm prompted the establishment of several mental health–promoting initiatives including a 24-hour mental health hotline (MHS, Barbados, n.d.).

DETERMINANTS OF HEALTH

HEALTH BEHAVIORS AND METABOLIC RISK FACTORS

Metabolic risks are main drivers of death and disability in Barbados, accounting for five of the top 10 risk factors overall in 2011 and 2021. The top three risk factors were hyperglycemia, obesity, and hypertension. Behavioral risk factors accounted for four of the top 10 risks, including alcohol and tobacco use and dietary risk (overnutrition). These risk factors are linked to NCD burden. Malnutrition (undernutrition) has declined remarkably from 2011 to 2021, demonstrating Barbados' effectiveness in addressing the social determinants of health (Institute for Health Metrics & Evaluation, n.d.).

ENVIRONMENTAL FACTORS

As a SIDS lying within the North Atlantic hurricane zone, Barbados is highly vulnerable to external shocks including direct and indirect climate-induced impacts operating at the intersection of human health and the environment (CIA, 2024). Accordingly, the MHW has a designated Climate Change and Health Programme with identified priority climate resilience targets including attainment of the PAHO SMART Hospitals standard for its healthcare facilities. The MHW's Health Action Plan converges with the overall National Action Plan, outlining a multisectoral approach to address climate and disaster vulnerability (MHW-Barbados, n.d.). Barbados is the headquarters for several regional health, disaster, and security organizations including the PAHO office for the Eastern Caribbean and Barbados, the Caribbean Disaster Management Agency (CDEMA), and the Regional Security System (Ministry of Foreign Affairs and Foreign Trade, n.d.).

SOCIAL AND ECONOMIC FACTORS

Barbados' Human Development Index (HDI) score of 0.814 places the country in the very high HDI category and reflects the priority focus given to the human development areas of income, education, and health. All citizens in Barbados have access to free education up to the tertiary level. The adult literacy rate is 99.6%, and the gender development index of 1.008 ranks 12th of 189 nations globally (Barbados Statistical Service, n.d.). Between 2019 and 2020, the gross domestic product (GDP) per capita in Barbados decreased from $19,156,339.9 to $17,028; however, rebounded to $22,673 in 2023. The 2019 to 2023 trends are linked to the economic fallout from the COVID-19 pandemic and later recovery in the tourism and services-dependent economy of Barbados (MHW-Barbados, n.d.; World Bank Group, n.d.).

HEALTHCARE SYSTEM

EMERGENCE AND LEGAL FRAMEWORK

The emergence of the healthcare system in Barbados typifies the pattern in the Caribbean and can be considered in the context of the transitions and developments from the postemancipation to the current republic state. Between emancipation in 1838 and the 1960s, when many Caribbean states ushered in political independence, there was emphasis on curative services with centralized hospital-based care and more basic dispensary and visiting medical providers in rural areas. In the early 20th century, public health training and services emphasized infectious disease management over prevention. Emerging from the poor social conditions and ensuing unrest, the Moyne Commission Report of 1936 and the Stockdale Report of 1943 identified the need to address the underlying social determinants of health and provide a widened spectrum of care designed to promote health and deliver services at the community level. This prefaces the World Health Organization's Primary Health Care (PHC) strategy which was adopted by regional governments (Theodore & Edwards-Wescott, 2011).

The MHW has administrative and regulatory authority for the provision of public healthcare services, under the leadership of the Minister of Health, as outlined in the Health Services Act, Cap 44 of the laws of Barbados. The goals of the MHW are to promote health, effective delivery of healthcare services, and environmental sustainability through a suite of programs predicated on the principles of PHC and Universal Health Coverage (UHC). PHC and UHC strategies shape the delivery of multiple health service programs (MHW-Barbados, n.d.).

FINANCING MECHANISMS

The Barbados healthcare system is funded via direct, indirect, and **ad valorem** (value-based) taxes. In keeping with the mandate of UHC, the government health expenditures averaged about 3% of the GDP between 2015 and 2016, representing half of the 6% target recommendation in the PAHO strategy for universal healthcare access and coverage (PAHO, n.d.). While the government is the largest contributor to health expenditures in Barbados, followed by out-of-pocket expenditures, this contribution is projected to decline from 54.5% in 2011 to 40.3% in 2050, with an accompanying increase in out-of-pocket expenditures from 39% to 44.3% and voluntary health insurance from 6.6% to 15.5% (IHME, n.d.). The high-income status renders the country ineligible for overseas development aid; however, donors and nongovernmental organizations (NGOs) play a small but significant role in healthcare funding.

Future considerations include implementing a strengthened and more sustainable health financing model that reduces the potential burden of out-of-pocket spending and, hence, advances progress toward UHC. There is scope for an enhanced role for voluntary health insurance via funding of services complementary to the government-funded basket/essential healthcare package (MHW-Barbados, n.d.).

HEALTHCARE DELIVERY AND TRAINING

Healthcare cost, quality, and access can be understood in the context of Barbados' health service delivery model. All residents have the right to access services at the point of delivery. Public health services are provided across several programmatic areas, including the following:

- *PHC*: delivered via nine community-based ambulatory centers (**polyclinics**) and three smaller satellite clinics that offer a wide-range of curative and preventive services and are strategically located to be accessible via the major roadways
- *Acute, secondary, tertiary, and emergency care*: delivered at the **Queen Elizabeth Hospital** (QEH)
- Mental health
- Care of older adults and people living with disabilities
- *Other services*: covers pharmaceutical, laboratory, and environmental health and health promotion

Training of health professionals is a priority with undergraduate and postgraduate programs available in medicine and nursing. Furthermore, the government ensures quality via regulatory functions that include professional councils for medical, nursing, pharmacy, dental, and paramedical professionals charged to set conduct standards and oversee registration to practice. Inspection and licensing programs are in place for pharmacies, drug manufacturing plants, and residential care facilities that provide care for older adults (MHW-Barbados, n.d.).

ALLOPATHIC SERVICES

Allopathic medicine is a system where doctors, nurses, and other healthcare professionals provide care according to biomedical/Western medicine practices. The QEH is Barbados' lone accredited public acute, secondary, and tertiary care institution, which also serves as a teaching hospital for the University of the West Indies at Cave Hill, Barbados. This facility opened on November 14th,

1964 and has a current bed capacity of 519. A wide range of medical specialties such as internal medicine, emergency medicine, hematology, oncology, and surgical specialties such as general surgery, urology, cardiothoracic surgery, and neurosurgery are offered free at the point of care (MHW-Barbados, n.d.).

TRADITIONAL AND COMPLEMENTARY CARE

Barbados and the wider Caribbean have a rich history in the use of traditional practices to treat illnesses and promote health due to heavy influence from West African, East Indian, and Indigenous ancestry. However, in recent times the use of different ethnomedicines in Barbados has declined, which may be attributed to factors such as decreased numbers of plant species, lack of knowledge with successive generations on the use of medicinal plants, and the increased effectiveness of modern medicine (Cohall et al., 2012).

Barbados also has practitioners in acupuncture, traditional Chinese medicine (TCM), and chiropractic, naturopathic, and osteopathic medicine. These traditional healthcare practices are found primarily within the private healthcare system with limited offering in the public system, where through a partnership between the People's Republic of China and the Government of Barbados, TCM is offered in the QEH (QEH, 2024).

CONCLUSION

The Barbados healthcare system follows the principles of PHC. The MHW is committed to continued progress toward achieving UHC for all. However, there are challenges regarding sustainable healthcare financing in the context of the island's economic and geographical vulnerabilities and increasing production costs and increasing healthcare burden due to NCDs. There have been several initiatives on the island, including the Barbados Defence Force, which manages and operates a **Type 1 Field Medical Hospital** that can provide humanitarian care in the event of a natural or manmade disaster. Type 1 facilities are accredited to provide outpatient care, stabilization, and referral of major trauma cases (PAHO, n.d.). Another initiative is the leveraging of public/private partnerships for health, including the government's collaborations with a dialysis provider and the Heart and Stroke Foundation to provide services for NCD complications to a growing number of patients requiring advanced care (MHW-Barbados, n.d.).

LEARNING ACTIVITIES

CourseConnect

To access self-assessment questions and interactive, competency-based learning activities for this chapter, visit www.springerpub.com/courseconnect. See inside front cover and tear-out for CourseConnect details.

REFERENCES

Barbados Government Information Service. (2024). *COVID-19 situation report*. https://gisbarbados.gov.bb/

Barbados Statistical Service. (n.d.). *International indices on Barbados*. https://stats.gov.bb/international-indices/

Barbados Statistical Service. (2013). *Population and housing census 2010*. https://stats.gov.bb/wp-content/uploads/2020/03/2010-PHC-Report-Vol-1.pdf

Central Intelligence Agency. (2024). *Barbados—the world factbook*. www.cia.gov

Cohall, H., Scantlebury-Manning, T., Cadogan-McLean, C., & Willis-O'Connor, S. (2012). The impact of the healthcare system in Barbados (Provision of health insurance and the Benefit Service Scheme) on the use of herbal remedies by Christian churchgoers. *The West Indian Medical Journal, 16*(3), 258–263. https://doi.org/10.7727/wimj.2011.178

Commonwealth Network. (2013). *Barbados*. Commonwealth Year Book. https://commonwealthofnations.org/yb-pdfs/barbados_country_profile.pdf

Institute for Health Metrics and Evaluation. (n.d.). *Barbados*. https://www.healthdata.org/research-analysis/health-by-location/profiles/barbados

Ministry of Foreign Affairs and Foreign Trade. (n.d.). *Foreign affairs and foreign trade*. https://www.foreign.gov.bb/regional-orgs/

Ministry of Health & Wellness–Barbados. (n.d.). *Ministry of Health & Wellness*. https://www.health.gov.bb/

Ministry of Industry, Innovation, Science and Technology. (2024). *Demographics*. Barbados Integrated Government Portal. https://www.gov.bb/Visit-Barbados/demographics

Pan American Health Organization. (n.d.). *PAHO*. https://www.paho.org/en

The Queen Elizabeth Hospital. (2024). Traditional Chinese medicine used at the QEH. https://www.qehconnect.com/traditional-chinese-medicine-used-at-the-qeh/

Theodore, K., & Edwards-Wescott, P. (2011). An assessment of primary health care in the Caribbean pre and post Alma Ata Declaration and a way forward. *International Journal of Humanities and Social Science, 1*(8). https://www.ijhssnet.com/journals/Vol._1_No._8;_July_2011/1.pdf

UN Data Portal. (n.d.). *UN population division data portal: Interactive access to global demographic indicators*. United Nations. https://population.un.org/dataportal/home

UN Population Fund. (n.d.). *Data portal*. United Nations Population Fund. https://www.unfpa.org/data

Vision Nova Inc. (n.d.). *Health Ministry's updates on dengue fever, gastro and respiratory illnesses*. https://www.health.gov.bb/News/Press-Releases/Health-Ministry-s-Updates-On-Dengu

World Bank Group. (n.d.). *World Bank open data*. https://data.worldbank.org/

CHAPTER 19

DOMINICAN REPUBLIC

Maryellen D. Brisbois and Thomas Foley

INTRODUCTION

The Dominican Republic is an upper middle–income country that shares the Caribbean Island of Hispaniola with Haiti (Figure 19.1). It is divided into 31 provinces and a National District, where Santo Domingo, the country's capital, is located (Pan American Health Organization [PAHO], n.d.). Dominicans are considered healthier than their Haitian neighbors; however, unsanitary water, inadequate housing, healthcare access issues, economic crises, climate impacts, and poor nutrition undermine health conditions for many in the Dominican Republic. More than 40% of the population remain below the poverty line. Gender gaps in jobs and wages, shorter working lives, and higher rates of unemployment contribute to higher rates of poverty among women (World Bank Group, 2024). Despite these socioeconomic challenges, the Dominican Republic has a rapidly improving economy and provides universal healthcare coverage (PAHO, 2024).

GEOGRAPHY AND POPULATION

GEOGRAPHIC FEATURES

The Dominican Republic is classified as a small-island developing state (SIDS) located in the Caribbean. It has a land area of approximately 48,600 square kilometers (30,200 square miles),

FIGURE 19.1 A map of Hispaniola.

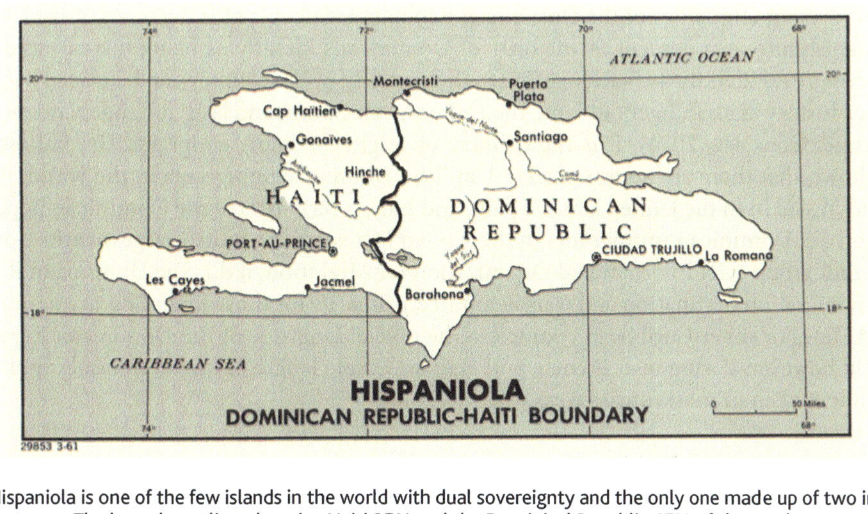

Note: Hispaniola is one of the few islands in the world with dual sovereignty and the only one made up of two independent states. The boundary, aligned to give Haiti 35% and the Dominical Republic 65% of the total area, runs generally north–south, crossing rather than paralleling the major mountain chains of the island. Completely demarcated, it is 224 miles in length, of which 96 miles consists of rivers.

Source: U.S. Department of State. (2020). *Hispaniola—Dominican Republic-Haiti boundary*. https://commons.wikimedia.org/wiki/File:Hispaniola_-_Dominican_Republic-Haiti_Boundary.jpg

occupying the eastern two thirds of the island of Hispaniola; Haiti occupies the remaining western one third. The Dominican Republic's coastline lies on the Atlantic Ocean and Caribbean Sea (Central Intelligence Agency [CIA], 2024). It is a renowned for its remarkable natural beauty, which includes

- the Central Cordillera and Cibao (La Vega Real) Mountain Ranges,
- the highest and lowest elevations in the West Indies (Mt. Duarte and Lake Enriquillo, respectively), and
- an extensive coastline with approximately 200 beaches such as the popular Playa Grande in Rio San Juan.

DEMOGRAPHICS

In 2023, the population of the Dominican Republic was approximately 11.3 million, making it the second most populous island country in the Caribbean behind Haiti. There were approximately 98.9 males to every 100 females. The life expectancy at birth for males was 70.53 years of age, while life expectancy at birth for females was 76.98 years. The Dominican Republic has experienced steady population growth during the 21st century; approximately 1% to 2% annually. However, the annual growth rate has been gradually declining.

During 2023, approximately 35.5% of the population was younger than 20 years old and 7.6% of the population was 65 years or older, making it one of the younger Caribbean countries. The median age in the Dominican Republic during 2023 was 27.7 years; an increase of nearly 7 years from 2000 when the median age was 21.1 years (UN Data Portal, n.d.). While the Dominican Republic is a relatively youthful Caribbean nation, it is beginning to undergo population aging.

Although the Dominican Republic traditionally had a large rural population, in the late-20th century it had one of the world's highest urbanization rates. Since the late 1990s, between 70% and 80% of the population shifted to urban dwelling (UN International Organization of Migration, n.d.; Wiarda & González, 2024).

Ethnicity, Race, and Language

The three major ethnicities of the Dominican Republic are people of Indigenous, mixed African, and SpanishEuropean descent. A majority of Dominicans identify as being mixed raced, while small minorities identify as Black or White. The diversity of the country can be traced back to its complex history as an Indigenous land, then a European colony, and lastly, an independent nation (Wiarda & González, 2024). It is the country of origin for many emigrants. Several estimates have shown that there are approximately 1 million Dominican emigrants in the world; the vast majority reside in in the United States, Spain, and Italy. Nearly 10% of the Dominican population lives abroad. Dominican immigrants in the United States are the fourth-largest Latin American immigrant group (UN International Organization for Migration, n.d.). The Dominican Republic is also a migration destination and transit country, primarily for those intending to migrate to the United States or other Caribbean countries. The official language of the Dominican Republic is Spanish; however, Portuguese, French, and Haitian Creole languages are commonly spoken and English is spoken in most tourist areas.

Sexual Orientation

There are a lack of data on the LGBTQI+ population in the Dominican Republic. While same-sex unions are not criminalized in the Dominican Republic, Dominicans who identify as LGBTQI+ are at an increased risk of being a victim of interpersonal violence (U.S. Department of State, 2022). The LGBTQI+ community, along with other marginalized groups, continue to face systematic discrimination in the Dominican Republic (Human Rights First, n.d.).

Religious Beliefs

More than 80% of the Dominican population belong to the Roman Catholic Church, which wields pronounced influence on cultural, political, and economic life. Nevertheless, the religious beliefs and practices of the rural populations are characterized by a blend of different forms or beliefs rooted in the culture of early historical Spanish and African communities. Evangelical groups, Judaism, and other religions account for a small segment of the population (Wiarda & González, 2024).

BRIEF COUNTRY HISTORY

The Indigenous Carib and Taino Arawak people established village-centered civilizations based on farming, fishing, hunting, and gathering on what is current day Hispaniola thousands of years prior to the arrival of Spanish colonizers in 1492. The Spanish originally established colonies on the north coast; however, reports of gold in the south led the Spaniards to abandon the northern outpost to establish the city of Santo Domingo on the southern coast in 1496. The Spanish ruled the island until the 17th century when French influence and settlement claims led to the western portion of Hispaniola being ceded to France in 1697, which resulted in the division of the island into two separate entities (current day Haiti and the Dominican Republic). The Haitians established the first independent nation in the Caribbean by defeating the French army. The Dominican Republic was the next sovereign Caribbean nation, declaring independence from the Spanish in 1821. However, it was quickly brough under Haitian rule via the Unification of Hispaniola. The Dominican Republic regained its independence from Haiti in 1844, reverted to Spanish rule in 1861, and reestablished independence from the Spanish in 1865 (Wiarda & González, 2024).

Since independence, Dominicans have experienced political and civil disorder, ethnic tensions, export-oriented booms and busts, long periods of military rule such as during the dictatorship of Rafael Trujillo from 1930 to 1961, and military interventions by the United States, most notably, from 1916 to 1924 and 1965 and 1966. U.S. military occupations of the Dominican Republic have, at times, strained relations between the two nations. The Dominican Republic has been moving toward a representative democracy since 1978, with the latest constitution disseminated in 2010. The constitution provides the foundation of progressing civil and economic rights in the Dominican Republic; along with the separation of power between the executive, legislative, and justice branches of the government (Wiarda & González, 2024).

HEALTH OUTCOMES

LIFE EXPECTANCY, LEADING CAUSES OF MORTALITY, AND LEADING MORBIDITY AND MORTALITY RISK FACTORS

In 2023, life expectancy at birth was 73.72 years in the Dominican Republic (UN Data Portal, n.d.). In 2021, the leading causes of death in the Dominican Republic were heart disease, stroke, COVID-19, neonatal disorders, diabetes mellitus, cirrhosis of the liver, chronic kidney disease, road injuries, and interpersonal violence. The leading morbidity and mortality risk factors during 2021 were malnutrition (undernutrition), hypertension, hyperglycemia, obesity, dietary risks (overnutrition), tobacco products, air pollution, elevated low-density lipoprotein (LDL) cholesterol, kidney disfunction, and alcohol abuse (Institute for Health Metrics and Evaluation [IHME], n.d.). Refer to Figures 19.2 and 19.3 for a list of the leading causes of mortality and leading risk factors in the Dominican Republic during 2011 and 2023.

In the Dominican Republic, nearly three out of every four deaths are caused by noncommunicable diseases (NCDs; 71%), which is consistent with the global average. The NCDs in the Dominican Republic that contribute to significant morbidity and mortality include heart

FIGURE 19.2 The leading causes of mortality in the Dominican Republic, 2011 and 2021.

Cause	2011 rank	2021 rank	Change in deaths per 100K, 2011–2021
Ischemic heart disease	1	1	↑ +22.8
Stroke	2	2	↑ +7.3
COVID-19	–	3	↑ +52.4
Neonatal disorders	3	4	↓ −10.5
Diabetes	6	5	↑ +6.3
Cirrhosis liver	7	6	↑ +4.3
Chronic kidney disease	10	7	↑ +4.7
Road injuries	4	8	↓ −1.0
Interpersonal violence	8	9	↓ −2.1
Hypertensive heart disease	11	10	↑ +1.7

● Communicable, maternal, neonatal, and nutritional diseases
● Noncommunicable diseases ● Injuries

Source: Institute for Health Metrics and Evaluation. (n.d.). *Dominican Republic, health data*. https://www.healthdata.org/research-analysis/health-by-location/profiles/dominican-republic

FIGURE 19.3 Leading morbidity/mortality risk factors in the Dominican Republic, 2011 and 2021.

Risk	2011 rank	2021 rank	Change in DALYs per 100K, 2011–2021
Malnutrition	1	1	↓ −1,132.5
High blood pressure	2	2	↑ +523.5
High fasting plasma glucose	3	3	↑ +659.7
High body mass index	4	4	↑ +624.4
Dietary risks	7	5	↑ +280.9
Tobacco	5	6	↑ +89.2
Air pollution	6	7	↑ +51.9
High LDL	8	8	↑ +261.0
Kidney dysfunction	10	9	↑ +225.2
High alcohol use	9	10	↑ +40.1

● Metabolic risks ● Environmental/occupational risks ● Behavioral risks

DALY, disability-adjusted life year; LDL, low-density lipoprotein.
Source: Institute for Health Metrics and Evaluation. (n.d.). *Dominican Republic, health data*. https://www.healthdata.org/research-analysis/health-by-location/profiles/dominican-republic

disease, stroke, diabetes mellitus, chronic kidney disease, and fatty liver disease. Communicable diseases and maternal, perinatal, and nutritional conditions account for approximately 13% of annual mortality. Common communicable diseases in the Dominican Republic are Dengue fever, malaria, cholera, amoebic dysentery, hepatitis, typhoid, rabies, diarrhea, skin infections, respiratory infections, HIV/AIDS, syphilis, and leptospirosis (Centers for Disease Control and

Prevention [CDC], 2024). In 2009, the CDC established an office in the Dominican Republic to collaborate with the country's Ministry of Health (MoH) in the following areas; HIV/AIDS, global health security, laboratory quality, surveillance, workforce development, emerging diseases and outbreak response, and other public health issues such as medical tourism. Notable improvements across these indicators have been made.

The COVID-19 pandemic in the Dominican Republic affected both the supply and demand for essential health services, especially at the beginning of the pandemic. Mobility restrictions and fear of infection in public places kept most people at home and away from health facilities. After the national presidential election in July 2020, new political leadership prioritized the reopening of the economy and effectively mobilized the country toward mass vaccination and testing. In the Dominican Republic, there were 660,790 confirmed COVID-19 cases and 4,384 deaths from COVID-19 January 22, 2020 to March 10, 2023 (Johns Hopkins University Coronavirus Resource Center, 2023).

INFANT, CHILD, AND MATERNAL MORTALITY

Despite being a high-middle income country, the Dominican Republic has concerning maternal, child, and neonatal mortality rates. The maternal mortality ratio (MMR) in 2020 was 107.3 maternal deaths per 100,000 live births (UN Population Fund, n.d.). Approximately 32 newborns per 1,000 live births died prior to their fifth birthday during 2023, which was just slightly below the 2023 global average of 36.3 deaths before age 5 per 1,000 live births. The infant mortality rate in the Dominican Republic during 2023 was 25.6 infant deaths per 1,000 live births. While infant mortality has declined by more than 10 infant deaths per 1,000 live births since the start of the 21st century, infant mortality in the Dominican Republic does not compare favorably with other high-middle income countries. Continued improvements in the prevention of infant mortality in the Dominican Republic is an area of need (UN Data Portal, n.d.).

Mental Illnesses

Mental, neurologic, substance use disorders, and suicide (MNSS) cause 16% of all disability-adjusted life years (DALYs) and 34% of all years lived with disability (YLDs) in the Dominican Republic. Common mental health conditions in the country include anxiety, depression, self-harm, somatic symptom disorder, headaches, substance use disorders (primarily alcohol abuse disorder), schizophrenia, bipolar disorders, and Alzheimer disease. Males are mostly affected by headaches and alcohol use and depressive disorders. Females are mostly affected by headaches and depressive and anxiety disorders (PAHO, n.d.).

DETERMINANTS OF HEALTH

HEALTH BEHAVIORS

Tobacco Use

Approximately 9% of all Dominican adults are current smokers. Of adults who smoke, 12.6% are males and 5.4% are females. While the prevalence of smokers in the Dominican Republic population has been declining during the 21st century, smoking continues to be a leading morbidity and mortality risk factor.

Nutrition

Poverty and inequality, coupled with the lack of diverse diets lie at the root of food insecurity and overlapping nutritional problems in the Dominican Republic, which suffers from recurrent natural climate shocks. According to the Global Climate Risk Index, it is one of the most vulnerable countries to climate change, leading to a weak agricultural structure. Nutrition problems in the Dominican Republic include

- chronic undernutrition, which affects 7% of children under 5 years;
- obesity; and
- anemia, which affects one in three women of reproductive age and approximately 60% of children between 6 and 11 months.

Despite nutritional challenges, the Dominican Republic produces much of its own food, as well as exports food. Agriculture accounts for about 1/8th of both the gross domestic product (GDP) and the workforce (Wiarda & González, 2024; UN World Food Program, 2024).

SOCIAL AND ECONOMIC FACTORS

Economy

The Dominican Republic has a mixed economy based largely on services (including tourism and finance), trade, manufacturing, telecommunications, and construction. Agriculture and remittances from the many Dominicans living abroad are also important aspects of the economy. Key agricultural production includes sugarcane, coffee, cacao, and tobacco (Wiarda & González, 2024). Over the last two decades, the Dominican Republic has been one of the fastestgrowing economies in the region. A combination of market-oriented structural reforms in the early 1990s and favorable external conditions have supported economic growth. In addition, prudent monetary and fiscal policy contributed to the Dominican Republic's macroeconomic stability (World Bank Group, 2024).

Educational Attainment

In the Dominican Republic, primary education is free and required for children age 7 to 14 years of age. The literacy rate in 2021 was approximately 99% (PAHO, n.d.; World Food Program USA, 2025). Enrollment in primary education from 2017 to 2023 was 92%. Enrollment in lower secondary education was 89%, while enrollment in upper secondary was 68%. Some children in isolated areas have limited access to education (UN Population Fund, n.d.).

Poverty

Over the past decades, the Dominican Republic has experienced sustained economic growth and stability; however, income distribution remains unequal among the population with poverty affecting over 40% and 10.4% living in extreme poverty. Most poor families live in urban areas, and 63% of impoverished families are headed by women. The unemployment rate in 2022 was 7.1%. Disaggregated by sex, the unemployment rate was 11.7% for women and 4.0% for men (PAHO, n.d.; World Food Program USA, 2025).

HEALTHCARE SYSTEM

The Dominican Republic has a two-tier healthcare system that includes government-sponsored free care available to all and private care with varying degrees of quality and out-of-pocket costs for supplies, medications, and hospital amenities. The government has prioritized universal access to health services as a fundamental principle in the design and overall planning of their national health strategy in order to mitigate healthcare inequities and health outcome disparities (PAHO, n.d.). The Dominican Republic has universal healthcare insurance as the government provides coverage to public hospitals that offer primary and tertiary care to Dominicans and residents. There is also a private hospital system that provides care, although private care can be expensive.

In 2020, public expenditures on health accounted for 3.24% of the GDP and 14.68% of total public expenditures, while out-of-pocket spending on health accounted for 24.65% of total health expenditures (PAHO, n.d.). In 2021, Dominican Republic's **Universal Healthcare (UHC) Service Coverage Index** was 77 on a scale of 0 for worst to 100 for best. The Dominican Republic's UHC Service Coverage Index score increased by 26 points from 2000 to 2021. The index is based on indicators measuring financial risk protection, access to quality essential healthcare services, and access to safe, effective, and affordable medicines and vaccines (World Health Organization [WHO], 2025).

Hospitals and trained medical personnel are available only in the larger cities and towns. In the rural areas, home remedies and traditional healers are often the only means of preserving or restoring health. Severely ill patients may be transported to nearby urban centers, where hospitalization is free; however, most families take that measure only in extreme cases, often when death is already imminent. In the Dominican Republic, public medical clinics and hospitals may lack basic resources and supplies, whereas private hospitals and doctors might offer a more comprehensive range of services but may require advance payment or proof of adequate insurance before providing medical services (CDC, 2024; Wiarda & González, 2024).

In the Dominican Republic, nurses are trained at accredited institutions with standards for both students and faculty. There is also a nursing council and opportunities for professional development and leadership roles; working conditions and hours are regulated. There were approximately 14,668 nursing, or 13.8 nurses per 10,000 people, in the Dominican Republic during 2020. There is an estimated shortage of 10,000 to 20,000 nurses projected for 2030, with few data regarding the interprofessional workforce that includes doctors, midwives, dentists, and pharmacists (WHO, 2020).

CONCLUSION

The Dominican Republic continues to face healthcare challenges. While there have been improvements in healthcare infrastructure and access, the Dominican Republic still struggles with high infant mortality rates, high prevalence of chronic diseases, and significant gaps in healthcare access between rural and urban areas. Additionally, the country faces high out-of-pocket payments that can result in healthcare inequities for marginalized groups. Despite challenges, the Dominican Republic government and private sector are working to strengthen the healthcare system, improve access to quality care, and address the social determinants of health.

LEARNING ACTIVITIES

CourseConnect >

To access self-assessment questions and interactive, competency-based learning activities for this chapter, visit www.springerpub.com/courseconnect. See inside front cover and tear-out for CourseConnect details.

REFERENCES

Centers for Disease Control and Prevention. (2024). *Yellow book*. https://wwwnc.cdc.gov/travel/yellowbook/2024/itineraries/dominican-republic

Central Intelligence Agency. (2024). *Dominican Republic—The world factbook*. www.cia.gov

Human Rights First. (n.d.). *Dominican Republic fact sheet: LGBT issues in the Dominican Republic*. https://humanrightsfirst.org/wp-content/uploads/2022/11/dominican-republic-fact-sheet.pdf

Institute for Health Metrics and Evaluation. (n.d.). *Dominican Republic*. https://www.healthdata.org/research-analysis/health-by-location/profiles/dominican-republic.

International Organization for Migration. (n.d.). *IOM: UN migration*. https://www.iom.int/

Johns Hopkins University Coronavirus Resource Center. (2023). *Dominican Republic*. https://coronavirus.jhu.edu/region/dominican-republic

Pan American Health Organization. (n.d.). *World Health Organization: Americas region.* https://www.paho.org/en

UN Data Portal. (n.d.). *UN population division data portal.* United Nations. https://population.un.org/dataportal/home/

UN Population Fund. (n.d.). *Data portal.* United Nations. https://www.unfpa.org/data

U.S. Department of State. (2023). *Country report on human rights practices: Dominican Republic.* https://www.state.gov/countries-areas/dominican-republic/

Wiarda, H. J., & González, N. L. (2024). *Dominican Republic.* Encyclopedia Britannica. https://www.britannica.com/place/Dominican-Republic

World Bank Group. (2024). *Dominican Republic: Country.* https://www.worldbank.org/en/country/dominicanrepublic

World Food Program USA. (2025). *Dominican Republic: Stable but starving.* https://www.wfpusa.org/place/dominican-republic/

World Health Organization. (2020). *State of the world's nursing.* https://apps.who.int/nhwaportal/Sown/Files?name=DOM

World Health Organization. (2025). *The Global Health Observatory: UHC service coverage index.* https://www.who.int/data/gho/data/indicators/indicator-details/GHO/uhc-index-of-service-coverage

CHAPTER 20

HAITI

Cathy F. Nickels-Herndon

INTRODUCTION

For many Haitians, access to necessary healthcare services can be difficult (Hashimoto et al., 2020). Political and economic challenges play a substantial role in limiting the delivery of health care in Haiti. While reading this chapter, it is important to consider the various factors that influence health and the provision of healthcare services in Haiti.

GEOGRAPHY AND POPULATION

GEOGRAPHICAL FEATURES

Haiti, officially known as the Republic of Haiti, shares the island of Hispaniola with the Dominican Republic (DR). Haiti is 27,750 square kilometers (17,243 square miles), making it the third largest Caribbean country. Haiti translates to the "Land of High Mountains" as it is the most mountainous Caribbean nation. However, due to deforestation, the country has experienced diminished agricultural activity that was once a key factor for economic growth (Macleod et al., 2024). The capital and most populous city of Haiti is Port-au-Prince, which is located in Haiti's southern region. A long fault line crosses south of Port-au-Prince accounting for several significant earthquakes, such as the 7.2 magnitude earthquake in August of 2021 that resulted in more than 2,000 deaths. The southern region of Haiti is also vulnerable to hurricanes and tropical storms (Roy & Labrador, 2024).

POPULATION

Size and Age Distribution

Haiti is the most populated country in the Caribbean. During 2023, the population of Haiti was approximately 11.7 million. Haiti has a growth rate of about 1.23%, and the Haitian population has increased by approximately 29% between 2000 and 2024. Haiti is also a young nation. In 2023, approximately 41% of the country was younger than 20 years, while less than 5% of the population was 65 years and older. Adults between the ages of 20 and 64 account for nearly 54% of the total population. The median age in Haiti during 2023 was 23.5 years, making Haiti the youngest of all Caribbean nations. Not surprisingly, Haiti has the highest birth rate in the Caribbean (UN Data Portal, n.d.).

Migration

In 2023, Haiti's crude rate of net migration was –5 per 1,000 persons (UN Data Portal, n.d.). After the assassination of President Jovenel Moise in 2021, Haiti's political leadership structure was thrust into extreme chaos. As a result, gang violence has grown substantially. Many sources, including mainstream media outlets and nongovernment organizations (NGOs), indicate that the capital city of Port-au-Prince is nearly completely overrun with gangs (Munch, 2024). The violence has caused many residents to attempt to flee the country. Seeking refuge, many Haitians have emigrated to the DR, southern Brazil (Tafner et al., 2023), Chile (McDonnell & Poblete, 2021), and the United States.

LGBTQ+ Population

In Haiti, population statistics are difficult to acquire on LGBTQ+ individuals. There are no laws or policies that recognize and protect LGBTQ+ individuals, and most religions practiced in the country only recognize male or female genders, complicating the ability to evaluate population diversity based on sexual orientation, sex, and gender (Crary, 2018).

Race and Ethnicity

Citizens of Haiti are predominately Haitian, although many individuals associated with missions or NGOs live there for extended periods. After the island's colonization in 1492, large numbers of African people were transported to the island as enslaved peoples by the French. As a consequence, some citizens of Haiti prefer to be acknowledged as "Haitian" while others prefer to recognize their African heritage as African–Haitian. Ethnically, most Haitians are Black with a small percentage (approximately 5%) being White (Central Intelligence Agency [CIA], 2024).

CULTURE

RELIGIOUS BELIEFS

Catholicism is the dominant religion of Haiti. Approximately 80% of the population are Catholic, with Protestant religions including Baptist practiced less commonly (CIA, 2024). Vodou is also a dominant religion in Haiti and is commonly practiced conjointly with Catholicism or other religions. In 2003, Vodou was delcared an official religion.

LANGUAGES

While Haitian Creole is spoken by approximately 95% of the population, French is taught in most schools. Both Haitian Creole and French are official languages in Haiti. Spanish and English are also spoken by a portion of the population, and these languages are becoming more commonly used (Macleod et al., 2024).

POLITICAL SYSTEM

The Haitian political system is rather complicated and has fluctuated repeatedly over time. While it is currently described as a Universal Suffrage system having an executive branch, including a president and prime minister, and legislative and judicial branches of government, it has been loosely governed as an autocracy and dictatorship in the past. The assassination of President Moise in 2021 caused governmental destabilization in Haiti. In 2024, a transitional presidential council was implemented in an attempt to stabilize the Haitian government. However, political instability and violence remain threats (Sanon & Coto, 2024).

HISTORICAL OVERVIEW

The island that Haiti shares with the DR was originally settled by the Taino people, who migrated from Central and South America several thousand years ago. During the late 15th and early 16th centuries, Spain claimed the island and named it La Espanola. However, settlement claims by the French led to the island being divided into two separate entities in 1697—the western portion ruled by the French (modern-day Haiti) and the eastern portion ruled by the Spanish (the modern-day DR). French colonists established sugar plantations, which were worked by enslaved Africans. The labor of the enslaved Africans made the French colony one of the wealthiest in the world (Roy & Labrador, 2024).

In 1804, an army of self-liberated Haitian slaves defeated Napoleon's French army, making Haiti the first independent nation in the Caribbean. Newly independent Haiti also became the first nation to abolish slavery. Since winning their independence in 1804, after 179 years of French rule, Haiti has struggled to develop a stable democracy and to garner the global respect it deserves based on its historical achievements. Out of fear of subsequent slave uprisings, the global community isolated Haiti, refusing to acknowledge their independent leadership and forcing them to pay reparations for defeating the French army. The global condemnation of Haiti caused near economic collapse. In 1825, France sought reparations for the loss of property, including slaves, as a result of the revolution, which created significant debt that Haiti still struggles to repay, impeding the growth of their economy and infrastructure (Council on Hemispheric Affairs [COHA], 2010).

Several struggles for power have occurred since independence, and fraud, corruption, and interference from other countries continually prevents Haiti from fully engaging in the global community. Haitians desire true democracy, but with each step forward, new barriers are thrown into their path. Recently, conflict has expanded profoundly, resulting in the growth of gangs to as many as 5,000 members. Much of this conflict evolved because of dissatisfaction with the installment of Ariel Henry as President following the assignation of former President Moise in 2021. In April of 2024 Henry stepped down, relegating leadership to a transitional council (Roy & Labrador, 2024).

HEALTH OUTCOMES

LEADING CAUSES OF MORTALITY

Due to poor record-keeping systems in Haiti, accurate statistics for health outcome measures are often based on indirect sources or generalizations (Fene et al., 2020). The Institute for Health Metrics and Evaluation (IHME; Figure 20.1) shares a comparison of leading causes of death in Haiti during 2011 and 2021. While noncommunicable diseases cause significant mortality in Haiti, the country still struggles to prevent mortality caused by neonatal issues and communicable diseases, which is reflective of a lower-income country with problems developing strong infrastructure. During 2021, the leading causes of death in Haiti were COVID-19, heart disease, stroke, neonatal disorders, diabetes, lower respiratory infections, HIV/AIDS, diarrheal diseases, congenital defects, and road injuries. In 2011, diarrheal diseases were the leading cause of death in Haiti (IHME, n.d.). While there were many contributing factors, the cholera outbreak following the earthquake in 2010 was a primary driver of the high incidence of diarrhea-related deaths in 2011. The susceptibility to natural and climate disasters presents challenges in protecting the health of Haitians.

MENTAL HEALTH

Since the earthquake of 2010, there has been increased awareness of challenges addressing and managing mental health concerns for Haitians. Violence, natural disasters, and poverty exacerbate mental health disorders with a dearth of psychiatrists, psychologists, and social workers serving the Haitian population (Cénat et al., 2021; Oscar, 2020). While services from these providers are limited, efforts have been initiated to bolster mental and social healthcare in Haiti.

In 2010, at the request of the Haitian Minister of Health, Partners in Health (a not-for-profit organization based in Boston, Massachusetts) assisted in creating a functional national mental health service (Raviola et al., 2020). Through this collaboration, patients have received tailored care for depression, epilepsy, psychotic disorders, trauma, and substance abuse disorders.

FIGURE 20.1 The leading causes of mortality in Haiti.

Cause	2011 rank	2021 rank	Change in deaths per 100K, 2011–2021
COVID-19	–	1	↑ +129.9
Ischemic heart disease	2	2	↑ +3.1
Stroke	3	3	↓ −3.6
Neonatal disorders	6	4	↓ −7.4
Diabetes	7	5	↑ +2.0
Lower respiratory infections	5	6	↓ −18.7
HIV/AIDS	4	7	↓ −37.4
Diarrheal diseases	1	8	↓ −70.9
Congenital defects	8	9	↓ −3.6
Road injuries	9	10	↓ −1.9

Communicable, maternal, neonatal, and nutritional diseases
Noncommunicable diseases   Injuries

Source: Institute for Health Metrics and Evaluation. (n.d.). *Haiti*. https://www.healthdata.org/research-analysis/health-by-location/profiles/haiti

INFANT AND MATERNAL MORTALITY

Haiti experiences significant infant and maternal mortality with the highest infant mortality rate in the Caribbean. In 2023, Haiti's infant mortality rate was 43.3 infant deaths per 1,000 live births (UN Data Portal, n.d.). Haiti also has the highest maternal mortality ratio in the Caribbean; in 2020 there were 350.4 deaths per 100,000 live births (UN Population Fund, 2024). Accessing quality prenatal and postnatal care has been a consistent concern for many Haitian women. It is common for women to work with a community healer, midwife, or even a neighbor to deliver a child. Because many communities do not have consistent medical resources, home births are common and caregivers likely ill-equipped to handle emergencies. Unsurprisingly, this can lead to infection and death for the mother, child, or both.

LIFE EXPECTANCY

Life expectancy in Haiti, influenced by poverty and political instability, is the lowest in the Caribbean. In 2023, life expectancy at birth in Haiti was 64.94 years, with women (at 68.3 years) experiencing 6.5 more years compared to men (61.73 years; UN Data Portal, n.d.).

DETERMINANTS OF HEALTH

LEADING MORBIDITY AND MORTALITY RISK FACTORS

While Haitians desire to achieve positive health outcomes, there are many factors that inhibit the ability of citizens to achieve optimal health. Haitians could be empowered by improved government and health systems and education that address leading morbidity and mortality risk factors. Figure 20.2 shows a comparison of the leading morbidity and mortality risk factors in Haiti during 2011 to 2021. The leading risk factors in Haiti during 2021 included malnutrition, air pollution, hypertension, water and sanitation hygiene (WaSH), hyperglycemia, dietary risks, high

FIGURE 20.2 Leading morbidity/mortality risk factors in Haiti.

Risk	2011 rank	2021 rank	Change in DALYs per 100K, 2011–2021
Malnutrition	1	1	↓ −6,929.0
Air pollution	3	2	↓ −902.3
High blood pressure	4	3	↑ +153.5
WaSH	2	4	↓ −5,945.1
High fasting plasma glucose	7	5	↑ +293.9
Dietary risks	6	6	↑ +142.9
High body mass index	8	7	↑ +332.6
Unsafe sex	5	8	↓ −1,151.1
High alcohol use	9	9	↑ +47.1
Kidney dysfunction	10	10	↑ +52.4

Metabolic risks   Environmental/occupational risks   Behavioral risks

DALYs, disability-adjusted life years; WaSH, water and sanitation hygiene.

Source: Institute for Health Metrics and Evaluation. (n.d.). *Haiti*. https://www.healthdata.org/research-analysis/health-by-location/profiles/haiti

body mass index, unsafe sex, alcohol use, and kidney dysfunction. The leading risk factors in Haiti are representative of a low-income country as they include a mix of socioenvironmental factors such as malnutrition and psychosocial behavioral factors such as alcohol abuse (IHME, n.d.).

SOCIAL DETERMINANTS

The social determinants of health significantly support or deter one's success in living healthfully throughout the lifespan. Many Haitians struggle to achieve optimal health because of the extreme influence the social determinants exert on health outcomes. Political instability and the frequency of natural and climatic disasters exacerbate the effects of the social determinants on Haitians (Roy & Labrador, 2024). Exploring the social determinants for Haitians illustrates barriers that exist and where improvements can be made to facilitate positive health outcomes.

Haiti is one of the poorest countries in the world. The gross domestic product (GDP) per capita in Haiti during 2023 was approximately $1,700. The estimated unemployment rate in 2022 was approximately 15% (World Bank Group, n.d.). While many Haitians report having some form of employment, including self-employment, underemployment is common. As noted previously, poverty is a substantial issue in Haiti with more than 50% of Haitians living below the poverty line (Roy & Labrador, 2024).

Formal education in Haiti is often a luxury. Those that attend school often come from families that can contribute in some way to pay for their education. There is no effective government funded "free" education system in Haiti although the Constitution allows for this service. International organizations, including those from the United States and Canada, provide and fund 90% of the schools in Haiti. Additionally, various mission or church organizations around the world sponsor schools throughout the country. Because not all individuals in Haiti have access to education, the literacy rate is approximately 53% (Schools for Haiti, 2022), which is one of the lowest literacy rates in the world.

ENVIRONMENTAL AND CLIMATE CHANGE ISSUES

Haiti is susceptible to environmental disasters such as earthquakes, hurricanes, tropical storms, cyclones, flooding, and mudslides. Haiti is also prone to severe effects from these disasters because of the political instability and lack of strong infrastructure rooted in historical mistreatment stemming from colonization, slavery, and outside influence postindependence. Deforestation and postdisaster epidemics further exacerbate the severity of effects experienced from environmental traumas. For example, the cholera outbreak that occurred after the 2010 earthquake led to thousands of additional deaths and prevented some aid workers from traveling to the country to lend assistance (Roy & Labrador, 2024).

THE HEALTHCARE SYSTEM

DELIVERY, FINANCE, INSURANCE, AND PAYMENT

While there is a government-funded national health care system in Haiti, it does not serve the population effectively. Often, patients seeking medical care are asked to pay for services at the time of treatment and to then seek reimbursement from the government. There is only a small percentage of the population that is able to provide upfront payments (Hashimoto et al., 2020). Haitians who are formally employed may receive health insurance coverage through their employer. It is common for many Haitians to consult with a healer or Vodou practitioner because of limited access and cost barriers to the allopathic healthcare system.

There are more than 900 medical service centers in Haiti (Le Ministère de la Santé Publique et de la Population, 2024). Haiti's Ministry of Health provides overall leadership of the healthcare system. Services can be accessed in hospitals, community clinics, dispensaries that are often run by nurses, and through services offered locally by nongovernmental organizations (NGOs), missionaries, or local centers of influence such as churches (A. Jean Baptiste, personal communication, May 31, 2024). Many clinics have inconsistent schedules and the provisions of healthcare services can be complicated by limited staff.

In Haiti, there are less than 0.23 physicians and 0.7 hospitals beds per 1,000 persons (CIA, 2024). Some hospitals, particularly in Port-au-Prince, have closed because of the growing gang violence (Munch, 2024). In addition, many healthcare providers have stopped going to their workplaces or fled Haiti because of safety concerns. Hospitals have been robbed of medical supplies and equipment, as well as structural elements of buildings. These factors leave many citizens without any access to healthcare services. Once the circumstances in Haiti improve, these institutions will require time to rebuild or repair their structures and obtain medical supplies and equipment.

HEALTHCARE TRAINING AND EDUCATION

According to the Haiti Ministry of Health (2022), there are approximately 84 schools that provide education in the health arena. However, there is still a shortage of trained healthcare providers. Trained providers are disproportionately located in urban areas near the large hospitals. In the rural areas, people often rely on local healers, Vodou practitioners, midwives, or other people in the community who may have undergone informal training.

HEALTHCARE COST, QUALITY, AND ACCESS

Data collection is an area of needed improvement in Haiti, including collecting data about healthcare expenditures. The Pan American Health Organization (PAHO) reported that public expenditure on health in 2020 accounted for approximately 4% of the total public expenditure. Out-of-pocket spending on health accounted for nearly 50% of the total health expenditure (PAHO, 2023). Healthcare costs can vary greatly depending on the community where care is sought and which type of facility and provider a person utilizes. Some hospitals and clinics ask patients to bring their own sterile gauze, bandages, and/or bedding, but not all patients can comply with the request. A variety of missions and NGOs in Haiti provide free healthcare services, attempting to curb out-of-pocket healthcare expenses for Haitians. Where healthcare services are available and affordable, patients can receive good quality care for a wide breadth of health concerns. Private hospitals, in particular, are known for providing high quality care and the widest care options (A. Jean Baptiste, personal communication, May 31, 2024). Healthcare staffing is a challenge in Haiti. The private hospitals tend to have better staffing when compared to the public hospitals and clinics.

CONCLUSION

Haiti is a remarkable island nation with beautiful beaches and mountains, rich history, and persevering people. The challenges Haiti faces as a result of colonization, slavery, fights for independence, disdain and alienation from other countries, fraud and corruption, and environmental disasters interfere with opportunities for progress. Haiti was a prosperous and powerful force in the Caribbean. How will Haitians regain that status?

An important principle of health planning is to consider the desires of the people who will be most impacted by interventions. This ideal expands to all aspects of developing and planning for improvement and success. The citizens of Haiti are clamoring for a legitimately elected democratic government that functions for the people. They want a country that promotes full health equity. Addressing the determinants of health, particularly the social determinants of health, is necessary to promote health equity in Haiti. Given the history of mistreatment toward Haiti by other countries, the global community should support Haiti in their efforts to build health equity. The best place for the global community to start providing support is to listen to the Haitian people.

LEARNING ACTIVITIES

CourseConnect

To access self-assessment questions and interactive, competency-based learning activities for this chapter, visit www.springerpub.com/courseconnect. See inside front cover and tear-out for CourseConnect details.

REFERENCES

Cénat, J. M., Harerimana, B., Michel, G., McIntee, S., Mukunzi, J. N., Hajizadeh, S., & Dalexis, R. D. (2021). The global challenge of providing mental health services in poverty: The situation of northern Haiti. *BJPsych International, 19*(1), 4–7. https://doi.org/10.1192/bji.2021.22

Central Intelligence Agency. (2024). *Haiti, The world factbook*. https://www.cia.gov/the-world-factbook/countries/haiti/#people-and-society

Council on Hemispheric Affairs. (2010). *The Haitian timeline: A history of military dictatorship and civil rule*. https://coha.org/military-dictatorship-in-haiti/

Crary, D. (2018, August 4). *In Haiti, slight progress for LGBT rights is seen as victory*. AP News. https://apnews.com/general-news-c5c51b84c9b5449d95d3f49ff47add59

Fene, F., Ríos-Blancas, M. J., Lachaud, J., Razo, C., Lamadrid-Figueroa, H., Liu, M., Michel, J., Thermidor, R., & Lozano, R. (2020). Life expectancy, death, and disability in Haiti, 1990–2017: A systematic analysis from the global burden of disease study 2017. *Revista Panamericana de Salud Pública, 44*, 2.

Haiti Ministry of Health. (2022). *List of recognized health science training institutions*. Republique D'Haiti, Ministere de la Santé Publique et de la Population. https://www.mspp.gouv.ht/documentation-sur-le-financement-de-la-sante/

Hashimoto, K., Adrien, L., & Rajkumar, S. (2020). Moving towards universal health coverage in Haiti. *Health Systems & Reform, 6*(1), e1719339. https://doi.org/10.1080/23288604.2020.1719339

Institute for Health Metrics and Evaluation. (n.d.). *Haiti*. https://www.healthdata.org/research-analysis/health-by-location/profiles/haiti

Macleod, M. J., Lawless, R., Girault, C. A., & Ferguson, J. A. (2024, May 23). *Haiti. Encyclopedia*. Britannica. https://www.britannica.com/place/Haiti

McDonnell, P. J., & Poblete, J. (2021, October 1). Haitians in Chile: Rough going for many prompts large-scale migration toward U.S. *Los Angeles Times*. https://www.latimes.com/world-nation/story/2021-10-01/chile-haitians-migration

Le Ministère de la Santé Publique et de la Population. (2024). *Carte sanitaire–Haiti cartographie* [Health map - Haiti mapping]. https://cartesanitaire.sisnu.net/cartographie

Munch, R. (2024, April). Chaos in Haiti. *Commonwealth, 151*(4), 6–7.

Oscar, J. W. (2020, November 13). *Accessing mental health care in Haiti: Challenges and opportunities*. Health Equity International. https://healthequityintl.org/stories/accessing-mental-health-care-haiti-challenges-and-opportunities

Pan American Health Organization. (2023). *Haiti*. Health in the Americas. https://hia.paho.org/en/countries-22/haiti-country-profile

Raviola, G., Rose, A., Fils-Aimé, J., Thérosmé, T., Affricot, E., Valentin, C., Daimyo, S., Coleman, S., Dubuisson, W., Wilson, J., Verdeli, H., Belkin, G., Jerome, G., & Eustache, E. (2020). Development of a comprehensive, sustained community mental health system in post-earthquake Haiti, 2010–2019. *Global Mental Health, 7*, e6. https://doi.org/10.1017/gmh.2019.33

Roy, D., & Labrador, R. C. (2024). *Haiti's troubled path to development*. Council on Foreign Relations. https://www.cfr.org/backgrounder/haitis-troubled-path-development

Sanon, E., & Coto, D. (2024, June 13). *Haiti's transitional council appoints new cabinet tasked with leading a country under siege by gangs*. AP News. https://apnews.com/article/haiti-new-cabinet-gangs-19fadbd9a84eeb79d854c7ed2ba2869c

Schools for Haiti. (2022). *Facts about Haiti*. https://schoolsforhaiti.com/facts-about-haiti/

Tafner, D. P., Nitschke, R. G., Tholl, A. D., Heidemann, I. T., Bellaguarda, M. L., & Marcon, S. S. (2023). Health promotion of Haitian immigrant families: Possibilities and barriers in everyday life in primary care. *Rev Rene, 24*, e83257. https://doi.org/10.15253/2175-6783.20232483257

UN Data Portal. (n.d.). *UN population division data portal: Interactive access to global demographic indicators*. United Nations. https://population.un.org/dataportal/home

UN Population Fund. (2024). *Data portal*. United Nations. https://www.unfpa.org/data

World Bank Group. (n.d.). *The World Bank open data*. https://data.worldbank.org/

PART VI: Health and Healthcare in Europe and North Asia

CHAPTER 21

OVERVIEW OF EUROPE AND NORTH ASIA

Anna Foucek Tresidder

GEOGRAPHY

Europe and North Asia (Figure 21.1) encompass a diverse range of countries with varying climates, landscapes, and demographic profiles. Europe comprises 50 countries and territories, of which 27 are members of the European Union (EU). Europe stretches from the Atlantic Ocean to the Ural Mountains, and encompasses a diverse range of regions, from the Scandinavian Peninsula to the Mediterranean coast. Europe generally has four well-defined seasons:

- *Spring:* mild temperatures, blooming flowers, and occasional showers
- *Summer:* warm to hot weather, sunny days, and popular tourist season
- *Autumn:* cool temperatures, colorful foliage, and occasional rain
- *Winter:* cold temperatures, with snow in many regions (National Oceanic and Atmospheric Administration [NOAA], 2023).

North Asia predominantly includes Russia's vast Siberian region and parts of Mongolia. This vastness contributes to diverse climates, landscapes, and natural resources, shaping the region's cultural and economic development. North Asia also experiences four seasons, but they tend to be more extreme due to its continental location:

- *Spring:* short and often unpredictable, with melting snow and fluctuating temperatures
- *Summer:* warm to hot, with long daylight hours and occasional rain
- *Autumn:* cool to cold, with colorful foliage and early snowfall in some areas
- *Winter:* harsh and cold, with long periods of snow and freezing temperatures (NOAA, 2023).

The geographical diversity impacts healthcare delivery, infrastructure, and service access across these regions.

BRIEF HISTORY

Historical events, economic changes, and political shifts have shaped the development of healthcare systems in Europe and North Asia. The origins of modern European healthcare can be traced back to the 19th and early 20th centuries with the establishment of social health insurance schemes in Germany under Otto von Bismarck. The post-World War II era saw the expansion of welfare states, with many European countries adopting comprehensive public health systems. The creation of the EU has further influenced healthcare policies through regulations and funding initiatives aimed at reducing disparities and promoting collaboration across member states (European Commission, 2023). In North Asia, the healthcare system evolved from the Soviet-era model, which was characterized by centralized, state-run healthcare. The collapse of the Soviet Union in 1991 led to significant reforms, transitioning toward a more decentralized system with varying degrees of privatization and public involvement. In this region, the healthcare systems have also undergone significant changes, transitioning from a centralized model to a more mixed system with both public and private components (Miranda, 2022).

FIGURE 21.1 Europe and North Asia.

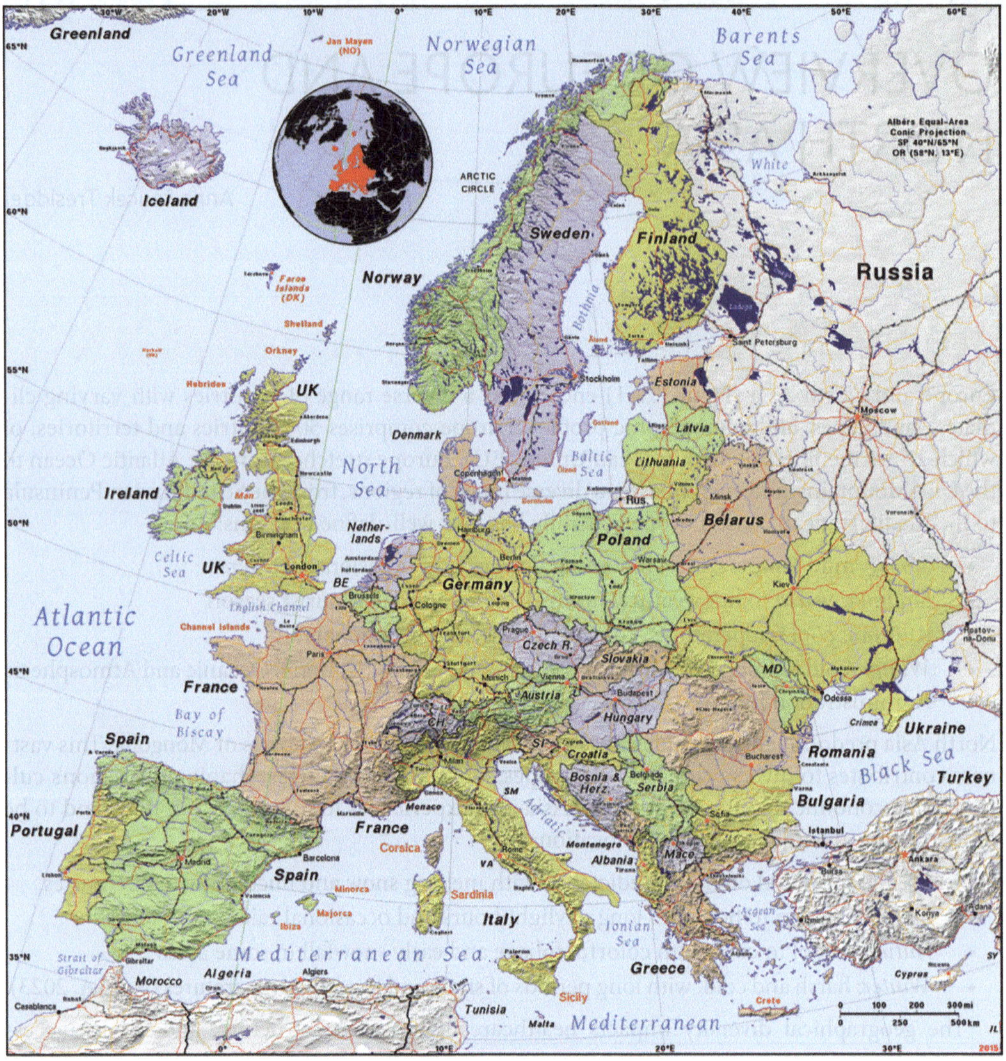

Source: Macky, I. (n.d.). *Europe*. http://ian.macky.net/pat/map/euro/euro.html

POPULATION

Europe is home to approximately 747 million people as of 2024 (Central Intelligence Agency [CIA], 2024). The population density is high in Western and Southern Europe, while Eastern Europe and Northern Europe have lower densities. Europe faces challenges such as an aging population, with a growing proportion of older individuals requiring healthcare services. Additionally, migration patterns have influenced demographic profiles and healthcare needs (European Commission, 2023).

North Asia, primarily Russia, has a population of about 145 million people (CIA, 2024). The region is characterized by low population density in vast areas, particularly in Siberia. North Asia also faces demographic challenges, including a declining population due to low birth rates and high mortality rates, again particularly in Russia. Mongolia, with a population of approximately 3.5 million (CIA, 2024), faces different challenges, including rural–urban migration and a younger population demographic.

SOCIOECONOMIC FACTORS

The European healthcare landscape is marked by a high level of social protection, with many countries offering universal healthcare coverage. Socioeconomic disparities exist, particularly between Eastern and Western Europe. Wealthier countries generally provide more comprehensive and accessible healthcare services. Issues such as healthcare funding, affordability, and efficiency vary, with some countries experiencing challenges related to healthcare spending and resource allocation.

In North Asia, economic disparities among regions significantly impact healthcare access and quality. Wealthier urban areas like Moscow and St. Petersburg have better healthcare facilities compared to rural areas. Economic reforms and shifting government priorities have influenced healthcare funding and service delivery. In Mongolia, socioeconomic factors such as poverty and rural isolation affect access to healthcare services. Economic development efforts are ongoing to address these disparities and improve healthcare infrastructure.

HEALTH OUTCOMES

European countries generally exhibit high health outcomes with low infant mortality rates and high life expectancy (Table 21.1). However, there are notable disparities among countries and regions. Western and Nordic countries tend to have higher health outcomes due to well-funded healthcare systems and higher standards of living. Eastern European countries face challenges such as higher rates of chronic diseases and lower life expectancy, influenced by socioeconomic factors and historical context. The EU has established directives and regulations that promote harmonization and cooperation among member states, leading to improved access to healthcare, standardized quality standards, and enhanced patient mobility. For instance, the **European Health Insurance Card (EHIC)** allows EU citizens to receive necessary healthcare while traveling within the EU, ensuring continuity of care regardless of location (European Commission, 2023).

In North Asia, health outcomes show significant regional disparities. Major health challenges like high mortality rates from noncommunicable diseases, such as cardiovascular diseases and cancer, contribute to a lower life expectancy than Western Europe (Table 21.1). Efforts to address these issues include healthcare reforms and initiatives aimed at improving preventive care and treatment. Mongolia has made progress in health outcomes, with improvements in life expectancy and reductions in infant mortality, though challenges remain in addressing healthcare access in remote areas and managing communicable diseases (Miranda, 2022).

The healthcare systems of Europe and North Asia are shaped by a combination of historical evolution, geographic diversity, population dynamics, and socioeconomic factors. While Europe benefits from a generally high standard of healthcare with variations among countries, North Asia faces significant challenges related to regional disparities and transitioning healthcare systems. Addressing these challenges requires ongoing reforms, investment, and targeted policies to improve health outcomes and ensure equitable access to healthcare services. Our authors represent the European countries of Portugal, Spain, and the United Kingdom. For North Asia, the country of Georgia is profiled.

LEARNING ACTIVITIES

CourseConnect

To access self-assessment questions and interactive, competency-based learning activities for this chapter, visit www.springerpub.com/courseconnect. See inside front cover and tear-out for CourseConnect details.

TABLE 21.1 HEALTH OUTCOMES FOR EUROPE AND NORTH ASIA

REGION/ COUNTRY	LIFE EXPECTANCY AT BIRTH (2021)	INFANT MORTALITY RATE (2021)	MATERNAL MORTALITY RATIO (2021)	LEADING CAUSE OF MORTALITY (2021)
Europe	81.5 years	3.1 per 1,000 live births	13 per 100,000 live births	Cardiovascular diseases
United Kingdom	82.5 years	3.6 per 1,000 live births	6.0 per 100,000 live births	Heart disease
Germany	81.8 years	3.3 per 1,000 live births	5.5 per 100,000 live births	Heart disease
France	83.1 years	3.1 per 1,000 live births	8.0 per 100,000 live births	Heart disease
Italy	82.3 years	2.8 per 1,000 live births	7.5 per 100,000 live births	Heart disease
Spain	83.0 years	2.9 per 1,000 live births	4.5 per 100,000 live births	Heart disease
Poland	77.2 years	4.8 per 1,000 live births	11.0 per 100,000 live births	Cardiovascular diseases
Portugal	81.07 years	2.2 per 1,000 live births	12.0 per 100,000 live births	Stroke
North Asia	73.2 years	12.9 per 1,000 live births	127 per 100,000 live births	Heart disease
Russia	71.9 years	7.1 per 1,000 live births	25.4 per 100,000 live births	Cardiovascular diseases
Mongolia	71.5 years	33.2 per 1,000 live births	135.0 per 100,000 live births	Respiratory infections
Georgia	75.6 years	9.0 per 1,000 live births	33.9 per 100,000	Cardiovascular diseases

Sources: Centers for Disease Control and Prevention. (2021). *Leading causes of death*. https://www.cdc.gov/ncbddd/leading-causes-of-death.html; Central Intelligence Agency. (2024). *Infant mortality rate—The world factbook*. www.cia.gov/the-world-factbook/field/infant-mortality-rate/country-comparison/; UN Population Fund. (2023). *Maternal mortality*. https://www.unfpa.org/maternal-mortality; World Health Organization. (2023). *Global health estimates: Life expectancy and leading causes of death*. https://www.who.int/data/gho

REFERENCES

Centers for Disease Control and Prevention. (2021). *Leading causes of death*. https://www.cdc.gov/ncbddd/leading-causes-of-death.html

Central Intelligence Agency. (2024). *Infant mortality rate—The world factbook*. www.cia.gov/the-world-factbook/field/infant-mortality-rate/country-comparison/

European Commission. (2023). *Health in the EU*. https://ec.europa.eu/health/health_policies/health_data_en

Miranda, D. (2022, September 13). *Challenges, progress, opportunities: European and Central Asian health systems.* https://eurohealthobservatory.who.int/news-room/news/item/13-09-2022-challenges-progress-opportunities-european-and-central-asian-health-systems

National Oceanic and Atmospheric Administration. (2023). *Global weather.* www.noaa.gov/jetstream/global

UN Population Fund. (2023). *Maternal mortality.* https://www.unfpa.org/maternal-mortality

World Health Organization. (2023). *Global health estimates: Life expectancy and leading causes of death.* https://www.who.int/data/gho

CHAPTER 22

GEORGIA

Nino Paichadze

INTRODUCTION

The Republic of Georgia, a former Soviet republic, has a highly urban and relatively diverse population with rich culture and traditions. Since declaring independence in 1991, Georgia has achieved improvements in population health and its healthcare system. This chapter provides context for these changes, reviews key population health outcomes and their determinants, and describes the current state of the healthcare system. Georgia's hybrid healthcare system (combining elements of public and private medical care) is still undergoing significant reform, and it remains to be seen how effective these changes will be in meeting the needs of the population and delivering quality care.

GEOGRAPHY AND POPULATION

GEOGRAPHICAL FEATURES

Georgia, an upper-middle–income country in the World Health Organization (WHO) European region, spans an area of 69,700 square kilometers (43,300 square miles) and is located on the eastern shore of the Black Sea (Central Intelligence Agency [CIA], 2024; WHO, 2024). It is bordered by Russia and the Greater Caucasus Mountains to the north, and Turkey, Armenia, and Azerbaijan to the south. The major rivers include the Mtkvari (Kura), Rioni, Enguri, and Alazani. The landscape is punctuated with the snow-covered peaks and glaciers of the Greater and Lesser Caucasus Mountains where the summits are as high as 5,000 meters (16,400 feet). Georgia has a diverse climate, with humid subtropical weather in western regions and a continental climate in the east (World Bank Group, 2021).

DEMOGRAPHIC FEATURES

The current population of Georgia is 3.7 million and is projected to decrease by 9.6% by 2050 (WHO, 2024). Georgia has a relatively young population with a low proportion of older people which is predicted to change as the population ages over the next 30 years (WHO, 2024). The current share of persons age 0 to 14 years is 15.0%; the working age population (15 to 64 years is 71.7%; while those 65 years and older comprise 13.3% (WHO, 2024). The fertility rate, which increased from 1.59 per 1,000 women in 2004 to 2.20 in 2015, was 2.06 per 1,000 women in 2022 (United Nations, 2024). The reasons for this increase are not entirely clear but likely reflect economic changes, government policies, and changing social norms.

ETHNIC GROUPS, RELIGION, AND LANGUAGE

The ethnic, religious, and linguistic composition of Georgia is diverse and has been shaped by its over 2,500-year history, with influxes of different ethnic groups from neighboring countries. Over 86.6% of the population are Georgians, 6.3% Azeri, 4.5% Armenians, and 2.3% other (CIA, 2024). In this Eastern Orthodox Christian country, 83.5% of the population are Christians and 10.7% Muslim (CIA, 2024). Georgian, a Kartvelian language, is the official and most widely spoken language (87.6% of the population); other languages spoken in the country include Azeri, Armenian, and Russian (CIA, 2024).

RURAL/URBAN

Georgia is highly urbanized with 61.0% of the population living in urban areas (National Statistics Office of Georgia [Geostat], n.d.). Over one third of Georgians live in the capital city of Tbilisi which has a population of 1.3 million. Other major cities include Batumi (population 183,181) in the southwest, Kutaisi (population 178,338) in the west, and Rustavi (population 130,100) in the southeast (Geostat, n.d.).

MIGRATION

After the disintegration of the Soviet Union, migration from Georgia has increased due to: (a) ethnic minorities returning to their countries of origin, (b) better socioeconomic conditions, and (c) wars, conflict, and political unrest (Bogishvili, 2021). Currently more than 861,000 Georgians live outside of the country (UN Department of Economic and Social Affairs [UNDESA], 2020). The value of remittances received in Georgia has been growing and in 2022 reached $3.85 billion and represented 15.6% of the gross domestic product (GDP; World Bank Group, n.d.).

CULTURE AND TRADITIONS

Georgian culture is deeply rooted in traditions of hospitality, winemaking, folk arts, literature, and distinctive architectural styles that have been preserved over centuries (National Geographic, 2018). Winemaking in Georgia dates back over 8,000 years and is deeply ingrained in the national culture and identity. Ancient winemaking traditions involve unique methods like fermenting wine in *qveri* (large clay vessels buried in the ground) and is included on the UNESCO Intangible Cultural Heritage list (UNESCO, n.d.).

POLITICAL SYSTEM

Georgia has a multiparty political system, with the ruling party and several other parties represented in Parliament (Kakhishvili et al., 2021). The country is a semipresidential republic where the president is the head of state, elected by direct popular vote for a 5-year term (CIA, 2024). The president shares power with the prime minister who is the head of government and leads the executive branch. The prime minister is nominated by the president and approved by the Parliament (CIA, 2024). The Cabinet of Ministers is appointed by the prime minister and is responsible for most executive functions and reports to the legislature (CIA, 2024).

BRIEF COUNTRY HISTORY

The region of Georgia once encompassed the ancient kingdoms of Colchis in the west and Iberia (Kartli) in the east (Curtis, 1994). The area was under Roman influence in the first centuries CE and Christianity became the state religion of both kingdoms by the middle of the fourth century. A Georgian golden age from the 11th to the 13th centuries was short-lived as the Mongols invaded the country in 1236. Subsequently, there was a period of contention between the Ottoman and Persian empires over influence in the region. In the 19th century, Georgia was annexed by the Russian Empire; it declared independence for a short period of time (1918–1921) following the Russian Revolution and subsequently became part of the Soviet Union until it regained independence on April 9, 1991.

Post-Soviet Georgia has faced territorial conflicts with the regions of Abkhazia and South Ossetia, who were backed by Russia. The regions declared independence after wars in the early 1990s (Wolff, n.d.). In 2008, Russia invaded Georgian territory in South Ossetia (North Atlantic Treaty Organization [NATO], 2024). While the United Nations and all but six Member States recognize these territories as part of Georgia, as of 2022 20% of Georgian territory is occupied by

Russia and 292,856 people are internally displaced (United Nations, 2023). Despite the challenges, Georgia has pushed for closer ties with the West, becoming one of NATO's closest partners and receiving EU candidate status in 2023.

HEALTH OUTCOMES

LIFE EXPECTANCY

Life expectancy at birth in Georgia has improved from 69.4 years in 2000 to 71.2 years in 2021 (WHO, 2024). There are significant gender disparities, with life expectancy for females at 75.6 years compared to only 66.9 years for males (WHO, 2024). Although Georgia lags behind some European nations where life expectancy is currently 76.3 years, its upward trajectory can be attributed to improvements in areas like healthcare access, nutrition, living standards, and economic development since 1991 (WHO, 2024).

LEADING CAUSES OF MORTALITY

Noncommunicable diseases (NCDs), accounting for 93% of all deaths and 25% of premature mortality, are the leading cause of morbidity and mortality in Georgia (WHO, n.d.). After COVID-19, which claimed over 17,000 lives throughout the pandemic (Johns Hopkins Coronavirus Resource Center, 2023) and was the top cause of death in 2021, the main causes of deaths per 100,000 population were stroke, ischemic heart disease, and hypertensive heart disease (Figure 22.1; Institute for Health Metrics and Evaluation [IHME], 2023). These three leading causes were the same for both men and women and have remained the same since 1990 (IHME, 2023).

MENTAL HEALTH

Mental health disorders were responsible for 154 deaths per 100,000 population and were among the top 10 causes of hospitalizations in 2021 (National Center for Disease Control and Public Health [NCDC], 2021). The incidence rate was 119.8 per 100,000 population including 109.5 per 100,000 among children (NCDC, 2021). Suicide mortality was 9.2 per 100,000 in 2019 (WHO, 2024).

COMMUNICABLE DISEASES

Since 1991, tuberculosis (TB) has emerged as a major public health problem in Georgia. Despite significant progress in combatting the burden, in 2019 the incidence rate was 74 per 100,000 population and mortality rate was 4.1 per 100,000 population (End TB, n.d.). An estimated 12% of new cases and 32% of previously treated cases were multidrug-resistant, rifampicin-resistant TB (Treat, n.d.).

Georgia is a low HIV epidemic country with prevalence of 0.4% in the adult population (UN AIDS, 2020) with most HIV cases concentrated among people who inject drugs (PWID), men who have sex with men (MSM) and female sex workers (FSW) and their partners. Georgia has exemplary achievements: In 2019, MSM and FSW cases had 91% antiretroviral (ARV) coverage among diagnosed people; viral suppression rates of 97% among those on treatment; and 64% of PWID cases living with HIV (UN AIDS, 2020).

MATERNAL AND INFANT MORTALITY

The maternal mortality ratio in Georgia has improved from 52.8 deaths per 100,000 live births in 2000 to 27.6 deaths per 100,000 live births in 2020 (WHO, 2024). However, maternal mortality is still higher than the regional average (13.2 per 100,000 live births in Europe). The trend for infant mortality rate is similar with a decrease from 31.7 per 1,000 live births in 2000 to 8.5 per 1,000 live births in 2020 (UNICEF, n.d.). Despite recent improvements, there is further need to ensure broad availability of emergency obstetric care and newborn care and to increase the quality of that care.

FIGURE 22.1 Top 10 causes of deaths in Georgia per 100,000 population, 2021.

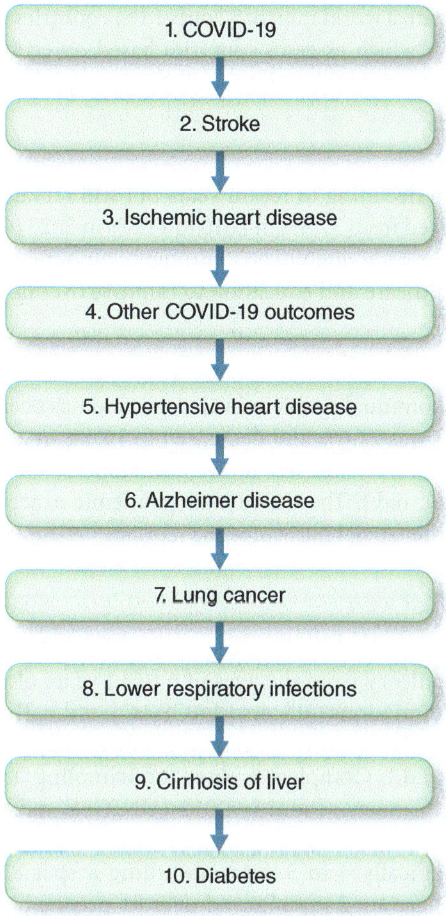

Source: Institute for Health Metrics and Evaluation. (2023). *Georgia quick facts*. https://www.healthdata.org/research-analysis/health-by-location/profiles/georgia

QUALITY OF LIFE INDEX

Quality of life in Georgia is improving since early 2010s. The UN Development Programme's (UNDP) **Human Development Index (HDI)** calculates achievement in three dimensions of human development: a long and healthy life, access to knowledge, and a decent standard of living. The HDI value for Georgia for 2022 was 0.814 which is classified as very high development with a rank of 60 out of 193 countries. This is slightly below its neighbors of Russia (ranked 56) and Turkey (45), but above Armenia (ranked 76) and Azerbaijan (89; UNDP, 2024).

DETERMINANTS OF HEALTH

ECONOMIC PROFILE

Georgia is a small transitional market economy which has made important reductions in poverty and gains in income over the past decade. The gross domestic product (GDP) was $24.78 billion in 2022 while the GDP per capita was $6,675 (World Bank Group, n.d.). Since 2003, Georgia has implemented broad economic reforms to liberalize its economy and attract foreign investment, but challenges still persist, such as high unemployment and reliance on remittances, meaning the money is being sent from other countries to family and friends residing in Georgia. Georgia's economy is considered moderately free with a world rank of 32 out of 184 countries by the Heritage Foundation's Index of Economic Freedom which assesses countries based on economic determinants such as property rights, tax burden, investment freedom, and other measures (Heritage Foundation, 2023).

POVERTY

Poverty in Georgia has been declining in recent years but still remains a challenge. The national absolute poverty rate decreased from 37.3% in 2010 to 11.8% in 2023 (Geostat, n.d.). The Georgian government aims to continue reducing poverty through economic growth, targeted social policies, and investments in healthcare and education to improve overall well-being.

UNEMPLOYMENT

Unemployment has been a continual problem in Georgia and has been a driver of migration. The unemployment rate in 2017 was 21.6% and decreased to 16.4% in 2022; however, it was as high as 20.6% in 2021 (Geostat, n.d.). Of those who were unemployed, 38.5% were unemployed for 12 months or more (Geostat, n.d.). The COVID-19 pandemic exacerbated general poverty and unemployment as well as other social hardships in Georgia.

EDUCATION AND LITERACY

Georgia has made significant strides in improving education and literacy rates in recent decades. Education is free and compulsory from the ages of 6 to 14 years old (American Association of Collegiate Registrars and Admissions Officers [AACRAO], n.d.). The system consists of 6 years of primary school, 3 years of basic (lower secondary) education, and 3 years of upper secondary education (AACRAO, n.d.). Completion rates for schooling are high with 100% of both girls and boys completing primary school in 2018 (UNICEF, n.d.). Literacy among children 15 to 24 years is also high with 100% of both girls and boys being literate (UNICEF, n.d.). University programs are typically 4 to 5 years, awarding a specialist's diploma or bachelor's degree (AACRAO, n.d.). There are 24 public and over 81 private higher education institutions in the country (AACRAO, n.d.).

NUTRITION

Undernutrition is not widespread; in 2018, among children under 5 years of age, 2.1% were underweight and 5.8% had stunted growth (National Statistics Office of Georgia, 2019). However, anemia is a much bigger problem, affecting 27.5% of women of reproductive age and 24.6% of children under 5 years in 2019, indicating micronutrient deficiencies (WHO, n.d.). In addition, 34.7% of adults (33.3% men and 34.9% of women) were classified as obese in 2022 (WHO, n.d.). Childhood obesity is also a growing concern, with 10.1% of those 5 to 19 years old being obese (WHO, n.d.).

LEADING RISK FACTORS FOR MORTALITY

The top three leading risk factors for deaths per 100,000 are high blood pressure, dietary risks, and tobacco use (Figure 22.2; IHME, 2023). Not surprisingly, almost all top 10 risks are health behaviors associated with the highest cause of death in Georgia—NCDs. Among Georgians over age 15, 32.0% are current tobacco users and 18.5% participate in heavy episodic drinking (WHO, n.d.). Sixty-six percent of adults are currently overweight and 35.0% are classified as obese. There are also gender disparities, with men having higher tobacco and alcohol use. The Georgian government enacted an NCD national strategy and action plan in 2017 and has some policies in place to limit tobacco demand, reduce harmful use of alcohol, and improve healthy diets, but more action is still needed.

FIGURE 22.2 Top 10 risk factors for deaths in Georgia per 100,000 population, 2021.

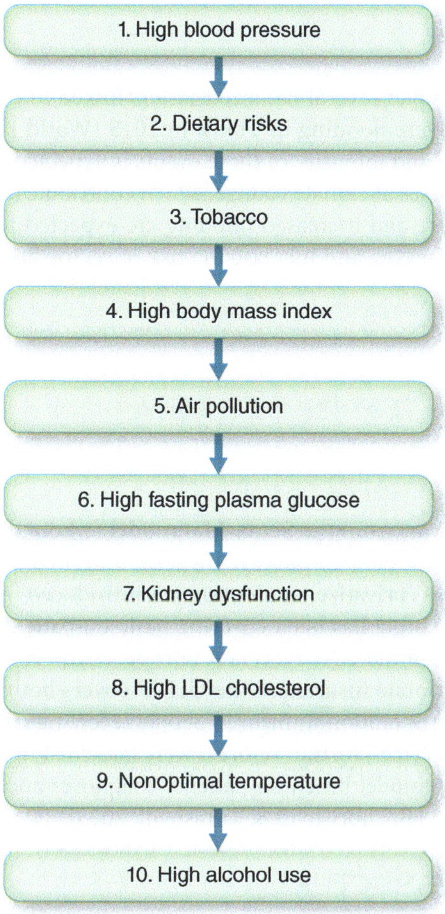

LDL, low-density lipoprotein.

Source: Institute for Health Metrics and Evaluation. (2023). *Georgia quick facts.* https://www.healthdata.org/research-analysis/health-by-location/profiles/georgia

SOCIAL JUSTICE

Introduction of the Universal Health Care Programme (UHCP) in 2013 marked a radical shift toward Universal Health Coverage (UHC), aiming to include the uninsured population. By 2017, over 90% of the population was covered by the UHCP, reflecting a significant stride toward equitable healthcare access (WHO Regional Office for Europe [WHO/Europe], 2020). Despite increased investment, public health expenditure remains low at 2.24% of total government health spending as of 2015 (WHO/Europe, 2020). High medication costs place a significant financial burden on the population. In 2017, pharmaceuticals accounted for 38% of health expenditures, with 27.8% of households reporting medication costs as their primary financial concern (WHO/Europe, 2020). The UHCP has increased health service utilization, particularly in rural areas and among the poorest households. In 2017, care-seeking behavior increased from 70.9% to 77.8% in the poorest quintile (WHO/Europe, 2020), narrowing the gap with wealthier groups. However, geographical variations persist, with rural residents facing greater challenges in accessing care. Georgia's health system reforms and UHC's efforts reflect significant strides towardsocial justice, yet persistent inequalities and systemic inefficiencies highlight the need for continued focus on equitable health access and outcomes.

CLIMATE CHANGE

In recent years, Georgia has had several natural disasters linked to changing climate such as the the drought of 2000 and severe flooding in Tbilisi in 2015 (World Bank & Asian Development Bank, 2021). The frequency and intensity of these events is expected to increase in the future. In addition to the economic losses of climate change, which contribute to higher poverty and unemployment, rising temperature and increased flooding are expected to lead to heat-related mortality, exacerbate existing diseases, and increase the risk of vector-borne diseases such as malaria within the country.

HEALTHCARE SYSTEM IN GEORGIA

HEALTHCARE DELIVERY AND FINANCING

The health system moved away from the **Semashko model** (where the healthcare system is centralized, state-run, and facilities are all publicly owned), inherited at independence, and is now decentralized. The system was privatized under reforms introduced from 2007 to 2012 and, since 2013, the government of Georgia has been covering basic outpatient, inpatient, and emergency services to all citizens through the UHCP (WHO/Europe, 2020). A small number of individuals benefit from private or corporate insurance. The UHCP covers both primary healthcare (PHC) and specialty care, with over 2 million uninsured people receiving coverage under this program. To encourage use of PHC services, further reforms were launched in 2021 with a revised benefits package and a new funding model based on patients' diagnoses and other factors (age, gender, etc.) was introduced in 2023 (Bochorishvili & Kurashvili, 2023).

HEALTHCARE INFRASTRUCTURE

In 2021, Georgia had 269 inpatient hospital facilities and 2,272 outpatient facilities (**polyclinics**, rural doctor's offices, etc.; NCDC, 2021). These facilities are primarily private, for-profit entities with the exclusion of rural ambulatories and medical centers in some hard-to-reach locations which are public (WHO/Europe, 2022). There were 556 hospital beds per 100,000 population and 80% of those beds were private (WHO/Europe, 2022). A limited number of specialty hospitals (such as for TB or psychiatry) are publicly owned and run (WHO/Europe, 2022).

The healthcare workforce is characterized by an excess of doctors, a lack of nurses, and uneven geographic distribution of providers. There were 56.1 medical doctors per 100,000 population in 2022, higher than the European average of 37.6 per 100,000 (WHO, 2024). Nurses (and midwives) number only 59.8 per 10,000 population in Georgia and 82.6 per 10,000 population on average in Europe (WHO, 2024).

HEALTHCARE TRAINING AND EDUCATION

Despite prioritizing bachelor's degree education, the number of nurses completing higher education between 2018 and 2021 decreased annually, while vocational nursing program enrollments remained high (State Audit Office of Georgia [SAO], 2023). In 2021, 15.2% of nurses were of retirement age, and new graduates constituted only 2.6% of the incoming workforce (SAO, 2023). Postgraduate medical education and certification mechanisms have several shortcomings; quality assessments are not conducted during qualification and certification tests, and updates to these tests are infrequent. Since 2018, the Ministry has been implementing continuous medical education (CME) in Georgia to ensure improvement of medical personnels' qualifications. However, participation in CME programs is low. Only 43% of doctors participated in CME from 2018 to 2021 (SAO, 2023).

HEALTHCARE COST, ACCESS, AND QUALITY

Georgia's spending on health has increased due to the UHCP but is still low by comparison to the region. Public spending on health was 2.7% of the GDP in 2019, well below the European average of 5.0% (WHO, 2023; WHO/Europe, 2022). Average health spending per capita was $970 compared to $3,225 in the region. The per-capita health spending breakdown is 41.0% public spending, 46.8% out-of-pocket spending, and small amounts allocated to private health insurance and other spending. With reforms, the share of public spending has increased while out-of-pocket spending decreased. However, out-of-pocket spending as a percentage is still high compared to the region and represents an important burden. Spending on outpatient medications, which were not part of the 2013 reform, is also a constraint.

Access to healthcare is limited by these high out-of-pocket costs, but there have been some increases in healthcare usage since the 2013 reforms. The number of encounters with outpatient facilities was 3.2 per capita in 2014 and increased to 4.4 per capita in 2021 (WHO/Europe, 2022). This is still low compared to 6.0 per capita in the European region (WHO/Europe, 2022). Inpatient use has also increased since 2014 when the bed occupancy rate was 188.3 and has improved to 201.2 in 2021 (WHO/Europe, 2022).

GAPS IN CARE

Georgia's healthcare system faces several critical gaps in care including financial barriers, workforce imbalances, fragmented PHC systems, issues in managing communicable diseases and NCDs, equity issues, and regional disparities and health information systems. The PHC system in Georgia is fragmented, offering poor value for the money compared to specialist or hospital care. PHC providers are paid a fixed rate per patient, incentivizing them to refer higher-risk patients to hospital care, which is reimbursed based on activity (WHO/Europe, 2020). This creates a preference for ambulance and inpatient care, further straining the healthcare system. The UHCP has improved access to healthcare for many households near the poverty line, but significant geographic disparities remain (WHO/Europe, 2020). Limited public sector coverage of outpatient medicines forces patients to pay out-of-pocket for drugs, increasing the risk of impoverishment and creating barriers to timely preventive care (WHO/Europe, 2020). This reliance on costly hospital and emergency care services further highlights the gaps in the healthcare system.

The healthcare data collection process in Georgia is highly fragmented, data collected in one part of the system are not easily accessible or usable in another (WHO/Europe, 2023). There are currently 188 different forms used in PHC facilities, many of which collect overlapping data (WHO/Europe, 2023). This redundancy not only consumes valuable time and resources but also leads to inconsistencies and errors in data recording.

HEALTHCARE PRACTICES

TRADITIONAL AND COMPLEMENTARY CARE

Georgia has a rich history of traditional medicine, with written medical records dating back to the 10th century. Today, the use of complementary and alternative medicine (CAM) is common in Georgia, although comprehensive data are scarce. CAM users in Georgia are generally disappointed with conventional medicine and seek more natural remedies (Nadareishvili et al., 2019) They report high satisfaction with CAM and do not often share their use of CAM with conventional medical providers (Nadareishvili et al., 2019).

HEALTHCARE INNOVATIONS

Digital Health

In recent years, the country has taken steps to build digital capacity through telemedicine and digital health solutions. Recent reforms identify digital solutions as a key component and the COVID-19 epidemic reinforced this need. As part of this effort, internet connections were established at 1,000 rural ambulatories (Zoidze et al., 2021). The UHCP has made significant progress in digital health and healthcare innovation, although the program's electronic data systems primarily monitor service uptake for financial processes rather than clinical quality. The NCDC manages electronic cancer screening registries and had documented screenings for over 80,000 individuals by 2021, and an immunization registry that recorded vaccinations for 90% of children under 5 years by 2022 (Machl, 2024).

CONCLUSION

Georgia has seen important improvements in the last 20 years in life expectancy and maternal mortality among other indicators; however, it lags behind the European region on many measures of population health. Like many countries, Georgia is struggling with the growing crisis of noncommunicable diseases and will need to address the high prevalence of risk factors in order to improve health outcomes. The country faces several important challenges to its healthcare system such as improving rural population health, reducing out-of-pocket costs, and improving health system performance, all of which need to be addressed to improve the overall health status of the country.

LEARNING ACTIVITIES

CourseConnect

To access self-assessment questions and interactive, competency-based learning activities for this chapter, visit www.springerpub.com/courseconnect. See inside front cover and tear-out for CourseConnect details.

REFERENCES

American Association of Collegiate Registrars and Admissions Officers. (n.d.). *Georgia*. https://www.aacrao.org/edge/country/georgia

Bochorishvili, E., & Kurashvili, S. (2023). *Georgia's healthcare sector*. Galt & Taggart. https://galtandtaggart.com/files/galt/georgias-healthcare-sector-overview_eng_may-23.pdf

Bogishvili, D. (2021). *Migration and its impacts on Georgia*. Centre for East European and International Studies (ZOiS). https://www.zois-berlin.de/en/publications/migration-and-its-impacts-on-georgia

Central Intelligence Agency. (2024). *The world factbook*. https://www.cia.gov/the-world-factbook/countries/georgia/

Curtis, G. E. (1994). *Georgia: A country study*. Library of Congress.

End TB. (n.d.) *End TB: Georgia*. https://endtb.org/georgia

Heritage Foundation. (2023). *Economic freedom country profile: Georgia*. https://www.heritage.org/index/pages/country-pages/georgia

Institute for Health Metrics and Evaluation. (2023). *GBD compare*. https://vizhub.healthdata.org/gbd-compare/

Johns Hopkins Coronavirus Resource Center. (2023). *Georgia*. https://coronavirus.jhu.edu/region/georgia

Kakhishvili, L., Keshelava, D., Papava, G., & Sichinava, D. (2021). *Georgia's political landscape: Diversity, convergence, and empty spots*. Friedrich-Ebert-Stiftung. https://southcaucasus.fes.de/news-list/e/georgias-political-landscape

Machl, S. (2024). *Telemedicine: Bridging a healthcare gap in Georgia*. https://georgia.un.org/en/258633-telemedicine-bridging-healthcare-gap-georgia

Nadareishvili, I., Pkhakadze, G., Tskitishvili, A., Bakuradze, N., & Lunze, K. (2019). Georgia's healthcare system and integration of complementary medicine. *Complementary therapies in medicine, 45*, 205–210. https://doi.org/10.1016/j.ctim.2019.06.016

National Center for Diseases Control and Public Health. (2021). *Health care statistical yearbook 2021 Georgia*. National Center for Diseases Control and Public Health.

National Geographic. (2018). *Eight surprising Georgian traditions*. https://www.nationalgeographic.com/travel/article/sponsor-content-8-surprising-georgian-traditions

National Statistics Office of Georgia. (n.d.). *Statistics*. https://www.geostat.ge/en

National Statistics Office of Georgia. (2019). *Georgia multiple indicator cluster survey 2018, survey findings report*. National Statistics Office of Georgia.

North Atlantic Treaty Organization. (2024). *Relations with Georgia*. https://www.nato.int/cps/en/natohq/topics_38988.htm

State Audit Office of Georgia. (2023). *Efficiency audit report: Professional development and efficiency of medical personnel*. State Audit Office of Georgia. https://sao.ge/en/

UN AIDS. (2020). *Country progress report—Georgia*. https://treattb.org/trial-sites/georgia/

United Nations. (2023). *Status of internally displaced persons and refugees from Abkhazia, Georgia, and the Tskhinvali region/South Ossetia, Georgia (A/77/870)*. https://undocs.org/Home/Mobile?FinalSymbol=A/77/870&Language=E&DeviceType=Desktop&LangRequested=False

United Nations. (2024). *UN data portal*. https://population.un.org/dataportal/home

UN Department of Economic and Social Affairs. (2020). *International migrant stock 2020*. https://www.un.org/en/desa/products/un-desa-databases

UN Development Programme. (2024). *Human development reports: Georgia*. https://hdr.undp.org/data-center/specific-country-data#/countries/GEO

UNESCO. (n.d.). *Ancient Georgian traditional qvevri wine-making method*. https://ich.unesco.org/en/RL/ancient-georgian-traditional-qvevri-wine-making-method-00870

UNICEF. (n.d.). *Country profiles: Georgia*. https://data.unicef.org/country/geo/

Wolff, S. (n.d.). *Georgia: Abkhazia and South Ossetia*. https://pesd.princeton.edu/node/706

World Bank Group. (n.d.). *World Bank open data*. https://data.worldbank.org/

World Bank Group. (2021). *World Bank climate change knowledge portal*. https://climateknowledgeportal.worldbank.org/country/georgia/climate-data-historical

World Bank & Asian Development Bank. (2021). *Climate risk country profile: Georgia*. World Bank and Asian Development Bank.

World Health Organization. (n.d.). *NCD data portal: Georgia*. https://ncdportal.org/CountryProfile/GHE110/GEO

World Health Organization. (2023). *Global health expenditure database*. https://apps.who.int/nha/database/Home/Index/en

World Health Organization. (2024). *Indicators*. https://data.who.int/indicators

WHO Regional Office for Europe. (2020). *Health and sustainable development: Progress in Georgia*. https://iris.who.int/handle/10665/359543

WHO Regional Office for Europe. (2022). *Health systems in action: Georgia*. https://eurohealthobservatory.who.int/publications/i/health-systems-in-action-georgia-2022

WHO Regional Office for Europe. (2023). *WHO COVID-19 response program: Report development on mapping of health data systems in Georgia. https://iris.who.int/handle/10665/359543*

Zoidze, A., Gabunia, T., & Ekberg, A. (2021). *Georgia: From crisis to opportunity: Advancing primary health care reform amid the COVID-19 pandemic*. WHO Regional Office for Europe.

CHAPTER 23

GREAT BRITAIN

Daniel C. Ehlke

INTRODUCTION

The United Kingdom of Great Britain and Northern Ireland (Figure 23.1) is an amalgam of nations (England, Scotland, Wales, and Northern Ireland) under a single head of state (currently King Charles III). It is a relatively densely populated realm, spread primarily across parts of two large islands. Its health sector is dominated by the National Health Service (NHS), a government owned and operated health system that is free to patients at the point of service. Founded in 1949, the NHS has become an institution many consider integral to British identity, and aspects of it have been copied in health systems around the world. Known as a birthplace of the sports of football (soccer), golf, and cricket, the British Isles was also a seminal site in the history of public health, with the early epidemiologic investigations of John Snow (Seaton, 2023).

GEOGRAPHY AND POPULATION

The country is comprised of a large, central island (known as Great Britain), on which is situated England, Wales, and much of Scotland. The northernmost portion of a neighboring (large) island to the east comprises Ireland, a part of the United Kingdom (the rest of that island constitutes the separate nation of Ireland Northern). A series of smaller islands to the north (most notably the Shetland and Orkney Islands) form part of Scotland. In terms of physical size, around three quarters of the land area could fit within the American state of Ohio. The total land area amounts to around 94,000 square miles.

DEMOGRAPHIC CHARACTERISTICS

The United Kingdom is home to a diverse population, itself partly one of the legacies of its imperial past. The national population is estimated at 69,138,000 as of 2024 (UN Data, 2024). Of that total population, nearly 10 million reside in the capital city of London. When it comes to the constituent parts of the United Kingdom, England accounted for 84.4% of the total population, Scotland 8.2%, Wales 4.6%, and Northern Ireland 2.8% (Central Intelligence Agency [CIA], 2024).

AGE

British society is aging, although the proportion of the population between infancy and 14 years remains flat. From 2010 to 2021, the percentage of those over the age of 60 years rose from 22.6% to 24.7%, while the percentage of children (age 0 to 14) remained just about steady, ranging between 17.5% and 17.6% years. Also remaining steady during the 11 years after 2010 was the nation's fertility rate, which was 1.9 per 1,000 in 2010, and 1.8 per 1,000 in both 2015 and 2021 (UN Data, 2024). The country continues to be enriched by those arriving from overseas; it was estimated that those with an initial background as international migrants came in at 7.1 million in 2010, rising to 9.4 million in 2021, even as the number of refugees has declined, from 253,000 (2010) to 192,000 (UN Data, 2024).

FIGURE 23.1 Map of the United Kingdom.

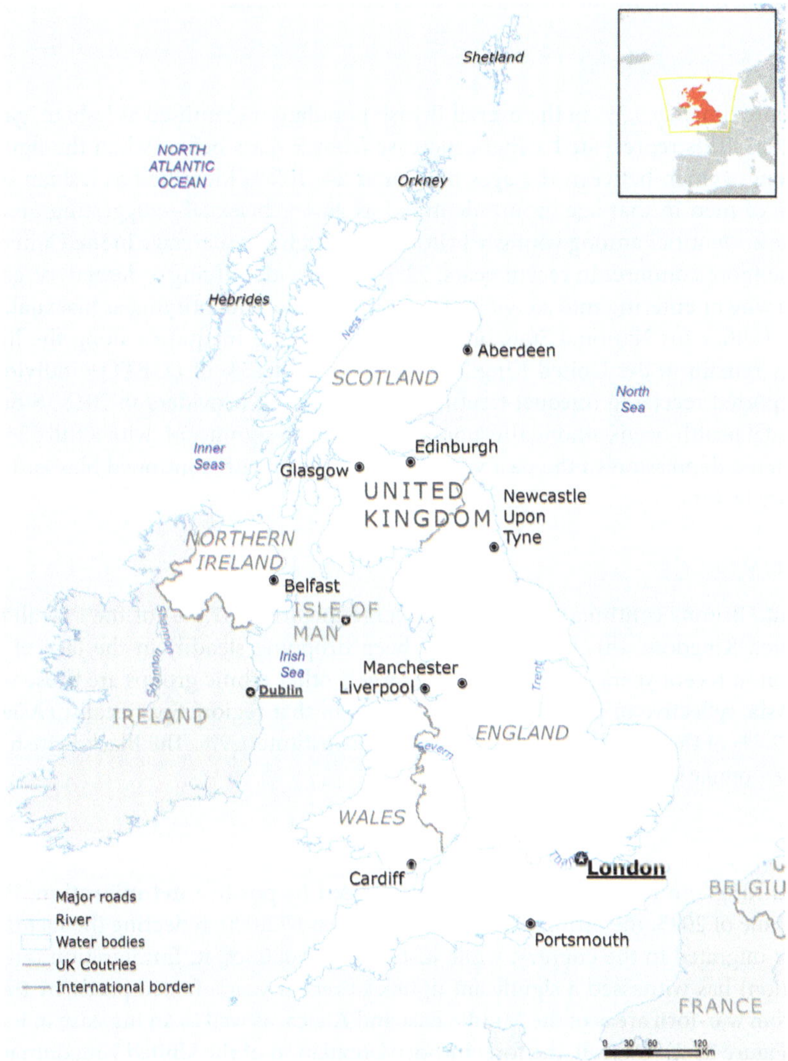

Source: European Commission. (n.d.). *Maps*. ERCC Portal. https://erccportal.jrc.ec.europa.eu/ECHO-Products/Maps

URBAN/RURAL

As of 2022, the urban population of the United Kingdom is estimated to be 56.5 million, while the rural population stands at 10.5 million. While the urban population has, in recent years, continued to grow on an annual basis, the rural population has witnessed a slow decline and, indeed, has remained fairly flat for decades (e.g., the rural population stood at 11.3 million in 1960). Though the United Kingdom's population is skewed toward urban areas, the country nonetheless contains vast expanses of countryside and sparsely populated regions, particularly in the north and west.

SEX AND GENDER

In the United Kingdom, there are 97.8 males for every 100 females. According to 2021 estimates, there were 262,000 transgender individuals in England and Wales, accounting for around 0.5% of the overall population (Office for National Statistics, 2021). The Scottish census does not currently contain information specific to transgender individuals, with a 2022 court decision allowing those identifying as trans to choose the gender to which they identify, including cases in which that differs from the information on one's birth certificate.

SEXUAL ORIENTATION

Overall, approximately 3.3% of the overall British population identified as lesbian, gay, or bisexual as of 2022. This represented a slight increase from 5 years before when the figure stood at 2.1%. Among women between the ages of 16 and 24, 10.6% identified as lesbian or bisexual, while 7.9% of men in that age group identified as gay or bisexual—suggesting greater acceptance of these identities among younger Britons. Although gay marriage in the United Kingdom has become more common in recent years, 72% of those identifying as lesbian or gay reported never marrying or entering into a civil partnership. For those identifying as bisexual, that figure was 82.9% (Office for National Statistics, 2022). Healthcare inequities along the lines of sexual identity remain in the United Kingdom: An estimated 13% of LGBTQ+ individuals in the country reported receiving unequal treatment by healthcare providers in 2018 (Stonewall UK, 2018). Mental health needs among this population are also significant, with a full 52% reporting having suffered depression in the past year (2017 to 2018), with continued bias and stigma key contributory factors.

ETHNICITY/RACE

While White Britons continue to constitute a large majority (87.2%) of the overall population of the United Kingdom, this proportion has been dropping steadily in the face of substantial immigration in recent years and decades. The largest other ethnic groups are those with origins in South Asia, reflective of past British **colonialism** in that region. Specifically, (Asian) Indians constitute 2.3% of the population, while Pakistanis constitute 1.9%. The Black British/Caribbean share of the population is 3% (CIA, 2024).

IMMIGRATION

The United Kingdom remains a country characterized by positive **net migration**. For the year ending in June of 2023, the estimated net migration was 672,000, reflecting the fact that 1.2 million people migrated to the country, while just over 500,000 left it. Immigration (and therefore net migration) has witnessed a significant uptick in recent years, fueled partly by the arrival of refugees from war-torn areas of the Middle East and Africa, as well as an increase in international students (Figure 23.2). Overall, the foreign-born population of the United Kingdom is estimated to be around 14% (The Migration Observatory, 2024). These individuals come to the country with unique healthcare needs, and will require a continued emphasis on **cultural competency** in the provision of care.

CULTURAL BELIEFS

RELIGION

Despite strong cultural roots in the Christian tradition, adherence to Christian faiths in the United Kingdom has been steadily decreasing over time. In England and Wales, the 2021 census marked the first time reported Christian religious affiliation fell below 50%, settling at 46.3%, down from 59% 10 years before. Thirty-seven percent of the English and Welsh populations reported no faith tradition while Muslims comprised 6.5% of the total and Hindus 1.5% (Office of National Statistics, 2021). Religious data for Scotland were reported in a separate census, but there data are broadly similar with 54% reporting Christian affiliation, 36% reporting no faith tradition, and approximately 1.5% reporting affiliation to Islam (Scotland's Census, 2021b).

FIGURE 23.2 Changes in UK migration.

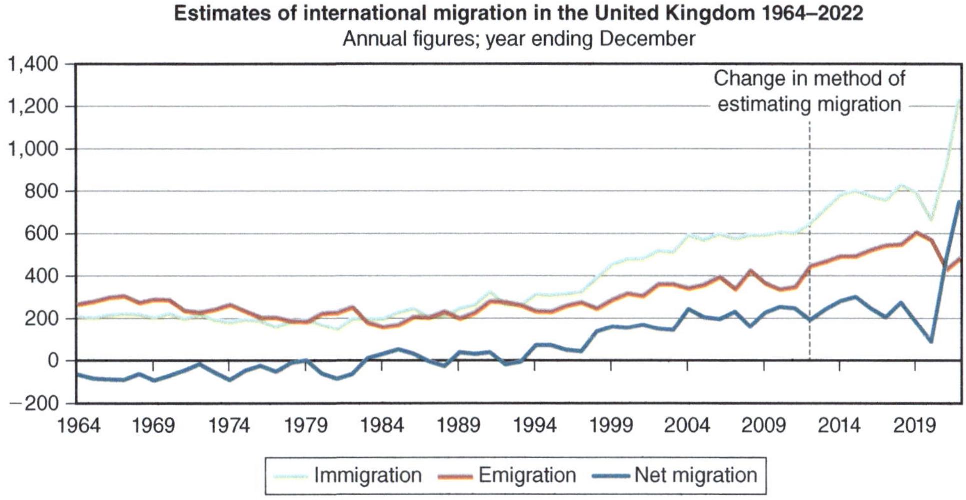

Source: Office for National Statistics. (n.d.). *ONS—Office for National Statistics.* https://www.ons.gov.uk/

LANGUAGES

The primary language spoken across the United Kingdom is English. A Germanic language, English is also heavily influenced by the Romance languages, particularly French. "Indigenous" Celtic languages like Scottish, Gaelic, and Welsh continue to be spoken in portions of the British Isles. Approximately 91% of the population of England and Wales (amounting to 52.6 million) reported English as their primary means of communication in 2024 (Statista, 2024). A similar proportion of Scots (92.8%) 3 years and older reported only speaking English at home (Scotland's Census, 2021a). The most common language other than English in England and Wales was Polish; 1.1% and 0.5% of Scots reported speaking Scottish and Gaelic at home, respectively.

POLITICAL SYSTEM

The roots of the British Parliament stretch back to at least the 14th century. Until the 17th century, monarchs retained significant political prerogatives. Since the "Glorious Revolution" of 1689, royal power has steadily eroded, with the process accelerating during the 19th century. Today, the country is a constitutional monarchy and all practical governing authority at the national level resides in Parliament. Though the United Kingdom is a unitary system, with subnational government retaining few significant powers, localities have historically played a key role in purchasing community health services for residents within the context of the NHS.

HISTORICAL CONSIDERATIONS

The presence of a powerful national legislature with traditionally strong party discipline, joined with a first-past-the-post electoral system that tends to produce large governing majorities, makes dramatic change easier to enact in the United Kingdom, in contrast to the United States and certain other countries. This likely explains in part how a country with broadly similar cultural traditions to that of the United States adopted such a dramatically different healthcare system.

HEALTH OUTCOMES

TOP CAUSES OF DEATH

The leading causes of death in the United Kingdom include Alzheimer disease (145 per 100,000 population); ischemic heart disease (106 per 100,000); lower respiratory infections (60 per 100,000); stroke (56 per 100,000); trachea, bronchus, and lung cancers (53 per 100,000); chronic obstructive pulmonary disease (COPD; 49 per 100,000); colon and rectal cancers (27 per 100,000); prostate cancer (20 per 100,000); breast cancer (19 per 100,000); and lymphomas/multiple myeloma at 14/100,000 (World Health Organization [WHO], 2023). Reflecting generally positive health outcomes nationwide, many of these afflictions can be associated with old age.

MENTAL HEALTH

Britain spends a greater proportion of its overall health investment on mental health than certain peer nations, including the United States (Stanton, 2014). In recent years, health officials have sought to increase the accessibility of psychological ("talking") therapies within the NHS, with an eye toward broadening participation in such programs and decreasing wait times. As a result, in 2023, 89% of those completing a course of "talking therapies" waited under 6 weeks before the first session commenced, beating the relevant government target. Nonetheless, the number of young people suffering from depression has risen in recent years (UK Parliament, 2024).

INFECTIOUS DISEASE

As in many other countries, the United Kingdom has seen considerable success in limiting the spread of infectious diseases in recent decades, though the nation was hit relatively hard by COVID-19 during its most acute phase from 2020 to 2022. To take several examples, there were still over 65,000 cases of whooping cough reported nationwide in 1982; by 2021, cases had dwindled to a mere 521. In 1982, 94,000 cases of measles were reported; by 2021, this number was down to 360 (UK Health Security Agency, 2022).

As of April 2024, the United Kingdom had reported a total of 24,910,387 COVID-19 cases. While case growth was most dramatic from the second half of 2021 through April 2022, when they grew from around 9 million to 21 million, new cases have declined significantly since late 2022, with fewer than 1 million newly diagnosed during that latter timeframe. The government of then prime minister Boris Johnson faced considerable criticism for its relatively laissez-faire approach to the disease in its earlier phases, and the explosion in new cases during this period placed severe strains on the NHS and overall health system, from which it has arguably yet to recover (Worldometer, 2024).

NONCOMMUNICABLE DISEASE

While significant progress has been made in combatting infectious disease across the United Kingdom, noncommunicable disease (NCD) remains a substantial burden nationally. Overall, 89% of deaths in the country can be attributed to NCDs, with heart disease and stroke representing particularly potent threats (Robbins et al., 2021). As in other nations, the British population also struggles with diabetes. An estimated 7% of adults suffer from type 2 diabetes, and 12% of English adults are considered to be prediabetic (Office for National Statistics, 2024).

INFANT AND MATERNAL MORTALITY

During the period between 2020 and 2022, the maternal mortality ratio for the United Kingdom was 13.41 per 100,000 population. As in some other Western nations, there is a significant gap when it comes to maternal mortality risks between White and Black Britons. For Black Britons, the maternal mortality ratio is just under three times greater than that for their White compatriots

(National Perinatal Epidemiology Unit [NPEU], 2024). The infant mortality rate in the country has remained quite low for a number of years. It was last reported to be 3.71 per 1,000 live births in 2022, down from 30 per 1,000 live births in 1950, a few years after the NHS was established (UN Inter-agency Group for Child Mortality Estimation, 2023).

LIFE EXPECTANCY

Overall life expectancy in the United Kingdom was 80.1 as of 2021. With the onset of COVID-19, this represented a drop from a high of 81.4 in 2019. Measured by sex, male life expectancy was 78.3 (down from 79.8 in 2019), and female life expectancy was 81.9 (up from 80.3 in 2019). These figures place the United Kingdom a bit above the United States, but below countries particularly known for population longevity, like Japan (WHO, 2024). Avoidable mortality rates in the United Kingdom are somewhat higher than certain peer nations, at 119 per 100,000 population. This compares to 83 per 100,000 in Japan—but 177 per 100,000 in the United States (Anandaciva, 2023).

DETERMINANTS OF HEALTH

NATIONAL AND PER-CAPITA GROSS DOMESTIC PRODUCT AND POVERTY RATES

The United Kingdom is a relatively wealthy country from a global perspective, although recent years have witnessed growing economic woes, giving rise to increases in such social ills as homelessness. In 2022, the national gross domestic product (GDP) was $3.1 trillion, with a per-capita GDP of $46,125 of the overall labor pool. For 2022 to 2023, the absolute poverty rate (measured as the number falling below 60% of median income in the base year of 2010 to 2011), stood at 12 million, or 18%. The total represented an increase of 600,000 over the previous year, the largest such rise in 30 years (Cuffe, 2024). The past few years also saw a significant increase (by 2.5 million) in food insecurity during the same period (UK Parliament, 2024).

EDUCATION AND LITERACY RATES

As of 2022, around half of British adults had some collegiate academic training, one of the higher rates among European nations (Statista, 2024). That year, 57% of those between 25 and 34 years of age held a upper secondary, college or university degree, up from 29% in 2000 (and somewhat above the Organisation for Economic Cooperation and Development [OECD] average of 48% (OECD, 2022). Some gaps, however, remain to be addressed in education; despite a national headline literacy of 99% (one of the highest in the world), around 16% of Britons were reported as having "very poor" literacy skills (National Literacy Trust, 2024).

UNEMPLOYMENT RATES

According to World Bank estimates, the British unemployment rate in 2023 was around 4.4%, a fairly significant uptick from 2022 which was 3.7%. Nonetheless, this was still well below the 2021 figure of 4.8%, during the height of the COVID-19 pandemic, and far lower than levels reached in the early 1990s, when unemployment was estimated to be closer to 11% (World Bank Group, 2024).

HEALTH BEHAVIORS

SMOKING

Overall across the United Kingdom, 12.9% of adults were reported to be smokers in 2022. This represented a significant drop from 46% of adults in 1974, when smoking rates began to be surveyed on an annual basis. Smoking in the country appears to have peaked in the late 1940s (around the founding of the NHS); in 1948, approximately 85% of British men reported smoking. NHS education campaigns over time as well as cultural stigmatization of smoking have contributed to this significant decline (Action on Smoking and Health, 2023).

FOOD/NUTRITION

The British diet has not historically been known for its variety or particular healthfulness. This is borne out by data from the latest Global Nutrition Report, which notes that the country is "off course" when it comes to hitting major nutritional targets among infants, young children, and mothers. To take one example, 7% of British infants are reported to have low birth weight. National intake of fruits and vegetables falls well below targets, while fish and red meat consumption is significantly above target levels (Global Nutrition Report, 2022). Appropriately for an island nation, fish forms a central part of the British diet, with "fish and chips" traditionally considered something akin to a national meal.

ENVIRONMENTAL AND CLIMATE CHANGE ISSUES

Like many countries around the world, the British people face a grave threat from climate change. Impacts are expected to take the form of increased temperatures, in turn leading to a rise in cases of heat exhaustion and heat stroke, as well as greater precipitation, which could, in turn, contribute to flooding and health impacts surrounding compromised water supplies. While it is difficult to attribute any particular weather event to climate change, the summer of 2022 featured record-breaking heat, with temperatures reaching 40°C (104°F) for the first time since record-keeping began. Climate change is expected to make such instances of extreme heat more common (Gov.uk, 2023).

HISTORICAL/THEORETICAL BACKGROUND OF HEALTHCARE

HEALTHCARE DELIVERY, FINANCE, INSURANCE, AND PAYMENT

The landmark election of 1945 brought to power a strongly progressive Labour Party government led by Clement Attlee. The Attlee government quickly set to work operationalizing elements of the Beveridge Report by developing a government-led, comprehensive, and free at the point of service NHS. The advent of the NHS involved effectively nationalizing the nation's hospitals, and entering into a direct economic relationship with its physicians. After several years of planning and preparation, the NHS officially came into being in 1948.

The Conservative government of Margaret Thatcher (prime minister from 1979 to 1991) sought to introduce greater competition within the NHS, both as a result of ideological commitments, and a desire to make the healthcare system more responsive to patients. This led to the development of the **internal market**, marked by a **purchaser–provider split**, in which hospitals would compete for patients referred to them by general practitioners (GPs) and certain local government bodies. With the return of the Labour Party to government under Tony Blair (prime minister from 1997 to 2008), some elements of the internal market were rolled back, but an emphasis on greater service responsiveness remained, now manifested by the imposition of numerous government performance targets for providers, as well as the establishment of the **National Institute for Health and Clinical Excellence (NICE),** a regulatory body charged with assessing clinical interventions for effectiveness (and recommending them for inclusion within NHS institutions). Under the NHS, remuneration for physicians and other health professionals have evolved over time. Today, doctors are paid under a mix of capitation (payment tied to patient lists, or number of patients) and performance-based compensation (Commonwealth Fund, 2020).

Conservative governments in the 2010s and 2020s have emphasized integration of care, and increased roles for private actors within the NHS. These developments culminated in the establishment of **integrated care systems**, 42 in number across England. These are alliances comprised of NHS institutions, representatives from local government, and private bodies involved in healthcare charged with improving overall population health and improving efficiency. They bear some resemblance to accountable care organizations recently introduced in the United States.

While the NHS in England has evolved considerably with changes in government in recent decades, these changes have penetrated the other nations within the United Kingdom unevenly. The government role remains preponderant, and a high degree of centralization remains the rule in the Scottish NHS. In Northern Ireland, the health system does not even go by the name "NHS"; it is known as Health and Social Care Northern Ireland. As the name implies, it brings together health and social care services, the latter of which are still largely the responsibility of local governments in other parts of the country.

HEALTHCARE PRACTICES

Healthcare in the United Kingdom is marked by strict gatekeeping. Each individual is required to register with a GP in the community. That GP, then, must provide any necessary referrals to more specialized care. Waiting times for specialty care (particularly procedures considered elective) can be long and have been growing longer in recent years. Many physicians attract private patients with the lure of cutting waiting times, which decreases any incentive to collectively work toward bringing those waiting times down. Britons may opt to purchase private health insurance to reduce wait times and for various other perks, but the private market remains relatively small.

Growing waiting lists have helped to fuel some popular discontent toward the NHS in recent years (Figure 23.3). Chronic staffing shortages and revelations of poor conditions and negligence

FIGURE 23.3 National Health Service waiting list times in England from 1949 to 2021.

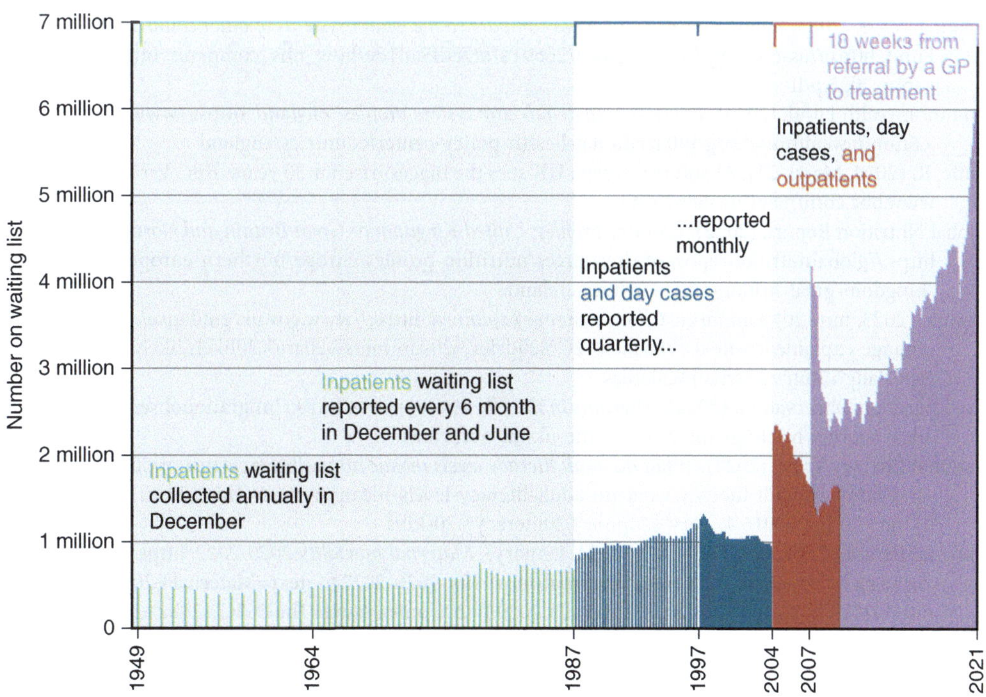

Note: Nuffield Trust analysis of data from NHS England and the Department of Health.

Source: Appleby, J. (2022, March 11). *Chart of the week: How has the waiting list changed over the years?* Nuffield Trust.

have taken a severe toll on morale within the NHS—leading to perceptions of what some have dubbed a state of "perma-crisis." Moreover, in recent years the United Kingdom has lagged when it comes not only to medical staffing, but also to infrastructure, with fewer MRI and CT scanning equipment (and, indeed, hospital beds) than many peer nations (Anandaciva, 2023).

NICE must approve services and products used within the NHS (and therefore readily available). The agency has proven reluctant to approve procedures associated with traditional and complementary medicine. The overwhelming stress within the NHS has been on implementing the Western biomedical paradigm.

CONCLUSION

While the NHS has long been an object of national pride, and international acclaim, years of underinvestment combined with the inevitable strains associated with the COVID-19 pandemic have created a climate of crisis around the institution. Future governments would do well to ensure the NHS is properly resourced if it is to perform effectively in future.

LEARNING ACTIVITIES

CourseConnect >

To access self-assessment questions and interactive, competency-based learning activities for this chapter, visit www.springerpub.com/courseconnect. See inside front cover and tear-out for CourseConnect details.

REFERENCES

Action on Smoking and Health. (2023, October). *Smoking statistics fact sheet.* https://ash.org.uk/uploads/Smoking-Statistics-Fact-Sheet.pdf?v=1697728811

Anandaciva, S. (2023, June). *How does the NHS compare to the health systems of other countries?* Kings' Fund. https://assets.kingsfund.org.uk/f/256914/x/7cdf5ad1de/how_nhs_compares_other_countries_abpi_2023.pdf

Commonwealth Fund. (2020). *International health care system profiles: England.* https://www.commonwealthfund.org/international-health-policy-center/countries/england

Cuffe, R. (2024, March 21). Absolute poverty: UK sees the biggest rise for 30 years. *BBC Verify.* https://www.bbc.com/news/uk-68625344

Global Nutrition Report. (2022). *Country profiles: United Kingdom or Great Britain and Northern Ireland.* https://globalnutritionreport.org/resources/nutrition-profiles/europe/northern-europe/united-kingdom-great-britain-and-northern-ireland/

Gov.uk. (2023, June 20). *Guidance: Climate change explained.* https://www.gov.uk/guidance/climate-change-explained#:~:text=Warmer%2C%20drier%20summers%20are%20likely,likely%2C%20especially%20in%20urban%20areas

The Migration Observatory. (2024). *Migrants in the UK: An overview.* https://migrationobservatory.ox.ac.uk/resources/briefings/migrants-in-the-uk-an-overview/

National Literacy Trust. (2024). *What do adult literacy levels mean?* https://literacytrust.org.uk/parents-and-families/adult-literacy/what-do-adult-literacy-levels-mean/#:~:text=This%20survey%20found%20that%2016.4,' very%20poor%20literacy%20skills'

National Perinatal Epidemiology Unit. (2024, January). *Maternal mortality 2020-2022.* https://www.npeu.ox.ac.uk/mbrrace-uk/data-brief/maternal-mortality-2020-2022#:~:text=Maternal%20mortality%20rates%20UK%202020%2D2022,-Overall%20293%20women&text=Thus%2C%20in%20this%20triennium%20272,%25%20CI%2011.86%2D15.10)

Office for National Statistics. (2021). *First census estimates on gender identity and sexual orientation.* https://www.ons.gov.uk/news/news/firstcensusestimatesongenderidentityandsexualorientation

Office of National Statistics. (2021). *Religion, England and Wales: Census 2021.* https://www.ons.gov.uk/peoplepopulationandcommunity/culturalidentity/religion/bulletins/religionenglandandwales/census2021

Office for National Statistics. (2022, November 29). *Religion, England and Wales: Census 2021.* Census 2021. https://www.ons.gov.uk/peoplepopulationandcommunity/culturalidentity/religion/bulletins/religionenglandandwales/census2021

Office for National Statistics. (2024, February 19). *Risk factors for pre-diabetes and undiagnosed type 2 diabetes in England: 2013 to 2019.* https://www.ons.gov.uk/peoplepopulationandcommunity/healthandsocialcare/healthinequalities/bulletins/riskfactorsforprediabetesandundiagnosedtype2diabetesinengland/2013to2019

Organisation for Economic Co-operation and Development. (2022). *Education at a glance 2022: United Kingdom.* https://www.oecd-ilibrary.org/sites/2d088c0c-en/index.html?itemId=/content/component/2d088c0c-en

Robbins, A. J., Fowler, A. J., Haines, R. W., Pearse, R. M., Prowle, J. R., & Puthucheary, Z. (2021). Emergency hospital admissions associated with non-communicable diseases 1998-2018 in England, Wales and Scotland: An ecological study. *Clinical Medicine, 21*(2), e179–e185. https://doi.org/10.7861/clinmed.2020-0830

Scotland's Census. (2021a). *Languages.* https://www.scotlandscensus.gov.uk/census-results/at-a-glance/languages/

Scotland's Census. (2021b). *Religion.* https://www.scotlandscensus.gov.uk/census-results/at-a-glance/religion/

Seaton, A. (2023). *Our NHS: A history of Britain's best-loved institution.* Yale University Press.

Stanton, E. (2014). The case for change for British mental healthcare. *The Lancet, 107*(4), 135–137. https://doi.org/10.1177/0141076814522144

Statista. (2024). *Languages in the UK: Statistics & facts.* https://www.statista.com/topics/2288/languages-in-the-united-kingdom/

Stonewall UK. (2018, November). *LGBT in Britain—Health (2018).* https://www.cia.gov/the-world-factbook/countries/united-kingdom/

UK Health Security Agency. (2022, December 12). *Notifiable diseases: Historic annual totals.* https://www.gov.uk/government/publications/notifiable-diseases-historic-annual-totals

UK Parliament. (2024, April 8). *Poverty in the UK: Statistics.* https://commonslibrary.parliament.uk/research-briefings/sn07096/

UN Data. (2024). *United Kingdom.* https://data.un.org/en/iso/gb.html

UN Inter-agency Group for Child Mortality Estimation. (2023). *Infant mortality rate-total, United Kingdom of Great Britain and Northern Ireland.* https://childmortality.org/all-cause-mortality/data?indicator=MRY0&refArea=GBR

World Bank Group. (2024, February 6). *Unemployment, total, United Kingdom.* https://data.worldbank.org/indicator/SL.UEM.TOTL.ZS?locations=GB

World Health Organization. (2023). *Health data overview for the United Kingdom of Great Britain and Northern Ireland.* https://data.who.int/countries/826

World Helath Organization. (2024). *Health data overview for the United Kingdom of Great Britain and Northern Ireland.* https://data.who.int/countries/826

Worldometer. (2024, April 13). *United Kingdom: Coronavirus cases.* https://www.worldometers.info/coronavirus/country/uk/

CHAPTER 24

PORTUGAL

Maryellen D. Brisbois and Helder Rocha Pereira

INTRODUCTION

The history of Portugal's foundation dates to 1147 and since then, the country has maintained relative stability in terms of its territorial dimension, its identity as a country, as well as its stability across religious, cultural, and linguistic contexts. As a European country, Portugal is in the far west of the "Old Continent," with an Atlantic inclination on the eastern side of the continent. The opening of maritime and trade routes, from the 15th and 16th centuries onward, initially with Africa and later with Brazil, India, and Southeast Asia, is one of the milestones that most demonstrated Portugal's history and relations with the world. In fact, this marked the beginning of a period not only of expanding knowledge and contact with new cultures and trade, but also an era of colonization of countries that lasted until the mid-1970s (Shercliff et al., 2024). Portugal is geographically distant from other major European cities and authorities; consequently, it is also separated from the decision-making political centers that may affect the country and its unique people. After cycles of greater isolation that included the ousting of a long authoritarian regime in 1974 and subsequent integration, Portugal is now a stable democratic republic, welcomed into the European Union (EU) in 1986, formerly the European Economic Community. These changes shifted Portugal toward an open and democratic regime and deepened models of assistance and education, within the tradition of European social models, which have shaped its recent history.

GEOGRAPHY AND POPULATION

GEOGRAPHIC FEATURES

Portugal has a surface area of 92,230 square kilometers (35,610 square miles) and, despite its small size, it has considerable geographical differences (Figure 24.1). The country is made up of a continental territory in mainland Europe and two archipelagos in the Atlantic Ocean: the Madeira Archipelago, with two main inhabited islands, and the Azores Archipelago with nine inhabited islands (Shercliff et al., 2024). These two island regions are currently autonomous regarding health, education, and government administration. This means that national policy plans can be implemented in the two island regions that are separate from the country.

In geographical terms, Portugal has a single land border with Spain (to the north and east) and the Atlantic Ocean (to the south and west). The north and center of the country have the main mountainous structures, with frequent precipitation. The southern part of the country is characterized by flatter areas, summers with high temperatures and more frequent periods of little rainfall and drought. Most of the population is concentrated on the country's coastline, with the interior having a dispersed population and much lower population density.

DEMOGRAPHIC FEATURES

The total population of Portugal in 2022 was 10.4 million (World Bank Group, 2024). Between 2001 and 2022, these figures remained relatively stable, with a population increase of around

FIGURE 24.1 Map of Portugal in mainland Europe.

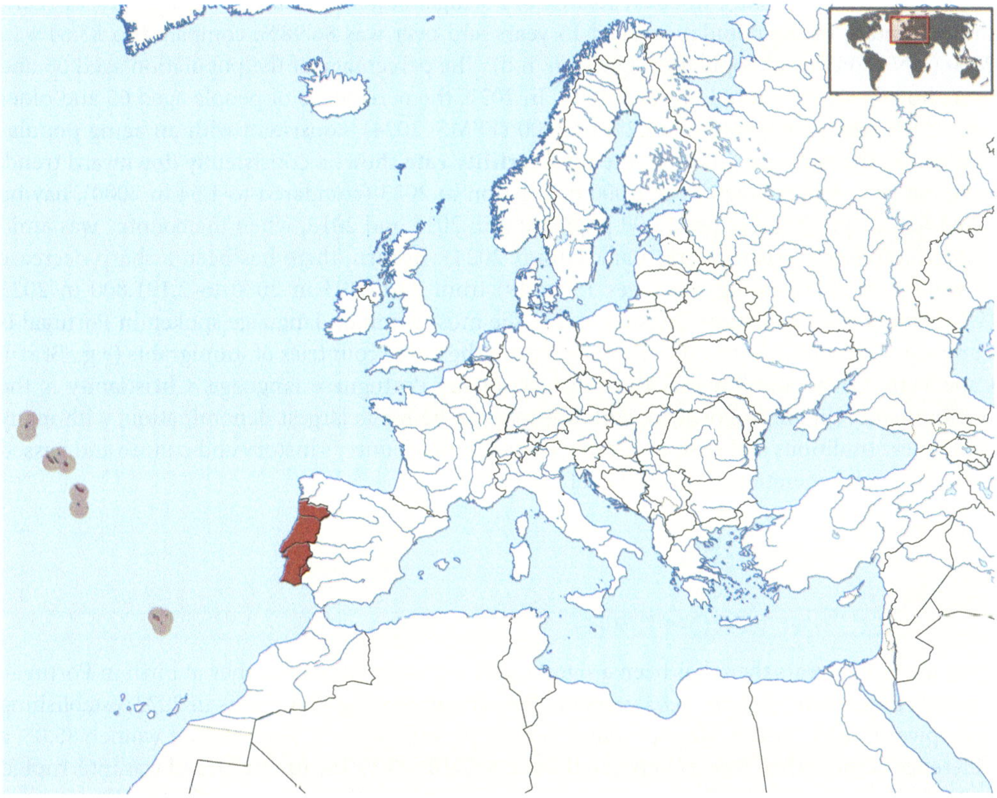

Source: Travail Personnel. (2011). *Image of Portugal*. https://fr.m.wikipedia.org/wiki/Fichier:Portugal_in_Europe_%28extended%29_%28special_marker%29.svg

0.79% between the two periods. Regarding gender, 52.3% of the population are categorized as female and 47.7% as male (Francisco Manuel dos Santos Foundation [FFMS], 2024). Data regarding statistics for the LGBTQ+ population in Portugal were not readily available; however, Portugal is recognized as one of 17 countries of the Organisation for Economic Co-operation and Development (OECD, 2020) that have the most legal protections for sexual and gender minorities. Portugal is largely considered one of the most LGBTQ+ friendly destinations to live and visit in the world (OECD, 2020). The foreign population living in Portugal in 2022 corresponds to 7.5% of the total resident population (in 2000 it corresponded to 2%; in 2010 to 4.2%; and in 2020 to 6.4% [FFMS, 2024]). By nationality, the five most significant immigrant communities are Brazil (30.7%), the United Kingdom (5.8%), Cape Verde (4.7%), India (4.5%), and Italy (4.1%). This trend, although growing, has fluctuated over the years according to economic cycles (Serviço de Estrangeiros e Fronteiras [SEF], 2023). This can be seen in the variation in total net migration (number of immigrants minus the number of emigrants). In 2021 the balance was 27,295; in 2020, 63,195; in 2021, −11,820; and in 2000, 63,195 (UN Data Portal Population Division, n.d.). Of Portugal's total surface area, 4165.14 square kilometers (1,608 square miles) are considered urban land areas. There is a growing tendency in the country for the population to move to urban areas. In 2000, the urban population was approximately 5.6 million, in 2015 6.5 million, and in 2022 approximately 7 million people (World Bank Group, 2024). The distribution of the population by age, as in many Western countries, is showing signs of aging. The median age of the population increased from 36.7 years to 45.8 years in 2023 (UN Data Portal Population Division, n.d.). In 2023, 13.18% of Portugal's total population was age 0 to 14 years; the percentage of the population aged 15 years and over was 86.98%, compared to 83.64% in 2000 (UN Data Portal Population Division, n.d). The percentage of the population aged 65 and over shows a steady annual upward trend. In 2022, the percentage of people aged 65 and older was 23.8% when compared to 16.2% in 2000 (FFMS, 2024), consistent with an aging population across the globe. In addition, the **total fertility rate** shows a consistently downward trend, standing at 1.38 pregnancies per 1,000 population in 2023 (compared to 1.54 in 2000), having fallen to 1.21 pregnancies per 1,000 population in 2011 and 2013, when the country was amid a severe economic crisis (World Bank Group, 2024). In turn, there has been a sharp decrease in women of childbearing age (ages 15 to 49) from 2,612,393 in 2000 to 2,191,800 in 2023 (UN Data Portal Population Division, n.d.). The most common language spoken in Portugal is European Portuguese, with other languages from the home countries of immigrants (e.g., Brazil, Cape Verde), who speak a variety of dialects of the Portuguese language. Christianity is the predominant religion in Portugal, with Catholicism being its largest denomination, with many Portuguese traditions and customs deeply rooted in the country's history and culture and passed down through generations (Shercliff et al., 2024).

HEALTH OUTCOMES

LIFE EXPECTANCY FROM BIRTH

Over the last 75 years there has been a significant increase in life expectancy at birth in Portugal, from 58.48 years in 1950, to 76.83 years in 2000, and exceeding 82.42 years in 2023, establishing this upward trend. Today, life expectancy at birth for men is 79.53 years and for women 85.06, a difference of more than 5 years between the sexes (Table 24.1) The upward trend was interrupted in 2020 and 2021 to 81.05 years and 81.04 years, respectively, likely related to the COVID-19 pandemic (UN Data Portal Population Division, n.d.).

TABLE 24.1 POPULATION, LIFE EXPECTANCY, AND INFANT MORTALITY RATES IN PORTUGAL, 1990–2023

	1990	2000	2010	2020	2023
Population	9.99 million	10.28 million	10.58 million	10.37 million	10.43 million
Life expectancy at birth in years	74.3	76.8	80.1	81.4	82.4
Life expectancy at birth in years (male)	70.8	73.3	76.7	78.4	79.4
Life expectancy at birth in years (female)	77.8	80.4	83.2	84.2	85.1
Infant mortality (per 1,000 live births)	10.9	5.7	2.6	2.4	2.6

Source: Adapted from UN Data Portal. (n.d.). *UN population division data portal*. United Nations. https://population.un.org/dataportal/home/.

LEADING CAUSES OF MORTALITY

The main causes of death in Portugal are related to noncommunicable diseases (NCDs). In ranking the top 10 causes of death in 2021 by the Institute for Health Metrics and Evaluation (IHME, n.d.), eight noncommunicable conditions and two communicable diseases are included in this ranking, one being COVID-19 (which is directly related to the period in which the ranking was measured). Despite that, the leading causes of death in 2021 were: (a) stroke; (b)COVID-19; (c) ischemic heart disease; (d) Alzheimer disease; (e) lower respiratory infections; (f) chronic obstructive pulmonary disease (COPD); (g) chronic kidney disease; (h) lung cancer; (i) colorectal cancer; and 9j) diabetes. In Portugal in 2022, diseases of the circulatory system were the cause of 26.5% of deaths; malignant tumors 22.4%; diseases of the respiratory system 9.7%; diseases of the digestive system 4.3%; and COVID-19 6.2%—a decrease from 10.4% in 2021 (FFMS, 2024). Overall, cancer was the second leading cause of death in Portugal (OECD, 2023). The impact of COVID-19 in Portugal, according to data monitored by the Coronavirus Resource Center at Johns Hopkins University and Medicine collected through October 2023, were 5,570,473 confirmed cases and 26,266 deaths. Data from the vaccination campaigns in Portugal showed 9,780,727 people (95.92% of the population) received at least one dose of vaccine (Johns Hopkins Corona Virus Resource Center, 2024).

INFANT AND MATERNAL MORTALITY

The infant mortality rate (number of deaths of infants under 1 year per 1,000 live births) in Portugal was one of the country's most problematic health indicators in the 1960s, with figures above 70 per 1,000 live births at the start of the decade (FFMS, 2024). This led to the promotion of local maternal and child healthcare programs with positive results. In 2000, the infant mortality rate was 5.6 per 1,000 live births, with a downward trend in subsequent years to 2.5 deaths in 2010, 2.4 deaths in 2020, and 2.4 deaths in 2023 (FFMS, 2024). The maternal mortality ratio (number of women who die during pregnancy or after childbirth per 100,000 live births) in 1960 was 115.5 maternal deaths per 100,000 and in 2021 it had declined to 8.8 deaths per 100,000. However, since 2000 this figure has fluctuated between 2.7 deaths per 100,000 in 2005 and 20.1 in 2020 (FFMS, 2024).

MENTAL ILLNESSES

The prevalence of mental health disorders in Portugal are among the highest in the European Union (EU). It is estimated that in 2019 more than 2.25 million people, 22% of the population, suffered from a mental health disorder, which was higher than the EU at 6.7% overall. Of these, anxiety disorders (9%), depressive disorders (6%), and those related to alcohol and drug use disorders (4%) were the most prominent (OECD/European Observatory on Health Systems and Policies, 2023). Mental health issues among higher education students have also come under the spotlight. Amaro et al. (2024) documented that mild to severe anxiety symptoms were reported by 75% of the participants, with approximately 20% reported having been previously diagnosed with a mental disorder, as opposed to 38.7% after the pandemic with 23% of participants reported taking medication for reasons related to mental health.

DETERMINANTS OF HEALTH

Portugal is included among the **high-income group** countries. In 2022, the gross domestic product (GDP) of Portugal was $255.2 billion. In the same year, the GDP per capita was $24,515.3. Between the year 2000 ($11,526.4 per capita) and 2008 ($24,949 per capita) there was an accelerated growth in GDP with fluctuations in 2010, 2012, and 2015 that align with the performance of the global economy (World Bank Group, 2024). Over the past 7 years, the percentage of unemployed people in Portugal has risen since 2000 (3.8%) to a peak of 16.2% in 2013. Since then, it had fallen sharply until 2019. In 2019, the unemployment rate was approximately 6% (World Bank Group, 2024).

HEALTH BEHAVIORS

There is a rank of 10 risk factors that contributed to death or disability in 2021 in Portugal, according to IHME (n.d.) data. There were three behavioral factors that include tobacco (number 4), dietary risks (5), and high alcohol use (6). Five other factors were categorized and ranked as metabolic risks: high plasma fasting glucose (number 1), high body mass index (2), high blood pressure (3), kidney dysfunction (7), and elevated low-density lipoprotein (LDL; 8). The last two risk factors were occupational or environmental/occupational: occupational risks (number 9) and nonoptimal temperature (10; IHME, n.d.). In 2019, 30% of all deaths in the country could be attributed to behavioral risk factors including tobacco use, alcohol consumption, diet-related risks, and low physical activity (OECD/European Observatory on Health Systems and Policies, 2023).

Tobacco Use

In 2019, the daily number of smokers of cigarettes were lower in Portugal when compared to the EU. In Portugal, the total percentage of smokers was 11.5%: Those that smoked fewer than 20 cigarettes per day was 7.5%, those that smoked 20 or more cigarettes per day was 4.0%. EU data showed 18.4% of the population were cigarette smokers, with 12.6 smoking fewer than 20 cigarettes per day and 5.9% smoking 20 or more cigarettes daily. Males in Portugal smoked less than those living in the EU, at 16.4% overall in Portugal, and 22.3% across the EU. Females had similar data to males with a total of 7.2% smoking daily in Portugal, and 14.8% in the EU in 2019 (Eurostat, n.d.).

Poor Dietary Intake

The major unhealthy food-related behaviors of the Portuguese population include high consumption of red and processed meat, low consumption of whole grains, and high sodium intake. Despite the wide availability of vegetables and fruits, daily consumption is below the recommended levels. These behaviors may reduce lifespan and health quality (Gregório et al., 2023). The prevalence of overweight children under 5 years of age is 7.1% and Portugal is "on course" to prevent that figure from increasing. Portugal has shown limited progress toward achieving the diet-related NCD targets. Nearly 23.5% of adult women age 18 years and over and 23.2% of adult men are currently living with obesity. Although Portugal's obesity prevalence is lower than the regional average of 25.3% for women and 24.9% for men, diabetes is estimated to affect 5.5% of adult women and 9.7% of adult men (Global Nutrition Report, 2024).

Physical Inactivity

Portugal has the lowest level of physical activity in Europe and a high level of sedentary lifestyle, although there are national physical activity recommendations for all age groups including children 0 to 5 years, children and adolescents 6 to 17, adults 18 to 64, older adults 65 years and older, and pregnant and breastfeeding women. National guidelines do not include frail/elderly persons age 85 years and older, and persons facing disability or chronic illness. According to the World Health Organization's (WHO) Portugal Physical Activity Factsheet (2021), it was estimated the prevalence of sufficient physical activity levels from persons aged 15 to 65 years ranged from 16.6% to 32.6% with the lowest percentage in those aged 55 to 65 and highest (32.6%) among those in the 15 to 54 age category (WHO, 2021).

Alcohol Abuse

Portugal has one of the highest levels of alcohol consumption in the EU, with 12 liters of pure alcohol consumed per capita per year,roughly equivalent to 2.5 bottles of wine or 4.6 liters of beer per week per person age 15 years and older. Based on current consumption patterns in Portugal, OECD simulations estimate that disease and injury caused by drinking more than1 to 1.5 drinks per day lead to treatment costs equal to 2.3% of health expenditure and a reduction in workforce productivity (OECD, 2021).

SOCIAL AND ECONOMIC FACTORS

Educational Attainment

The educational attainment level of Portugal's adult population (age 25 to 64) per 2021 data noted that 41% had not finished high school, 28% had some college, and 31% were working toward a degree. When considering the specific age group between 25 and 34 years in 2021, 17% of this group did not have a high school diploma which represents a sharp decrease from 44% in 2011; 36% had some college (29% in 2011), and 47% were working toward a degree (27% in 2011). This development trend points to convergence toward the OECD average values within 10 years for this age group (OECD, 2022). The compulsory age for school attendance starts at 6 years and lasts until the age of 18. Sixty-one percent of young people between the ages of 18 and 24 remain in full- or part-time educational programs at college levels (above the OECD average of 54%). In turn, only 5% of these students complement their studies with some form of work which falls below the OECD average of 17% (OECD, 2022).

Poverty

The at-risk-of-poverty threshold varies over time and differs according to the country being analyzed. The threshold can be considered as the value below which someone is considered to have a low income compared to the rest of the population (FFMS, 2024). In Portugal in 2022, this amount was set at approximately $7,200. When analyzing the risk of poverty in 2022, 41.8% of the population is identified as at poverty risk before government assistance. This assistance may include monthly income for families at risk, housing support, support for caregivers at home, meals and supplies for school-age children, and free daycare. This figure drops to 20.7% of the population after government assistance, which indicates a significant role for the state in mitigating the risk of more aggravated situations of poverty. When analyzing by age group before supplemental governmental services, the risk of poverty reaches more than 80% of people over 65, a figure that drops to 17.1% after government assistance (FFMS, 2024).

HUMAN DEVELOPMENT

The UN Development Program (2025) offers a definition: "Human development is about expanding the richness of human life rather than simply the richness of the economy. It focuses on people and their opportunities and choices." The Human Development Index (HDI) is based on dimensions and indicators related to a long and healthy life, access to knowledge and the capacity for a decent standard of living (https://hdr.undp.org/). Between 1990 and 2022, Portugal's HDI grew from 0.703 to 0.874 (an increase of 24.3%) which classifies Portugal at a very high level on a scale of 0 to 1. Portugal ranks 42 out of 193 countries as related to life expectancy, education, and per-capita income indices. For the same years, Portugal ranked below Spain (0.911) and Finland (0.942) in the EU and (0.927) in the United States (United Nations Human Development Reports [UNHDP], 2024).

The **Gender Inequality Index (GII)** evaluates gender gaps in three dimensions and compares inequality between women and men considering reproductive health (as measured by maternal mortality ratio and adolescent birth rates), empowerment (as measured by the share of parliamentary seats and education), and the labor market (as measured by labor force participation rates). Portugal has a GII value of 0.076 and is in 21st place out of 166 countries (in 1990 it was

26th). In 2022, the maternal mortality ratio was 11.8 deaths per 100,000 live births; the **adolescent birth rate** was 7.1 births per 1,000 women age 15 to 19; seats in Parliament were 37% (gender gap, 26.1%); population with at least some secondary education (age 25 and older) was 59.7% for women (gender gap, 2.2%); labor force participation rate (age 15 and older) 54.7% for women (gender gap, 8.4%). When compared to the same countries for the same year, Portugal ranks above countries for their GII such as Spain (0.059) and Finland (0.032) in the EU and above the United States (0.180) in the world context (UNHDP, 2024).

HEALTHCARE SYSTEM

Before 1979, healthcare in Portugal was dispersed, with the state taking on a supplementary role in some areas of public health considering the poor health situation of the population. There were organized forms of healthcare for workers and their families, as well as national projects and institutes aimed at addressing more problematic areas (e.g., trends in infant mortality). The National Health System (NHS) was created in 1979, giving concrete expression to the right to health protection, the provision of comprehensive healthcare, and access to all Portuguese citizens regardless of their economic and social status, as assumed and made explicit in Portugal's Constitution (Serviço Nacional de Saíde [SNS], 2024). The NHS is made up of a network of different hospitals, health center groupings (within the scope of primary healthcare), and different institutes (e.g., National Institutes of Emergency Medicine, Blood and Transplantation, and Public Health). The NHS network works in an articulated manner with universal health coverage and access that are mostly free of charge (SNS, 2024).

FINANCING AND INSURANCE

According to the IHME, health spending in Portugal in 2021 was $2,481 per person. Of this, $193.36 corresponds to prepaid private spending, $720.50 for out-of-pocket spending, and the remaining $1567.50 to government health spending (IHME, n.d.). In 2021, public financing of health expenditures was 63.2%, which is well below the EU average of 81.1% (OECD, 2023). The weight of voluntary health insurance (VHI) in 2021 was 7.8% (up from 4.4% when compared to the figure for the EU). This indicates a growing trend in this type of financing in line with the development of private health structures. The expenditure on health in 2021 was 11.1% of GDP (again in line with the EU). In 2021, 44% of Portugal's health budget was allocated to outpatient care, which reflects a concentration of the care system in primary care (OECD, 2023).

DELIVERY

Facilities

The NHS is primarily responsible for providing hospital care and overseeing 114 of the country's 219 hospitals. This public network provides two thirds of the available hospital beds and is responsible for 70% of patient admissions (OECD, 2023). The density of hospital beds per 1,000 inhabitants is relatively low at 3.5 compared to the EU average of 4.8 beds. According to national data, there are around 200 beds in hospitals per 100,000 inhabitants, a figure that has remained stable over the last decade (FFMS, 2024). The primary healthcare network is widespread across the territory and in 2020, 91.6% of the population had access to a primary healthcare physician, with 86.3% of the population also havingaccess to a family nurse (Direção Geral de Saúde, 2022).

Providers

In 2021, Portugal had 5.6 doctors per 1,000 inhabitants (higher than the EU average) and 7.4 nurses per 1,000 inhabitants, which, despite the increase in the number of recent nurse graduates, this figure is still 13% lower than the EU average (OECD, 2023). The distribution of human resources is also uneven: 70% of resources are concentrated in Lisbon, the capital, and in the northern region, which accounts for 62% of the population (OECD, 2023). The NHS hospitals in 2022 had an increase in healthcare personnel to 114,425, from 87,293, with 19.6% being doctors, 35.5% nurses, and 7.2% diagnostic and laboratory staff (FFMS, 2024).

TRADITIONAL AND COMPLEMENTARY CARE

The World Health Organization recognizes that traditional and complementary medicine is a vital part of the global healthcare system. Use of complementary care has become widespread in the last two decades, with use in general populations worldwide ranging from 9.8% to 76%. Across the EU, the unadjusted weighted estimates for use of complementary care over the past 12 months in the surveyed countries ranged from 10% in Hungary, to approximately 40% in Germany and Switzerland (Kemppainen et al., 2018). In Portugal, approximately 14.1% of persons who were surveyed had utilized complementary care in the prior year. Legislation in Portugal for traditional and complementary care launched in 2003, with regulations and attempted implementation in 2013 and 2019; from the start, however, it has been controversial (Santos & Mendes, 2020).

ACCESS, QUALITY, AND COST

Challenges across the Portuguese healthcare system consist of long wait times for some services, limited availability of specialized services, complex bureaucratic processes, shortage of healthcare professionals, and an aging population (OECD/European Observatory on Health Systems and Policies, 2023).

OECD data regarding five key indicators related to trends in population health and health system performance demonstrate that Portugal performs better than the OECD average on: (a) 42% of indicators related to health status, (b) 75% of indicators related to risk factors, (c) 55% of indicators related to quality of care, (d) 30% of indicators related to access to care, and (e) 30% of indicators related to health system resources. In looking more closely at access, the Portuguese population is covered for a set of core health services, with 63% of the population satisfied with the availability of quality healthcare that included primary care, safe prescribing, and preventive care data, and only 2.3% of the population reporting unmet needs. Financial coverage associated with the healthcare system in Portugal was at 63%, with some out-of-pocket spending higher than the OECD average which may negatively impact vulnerable groups (OECD/European Observatory on Health Systems and Policies, 2023).

CONCLUSION

The Portuguese healthcare system is a publicly funded system that provides universal health coverage for all citizens with a focus on primary care through a strong network of family doctors and community health centers. The strengths of the National Health System are high-quality healthcare services with broad coverage and access, and low out-of-pocket costs. Data indicate Portugal's healthcare system is performing well with quality outcomes in infant mortality, life expectancy, and management of noncommunicable diseases. Like many countries, Portugal faces challenges related to an aging population and rising health costs. Overall, the Portuguese healthcare system is considered one of the best in the world, with a strong focus on universal access, comprehensive benefits, and high-quality care.

LEARNING ACTIVITIES

CourseConnect

To access self-assessment questions and interactive, competency-based learning activities for this chapter, visit www.springerpub.com/courseconnect. See inside front cover and tear-out for CourseConnect details.

REFERENCES

Amaro, P., Fonseca, C., Afonso, A., Jacinto, G., Gomes, L., Pereira, H., José, Silva, C., Lima, A., Arco, H., Nabais, J., Lopes, M., Pereira, A., Fragoeiro, I., & Pinho, L. (2024). Depression and anxiety of Portuguese university students: A cross-sectional study about prevalence and associated factors. *Depression and Anxiety,* 1–14. https://doi.org/10.1155/2024/5528350

Direção Geral de Saúde. (2022). *Plano nacional de saúde 2030* [National health plan 2030 of Portugal]. DGS, Lisboa. https://pns.dgs.pt/

Eurostat. (n.d.). *Database.* https://ec.europa.eu/eurostat/web/main/data/database

Fundação Francisco Manuel dos Santos. (2024). *PORDATA—Statistics about Portugal and Europe.* http://www.pordata.pt

Global Nutrition Report. (2024). *Country nutrition profiles.* Portugal. https://globalnutritionreport.org/resources/nutrition-profiles/europe/southern-europe/portugal/

Gregório, M., Henriques, A., Freitas, M. G., Mestre, R., Teixeira, D., Salvador, C., & Graça, P. (2023). *Programa nacional para a promoção da alimentação saudável 2022–2030* [National programme for the promotion of healthy eating 2022–2030]. Direção-Geral da Saúde, Lisboa, Portugal.

Institute for Health Metrics and Evaluation. (n.d.). *Portugal. Quick facts.* https://www.healthdata.org/research-analysis/health-by-location/profiles/portugal#main-content

Johns Hopkins Corona Virus Resource Center. (2024). *Portugal overview.* https://coronavirus.jhu.edu/region/portugal

Kemppainen, L. M., Kemppainen, T. T., Reippainen, J. A., Salmenniemi, S. T., & Vuolanto, P. H. (2018). Use of complementary and alternative medicine in Europe: Health-related and sociodemographic determinants. *Scandanavian Journal of Public Health, 46*(4), 448–455. https://doi.org/10.1177/1403494817733869

Organisation for Economic Co-operation and Development. (2020). *Over the rainbow*? The road to LGBTI inclusion. https://www.oecd.org/portugal/OECD-LGBTI-2020-Over-The-Rainbow-PORTUGAL.pdf

Organisation for Economic Co-operation and Development. (2021). *Preventing harmful alcohol use.* OECD Health Policy Studies, OECD Publishing, Paris. https://doi.org/10.1787/6e4b4ffb-en

Organisation for Economic Co-operation and Development. (2022). *Education at a glance 2022:OECD indicators.* OECD Publishing, Paris. https://doi.org/10.1787/3197152b-en

Organisation for Economic Co-operation and Development. (2023). *EU country cancer profile: Portugal 2023.* EU Country Cancer Profiles, OECD Publishing, Paris. https://doi.org/10.1787/2f84bf79-en

Organisation for Economic Co-operation and Development/European Observatory on Health Systems and Policies. (2023). *Portugal: Country health profile 2023.* State of Health in the EU, OECD Publishing, Paris/European Observatory on Health Systems and Policies, Brussels. https://www.oecd.org/els/portugal-country-health-profile-2023-069af7b1-en.htm

Santos, R., & Mendes, C. (2020). Traditional and complementary medicine legislation in Portugal—Progress, challenges and flaws. *European Journal of Integrative Research, 35*,101104. https://doi.org/10.1016/j.eujim.2020.101104

Serviço de Estrangeiros e Fronteiras. (2023). *Relatório de imigração, fronteiras e asilo, 2022* [Annual report on migration and ssylum 2022]. Serviço de Estrangeiros e Fronteiras, Oeiras. https://www.sef.pt/pt/Documents/RIFA2022%20vF2a.pdf

Serviço Nacional de Saíde. (2024). *Saiba como nasceu o Serviço Nacional de Saúde e quais os desenvolvimentos dos últimos 40 anos* [Learn how the National Health Service was created and what developments have taken place over the last 40 years]. https://www.sns.gov.pt/sns/servico-nacional-de-saude/historia-do-sns/

Shercliff, J., Amaral, I., Wheeler, D., Opello, W., Smith, C., Livermore, H., & Kaplan, M. (2024). *Portugal.* Encyclopedia Britannica. https://www.britannica.com/place/Portugal

UN Data Portal Population Division. (n.d.). *UN population division data portal. Interactive access to global demographic indicators.* https://population.un.org/dataportal/home?df=ee11c4e5-9d68-40e5-a533-a7f5b0e9b381

UN Development Program. (2025). *Human development reports.* https://hdr.undp.org/system/files/documents/global-report-document/hdr2025reporten.pdf.

United Nations Human Development Reports. (2024). *Portugal.* https://hdr.undp.org/data-center/specific-country-data#/countries/PRT

World Bank Group. (2024). *Portugal.* https://data.worldbank.org/country/portugal

World Health Organization. (2021). *Portugal physical activity. Factsheet 2021.* https://cdn.who.int/media/docs/librariesprovider2/country-sites/physical-activity-factsheet---portugal-2021.pdf?sfvrsn=d8fac7be_1&download=true

CHAPTER 25

SPAIN

Antoinette Francher-Donald and Amy Dawson

GEOGRAPHICAL FEATURES

FEATURES, DIVISIONS, AND POPULATION SIZE

Spain, a country in Western Europe approximately the size of Texas, is inhabited by more than 47 million people. Prominent geographic features include the Mediterranean Sea and Pyrenees Mountains. Spain enjoys a long growing season, mild climate, diverse agricultural products, and a connected transportation system through roads and public transportation. The principal land mass is the Iberian Peninsula bordered on the north by the Pyrenees Mountains; by the Mediterranean Sea to the south and east with a small land border with Gibraltar; with France, Andorra, and the Bay of Biscay to the north and northeast; and with Portugal and the Atlantic Ocean to the west and northwest. As of 2024, Spain ranked 32nd with 0.57% of the world's population (Macrotrends, 2024; La Moncloa, 2025).

AGE DISTRIBUTION, MEDIAN AGE, AND BIRTH RATES

Since the beginning of this century, Spain has experienced drastic decreases in all age groups under 45 years of age and now has a median age of 44.8 years. Due to death and migration rates, Spain's overall population is projected to decline and populations in age groups over age 45 years will continue to increase. Population age structure is critical to a nation's socioeconomic issues and can impact health, economic and political issues; thus, the Spanish government is currently studying the impacts of the aging population and evaluating the investments required to support its current population and recruit and retain younger citizens. Age structure can also impact health, economic and political issues, and the slow growth of a young adult population may cause workforce gaps. Over the past decade, the Spanish birth rate has dropped by nearly 25%. This decline has left Spain with the second lowest fertility rate in the European Union (EU). Spain has a 1.19 live births per female compared to the EU average of 1.53, both far short of the 2.1 births at which existing population levels would be maintained (IndexMundi, 2017; World Bank Group, 2023).

URBAN AND RURAL POPULATIONS

In 2023, Spain's urban population was 81.6% of the total population—an approximate 12% increase since 1974. In many of the urban areas, the rich ethnic culture, night life, and walks on the beach are part of a native Spaniard's experience. Perhaps the most famous and unique cultural event in Spain, **Las Fallas** is a regional festival in Valencia, held in March to celebrate the arrival of spring, with parades, food, fireworks, and burning of the *ninots* (satirical or humorous monuments made by the locals). Spain's rural population has declined slightly, but its countryside has given rise to fruitful vegetation, wildlife, and minerals. Spain is known for citrus fruit, olives, and figs (Macrotrends, 2024).

SEX AND GENDER

In 2023, Spain's female population represented 51% (24,361,595) and males 49% (23,416,745) of the total population. Although, Spain is one of 17 countries in the Organisation for Economic Co-operation and Development (OECD) that is responsive to inclusivity of the transgender population, Spain's Instituto Nacional de Estadística (INE) does not currently track transgender residents (INE, 2024).

RACIAL AND ETHNIC GROUPS

Spain is steeped in cultural heritage from a blend of persons from Western and Eastern Europe and Northern Africa with an emphasis from places such as Rome, Germany, Czechia, and Iberia. The largest ethnic groups in Spain are Castilians, Catalans, Basques, Galicians, and Valencians (La Moncloa, 2025).

CULTURAL ELEMENTS

RELIGIONS

Spain is known for its iconic and symbolic architecture and cathedrals. One such Catholic masterpiece is Basilica de La Sagrada Familia or "Basilica of the Holy Family." The Catholic Church in Spain has a long history and is still the largest religion in Spain today. A 2022 survey indicated that 56% of respondents identified as Catholics contrasting a 2017 survey that reported 71.5% identified as Catholic. Spain is home to many other religious affiliations, including Muslim, Protestant, and Buddhist, as well as nonbelievers, agnostics, and atheist residents (U.S. Department of State [DoS], 2022).

LANGUAGES

Spain has four languages spoken by its population: Castilian Spanish (99% speak Casrilian as a first or second language), Catalan (15% to 20%), Galician (5% to 7%), and Basque (2% to 3%; INE, 2024). Each of these languages has its distinctive history, culture, and literature that have had enormous impact on Spain's traditions that still thrive today. Additionally, Spain is host to numerous regional dialects, such as Andalusian, Murcian, and Extremaduran (Navarro, 2022).

POLITICAL SYSTEMS

Spain is classified as democratic constitutional monarchy known as a parliamentary monarchy, with the monarch as the head of government andas prime minister and head of state. The current political system in Spain has been in place since *La Transición* in the late 1970s when the country moved from a dictatorship to a democracy after decades of General Francisco Franco's military rule (Karacs, 2025).

IMPORTANT TRADITIONS, PRACTICES, EVENTS, AND LEISURE PURSUITS

At the national level, the most important holidays are Holy (or Maundy) Thursday, Good Friday, Easter Monday, Corpus Christi, the Feast of Saint James (July 25), and All Saints' Day (November 1). The most important day of the Christmas period, and the day on which children receive presents, is the Day of the Three Kings or the Epiphany (January 6). Since 1978 the official national holiday has been Constitution Day on December 6 (O'Callaghan & Viguera, 2025).

Spain's most famous traditions include enjoying tapas, flamenco (form of music), and soccer, which is known as *fútbol* and is Spain's national sport. Spaniards also enjoy strolling, watching television, listening to music, reading, and surfing the internet (Sublime Spain, 2025).

HEALTH OUTCOMES

TOP 10 CAUSES OF DEATH FOR WOMEN IN SPAIN

The top 10 causes of death for women in Spain include Alzheimer disease and other dementias, ischemic heart disease, stroke, colon and rectal cancers, breast cancer, lower respiratory infections, hypertensive heart disease, chronic obstructive pulmonary disease, kidney diseases, and trachea, bronchus, and lung cancers (World Health Organization [WHO], 2025).

TOP 10 CAUSES OF DEATH FOR MEN IN SPAIN

The top 10 causes of death for men in Spain include ischemic heart diseas trachea, bronchus and lung cancers, Alzheimer disease and other dementias, chronic obstructive pulmonary disease, stroke, colon and rectal cancers, lower respiratory infections, prostate cancer, kidney disease, and bladder cancer (Figure 25.1; WHO, 2025).

MENTAL HEALTH

According to a 2021 survey, nearly half of Spaniards expressed concerns that the COVID-19 pandemic could have a negative long-term impact on their mental health—a figure that is slightly above the global average. In 2020, approximately 7.2% of women and 3.2% of men were diagnosed with depression with older residents being the group most affected. When it comes to anxiety, nearly 8.1% of women and 3.5% of men suffered from the condition with more than 11.3% and 4.4% for senior groupings, respectively. The real dominance of these illnesses is expected to increase (Statista, 2024).

INFECTIOUS DISEASES

Some of the most common infectious diseases among the adult population are pseudomembranous colitis, AIDS, pneumonia, genital herpes, genital warts, hepatitis A, hepatitis B, hepatitis C, HIV, tuberculosis, candidiasis (López-Cuadrado et al., 2014).

INFANT AND MATERNAL MORTALITY

The infant mortality rate is an indicator of a nation's health. Generally, the countries with the lowest mortality rates have some of the highest life expectancy averages. Spain's infant mortality rate is one of the lowest in the world. In 2024, Spain realized an infant mortality rate of 1.955 deaths per 1,000 live births (Figure 25.2).

Spain's maternal mortality ratio is 3.47 in 100,000 live births and that rate has remained steady over the last 20 years. The most common cause of maternal death was hypertensive disorders of pregnancy (INE, 2024).

LIFE EXPECTANCY

Infant mortality and life expectancy are connected. In terms of health, Spaniards are expected to live until age 84, which is more than 10 years greater than global life expectancy. Spaniard women's life expectancy is 86.2 years and men's life expectancy is 80.3. According to WHO, the global life expectancy as of 2016 was 72.0 years: 74.2 years for females and 69.8 years for men (Macrotrends, 2024).

QUALITY OF LIFE INDEXES

Quality of life consists of a multitude of variables including housing, income, and community engagement. According to OECD's Better Life Index Study, Spaniards were less likely to be satisfied with life than other countries. Although Spain underperforms in life satisfaction and job dimensions, Spain performs well in areas such health and safety. Some key findings include 81.4% of Spaniards on average feel safe walking alone at night and the average homicide rate is 0.7, compared to OECD rates of 74% to 2.6, respectively. Additionally, full-time employees spend two thirds of their day on personal care according to the OECD Better Life Index (OECD, 2024).

FIGURE 25.1 Important health-related and healthcare-related statistics for Spain, 2024.

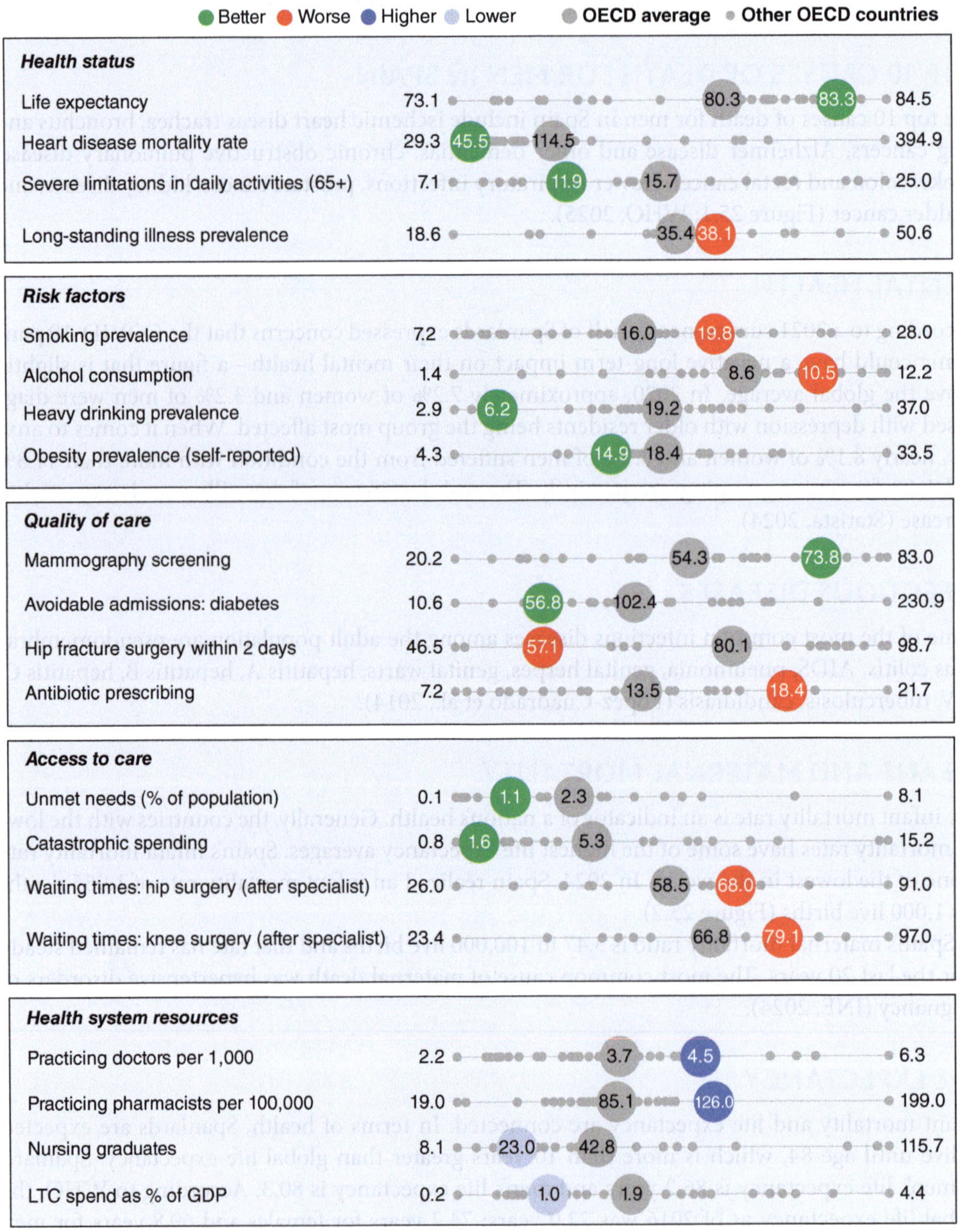

GDP, gross domestic product; LTC, long-term care; OECD, Organisation for Economic Co-operation and Development.

Source: Organisation for Economic Co-operation and Development. (2024). *Spain*. https://www.oecd.org/spain/health-at-a-glance-Spain-EN.pdf

DETERMINANTS OF HEALTH

NATIONAL AND PER-CAPITA GROSS DOMESTIC PRODUCT AND POVERTY RATES

Spain's gross domestic product (GDP) continues to improve. In 2023, Spain's national GDP was $1,580,741 million and per-capita GDP was $32,530, ranking it 14 out of 196 and 77 out of 196

FIGURE 25.2 Spain's ranking among European nations in infant mortality rate, 2024.

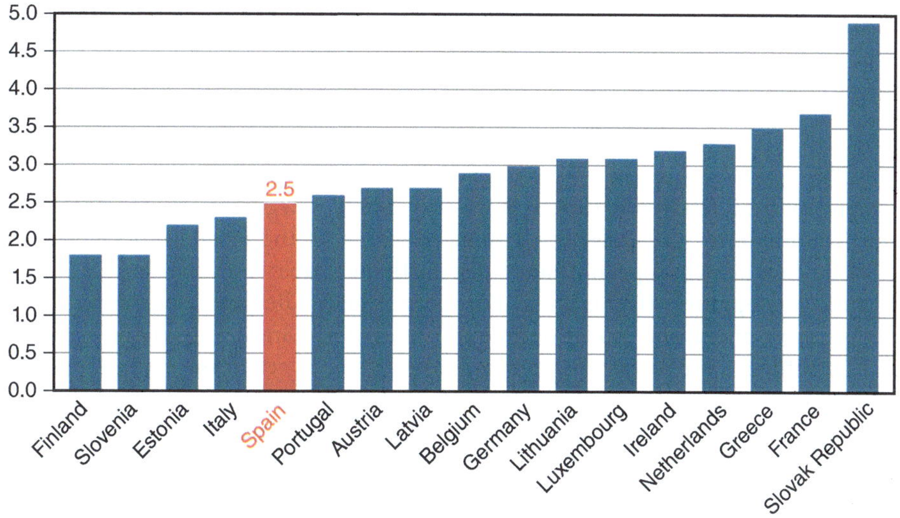

Source: Organisation for Economic Co-operation and Development. (2024). *Infant mortality rates*. https://www.oecd.org/en/data/indicators/infant-mortality-rates.html

countries, respectively. Spain's food insecurity and poverty are continuing problems. According to Eurostat, Spain's Risk of Poverty rate was 20.40%. Poverty can be cyclical, with lack of access to education, healthcare, and job opportunities perpetuating the inability to improve financial situations. Groups most at risk of living in poverty or who currently live in poverty are children, women, and older populations (World Bank Group, 2025).

EDUCATION AND LITERACY RATE

Education

Spain's early childhood school enrollment rate continue to increase and is higher than the OECD and the EU25 enrollment rate averages. Of Spaniard children under 2 years of age, 24.7% attend school compared to 18% and 11.8% of the OECD and the EU25 enrollments, respectively. The rate of enrollment for Spaniards age 15 to 19 is 87.9% and nearly half of Spaniards between 25 and 34 years of age have achieved higher education, which is above the European average (La Moncloa, 2025).

Literacy

The adult literacy rate is the percentage of people age 15 and higher who can both read and write. According to a 2020 Trend Economics report, 98.5% of Spanish adults were literate. Spain's literacy has been relatively consistent and is far higher than that of the U.S. rate of 79% (Macrotrends, 2024).

UNEMPLOYMENT RATES

The unemployment rate in Spain is high at 11.6% relative to the rest of the European Union's 6.5%, placing it at 19 out of 20 countries in the G20. Unemployment is higher for young adults, resulting in a delayed entry into the workforce. The high rates of unemployment are attributed to temporary contracts especially in the tourism and hospitality sectors which are very large, as well as overall poor national productivity. Actions taken to curb unemployment include labor reform in 2022 limiting temporary contracts. Immigration of skilled labor can temporarily increase unemployment rates of Spain's citizens but increases overall national productivity. Although unemployment rates are high, the levels are expected to remain stable while productivity growth strategies are implemented (OECD, 2024).

FOOD/NUTRITION

Spain has abundant production of a variety of fruits, vegetables, legumes, grains, meats, fish, and olive oil. Traditionally, Spain has been associated with both the Mediterranean diet pattern as well as the Southern European Atlantic diet. Both diets are rich in olive oil, fish, fruits, vegetables, nuts, and legumes. The Southern European Atlantic diet also includes high consumption of potatoes, bread, and moderate amounts of dairy and meat. Current concerns are that the diet is shifting more toward pre-prepared meals and sweets resulting in increasing rates of overweight, obesity, cancer, and cardiovascular disease. There may also be a negative environment impact in the dietary shift as meat-based diets are associated with higher water needs and increased carbon production (Serra-Majem et al., 2004; Varela-Moreiras et al., 2010).

HEALTH BEHAVIORS

Spain culture reinforces many positive health behaviors. Work is interrupted in the middle of the day for up to 3 hours to have the main meal of the day and even though most do not nap, it is also the time of the traditional "siesta" during the high heat of the day. Shops and businesses open again from about 4 to 7 pm and a late meal is served about 9 to 10 pm. There is a high emphasis on being outside, mingling, socializing, drinking coffee or an alcoholic beverage with snacks (tapas) in the late afternoon or evening before dinner. Vigorous physical activity of over 150 minutes a day is followed by 65% of the population and 50% of the population consumes adequate fruit and vegetables daily. Only 15% of Spain's citizens smoke but 70% drink alcohol daily and 95% sleep more than 6 hours a night (Lopez-Bueno et al., 2020).

Healthy behaviors are highly correlated with high subjective well-being scores in Spain. Average life satisfaction was rated 7.3 out of 10, correlated with a household income over $2,500 month. The typical Spanish diet includes intake of more fish and fruit than its Western counterparts. It also contains less meat and sweets. There are more home-cooked meals consumed with family and friends, more exercise, and more socialization. Health and happiness rating correlate with the life satisfaction score (Cabiedes-Miragaya et al., 2021).

TOP 10 MORTALITY RISK FACTORS

Spain's top 10 mortality risk factors mirror those of high-income countries for tobacco use, high blood pressure, overweight and obesity, low levels of physical activity, elevated blood sugar, elevated cholesterol, low fruit and vegetable ingestion, poor urban air quality, and high alcohol consumption (WHO, 2009). Tobacco rates are high at 27.7% and account for 11% of excess mortality (WHO, 2025). Hypertension afflicts 33% of the population but only 57% are treated, so hypertension is responsible for 10% of deaths per year (Banegas et al., 2024). Obesity rates have stabilized over the last few years at 17% of adults. Adults with sedentary lifestyles are relatively low at 31% for men and 42% for women and have been decreasing over the past 20 years (WHO, 2025).

Incidence of diabetes by oral glucose tolerance test is 11.5 per 1,000 person-years and contributes to cardiovascular mortality and stroke (Rojo-Martínez et al., 2020). Adherence to the Mediterranean diet has been shown to decrease cardiovascular mortality. This diet is rich in fruits, vegetables, fish, whole grains and olive oil while simultaneously limiting sweets and consumption of red meat (Aleman et al., 2016).

SOCIAL JUSTICE AND HUMAN RIGHTS ISSUES

Spain has an expanded view of what constitutes a human right when it comes to social definitions such as adequate food and housing, right to education and right to work. There are public demonstrations when families are removed from a home for failing to pay rent or for squatting illegally in a home when they have no adequate alternative (Díaz-Parra & Mena, 2015). Spain has a generous system of social insurance and social assistance that reduces the effective poverty rate by 55% to 14.3% in 2023 for the total population. The effect on native Spaniards is twice as high as immigrants—with 28% reduction in poverty for immigrants and 45% for native populations. Other vulnerable populations include young people up to age 24, those with disabilities, and older Spaniards. A recent initiative aimed at eliminating child poverty was announced early in 2024 (La Moncloa, 2024).

Vulnerable ethnic minorities include the Roma people throughout Western Europe. There are roughly 10 million Roma in Europe and nearly 1 million in Spain. Originally part of Northern India roughly 600 years ago, the Roma have faced discrimination and poverty in Europe. A specific national strategy was initiated in 2012 through 2020 for inclusion and improvement in educational, economic, and health outcomes for the Roma people (Fernández-Feito et al., 2019). Social acceptance of sexual diversity in Spain is high at 89%; however, according to the EuroQual-5 dimensions-5 levels in Barcelona, persistent inequities are seen among women attracted to the same sex, but not men (Marti-Pastor et al., 2022).

ENVIRONMENTAL AND CLIMATE CHANGE ISSUES

Spain struggles with lack of rain, soil erosion, and overuse of groundwater and desertification which threatens most of the arable land. A Spanish Plan of Action to Combat Desertification has been enacted to study alternatives to current land and crop management to protect against the effects of climate change (Martínez-Valderrama et al., 2016). Spain is known for its olive production, so olive groves are used as targets to study the effect of climate change and land use policies on preservation of land productivity (Arenas-Castro et al., 2020).

HISTORICAL/THEORETICAL BACKGROUND OF HEALTHCARE

Spain was led by the dictator Franco with resulting poverty and oppression until 1975. In 1978 a new democratic constitution was enacted which included hospital reform and later, universal coverage of publicly financed healthcare. This revolution in healthcare was 30 years behind the rest of Europe, which had implemented changes after World War II. During the overhaul of its healthcare system, Spain placed particular emphasis on the development of primary care and careful placement of primary care centers to be accessible to all of Spain's population—both urban and rural. The primary care centers are fully equipped as urgent care centers with labs, x-ray equipment, immunizations, and outpatient services. Specialty services are by referral and may be located in specialty hospitals (WHO, 2025).

WHO has recognized the efficiency of the Spanish health system as one of the best among the OECD countries, achieving universal health coverage at a cost of $4,432 per person per year. In contrast, the most expensive system is the United States with no universal health coverage yet a cost of $12,012 per person per year in 2021 (Figure 25.3; WHO, 2025). Spain approaches healthcare training and delivery in a systematic fashion, setting quotas at a national level for the number of positions available for a variety of health disciplines to improve healthcare efficiency and quality while managing costs. Strengths include the low cost, high quality, and comprehensive coverage of health services with appropriate physical distribution of services. Detractors include wait times for nonurgent procedures, rise in variability between autonomous regions in quality indicators such as antibiotic prescribing, low ratio of nurses, and persistently high levels of smoking. Spain incorporated social determinants of health into the new plan for healthcare quality starting in 2010 (WHO, 2025).

FIGURE 25.3 Spain's ranking in health spending, with sources of payments, 2024.

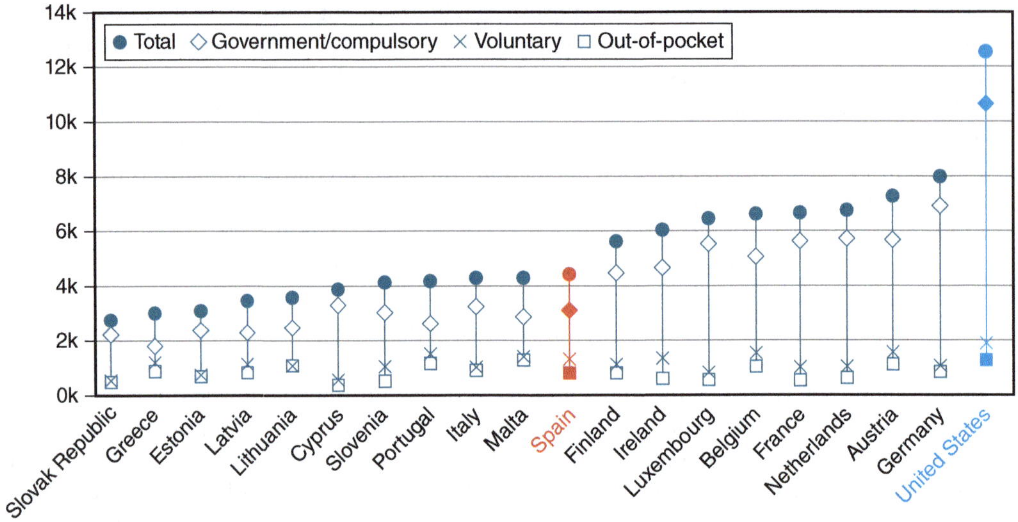

Source: Organisation for Economic Co-operation and Development. (2024). *Health spending*. https://www.oecd.org/en/data/indicators/health-spending.html

HEALTHCARE DELIVERY, FINANCE, INSURANCE, AND PAYMENT

Healthcare delivery is assigned to the autonomous regions in Spain. Local primary care centers are accessible within 30 minutes, reflecting a well-distributed primary care system. Public healthcare funding is used for public health centers, emergency care, and hospital systems. Medication cost is partially shared by patients, but thousands of medications have negotiated prices with the Spanish government, controlling costs. Private physicians, clinics, and hospitals are also available which can be paid for out-of-pocket or with private insurance. Some communities provide their own mutual insurance for the population, receive public funding at a specified amount, and then run private facilities paid for by public healthcare money. This allows the facility to have more control of the management of the funds, to have more freedom to increase wages for healthcare workers, to provide privately funded services alongside publicly funded services, and to increase efficiency (WHO, 2025).

HEALTHCARE TRAINING AND EDUCATION

Healthcare training is competitive and nearly free in public universities. There are new specialties being added to both nursing and physician training, such as family and community care, pediatrics, geriatrics, mental health, forensics, genetics, emergency medicine, and infectious diseases. New technology is being used for simulations and development of critical thinking (Balz & Forjan, 2023; WHO, 2025).

HEALTHCARE COST, QUALITY, AND ACCESS

Spain spends less on healthcare than other countries in the EU and less than other wealthy countries in the OECD. The current percentage of GDP on healthcare is 10.2%, slightly higher than the EU average due to the lower GDP in Spain (OECD, 2024). Spain enacted austerity measures in the publicly funded health system in 2013 due to an economic downturn. During that time healthcare quality suffered with increases in wait times for primary care, specialty care, and nonemergency services (WHO, 2025).

GAPS IN CARE OR HEALTHCARE SHORTAGE AREAS

Spain has a high physician-to-population ratio but a low nurse ratio, with expected shortages of physicians, nurses, and other health professionals over the next decade due to emigration and retirement. A new registry is being implemented to help forecast healthcare worker shortages. New strategies are being discussed at the national level to increase the supply of healthcare professionals, including bringing in professionals from other countries, increasing wages to retain nationally trained staff, and increasing the number of graduates (Bernal-Delgado et al., 2024).

CONCLUSION

Presently, Spain is ranked as the fourth most populous country in the EU. Although the birth rate continues to decline, Spain's total population in 2025 is expected to exceed 52 million. One of the potential contributors to the population increase is average longer life expectancy. A Spaniard women's life expectancy has reached 86.2 years of age and men's 80.3 years of age. The largest populations cohort in 2050 will be those in their early 40s and early 70s. Present data support that Spain will have more than 75,500 women 100 years of age or older (Statista, 2024).

LEARNING ACTIVITIES

CourseConnect

To access self-assessment questions and interactive, competency-based learning activities for this chapter, visit www.springerpub.com/courseconnect. See inside front cover and tear-out for CourseConnect details.

REFERENCES

Aleman, J. A., Zafrilla Rentero, M. P., Montoro-García, S., Mulero, J., Perez Garrido, A., Leal, M., Guerrero, L., Ramos, E., & Ruilope, L. M. (2016). Adherence to the "Mediterranean diet" in Spain and its relationship with cardiovascular risk (DIMERICA study). *Nutrients, 8*(11), 680. https://doi.org/10.3390/nu8110680

Arenas-Castro, S., Gonçalves, J. F., Moreno, M., & Villar, R. (2020). Projected climate changes are expected to decrease the suitability and production of olive varieties in southern Spain. *Science of the Total Environment, 709*, 136161. https://doi.org/10.1016/j.scitotenv.2019.136161

Balz, A., & Forjan, M. (2023). Technology enhanced training in medical multi-user scenarios. In O. Viberg, I. Jivet, P. J. Muñoz-Merino, M. Perifanou, & T. Papathoma (Eds.), *Responsive and sustainable educational futures: 18th European Conference on Technology Enhanced Learning, EC-TEL 2023, Aveiro, Portugal, September 4–8, 2023, Proceedings*. Springer-Verlag. https://doi.org/10.1007/978-3-031-42682-7_61

Banegas, J. R., Sánchez-Martínez, M., Gijón-Conde, T., López-García, E., Graciani, A., Guallar-Castillón, P., García-Puig, J., & Rodríguez-Artalejo, F. (2024). Numerical values and impact of hypertension in Spain. *Revista Española de Cardiología (English Edition), 77*(9), 767–778. https://doi.org/10.1016/j.rec.2024.03.011

Bernal-Delgado, E., Angulo-Pueyo, E., Ridao-López, M., Urbanos-Garrido, R. M., Oliva-Moreno, J., García-Abiétar, D., & Hernández-Quevedo, C. (2024). *Spain: Health system summary, 2024*. European Observatory on Health Systems and Policies, WHO Regional Office for Europe.

Cabiedes-Miragaya, L., Diaz-Mendez, C., & Garcia-Espejo, I. (2021). Well-being and the lifestyle habits of the Spanish population: The association between subjective well-being and eating habits. *International Journal of Environment Research and Public Health, 18*(4), 1553. https://doi.org/10.3390/ijerph18041553

Díaz-Parra, I., & Mena, J. C. (2015). Squatting, the 15-M movement, and struggles for housing in the sontext of the Spanish social crisis. *Human Geography, 8*(1), 40–53. https://doi.org/10.1177/194277861500800103

Fernández-Feito, A., Pesquera-Cabezas, R., González-Cobo, C., & Prieto-Salceda, M. D. (2019). What do we know about the health of Spanish Roma people and what has been done to improve it? A scoping review. *Ethnicity & Health, 24*(2), 224–243. https://doi.org/10.1080/13557858.2017.1315373

IndexMundi. (2017). *Spain*. https://www.indexmundi.com/facts/spain#Health

Instituto Nacional de Estadística. (2024). *Tasas de actividad por sexo y grupo de edad* [Activity rates by sex and age group]. https://www.ine.es/jaxiT3

Karacs, S. (2025). *The Spanish government: Politics in Spain*. https://www.expatica.com/es/living/gov-law-admin/spain-government-106928/

La Moncloa. (2024). *The government of Spain approves new basic material assistance programme for the most vulnerable families*. https://www.lamoncloa.gob.es/lang/en/gobierno/councilministers/paginas/2024/20240123_council.aspx

La Moncloa. (2025). *Spain's geography*. https://www.lamoncloa.gob.es/lang/en/espana/historyandculture/geography/paginas/index.aspx

Lopez-Bueno, R., Calatayud, J., Casana, J., Casajus, J. A., Smith, L., Tully, M. A., Andersen, L. L., & Lopez-Sanchez, G. F. (2020). COVID-19 confinement and health risk behaviors in Spain. *Frontiers in Psychology, 11*, 1426. https://doi.org/10.3389/fpsyg.2020.01426

López-Cuadrado, T., Llácer, A., Palmera-Suárez, R., Gómez-Barroso, D., Savulescu, C., González-Yuste, P., & Fernández-Cuenca, R. (2014). Trends in infectious disease mortality rates, Spain, 1980–2011. *Emerging Infectious Diseases, 20*(5), 782–789. https://doi.org/10.3201/eid2005.131528

Macrotrends. (2024). *Spain population 1950-2024*. https://www.macrotrends.net/global-metrics/countries/esp/spain/population

Marti-Pastor, M., German, D., Perez, G., Bartoll, X., Diez, E., Pont, A., Garín, O., Alonso, J., Hernandez, G., & Mayoral, K. (2022). Health inequalities by sexual orientation: Results from the 2016–2017 Barcelona health survey. *LGBT health, 9*(7), 496–511. https://doi.org/10.1089/lgbt.2021.0171

Martínez-Valderrama, J., Ibáñez, J., Del Barrio, G., Sanjuán, M. E., Alcalá, F. J., Martínez-Vicente, S., Ruiz, A., & Puigdefábregas, J. (2016). Present and future of desertification in Spain: Implementation of a surveillance system to prevent land degradation. *Science of the Total Environment, 563*, 169–178. http://doi.org/10.1016/j.scitotenv.2016.04.065

Navarro, I. (2022). *Sensational Spain: Languages of Spain*. https://sensationalspain.com/languages-in-spain/

O'Callaghan, J. F., & Viguera, M. J. (2025). *Spain: Cultural life*. Britannica. https://www.britannica.com/place/Spain/Festivals-and-holidaysstivals

Organisation for Economic Co-operation and Development. (2024). *OECD economic outlook*. https://www.oecd.org/en/publications/2024/12/oecd-economic-outlook-volume-2024-issue-2_67bb8fac/full-report/spain_99cebb3f.html

Rojo-Martínez, G., Valdés, S., Soriguer, F., Vendrell, J., Urrutia, I., Pérez, V., Ortega, E., Ocón, P., Montanya, E., & Menéndez, E. (2020). Incidence of diabetes mellitus in Spain as results of the nation-wide cohort di@ bet. es study. *Scientific Reports, 10*(1), 2765. https://doi.org/10.1038/s41598-020-59643-7

Serra-Majem, L., Ribas, L., Ngo, J., Ortega, R. M., García, A., Pérez-Rodrigo, C., & Aranceta, J. (2004). Food, youth and the Mediterranean diet in Spain. Development of KIDMED, Mediterranean Diet Quality Index in children and adolescents. *Public Health Nutrition, 7*(7), 931-935. doi: 10.1079/phn2004556. PMID: 15482620.

Statista. (2024). *Mental health in Spain*. https://www.statista.com/study/91617/mental-health-in-spain/

Sublime Spain. (2025). *Leisure in Spain: 5 of the best activities*. https://www.sublimespain.com/leisure-in-spain/

U.S. Department of State. (2022) *Spain*. https://www.state.gov/reports/2022-report-on-international-religious-freedom/spain/

Varela-Moreiras G, Avila, J, M., Cuadrado, C., del Pozo, S., Ruiz, E., & Moreiras, O. (2020). Evaluation of food consumption and dietary patterns in Spain by the food consumption survey: Updated information. *European Journal of Clinical Nutrition, 64*(Suppl 3), S37-S43. doi: 10.1038/ejcn.2010.208. PMID: 21045847.

World Bank Group. (2023). *Birth rate, crude (per 1,000 people) - Spain*. https://data.worldbank.org/indicator/SP.DYN.CBRT.IN?locations=ES

World Bank Group. (2025). *Understanding poverty*. https://www.worldbank.org/en/topic/poverty/overview

World Economics. (2021). *Spain GDP economic data*. https://www.worldeconomics.com/Country-Size/spain.aspx

World Health Organization. (2009). *Global health risks: Mortality and burden of disease attributable to selected major risks*. https://www.who.int/publications/i/item/9789241563871

World Health Organization. (2025). *World health statistics: Spain [country overview]*. data.who.int

PART VII: Health and Healthcare in North and West Africa

CHAPTER 26

OVERVIEW OF NORTH AND WEST AFRICA

Inijesu Taiwo and Thomas Foley

GEOGRAPHY

North and West Africa are ecologically diverse regions that include the water-scarce drylands of the Sahara Desert, the Atlas Mountains, the Niger River, long coastal areas, and thriving tropical forests. North Africa includes seven primarily desert nations along the North Atlantic Oceans and Mediterranean and Red Seas. The countries of North Africa are Algeria, Egypt, Libya, Morocco, Sudan, Tunisia, and Western Sahara. West Africa includes coastal countries along the Atlantic Ocean and countries that span the rain forests and into the drylands of the desert. The 16 countries that makeup West Africa are Benin, Burkina Faso, Cabo Verde, Cote d'Iviore, Gambia, Ghana, Guinea, Guinea Bissau, Liberia, Mali, Mauritania, Niger, Nigeria, Senegal, Sierra Leone, and Togo. Both West and North Africa are vulnerable to the effects of climate change. In the northern and eastern areas of West Africa and a majority of North Africa, desertification and drought are threats. Flooding is a threat along and near the coast of the southwestern part of West Africa (Berglee, 2016). Figure 26.1 (Ogbodo et al., 2023) is a map of West and North Africa.

BRIEF HISTORY

West and North Africa each have a rich tapestry of history influenced by diverse civilizations, trade networks, colonialism, and postindependence developments. In West Africa's precolonial era, powerful empires like the Ghana Empire, Mali Empire, Songhai Empire, and the Benin Empire were renowned for their wealth, trade, and cultural achievements. Early North Africa civilizations such as Ancient Egypt, Phoenicia, Carthage, and Numidia are celebrated for their contributions to art, architecture, and governance. Islamic expansion from the seventh century brought about Islamic dynasties and trade networks, shaping the region's culture and society (Akyeampong & Gates, 2012). However, European colonization from the 15th to 20th centuries led to resource exploitation, the trans-Atlantic slave trade, and significant cultural and economic harms to the people and civilizations of North and West Africa (Falola & Warnock, 2007). West and North African countries experienced a wave of independence during the decolonization movement in the 20th century. Postdecolonization, these countries continue to evolve with modern developments, political shifts, economic growth, social changes, and regional collaborations (Akyeampong & Gates, 2012).

POPULATION

In 2023, the population of West Africa was more than 440 million people. Nigeria, which is one of the world's most heavily populated countries, accounted for approximately half of West Africa's population. In 2023, Nigeria's population was approximately 224 million people. In

FIGURE 26.1 African regions map.

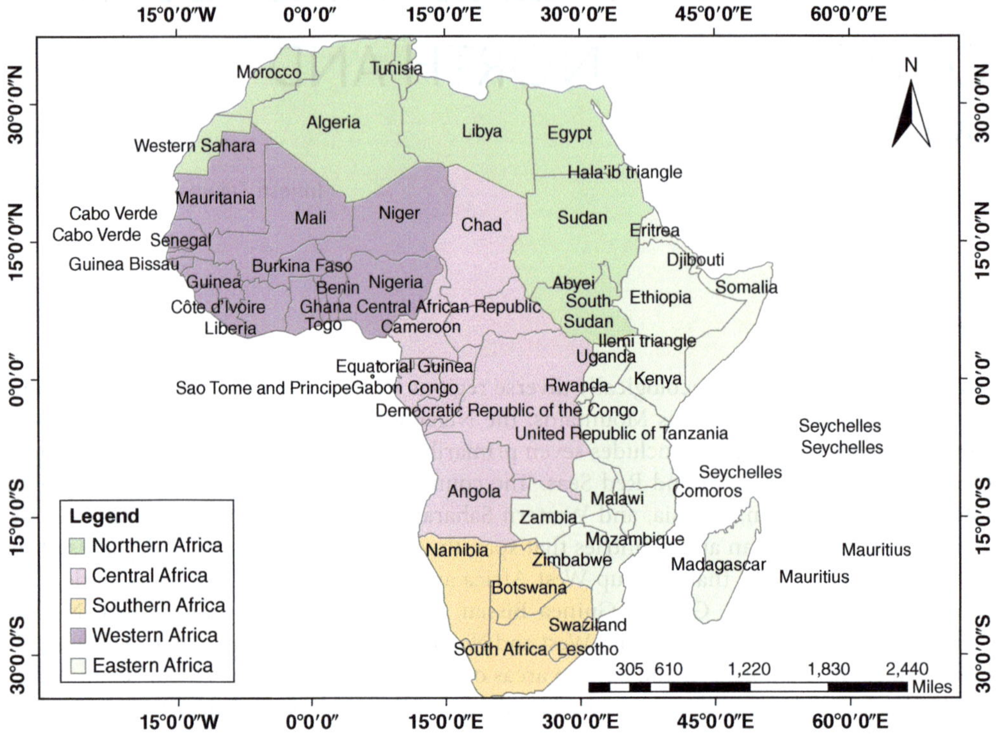

Note: South Sudan is considered a part of Eastern Africa as opposed to Northern Africa.

Source: Ogbodo, U. S., Liu, S., Feng, S., Gao, H., & Pan, Z. (2023). Trade-offs and synergies among 17 ecosystem services in Africa: A long-term multi-national analysis. *Remote Sens, 15*(14), 3588. https://doi.org/10.3390/rs15143588)

comparison, the population of the small West African island nation of Cabo Verde was approximately 599 thousand people. In 2023, North Africa's population was approximately 264 million. Egypt, with a population of approximately 113 million, accounted for 43% of North Africa's population. The disputed North African country Western Sahara, with a population of less than 600 thousand people, is one of the most sparsely populated countries in the world (UN Data Portal, n.d.).

While most of North African countries are undergoing population aging, West Africa is one of the youngest regions in the world. In 2023, the median age in West Africa was 17.3 years while the median age in North Africa was 27.2 years. Not surprisingly, given the younger population in much of West Africa, the birth rate is much higher when compared to North Africa. In 2023, the birth rate in West Africa was 35.3 births per 1,000 people while it was 22.3 births per 1,000 people in North Africa. Cabo Verde and Sudan are exceptions regarding regional norms. In 2023, Cabo Verde had a lower birth rate (16.4 births) and higher median age (27.4 years) in comparison to the rest of West Africa. Sudan had a higher birth rate (32.6 births) and lower median age (18.6 years) when compared to other North Africa countries (UN Data Portal, n.d.).

SOCIOECONOMIC FACTORS

While Algeria, Egypt, and Nigeria are the leading African economies with three of the wealthiest African gross domestic products (GDPs), North and West African countries struggle financially and include significant income disparities. In 2023, Libya had the highest per-capita GDP in the area at approximately $6,700. All other North and West African countries had per-capita GDPs less than $5,000 including Algeria, Egypt, and Nigeria. Eight countries had per-capita GDPs less than $1,000. The West African nation Sierra Leone had the lowest per-capita GDP at approximately $459. Educational attainment and literacy are problems in much of West Africa. Several West African countries such as Mali, Burkina Faso, and Niger have the lowest literacy rates in the world (World Bank Group, n.d.).

TABLE 26.1 HEALTH OUTCOMES IN NORTHERN AND WESTERN AFRICA

REGION / COUNTRY	LIFE EXPECTANCY AT BIRTH, 2023	INFANT MORTALITY, 2023	MATERNAL MORTALITY, 2020	LEADING CAUSE OF MORTALITY, 2021
North Africa	71.95 years	21.1	103	
Algeria	77.3	16	78	COVID-19
Egypt	70.81	16	17	Heart disease
Libya	73.25	8.9	72	Heart disease
Morocco	75.2	13.7	72	Heart disease
Sudan	66.1	36.9	270	Heart disease
Tunisia	76.94	11.9	37	COVID-19
Western Sahara	71.19	22.7	No data	No data
West Africa	57.57 years	58.9	754	
Benin	60.45	55	523	Malaria
Burkina Faso	60.57	46.1	264	Malaria
Cabo Verde	76.93	11.6	42	Heart disease
Cote d'Ivoire	60.11	56.2	480	Malaria
Gambia	64.12	26.7	458	COVID-19
Ghana	64.53	32.1	263	COVID-19
Guinea	59.55	64.5	553	COVID-19
Guinea-Bissau	60.56	51	725	COVID-19
Liberia	62.04	56	652	Malaria
Mali	60.03	53.8	440	Neonatal disorders
Mauritania	65.48	43.9	464	Stroke
Niger	62.93	40.4	441	Malaria
Nigeria	53.87	70.6	1,047	Neonatal disorders
Senegal	69.31	18.2	261	COVID-19
Sierra Leone	60.79	70.5	443	Malaria
Togo	61.82	43.1	339	Malaria

Sources: Institute for Health Metrics and Evaluation (n.d.). *Health research by location: Country profiles*. https://www.healthdata.org/research-analysis/health-by-location/profiles; UN Data Portal. (n.d.). *Population division data portal*. United Nations. https://population.un.org/dataportal/home/; UN Population Fund. (n.d.). *Data portal*. https://www.unfpa.org/data

HEALTH OUTCOMES

There are drastic health disparities when comparing West Africa to North Africa. From a regional perspective, West Africa has the lowest life expectancy at birth and the highest regional infant and maternal mortality in the world (UN Data Portal, n.d.; UN Population Fund, n.d.). Most West Africa countries still experience significant mortality from neonatal disorders, malaria, diarrheal diseases, HIV/AIDS, and tuberculosis (Institute for Health Metrics and Evaluation, n.d.). Cabo Verde is a regional exception as it experiences greater life expectancy at birth and lower infectious disease, infant, and maternal mortality when compared to other West Africa countries. In North Africa, Sudan is an exception as it experiences greater infant and maternal mortality and shorter life expectancy when compared to other countries in the northern region (UN Data Portal, n.d.). Table 26.1 describes key health outcomes in North and West Africa.

LEARNING ACTIVITIES

CourseConnect >

To access self-assessment questions and interactive, competency-based learning activities for this chapter, visit www.springerpub.com/courseconnect. See inside front cover and tear-out for CourseConnect details.

REFERENCES

Akyeampong, E. K., & Gates, H. L. (2012). *Dictionary of African biography*. Oxford University Press.

Berglee, R. (2016). *World regional geography*. University of Minnesota Libraries Publishing.

Falola, T., & Warnock, A. (2007). *Encyclopedia of the middle passage: Greenwood milestones in African American history* (1st ed.). Greenwood.

Institute for Health Metrics and Evaluation. (n.d.). *Health research by location: Country profiles*. University of Washington. https://www.healthdata.org/research-analysis/health-by-location/profiles

Ogbodo, U. S., Liu, S., Feng, S., Gao, H., & Pan, Z. (2023). Trade-offs and synergies among 17 ecosystem services in Africa: A long-term multi-national analysis. *Remote Sens, 15*(14), 3588. https://doi.org/10.3390/rs15143588

UN Data Portal. (n.d.). *UN population division data portal*. United Nations. https://population.un.org/dataportal/home/

UN Population Fund. (n.d.). *Data portal*. United Nations. https://www.unfpa.org/data

World Bank Group. (n.d.). *World Bank open data*. https://data.worldbank.org/

CHAPTER 27

EGYPT

Marwa Mamdouh Shaban and Mostafa Shaban

INTRODUCTION

Egypt's healthcare system is a mix of public and private providers, with the public sector playing a dominant role. The **Ministry of Health and Population (MoHP)** oversees the public healthcare system, which includes a network of hospitals, primary care clinics, and specialized facilities. In 2019, the government launched the **Universal Health Insurance (UHI)** program, which aims to provide comprehensive healthcare coverage to all Egyptians by 2032. The UHI is being implemented in phases, with the first phase covering eight governorates as of 2023 (Fasseeh, ElEzbawy, Adly, et al., 2022).

The government has also been investing in the modernization and expansion of the public healthcare infrastructure. This includes the construction of new hospitals, the upgrading of existing facilities, and the acquisition of advanced medical equipment. The private healthcare sector has been growing in recent years, driven by increased demand for quality healthcare services, especially among the middle- and upper-class populations. This has led to the establishment of numerous private hospitals, clinics, and diagnostic centers (Fasseeh ElEzbawy, Gamal, et al., 2022).

Egypt has been actively promoting medical tourism, leveraging its relatively affordable costs and the availability of qualified healthcare professionals. The country has seen an influx of patients from neighboring countries seeking medical treatment. The COVID-19 pandemic posed significant challenges to Egypt's healthcare system, leading to the expansion of testing capabilities, the establishment of dedicated treatment facilities, and the acceleration of the vaccination program (AbdelAziz & Kewina, 2022).

Overall, Egypt is making strides in improving its healthcare infrastructure and expanding access to quality healthcare services, although challenges such as regional disparities, limited resources, and the burden of noncommunicable diseases (NCDs) remain (Bohl et al., 2018).

IMPORTANCE OF UNDERSTANDING THE HEALTHCARE SYSTEM IN EGYPT

Understanding the healthcare landscape in Egypt is crucial for several reasons. First, the country's public–private mix of healthcare provision requires a comprehensive understanding of the roles, responsibilities, and interactions between the different stakeholders. This knowledge is essential for patients to navigate the system and access the appropriate healthcare services (Prashker, 1994). Additionally, the ongoing implementation of the UHI program represents a significant transformation of the healthcare system, and staying informed on its progress and implications is vital for policymakers, healthcare providers, and the public. Moreover, Egypt's ambitions to become a regional hub for medical tourism necessitate a thorough understanding of the country's healthcare capabilities, quality standards, and regulatory environment (Khalifa et al., 2022).

This information is crucial for both domestic and international patients, as well as healthcare investors and practitioners looking to engage with the Egyptian market. Finally, the healthcare system's ability to respond to public health emergencies, such as the COVID-19 pandemic, underscores the importance of continually monitoring and evaluating the system's resilience and adaptability. By understanding the nuances of Egypt's healthcare landscape, stakeholders can make informed decisions, contribute to the system's development, and ensure the provision of accessible and high-quality healthcare services for the population (Abd El Ghaffar et al., 2022).

HISTORICAL CONTEXT

Egypt's healthcare system has a long and complex history, shaped by various political, economic, and social factors over the decades. During the monarchy era prior to the 1952 revolution, the healthcare system was characterized by a predominantly private, fragmented, and urban-centric model, with limited access for rural and lower-income populations. Following the revolution, the government sought to expand public healthcare provision and establish a more centralized, state-led system. This included the nationalization of private hospitals and the creation of the Ministry of Health to oversee the public healthcare network. The 1970s and 1980s saw further investments in expanding primary healthcare services and the construction of new public hospitals, particularly in rural areas. However, the subsequent economic reforms and structural adjustment programs of the 1990s led to a decline in public healthcare spending and the gradual growth of the private sector (Abdou & Zaazou, 2013).

The early 2000s witnessed renewed efforts to improve healthcare access and quality, including the introduction of health insurance schemes and public–private partnerships. The ongoing UHI program, launched in 2019, represents the government's most ambitious attempt to date to achieve universal healthcare coverage and address the persistent inequities in the system. Understanding this historical evolution is crucial for contextualizing the current challenges and opportunities facing Egypt's healthcare landscape (Koohpayezadeh et al., 2021).

HEALTHCARE INFRASTRUCTURE

Egypt's healthcare infrastructure is a complex mix of public and private facilities, ranging from primary care clinics to specialized tertiary hospitals. The public healthcare system is the backbone of the country's overall healthcare provision, consisting of a network of MoHP hospitals, university-affiliated hospitals, and healthcare centers. These public facilities are often concentrated in urban areas, with more limited coverage in rural regions (Elsharkawy et al., 2022). In recent decades, there has been a gradual expansion of primary healthcare services, including the establishment of family health units and centers across the country. The private healthcare sector, on the other hand, has grown significantly, particularly in urban areas, catering to middle- and upper-income populations. This private system includes a diverse range of facilities, from small, private clinics to large, high-tech private hospitals. Additionally, Egypt has a significant number of nonprofit and charitable healthcare providers, which play an important role in serving the underserved communities. The ongoing UHI program aims to integrate the public and private sectors, improving access and quality of care for all Egyptians. However, challenges remain in ensuring an equitable distribution of healthcare resources and infrastructure, particularly in rural and underserved areas (Shouman et al., 2022).

Healthcare facilities in Egypt are classified as primary, secondary, or tertiary healthcare facilities. Primary healthcare facilities consist of a network of family health units and centers operated by the MoHP. These facilities provide basic preventive, curative, and rehabilitative services, including outpatient clinics, maternal and child health services, and community-based programs (AlSawahli & Heba, 2019). The primary care system also includes a growing number of private clinics and general practitioners, which serve as the first point of contact for many Egyptians. Secondary healthcare in Egypt is provided by general and district hospitals, which offer a wider range of inpatient and outpatient services compared to primary care facilities. These hospitals are typically larger, well-equipped facilities that can handle more complex medical cases. The secondary healthcare system includes both public hospitals run by the MoHP and private hospitals and clinics that cater to the middle- and upper-income populations (Fasseeh, ElEzbawy, Adly, et al., 2022).

At the top of the healthcare pyramid are Egypt's tertiary care facilities, which provide highly specialized and advanced medical services. These include university teaching hospitals, specialized national institutes (e.g., cancer, heart, neuroscience institutes), and some private hospitals with state-of-the-art equipment and expertise (International Finance Corporation, 2023). These tertiary centers serve as referral hubs, treating patients with complex or rare medical conditions that cannot be adequately managed at the primary or secondary levels.

This comprehensive healthcare infrastructure, spanning primary, secondary, and tertiary facilities, aims to provide Egyptians with a continuum of care. However, challenges remain in terms of equitable access, particularly in underserved rural areas, and ensuring high-quality services across all levels of the system (Shouman et al., 2021).

HEALTHCARE FINANCING

Overall, the coexistence of public and private healthcare facilities in Egypt reflects the country's efforts to address the diverse healthcare needs of its population, while also navigating the complexities of resource allocation and healthcare financing. Healthcare financing in Egypt is a complex and evolving landscape, involving a mix of public and private sources (Fasseeh, ElEzbawy, Adly, et al., 2022). The primary source of public healthcare funding in Egypt is the government's budget, channeled through the MoHP. This public spending accounts for a significant portion of the overall healthcare expenditure in the country. However, the level of public healthcare spending has fluctuated over the years, influenced by broader economic and fiscal considerations (Ismail, 2018).

SOURCES OF HEALTHCARE FUNDING: GOVERNMENT, PRIVATE, AND OUT-OF-POCKET

In recent years, the government has made efforts to increase its investment in the healthcare sector, particularly through the implementation of the UHI program. The UHI aims to expand population coverage and improve access to healthcare services, funded through a combination of government subsidies and mandatory contributions from individuals and employers. The private healthcare sector in Egypt is largely financed through out-of-pocket payments by individuals and households (Burke et al., 2018). This includes direct payments for services at private hospitals, clinics, and diagnostic centers, as well as the growing use of private health insurance plans. The private health insurance market in Egypt has been expanding, catering to middle- and upper-income populations. However, the coverage and penetration of private insurance remain relatively low compared with many other countries.

Despite the efforts to strengthen healthcare financing, Egypt continues to face several challenges, including high out-of-pocket expenditures, which can create barriers to healthcare access, especially for lower-income populations; insufficient public healthcare budgets to meet the growing demand for services; uneven distribution of healthcare resources and funding across different regions and populations; and fragmentation in the healthcare financing system, with a lack of integration between public and private sources. Addressing these challenges and achieving more equitable and sustainable healthcare financing remains a key priority for policymakers in Egypt. Ongoing reforms, such as the UHI program, aim to address these issues and move the country toward universal health coverage (Gaye et al., 2021).

Egypt has a complex and evolving landscape of health insurance coverage and schemes, comprising both public and private components. The primary public health insurance scheme in Egypt is the UHI program, which was launched in 2019 with the goal of achieving universal health coverage by 2032. The UHI system is designed to gradually expand coverage, starting with select governorates and gradually scaling up nationwide (Doshmangir et al., 2021). Under the UHI, beneficiaries are required to make monthly contributions based on their income level, with subsidies provided for lower-income individuals and families. The program aims to integrate both public and private healthcare providers, offering a comprehensive package of essential health services. In addition to the UHI, Egypt also has a social health insurance scheme managed by the Health Insurance Organization (HIO), which covers public sector employees, pensioners, and their dependents (Devi, 2018).

The private health insurance market in Egypt has been growing, catering primarily to the middle- and upper-income segments of the population. Private insurance plans are offered by both commercial insurance companies and some employers as part of their employee benefits. Private insurance plans typically provide coverage for a wider range of services, including access to private healthcare facilities, specialized treatments, and advanced diagnostic services. However, the cost of private insurance premiums can be a significant barrier for many Egyptians (World Economic Forum, 2023).

Despite the efforts to expand health insurance coverage, significant gaps remain in the overall system. As of 2023, it is estimated that only around 60% of the Egyptian population has some form of health insurance coverage, with the remaining 40% relying on out-of-pocket payments or limited access to public healthcare services. Key challenges in the health insurance landscape include uneven distribution of coverage, with lower enrollment rates in rural and lower-income areas; limited benefit packages and exclusions in some insurance plans; affordability issues, particularly for lower-income individuals and families; and fragmentation and lack of integration between public and private insurance schemes (World Bank Group, 2020).

Addressing these challenges and achieving universal health coverage remains a significant priority for the Egyptian government, as it seeks to ensure equitable access to quality healthcare for all its citizens. Egypt faces several key challenges in healthcare financing, which are hampering efforts to provide equitable and sustainable access to healthcare services for the population (Fasseeh, ElEzbawy, Adly, et al., 2022):

- *Insufficient public healthcare spending*: The level of public healthcare spending in Egypt, as a percentage of the overall government budget and gross domestic product (GDP), has historically been relatively low compared with many other countries. This limited public investment in the healthcare sector has constrained the ability to expand infrastructure, upgrade facilities, and improve the quality of services (Fasseeh, ElEzbawy, Adly, et al., 2022).
- *High out-of-pocket expenditures*: A significant portion of healthcare costs in Egypt are borne by individuals and households through out-of-pocket payments. This places a heavy financial burden on the population, especially the lower-income segments, and can create barriers to accessing necessary healthcare services.
- *Fragmented healthcare financing in Egypt*: Multiple public and private insurance schemes operate in parallel. This lack of integration and coordination can lead to inefficiencies, duplication of efforts, and challenges in ensuring comprehensive coverage and optimal resource allocation (Iqbal et al., 2022).
- *Uneven distribution of healthcare resources*: Both in terms of infrastructure and funding, distribution of resources is uneven across different regions of Egypt. This disparity between urban and rural areas, as well as between different governorates, exacerbates inequities in access to healthcare services.
- *Limited population coverage by health insurance*: Despite ongoing efforts to expand the UHI program, a significant portion of the Egyptian population, particularly in rural and low-income areas, remains uninsured or underinsured. This leaves many individuals vulnerable to the financial burden of healthcare costs (Frostad et al., 2022).
- *Insufficient investment in preventive and primary care*: The healthcare system in Egypt has traditionally been focused more on curative care, with a relatively lower emphasis on preventive healthcare and primary care services. This imbalance can lead to higher costs and poorer health outcomes in the long run.
- *Governance and management challenges*: Effective governance, coordination, and management of the healthcare financing system poses ongoing challenges, requiring improved data-driven decision-making, transparency, and accountability mechanisms. Addressing

these complex healthcare financing challenges will require a multifaceted approach, involving policy reforms, increased public investment, innovative financing mechanisms, and a focus on enhancing the efficiency and equity of the overall healthcare system in Egypt (Frostad et al., 2022).

HEALTHCARE WORKFORCE

The healthcare workforce in Egypt faces multifaceted challenges amid a growing population and evolving healthcare needs. As of recent reports, Egypt has made strides in expanding its healthcare infrastructure, yet disparities persist in access to quality care across urban and rural areas. The healthcare workforce, comprising doctors, nurses, and allied health professionals, grapples with issues such as inadequate training opportunities, uneven distribution of healthcare facilities, and low doctor-to-patient ratios compared with international standards. Efforts to address these challenges include government initiatives to increase medical school enrollments and enhance training programs. However, retention remains a concern due to factors like low salaries and limited career development opportunities. The COVID-19 pandemic has further highlighted the strain on healthcare workers, underscoring the need for sustainable workforce management and investment in healthcare infrastructure (Elkalamawi et al., 2021).

HEALTHCARE ACCESS AND UTILIZATION

As noted, Egypt has made significant strides in improving healthcare access and utilization over the past decade, but challenges remain. The country has a mixed public–private healthcare system, with a large public sector that provides subsidized care, as well as a growing private sector. Access to healthcare services has expanded, with the government working to increase the number of primary care facilities and hospitals, especially in rural and underserved areas. However, significant disparities in access persist between urban and rural populations, as well as between higher and lower socioeconomic groups (Katoue et al., 2022).

Utilization of healthcare services has also improved, with more Egyptians seeking care when needed. The government has implemented initiatives to increase health insurance coverage and reduce out-of-pocket spending. Still, many Egyptians, particularly those in the informal sector, lack adequate financial protection, leading to high rates of catastrophic health expenditures. Quality of care remains a concern, with issues such as shortages of medical supplies, uneven distribution of healthcare workers, and variable adherence to clinical standards. The government has been working to address these challenges through investments in infrastructure, workforce development, and quality improvement programs. Overall, Egypt has made progress in improving healthcare access and utilization, but more work is needed to ensure equitable and high-quality care for all Egyptians. Ongoing reforms and investments in the healthcare system will be crucial for achieving universal health coverage and better health outcomes (Biltagy & Hamdi, 2024).

HEALTHCARE QUALITY AND OUTCOMES

The quality of healthcare services in Egypt has been a significant concern, with variable standards of care across the public and private healthcare systems. While the government has made efforts to improve infrastructure and invest in healthcare worker training, many challenges remain in ensuring consistent and high-quality care (Food and Agriculture Organization, 2017).

One of the key issues affecting healthcare quality is the shortage and maldistribution of skilled healthcare professionals, particularly in rural and underserved areas. This shortage, coupled with suboptimal working conditions and limited resources, can lead to overburdened healthcare facilities, longer wait times, and compromised patient safety and outcomes. Furthermore, adherence to clinical guidelines and standards of care is not always consistent, with variations in diagnostic practices, treatment protocols, and patient management across different healthcare settings. This can result in suboptimal health outcomes and the perpetuation of health disparities, especially for certain patient populations (Balkhy, 2024).

Challenges in healthcare infrastructure, such as inadequate medical equipment, limited access to essential medicines, and poor maintenance of facilities, can also undermine quality of care. These resource constraints can hinder the ability of healthcare providers to deliver effective and timely treatment, leading to poorer health outcomes for patients. In recent years, the government has made efforts to address these quality issues, including implementing quality assurance frameworks, investing in healthcare workforce development, and strengthening supply chain management. However, more comprehensive and sustained efforts will be needed to ensure that all Egyptians have access to high-quality, patient-centered healthcare services that improve health outcomes and reduce disparities (Javed et al., 2021).

EMERGING TRENDS AND CHALLENGES

One prominent trend in Egypt's healthcare landscape is the growing prevalence of NCDs, such as cardiovascular diseases, diabetes, cancer, and respiratory illnesses. This epidemiologic shift, driven by factors like urbanization, unhealthy lifestyle habits, and an aging population, has placed increasing demands on the healthcare system. Addressing the rise of NCDs requires a comprehensive approach that goes beyond traditional curative care. The Egyptian government has recognized the need to strengthen primary healthcare, promote preventive measures, and enhance the management of chronic conditions. Initiatives such as the expansion of community-based screening programs and the integration of NCD care into primary healthcare services are under way (El-Saadani et al., 2021).

Another emerging trend is the increasing role of digital health technologies in improving healthcare quality and accessibility. The COVID-19 pandemic has accelerated the adoption of telemedicine, mobile health applications, and electronic health records. While still in the early stages, these digital innovations hold the potential to enhance patient–provider communication, facilitate remote monitoring, and improve the efficiency of healthcare delivery. However, the widespread implementation of digital health solutions faces several challenges, including the need for robust infrastructure, secure data management, and development of digital literacy among both healthcare providers and the general population. Addressing these barriers will be crucial for ensuring equitable access to the benefits of digital health technologies (Golinelli et al., 2020).

The healthcare workforce remains a critical challenge in Egypt, with persistent shortages of skilled healthcare professionals, particularly in rural and underserved areas. The government has made efforts to address this issue, such as expanding medical and nursing education programs and implementing incentives to attract and retain healthcare workers in remote regions. Nevertheless, more comprehensive strategies are needed to build a resilient and well-distributed healthcare workforce. As Egypt navigates these emerging trends and challenges, the government's commitment to universal health coverage and the continuous improvement of healthcare quality and patient safety will be crucial in ensuring that all Egyptians have access to high-quality, equitable, and responsive healthcare services (Khalil & Alameddine, 2020).

CONCLUSION

Egypt's healthcare system has made significant strides in expanding access and improving infrastructure, but challenges remain in areas such as healthcare financing, workforce management, and addressing regional disparities. The successful implementation of the UHI program and the continued investment in modernizing the healthcare system will be crucial in strengthening the overall healthcare landscape in Egypt.

LEARNING ACTIVITIES

CourseConnect

To access self-assessment questions and interactive, competency-based learning activities for this chapter, visit www.springerpub.com/courseconnect. See inside front cover and tear-out for CourseConnect details.

REFERENCES

Abd El Ghaffar, M. M., Salem, M. R., Al Soda, M. F., Abd El Razik, M. S., Tahoon, M. H., Tahoon, M. F., Eysa, B., Hegazy, A. E. E., Eleraky, A. E., Eltayar, A. A., Eldarandly, W. M. H. E. D., & Omran, D. (2022). COVID-19 pandemic preparedness in Egypt's teaching hospitals: A needs assessment study. *Frontiers in Public Health, 9*, 748666. https://doi.org/10.3389/fpubh.2021.748666

AbdelAziz, G., & Kewina, I. (2022). Medical tourism and Egypt's strategic vision 2030: Pull motivations that trigger the international patients' intention to vsit Egypt as a medical tourism hub. *The Academic Journal of Contemporary Commercial Research, 2*(2), 53–77. https://doi.org/10.21608/ajccr.2022.245006

Abdou, D. S., & Zaazou, Z. (2013). The Egyptian revolution and post socio-economic impact. *2013 proceedings of the Middle East Economic Association* (Vol. 15, pp. 92-115). https://meea.sites.luc.edu/volume15/pdfs/The-Egyptian-Revolution-and-Post-Socioeconomic-Impact.pdf

AlSawahli, H., & Heba. (2019). *Physicians' motivation in the Ministry of Health and Population—Egypt: Challenges and opportunities*. http://dar.aucegypt.edu/handle/10526/5657

Balkhy, H. (2024). Increasing access to healthcare in the Eastern Mediterranean region. *Eastern Mediterranean Health Journal, 30*(2), 91–92. https://doi.org/10.26719/2024.30.2.91

Biltagy, M., & Hamdi, M. (2024). Public health expenditure and household poverty: Case study of Egypt. *Future Business Journal, 10*(1), 7. https://doi.org/10.1186/s43093-023-00295-0

Bohl, D. K., Hanna, T. L., Scott, A. C., Moyer, J. D., Hedden, S. G., Conceição, P., Merlen, S., Mizra, T., & Wally, N. M. (2018). *Sustainable development goals report: Egypt 2030*. Josef Korbel School of International Studies, University of Denver.

Burke, S., Barry, S., Siersbaek, R., Johnston, B., Ní Fhallúin, M., & Thomas, S. (2018). Sláintecare—A ten-year plan to achieve universal healthcare in Ireland. *Health Policy, 122*(12), 1278–1282. https://doi.org/10.1016/j.healthpol.2018.05.006

Devi, S. (2018). Universal health coverage law approved in Egypt. *The Lancet, 391*(10117), 194. https://doi.org/10.1016/S0140-6736(18)30091-6

Doshmangir, L., Bazyar, M., Rashidian, A., & Gordeev, V. S. (2021). Iran health insurance system in transition: Equity concerns and steps to achieve universal health coverage. *International Journal for Equity in Health, 20*(1), 37. https://doi.org/10.1186/s12939-020-01372-4

Elkalamawi, E., Gamal, E., Hassan, H., & Salama, N. (2021). *Increasing the retention of the health workforce in Egypt: Improving work environments: A policy paper*. The Public Policy Hub. https://fount.aucegypt.edu/studenttxt/90/

El-Saadani, S., Saleh, M., & Ibrahim, S. A. (2021). Quantifying non-communicable diseases' burden in Egypt using state-space model. *PLoS One, 16*(8), e0245642. https://doi.org/10.1371/journal.pone.0245642

Elsharkawy, A., Salem, M. R., Asem, N., Ibrahim, W. K., Ramadan, E. G., Abdelaziz, M. A., Hashish, A., Elsayed, H., & Hassany, M. (2022). Perceived stigma and healthcare services in healthcare settings among people living with HIV in Egypt: A qualitative study. *Transactions of The Royal Society of Tropical Medicine and Hygiene, 116*(9), 868–873. https://doi.org/10.1093/trstmh/trac028

Fasseeh, A., ElEzbawy, B., Adly, W., ElShahawy, R., George, M., Abaza, S., ElShalakani, A., & Kaló, Z. (2022). Healthcare financing in Egypt: A systematic literature review. *Journal of the Egyptian Public Health Association, 97*(1), 1. https://doi.org/10.1186/s42506-021-00089-8

Fasseeh, A. N., ElEzbawy, B., Gamal, M., Seyam, A., Abourawash, A., George, M., Anwar, M., Amin, M., Khalifa, A. Y., Elshalakani, A., Hatem, A., Abdelhamid, S., Elsamouly, H., Fasseeh, N., Adel, R., Dawood, H., Abaza, S., & Kaló, Z. (2022). A roadmap toward implementing health technology. *Frontiers in Public Health, 10*, 896175. https://doi.org/10.3389/fpubh.2022.896175

Food and Agriculture Organization. (2017). *The future of food and agriculture: Trends and challenges.* https://openknowledge.fao.org/server/api/core/bitstreams/2e90c833-8e84-46f2-a675-ea2d7afa4e24/content

Frostad, J. J., Nguyen, Q. P., Baumann, M. M., Blacker, B. F., Marczak, L. B., Deshpande, A., Wiens, K. E., LeGrand, K. E., Johnson, K. B., Abbasi-Kangevari, M., Abdoli, A., Abolhassani, H., Abreu, L. G., Abrigo, M. R. M., Abu-Rmeileh, N. M., Adekanmbi, V., Agrawal, A., Ahmed, M. B., Al-Aly, Z., . . . Reiner, R. C. (2022). Mapping development and health effects of cooking with solid fuels in low-income and middle-income countries, 2000–18: A geospatial modelling study. *The Lancet Global Health, 10*(10), e1395–e1411. https://doi.org/10.1016/S2214-109X(22)00332-1

Gaye, Y.-E., Agbajogu, C., & El Oakley, R. (2021). COVID-19 on the Nile: Review on the management and outcomes of the COVID-19 pandemic in the Arab Republic of Egypt from February to August 2020. *International Journal of Environmental Research and Public Health, 18*(4), 1588. https://doi.org/10.3390/ijerph18041588

Golinelli, D., Boetto, E., Carullo, G., Nuzzolese, A. G., Landini, M. P., & Fantini, M. P. (2020). Adoption of digital technologies in health care during the COVID-19 pandemic: Systematic review of early scientific literature. *Journal of Medical Internet Research, 22*(11), e22280. https://doi.org/10.2196/22280

International Finance Corporation. (2023). *Country private sector diagnostic Egypt health sector deep dive realizing the full potential of a productive private sector.* https://www.ifc.org/en/insights-reports/2023/egypt-private-sector-diagnostic-health-sector-deep-dive

Iqbal, M., Feroz, A. S., Siddeeg, K., Gholbzouri, K., Al-Raiby, J., Hemachandra, N., Saleem, S., & Siddiq, S. (2022). Engagement of private healthcare sector in reproductive, maternal, newborn, child and adolescent health in selected Eastern Mediterranean countries. *Eastern Mediterranean Health Journal, 28*(9), 638–648. https://doi.org/10.26719/emhj.22.057

Ismail, S. A. (2018). The rocky road to universal health coverage in Egypt: A political economy of health insurance reform from 2005–15. *International Social Security Review, 71*(2), 79–101. https://doi.org/10.1111/issr.12167

Javed, A., Lee, C., Zakaria, H., Buenaventura, R. D., Cetkovich-Bakmas, M., Duailibi, K., Ng, B., Ramy, H., Saha, G., Arifeen, S., Elorza, P. M., Ratnasingham, P., & Azeem, M. W. (2021). Reducing the stigma of mental health disorders with a focus on low- and middle-income countries. *Asian Journal of Psychiatry, 58*, 102601. https://doi.org/10.1016/j.ajp.2021.102601

Katoue, M. G., Cerda, A. A., García, L. Y., & Jakovljevic, M. (2022). Healthcare system development in the Middle East and North Africa region: Challenges, endeavors and prospective opportunities. *Frontiers in Public Health, 10*, 1045739. https://doi.org/10.3389/fpubh.2022.1045739

Khalifa, A. Y., Jabbour, J. Y., Mataria, A., Bakr, M., Farid, M., & Mathauer, I. (2022). Purchasing health services under the Egypt's new Universal Health Insurance law: What are the implications for universal health coverage? *The International Journal of Health Planning and Management, 37*(2), 619–631. https://doi.org/10.1002/hpm.3354

Khalil, M., & Alameddine, M. (2020). Recruitment and retention strategies, policies, and their barriers: A narrative review in the Eastern Mediterranean Region. *Health Science Reports, 3*(4). https://doi.org/10.1002/hsr2.192

Koohpayezadeh, J., Azami-Aghdash, S., Derakhshani, N., Rezapour, A., Alaei Kalajahi, R., Sajjadi Khasraghi, J., Nikoomanesh, M., Sabetrohani, H., & Soleimanpour, S. (2021). Best practices in achieving universal health coverage: A scoping review. *Medical Journal of the Islamic Republic of Iran, 35*, 191. https://doi.org/10.47176/mjiri.35.191

Prashker, M. J. (1994). Health care research and policy studies. *Current Opinion in Rheumatology, 6*(2), 140–146. https://doi.org/10.1097/00002281-199403000-00004

Shouman, S., Emara, T., Saber, H. G., & Allam, M. F. (2021). Awareness and attitude of healthcare workers towards telehealth in Cairo, Egypt. *International Journal of Clinical Practice, 75*(6). https://doi.org/10.1111/ijcp.1412

Shouman, S., Emara, T., Saber, H. G., & Allam, M. F. (2022). Awareness and attitude of primary healthcare patients towards telehealth in Cairo, Egypt. *Current Medical Research and Opinion, 38*(6), 993–998. https://doi.org/10.1080/03007995.2022.2065141

World Bank Group. (2020). *Supporting Egypt's universal health insurance system project.* http://documents1.worldbank.org/curated/en/528341591123310893/pdf/Egypt-Supporting-Egypt-s-Universal-Health-Insurance-System-Project.pdf

World Economic Forum. (2023). *The global risks report 2023.* https://www.weforum.org/reports/global-risks-report-2023

CHAPTER 28

GHANA

Anika Daniels-Osaze and Anthony Seth Eshun

INTRODUCTION

The Republic of Ghana is an anglophone country in the Gulf of Guinea, West Africa. This chapter provides a comprehensive overview of healthcare in Ghana through an academic, historical, and cultural lens. The three main objectives of this chapter are to (a) discuss the structure of Ghana's healthcare and its delivery; (b) understand the determinants of health, health outcomes, and contributing factors; and (c) provide a cultural and social context for how medical treatment is administered to the population. We review the country's demographics, cultural beliefs, and various existing healthcare practices, and later introduce some innovative developments currently being used or in development.

GEOGRAPHIC CHARACTERISTICS

The Republic of Ghana has a total area of 238,540 square kilometers (148,222 square miles), with most of the land (about 69%) used for agriculture, 3% land use is urban areas, 35% forest, and 5% water areas. There are 16 regional divisions, with the country's capital, Accra, located in the Greater Accra region. These regions are subdivided into 216 administrative local districts. Accra and Kumasi, the capital city of the Ashanti region, are the most populous cities, with over 2.6 million and 3 million citizens, respectively (Sasu, 2023).

DEMOGRAPHIC FEATURES

Ghana's population, a dynamic mix of urban and rural residents, stands at 33,476,000. The country's urban population accounts for about 59% of the total, reflecting rapid urbanization. The male-to-female distribution is almost equal, with males accounting for 49.9% and females for 50.1%. Notably, Ghana boasts a youthful population, with the median age for both sexes being 20.7 years. This youthfulness presents a unique opportunity for future healthcare development. Over the past decade, the country has seen a steady decline in its crude birth rate, from 31.5 to 25.9 per 1,000 people, indicating a shift in the population dynamics (United Nations, 2024).

ETHNICITY/RACE

Ghana's population is a rich tapestry of over 100 ethnic groups, each contributing to the country's cultural diversity. This diversity is particularly pronounced in urban areas, which have become melting pots due to migration in search of employment. The Akans, the largest ethnic group, are settled in the southern and central parts of the country, while the Mole-Dagbani ethnic group in the northern region forms a significant portion of Ghana's population. The Ewes are situated around the Volta and the Ga-Dangbes in the capital city of Accra toward the east of Ghana. Less populated ethnic groups like the Guans are settled in the rainforest areas, with other smaller ethnic groups spread across northern Ghana (Sasu, 2023).

LANGUAGE

There are more than 80 languages spoken in Ghana. English is the most widely spoken language (50%–60% of the population), with the Akan language and its various dialects, which include Twi, Fante, Akwapem, Akyem, and Ahafo, being the most widely spoken local languages by over 9 million Ghanaians. Other local languages include the Ewe, Abron, and Dagbani languages, with approximately 3.8 million, 1.2 million, and 1.2 million speakers, respectively (Sasu, 2023).

RELIGION/SPIRITUALITY

Ghana is predominantly Christian (approximately 71.2% of the population), with Islam (approximately 20%) being the second, followed by traditional native religions and other beliefs, which form 9% of the population. The ethnic population closer to the Atlantic coast was influenced by Western education and Christianity during the colonial era. Northern ethnicities were less exposed to those influences and came under Islamic influence (U.S. Department of State, 2022).

BRIEF COUNTRY HISTORY

Ghana, the first sub-Saharan country to become independent from colonialism, is regarded as the cradle of democracy in West Africa. Originally known as Wagadu by ancient inhabitants, Ghana's history can be traced to the Ghana Empire, a powerful empire that spanned Mauritania, Mali, and Senegal from the sixth to the 13th centuries. Traditional healers administered health;,education was centered on apprenticeship, and the ruling chieftains administered justice systems. The arrival of the Portuguese, Dutch, and British to trade with coastal chieftains in Ghana marked a pivotal moment that would change the course of Ghana's history. Known as the Gold Coast due to its abundance of gold, the British exploited trade alliances and took control in the 19th century to extend their territories northward. They met significant resistance from the Ashanti kingdom, which emerged as the most powerful and wealthy of all the kingdoms after the collapse of the Ghana Empire, resulting in the Anglo–Ashanti wars. The Ashanti kingdom was defeated, marking the beginning of British colonial rule and the enslavement trade, which lasted a century. During this period, Ghana saw westernization of its culture, education, healthcare, politics, and religion (Tracing Center, 2012).

Growing discontent with colonial rule and a quest for independence arose, with many incidents of civil unrest. Ghana won its independence on March 6, 1957, resulting in the appointment of Osagyefo Dr Kwame Nkrumah as the first prime minister. The country reclaimed its traditional name, Ghana. Nkrumah's government was overthrown in 1966, beginning a series of coup d'états that would hamper Ghana's democratic and economic progress. In 1992, Ghana had its final transition from military to democratic rule with a new constitution in force (Tracing Center, 2012).

POLITICAL SYSTEM

Ghana is a multiparty republic with a constitutionally recognized president as head of state. The president and members of Parliament are elected for 4-year terms by universal adult suffrage. The Council of State serves as an advisory body to the president. The traditional political system is led by chieftains who governed before constitutional rule. Traditional rulers run parallel lines with the government as ceremonial figureheads who are respected as custodians of Ghana's traditional heritage. They play key leadership roles in regional integration, human rights advocacy, and local community development (Brittanica, n.d.).

HEALTH OUTCOMES

Despite a significant improvement in the healthcare system over the past two decades, Ghana still lags in meeting Sustainable Development Goal (SDG) targets for maternal and infant mortality and life expectancy. Substantial differences exist between rural and urban healthcare and health outcomes.

LIFE EXPECTANCY FROM BIRTH

The average life expectancy for Ghanaians is 66.3 years, with females having a higher life expectancy of 66 years and males having an average life expectancy of 61 years. Life expectancy has increased steadily from 57 years in the year 2000. An improved healthcare delivery system, food and water security, low cost of living, lifestyle modifications, and improved education account for Ghana's gradual demographic transition toward an ageing population (World Health Organization [WHO], 2023).

LEADING CAUSES OF MORTALITY

Ghana has seen a 38% decline in **mortality rates** attributable to the top 10 causes of death (Figure 28.1), from 625 per 100,000 population in 2000 to 288 per 100,000 in 2019. Causes of death from infectious diseases, maternal and perinatal conditions, and malnutrition, which accounted for 82% of these deaths in 2000, declined to 63% in 2019 (WHO, 2023). During 2023, the leading causes of death in Ghana were COVID-19, stroke, neonatal disorders, malaria, HIV/AIDS, lower respiratory infections, heart disease, tuberculosis, chronic kidney disease, and diabetes (Institute for Health Metrics and Evaluation, n.d.).

NONCOMMUNICABLE DISEASES VERSUS INFECTIOUS DISEASES

The rising incidence of chronic noncommunicable diseases (NCDs) compared to infectious diseases places excessive strain on resources required to improve Ghana's healthcare and health

FIGURE 28.1 Top 10 causes of death in Ghana 2011 and 2021.

Cause	2011 rank	2021 rank	Change in deaths per 100K, 2011–2021
COVID-19	–	1	↑ +84.8
Stroke	3	2	↓ −10.3
Neonatal disorders	2	3	↓ −32.7
Malaria	1	4	↓ −68.3
HIV/AIDS	4	5	↓ −19.3
Lower respiratory infections	5	6	↓ −19.1
Ischemic heart disease	6	7	↓ −0.3
Tuberculosis	7	8	↓ −10.3
Chronic kidney disease	10	9	↑ +0.7
Diabetes	11	10	↑ +0.0

● Communicable, maternal, neonatal, and nutritional diseases
● Noncommunicable diseases

Source: Institute for Health Metrics and Evaluation. (n.d.). *Health research by location: Country profiles*. https://www.healthdata.org/research-analysis/health-by-location/profiles

outcomes. The prevalence of the most common NCDs among adults in Ghana, cardiovascular disease, chronic kidney disease, and diabetes, have risen sharply, with about 65% of deaths associated with these NCDs. Ischemic heart diseases and strokes, which are sequelae of systemic hypertension and diabetes mellitus, accounted for 30% of all deaths among adults in 2019 compared to 14% in 2000. The incidence of systemic hypertension shows minimal variation between rural and urban areas. Despite a decline in infectious diseases like malaria, HIV/AIDS, and tuberculosis, these diseases remain among the top 10 causes of mortality in Ghana (WHO, 2023).

MORTALITY RATES

Infant Mortality

Infant mortality rates in Ghana over the past decade have declined from 40.7 per 1,000 live births in 2014 to 30 deaths per 1,000 live births in 2024 (United Nations, 2024). Sixty percent of deaths during the infant period occur within the perinatal period, with 92% of neonatal deaths occurring within the first week of life from complications of preterm births, neonatal infections, and birth asphyxia. There have been significant differences in infant mortality rates between rural and urban areas in Ghana, with babies born in rural areas twice more likely to die compared to urban areas. Infants whose mothers were teenagers without formal education beyond primary education had a higher risk of death (Adongo & Ganle, 2023).

Maternal Mortality

Over the past two decades, maternal mortality ratios (MMR) in Ghana have declined from 499 per 100,000 births in 2000 to 263 per 100,000 births in 2022 (World Bank Group, 2024). This has resulted from health policy reforms in healthcare infrastructure, essential medicines, and human resources. Policy amendments in 2003 by the Ghana Health Services (GHS) waived the payment of delivery fees by pregnant women at public health facilities. The free comprehensive maternal healthcare rolled out in 2008 under the **National Health Insurance Scheme (NHIS)** resulted in increased usage of facility delivery and postnatal care services across Ghana. Despite these significant improvements, Ghana is considered to have a high maternal mortality ratio (WHO, 2023), with deaths resulting from obstetric hemorrhage, hypertensive disorders in pregnancy, sepsis resulting from nonmedical abortions, respiratory tract infections, and HIV/AIDS. Maternal mortalities are considerably higher in rural areas, especially among women with low educational and socioeconomic status, compared to urban areas. The disparities in rural–urban maternal outcomes are due to a shortage of medical resources and financial constraints among patients (Adu et al., 2021).

MENTAL HEALTH

WHO (2022) has estimated that 13% of Ghanaians suffer from poor mental health. Lower socioeconomic status and educational levels are associated with a much higher risk for poor mental health. Women who lack education, a sustainable means of income, and social support systems (mainly resulting from violent intimate partnerships) are the most vulnerable. The risk of developing mental health problems does not seem to be affected by age or urban versus rural residency. Mood disorders (the most common being depression), substance abuse, and schizophrenia are the most prevalent mental health conditions, with many Ghanaians choosing spiritual healing through prayer camps and alternative traditional medicine over allopathic medicine (Nonvignon et al., 2020).

DETERMINANTS OF HEALTH

Economic stability, education, lifestyle, the environment, culture, and healthcare quality are crucial determinants of Ghanaians' health status. This section shows the relationship between these determinants and provides context.

ECONOMIC STABILITY

Extensive evidence supports that financially advantaged individuals have better health outcomes than their disadvantaged counterparts. Ghana has a gross domestic product (GDP) of $73.77 billion, and a per capita of $2,203.56 (World Bank Group, 2024). Ghana's Ministry of Health (MoH) receives less than 2% of its GDP allocated to healthcare, which falls significantly below the 15% threshold toward achieving universal healthcare. This percentage of GDP allocated to healthcare is expected to decline in the years ahead due to the ongoing economic crisis and high inflation rates that adversely affect budgetary allocations and expenditures within the health sector. Despite the economic challenges, Ghana's poverty rate has declined from 58.4% in 1987 to 25.2% in 2016 (World Bank Group, 2024) and lowered its unemployment rate to 3.56%, lower than Africa's average unemployment rate of 6.6% (Global Economic Data, 2023).

EDUCATION AND LITERACY

The Ghanaian government guarantees universal education through primary school, accounting for the country's high literacy rate. A better educated, literate population is associated with improved health status and outcomes. There has been a significant rise in literacy rates in Ghana from 57.9% recorded two decades ago to 80.38% as of 2020 (Macrotrends, 2024). However, education and adult literacy in Ghana have not always translated to superior personal health literacy. Low health literacy rates are common among older adults and rural dwellers due to differences in the social environment. Low health literacy leads to obesity, smoking, alcoholism, and antibiotic misuse, which results in poor health status and chronic illnesses (Amoah et al., 2022).

LIFESTYLE AND HEALTH BEHAVIOR

Lifestyle and behavioral risk factors such as inadequate fruit and vegetable intake, poor eating habits, physical inactivity, alcohol abuse, and tobacco use were associated with higher risks of NCDs. The increased consumption of highly processed foods, refined cereals, sugar-sweetened beverages, and an already extant carbohydrate-rich diet has contributed to the fivefold increase in obesity rates between 1980 and 2015, as well as the rising incidence of diabetes and dyslipidemias, particularly in urban areas (Laar et al., 2020). A surge in urbanization and digital technology has reduced the need for physical activity, contributing to a rising risk of NCDs (Boakye et al., 2023). Alcohol consumption has doubled over the past two decades, which could account for the rising incidence of liver diseases (Osei-Bonsu, 2017). The prevalence of smoking in Ghana is low (2.6%). Media campaigns against smoking and a strong cultural and religious dislike for smoking have contributed to its unpopularity in Ghana (Sasu, 2023).

ENVIRONMENT

Environmental pollution and climate-related events have a massive impact on health, with air pollution being the most critical environmental health hazard. Accra recorded an alarming increase in nitrogen oxide pollution, a marker of traffic emissions in cities, from about 25% in 2006 to 180% in 2021. It is currently ranked as the 45th most air-polluted city globally, with a moderate pollution index of 59 (IQAir, 2024). About 60% of water bodies in Ghana are polluted, with most of them in critical condition. Small-scale gold mining activities, locally known as "galamsey," carried out predominantly in Ghana's Ashanti, Eastern, Western, and Central regions, have polluted waterbodies with poisonous chemicals like cyanide, cadmium, and mercury. Research about the rising incidence of kidney diseases in Ghana has identified mercury poisoning from illicit small-scale mining activities as contributory (Ofori, 2024).

QUALITY OF HEALTHCARE

Ghana has seen a significant improvement in healthcare quality, with healthcare becoming more readily accessible than it was a decade ago. Ghana had a doctor-to-population ratio of one doctor to 6,500 people in 2020, a significant leap from a ratio of one to 17,899 people in 2005. Forty-two percent of all Ghana's doctors are in Accra alone, with up to 81.3% of all doctors concentrated in the mostly urban areas of five regions: Greater Accra, Ashanti, Central, Northern, and Volta regions (WHO, 2022). Economic hardships and poor incentives for health workers after the COVID-19 pandemic have resulted in many health professionals (mostly nurses) leaving Ghana to seek better work opportunities overseas.

CULTURAL CONTEXT

Ghana's culturally diverse population is accompanied by diverse belief systems that shape the way of life and the beliefs about health. Some beliefs divergent from scientific evidence are hardwired among some cultures, hampering quality health. Prior to colonialism, Ghanaian communities trusted their care to local priests who used divination to help cure the sick based on the concept that illness was due to metaphysical entities. It was believed that these illnesses were retribution for some wrongdoing or violation of a cultural norm and that good health was a reward for those who respected and followed cultural traditions (Abubakari et al., 2024). Some of these beliefs and practices are still held today. The practice of female genital mutilation among women in certain parts of northern Ghana as a remedy for sexual promiscuity is an example of a harmful practice that affects female sexual health adversely. However, there are positive examples of cultural influence on healthcare such as the practice of natural childbirth and the use of **herbal medicine** to treat certain ailments. It is common practice in Ghanaian culture to combine both traditional and orthodox approaches to healthcare. This has proved to be helpful in gaining the trust of the patient and has improved patient outcomes (Abubakari et al., 2024). Providing quality healthcare and reducing disparities require healthcare providers to respect the cultural beliefs and traditions of the patient while incorporating evidence-based medicines and interventions.

HEALTHCARE SYSTEM

OVERVIEW

Ghana's medical system is centered in the two largest cities, Accra and Kumasi. In 2003, the government introduced the NHIS, which eliminated the need for citizens to pay upfront for care, known as the "cash and carry system." The goal was to provide equitable access to healthcare services to all residents of Ghana. The National Health Insurance Authority (NHIA), established under the National Health Insurance Act of 2003, Act 650, is the governing body for the insurance plan and consists of 16 regional offices, one for each region. The GHS and the Christian Health Association of Ghana (CHAG) consist of government and quasigovernment hospitals and clinics. Some private facilities are available. Patients first see a primary care provider for routine evaluations and are referred to specialists for more complex health issues (Sackey & Amponsah, 2017).

FINANCING AND INSURANCE COVERAGE

According to the National Health Insurance Authority (2024), funding for the NHIS is provided by multiple sources, including the national budget, income and insurance taxes, NGO contributions, philanthropy, local resources, private donors, premiums, and private health insurance. The NHIS pays for hospitalizations, outpatient doctor visits, emergencies, oral health, eye care, maternity services, and certain approved medications. NHIS does not cover assisted reproduction, dialysis for chronic renal failure, organ transplants, cancer treatments (except cervical and breast cancer), heart or brain surgery other than those caused by accidents, conditions requiring treatment abroad or cosmetic surgery unrelated to trauma (see https://www.nhis.gov.gh/benefits for more details). The NHIS is billed monthly by participating hospitals for patients in the program. Premium amounts are determined based on income and are not charged to children under 18, adults over 70, pregnant women, or poor citizens. As of 2023, 68.6% of Ghana's population is covered by health insurance; 64.5% are men and 72.6% are women. Unfortunately, those in the lower income brackets and the sickest people are least likely to sign up for the program due to their inability to afford the premiums (Brenyah et al., 2023).

ACCESS TO HEALTHCARE

Ghana seeks to promote quality, accessible healthcare and easy transmission of healthcare information. The introduction of the NHIS to cover healthcare costs for all Ghanaians, along with widespread immunization programs and free maternal healthcare, increased access to skilled maternal services. The implementation of a national Hospital Management System used by government hospitals in Ghana to improve healthcare information storage and transmission throughout the country has also improved access to quality healthcare. However, enrollment in the NHIS is still relatively low due to poverty, with some patients complaining about bureaucracy regarding the NHIS registration process. Hospital wards and clinics are overcrowded, and the time allotted per patient is limited. For years, the number of hospital beds available has been low, with limited ambulance services and poor road networks hampering swift referral of patients between health facilities. There is a great need for medical assistance in rural areas. The need for health insurance in Ghana far exceeds the NHIS program's capacity to achieve its target of covering at least 95% of Ghanaians' health issues. The NHIA has experienced a fiscal deficit since 2010, adversely affecting the implementation of services by the NHIS, thus questioning its sustainability. Payment of insurance claims to healthcare facilities has been unreliable, resulting in patients paying higher out-of-pocket costs (Agbanyo, 2020).

PHARMACEUTICALS AND HERBAL MEDICINES

Medication coverage and expense are significant barriers in the healthcare system. For example, the NHIS covers only 47% of children's cancer medications. Patients and their families typically make out-of-pocket payments for medications not covered by the NHIS, which they usually cannot sustain, resulting in the stoppage of medications midway through treatment. Due to deeply ingrained cultural practices, many Ghanaians depend on scientifically unproven herbal home remedies for healthcare. As a result, the government commissioned research centers to study and test the effectiveness of traditional medicines in Ghana and created policies to support the development of herbal medicine clinics. At least 17 government-regulated facilities have licensed herbalists authorized to provide herbal medicine to clinics and hospitals. However, the NHIS does not cover certified herbal medicines, decreasing healthcare services utilization (Nketia, et al., 2022).

IMPROVEMENTS IN HEALTHCARE

Healthcare has significantly improved since the implementation of the NHIS. Out-of-pocket expenses have decreased, and the government has increased healthcare spending to improve services. Life expectancy has steadily increased since 1995. Community-based health planning and services (CHPS) are also increasing. The Ghana Essential Health Intervention Project (GEHIP) was established to reduce child mortality, particularly in rural areas, by improving the accessibility of child immunization and improved treatment of malaria, diarrhea, and acute respiratory diseases. The number of mothers registered in the NHIS increased after free maternal care was implemented (Bawah et al., 2019).

TECHNOLOGY AND INNOVATION

Modern technology is available in urban facilities, but small towns still need modern equipment and facilities to serve many patients. Nationwide, the availability of ventilators proved problematic during the height of the COVID-19 pandemic. However, several technological advancements are being considered in the Ghana health industry to improve overall services. Telemedicine is slowly being adopted and can advance access to medical care nationally. Electronic medical records have also improved healthcare services in the country. In 2017, the MoH facilitated the national implementation of the **Lightwave Health Information Management System** (LHIMS), which improved the efficiency of healthcare delivery and data protection (Agyemang et al., 2023). The "mHealth" mobile phone app, which has been slow to adopt due to socioeconomic factors, helps eliminate access issues and disparities in rural communities in Ghana (Peprah et al., 2020).

CONCLUSION

Ghana has made tremendous strides in promoting medical care in a moderately large and highly complex country. However, even with the current advances, the prevalence of NCDs will increase healthcare costs astronomically. Despite improving poverty, unemployment, and economic stability, Ghana must prioritize its health sector to improve health outcomes. Ghana has struggled to extend modern medical care to smaller towns and rural areas. Infections are common in rural areas, negatively impacting the health of women and children. An increase in the healthcare workforce, especially in rural areas, is critical. Universities and medical training programs must be expanded beyond the saturated, larger urban centers to provide more medical specialty training and to create incentives to retain physicians in the country. Technological innovations, such as LHIMS and telemedicine, can assist in increasing efficiency and access to healthcare and reduce healthcare disparities, particularly in rural areas of the country. Including certified herbal medicines on the NHIS medicine list as covered treatments can increase the use of medical facilities and patient adherence to treatment plans.

CASE STUDY

The authors of this chapter surveyed patients from one of the Catholic hospitals, Our Lady of Grace, in the Central Region from March to May 2024 to assess patient satisfaction with the NHIS healthcare system. We solicited feedback regarding the quality of care, healthcare, and costs; preference for herbal medicines; and ease of access to the healthcare facility. Results showed that 82% of the patients believe that orthodox healthcare is more accessible than traditional or complementary care; 63% felt that distance inhibits accessibility; 61% stated that the cost of travel is a burden; and over 70% believe that orthodox healthcare is expensive and limits accessibility. Approximately 80% were satisfied with the services provided, but only 58% of the patients felt that the NHIS adequately covered their healthcare costs. The survey document is provided in Figure 28.2.

FIGURE 28.2 Healthcare satisfaction survey administered to patients in two hospitals in the Central Region of Ghana.

SECTION A: DEMOGRAPHICS *(For section A, please underline which applies)*

Age: 15–35 years / 36–50 years / 51–70 years / >70 years **Employment Status:** Employed / Unemployed

Gender: M / F **Educational Status:** None / Informal / Primary / Secondary / Tertiary

Marital Status: Single / Married / Divorced / Widowed **Insurance Status:** NHIS / Private Insurance / Non-Insured

For sections B and C, please tick which applies

SECTION B:	BARRIERS TO HEALTHCARE		Yes	No
1	In your opinion, is orthodox healthcare more accessible than other traditional/complementary healthcare, e.g., herbal, homeopathy?			
2	Does the distance from your residence to your healthcare facility adversely impact accessibility?			
3	Is the cost of travel to your healthcare providers a burden and does it adversely impact accessibility?			
4	Does NHIS offer significant cost cuts to you when seeking healthcare? *(applies to NHIS subscribers)*			
5	Is the hospital waiting time short enough for you during hospital visits?			
6	Do you consider the cost of orthodox healthcare to be expensive thus limiting accessibility?			
7	Are you pleased with the customer care you receive from your healthcare providers?			
8	In your opinion, do these factors make orthodox healthcare inconvenient?	a. Lack of diagnostic resources		
		b. Scarcity of specialist services		
		c. Difficulty accessing emergency referral services		

SECTION C:	OPINIONS ON HEALTHCARE	Yes	No
1	In your opinion, does the NHIS scheme adequately cover your healthcare costs? *(applies to NHIS subscribers)*		
2	Are you open to considering paying for other insurance schemes to complement the NHIS?		
3	Do you consider or do you subscribe to other traditional and complementary care (herbal, homeopathy)?		

If yes, any reason? *(Tick which applies)*	They are cheaper ☐	They are effective ☐	They are very accessible ☐	Other reasons:
If not, any reason? *(Tick which applies)*	They are expensive ☐	They are ineffective ☐	They have not been validated ☐	Other reasons:

LEARNING ACTIVITIES

CourseConnect

To access self-assessment questions and interactive, competency-based learning activities for this chapter, visit www.springerpub.com/courseconnect. See inside front cover and tear-out for CourseConnect details.

REFERENCES

Abubakari, A.-K., Gross, J., Boateng, S. K., & Ansong, R. (2024). Cultural competency of nurses in a multicultural healthcare system in two regions of Ghana. *International Journal of Africa Nursing Sciences, 20*, 100728. https://doi.org/10.1016/j.ijans.2024.100728

Adongo, E. A., & Ganle, J. K. (2023). Predictors of neonatal mortality in Ghana: Evidence from 2017 Ghana maternal health survey. *BMC Pregnancy and Childbirth, 23*(1), 556. https://doi.org/10.1186/s12884-023-05877-y

Adu, J., Mulay, S., & Owusu, M. F. (2021). Reducing maternal and child mortality in rural Ghana. *Pan African Medical Journal, 39*, 263. https://doi.org/10.11604/pamj.2021.39.263.30593

Agbanyo, R. (2020). Ghana's national health insurance, free maternal healthcare and facility-based delivery services. *African Development Review, 32*(1), 27–41. https://doi.org/10.1111/1467-8268.12412

Agyemang, E., Esia-Donkoh, K., Adu-Gyamfi, A. B., Douri, J. B., Adoma, P. O., & Achampong, E. K. (2023). Assessing the efficient use of the Lightwave Health Information Management System for health service delivery in Ghana. *BMJ Health and Care Informatics, 30*(1), e100769. https://doi.org/10.1136/bmjhci-2023-100769

Amoah, P. A., Musalia, J., & Abrefa Busia, K. (2022). Health behaviors and health literacy: Questing the role of weak social ties among older persons in rural and urban Ghana. *Frontiers in Public Health, 10*, 777217. https://doi.org/10.3389/fpubh.2022.777217

Bawah, A., Awoonor-Williams, J., Asuming, P., Jackson, E., Boyer, C., Kanmiki, E., Achana, F., Akazili, J., & Phillips, J. (2019). The child survival impact of the Ghana essential health interventions program: A health systems strengthening plausibility trial in northern Ghana. *PLoS One, 14*(6), e0218025. https://doi.org/10.1371/journal.pone.0218025

Boakye, H., Atabila, A., Hinneh, T., Ackah, M., Ojo-Benys, F., & Bello, A. I. (2023). The prevalence and determinants of non-communicable diseases among Ghanaian adults: A survey at a secondary healthcare level. *PLOS ONE*. https://doi.org/10.1371/journal.pone.0281310

Brenyah, J. K., Dassah, E., & Yeboah, G. (2023). Social Protection supports and management of non-communicable diseases in Ghana: A qualitative cross-sectional perspective of health stakeholders. *Saudi Journal of Health Systems Research, 3*(1–4), 188–203. https://doi.org/10.1159/000531700

Brittanica. (n.d.). *Government and society*. https://www.britannica.com/place/Ghana/Government-and-society

Global Economic Data, Indicators, Charts and Forecast. (2023). *Ghana unemployment rate*. https://www.ceicdata.com/en/indicator/ghana/unemployment-rate

Institute for Health Metrics and Evaluation. (n.d.). *Health research by location: Country profiles*. https://www.healthdata.org/research-analysis/health-by-location/profiles.

IQAir. (2024). *2023 World air quality report*. https://www.iqair.com/world-air-quality-report

Laar, A., Barnes, A., Aryeetey, R., Tandoh, A., Bash, K., Mensah, K., Zotor, F., Vandevijvere, S., & Holdsworth, M. (2020). Implementation of healthy food environment policies to prevent nutrition-related non-communicable diseases in Ghana: National experts' assessment of government action. *Food Policy, 93*, 101907. https://doi.org/10.1016/j.foodpol.2020.101907

MacroTrends. (2024). *Ghana literacy rate 1960–2024*. https://www.macrotrends.net/global-metrics/countries/GHA/ghana/literacy-rate

National Health Insurance Authority. (2024). *Homepage*. https://www.nhis.gov.gh/nhia

Nketia, A., Nakua, E., Tetteh, A. W., Thomford, K. P., Boadu, K. O., & Thomford, A. K. (2022). Non-inclusion of certified herbal medicines in the National Health Insurance Scheme affects patient utilization of the integrated herbal medicine services in Ghana. *Traditional Medicine Research, 7*(4), 39. http://doi.org/10.53388/TMR20220911001

Nonvignon, J., Amissah, C. R., Agyemang, S. A., & Wong, B. (2020, February 22). *Benefit–cost analysis of mental health interventions in Ghana*. https://copenhagenconsensus.com. https://copenhagenconsensus.com/sites/default/files/gp_a4_mental_health_final.pdf

Ofori, S. A. (2024). Ecological study of galamsey activities in Ghana and their physiological toxicity. *Journal of Environmental Toxicology Research, 1*(1), 1–14. https://doi.org/10.59462/jetr.1.1.101

Osei-Bonsu, E. (2017). Prevalence of alcohol consumption and factors influencing alcohol use among the youth in Tokorni-Hohoe, Volta region of Ghana. *Science Journal of Public Health, 5*(3), 205. https://doi.org/10.11648/j.sjph.20170503.18

Peprah, P., Abalo, E. M., Agyemang-Duah, W., Budu, H. I., Appiah-Brempong, E., Morgan, A. K., & Akwasi, A. G. (2020). Lessening barriers to healthcare in rural Ghana: Providers and users' perspectives on the role of mHealth technology. A qualitative exploration. *BMC Medical Informatics and Decis, 20*(1), 27. https://doi.org/10.1186/s12911-020-1040-4

Sackey, F. G., & Amponsah, P. N. (2017). Willingness to accept capitation payment system under the Ghana national health insurance policy: Do income levels matter? *Health Economics Review, 7*(1), 38. https://doi.org/10.1186/s13561-017-0175-1

Sasu, D. D. (2023). *Topic: Ghana*. Statista. https://www.statista.com/topics/3029/ghana/#topicOverview

Tracing Center. (2012). *Ghana and the slave trade*. https://www.tracingcenter.org/resources/background/ghana-and-the-slave-trade/

United Nations. (2024). *Data portal population division*. https://data.un.org/

U.S. Department of State. (2022). *2022 Report on international religious freedom: Ghana*. https://www.state.gov/reports/2022-report-on-international-religious-freedom/ghana/#:~:text=Religious%20Demographyandtext=According%20to%20the%202021%20government,or%20have%20no%20religious%20beliefs

World Bank Group. (2024). *Ghana*. World Bank Open Data. https://data.worldbank.org/

World Health Organization. (2022). *Ghana*. https://data.who.int/countries/288

World Health Organization. (2023). *Analytical fact sheet*. https://files.aho.afro.who.int/afahobckpcontainer/production/files/iAHO_Maternal_Mortality_Regional_Factsheet.pdf

CHAPTER 29

NIGERIA

Inijesu Taiwo and Jerome A. Nenger

INTRODUCTION

Nigeria's healthcare system is a dynamic landscape reflecting the nation's historical, cultural, and economic complexities. This chapter delves into the intricate tapestry of healthcare delivery in Nigeria, from its traditional healing practices to the modern challenges and innovations shaping its future. As you engage with this chapter, it is crucial to consider the following questions: How has Nigeria's healthcare system evolved over time, blending traditional healing methods with modern medical practices? What are the primary challenges facing Nigeria's healthcare system today, and how do they impact healthcare access and outcomes?

GEOGRAPHY AND POPULATION

GEOGRAPHICAL FEATURES

Nigeria shares its borders to the north with Niger, to the east with Chad and Cameroon, to the south with the Gulf of Guinea of the Atlantic Ocean, and to the west with Benin (Figure 29.1). Not only is Nigeria expansive in landmass—exceeding that of the U.S. state of Texas—but it also holds the title of Africa's most populous nation (Kirk-Greene et al., 2024).

Nigeria is commonly referred to as the "Giant of Africa." The diversity of its peoples and languages, the expanse of its terrain, and the presence of oil and other natural riches all contributed to the origin of its name (Bala & Tar, 2020). It has a total surface area of 923,768 square kilometers (574,000 square miles). It consists of 36 states and the Federal Capital Territory of Abuja (Commonwealth Governance, 2014).

The Niger and Benue Rivers are the two main geographic features of the nation. The Niger River flows directly south from the two rivers, which together resemble the top arms of a flattened letter Y. As the rivers approach the Gulf of Guinea, they sprawl out into a vast and complex delta. The Niger Delta and the coastal waters contain most of Nigeria's oil reserves. With elevations reaching 2,419 meters (7,936 feet), the country's highest peaks are in the eastern highlands that border Cameroon. The Jos Plateau, located in east-central Nigeria, is a significant geographical feature characterized by its elevation, ranging from approximately 1,200 to 1,800 meters (3,937 to 5,905 feet) above sea level, with some peaks reaching altitudes as high as 1,780 meters (5,833 feet; Hemba et al., 2019).

DEMOGRAPHICS

With a total population of over 229.1 million (UN Data Portal, n.d.), Nigeria is the sixth most populated nation in the world and the most populous in Africa (Central Intelligence Agency [CIA], n.d.-a, n.d.-b). The population density has increased by over 140% between 1950 and 2024 (UN Data Portal, n.d.). Nigeria maintains a significant population growth rate of 2.4% (World Bank Group, n.d.), driven by a high fertility rate of approximately 5.2 children per woman (World Bank Group, n.d.). The Nigerian population displays diversity across age, gender, language, ethnicity, and other dimensions.

FIGURE 29.1 Map of Nigeria.

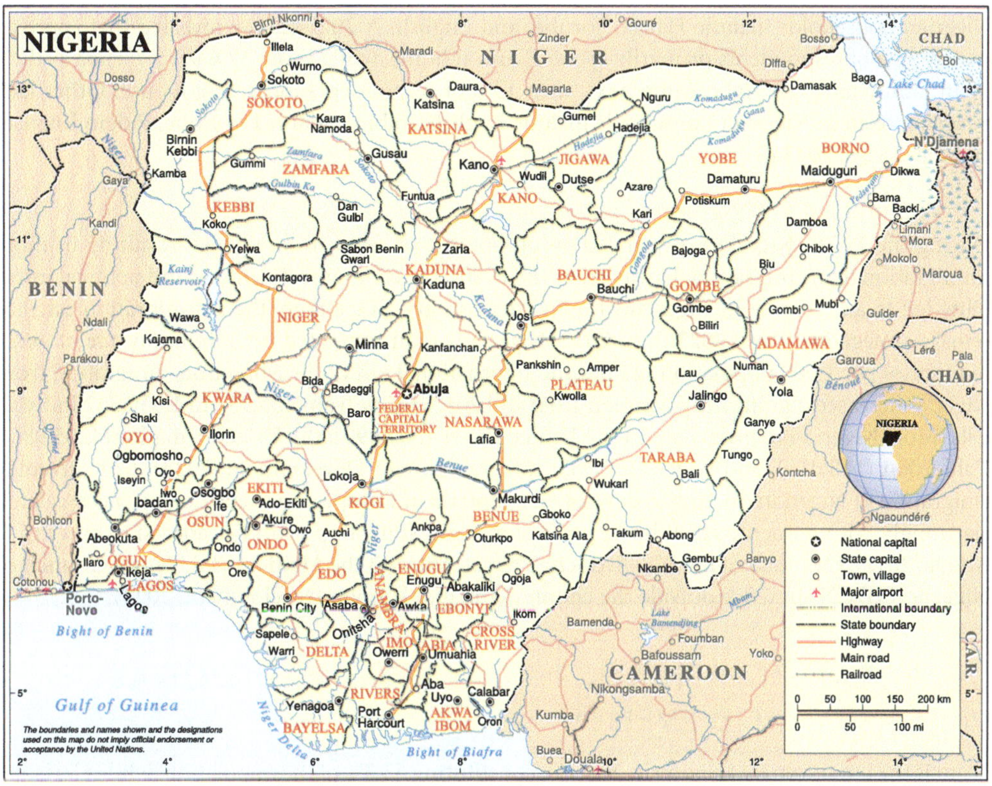

Source: Burmesedays. (2010). *Nigeria regions map*. https://commons.wikimedia.org/wiki/File:Nigeria_Regions_map.svg.

Age

The median age in Nigeria declined from 18.1 years in 1950 to 16.9 in 2020, but there is a projection for a twofold increase by 2100 (O'Neill, 2024b). According to World Bank Open Data, about 2.97% of Nigeria's population was 65 years of age or older in 2022, a slight decline from 1960 when the percentage was 3.33% (Trading Economics, n.d.). The nation boasts the world's largest youth population (Akinyemi, 2023), with 43.04% of the population aged 14 or younger and 53.98% between 15 and 64 years old in 2022 (O'Neill, 2024a).

Ethnicity/Tribe

Nigeria exhibits significant ethnic diversity, comprising over 250 distinct ethnic groups (World Factbook Glyph, n.d.). As of 2018 estimates, Nigeria's primary ethnic groups include the Hausa, Yoruba, and Igbo (Ibo). The Hausa ethnic group is estimated to comprise 30% of the nation's population and primarily speaks the Hausa language. Together, the Yoruba and Igbo (also called Ibo) ethnic groups constitute another 30% of Nigeria's population (Sasu, 2022). Other notable groups include the Edo, Fulani, Ibibio, Ijaw, Kanuri, and Tiv (CIA, 2021).

Language

Nigeria stands out as one of the world's most linguistically diverse countries, boasting a rich tapestry of over 500 languages (Translators Without Borders, 2022). The introduction of the English language to Nigeria occurred during the era of British colonial rule in the country (Chepkemoi,

2019). While English is the official language, it is less prevalent in rural regions and among those with limited education (Translators Without Borders, 2022). The main languages spoken in Nigerian households include Hausa, Yoruba, and English. A 2022 survey revealed that approximately 32% of respondents primarily spoke Hausa at home, while about 17% used Yoruba as their main family language. Igbo came next, with 13% of respondents indicating its use. Other languages spoken in Nigerian households include English, Ibibio, Fulani, Tiv, Nupe, Pidgin English, and Ijaw (Sasu, 2023a).

Immigration and Emigration

During the 1970s, Nigeria experienced an oil boom that drew in foreigners, resulting in more immigration than emigration. However, by the 1980s, the economic downturn and political instability led to an increase in Nigerians leaving the country. Since then, the net migration rate has remained negative (Sasu, 2023b). In 2022, Nigeria had an estimated net migration rate of −0.21 migrant(s) per 1,000 population. As per the International Office for Migration, emigration from Nigeria increased significantly between 1990 and 2013, rising from 465,932 to 1,030,322 individuals. Most Nigerian migrants are in the United States (309,699), the United Kingdom (203,980), Cameroon (148,076), and Niger (130,982; Integral Human Development, 2023). Concurrently, emigration of Nigerian doctors to developed countries in Europe and the Americas has escalated alarmingly, with numerous healthcare professionals pursuing opportunities abroad (Akinyemi & Atilola, 2012). Over half of the 72,000 doctors registered with the **Medical and Dental Council of Nigeria (MDCN)** practice outside the country (Integral Human Development, 2023).

CULTURAL SIGNIFICANCE: RELIGION, TRADITIONAL PRACTICES, AND EVENTS

Islam is the predominant religion in Nigeria, constituting 53.5% of the population, while Christian denominations make up approximately 45%, with Roman Catholicism as the largest branch at 10.6%. Other religions, including traditional worship practices, account for the remaining 0.6% (Sasu, 2023c). Nigeria observes three secular national holidays and various Muslim and Christian holidays, affecting government offices, businesses, and banks. Nigeria's cultural diversity is showcased through festivals like the Argungu festival, Osun festival, and the Calabar festival, highlighting traditional practices and cultural richness (iExplore, n.d.).

HEALTH OUTCOMES

Health outcomes in Nigeria have not improved significantly since 2021 despite increased spending. Compared to countries with similar or even lower health expenditure but better outcomes, it indicates the need for strengthening the health system and implementing targeted interventions. Addressing issues such as unsafe water sources, inadequate sanitation, malnutrition, and exposure to air pollution could lead to substantial improvements in population health (Angell et al., 2022).

LIFE EXPECTANCY AT BIRTH

Life expectancy in Nigeria has been improving gradually over the years (Lawanson & Umar, 2021). In the 1960s and 1970s, life expectancy in Nigeria was relatively low, with estimates ranging from the mid-30s to low 40s. By the 1990s, life expectancy had improved to approximately 47 to 50 years (World Bank Group, 2019). The current life expectancy for both sexes is 54.11 (UN Data Portal, n.d.). In Nigeria, life expectancy varies across regions and between genders. Men generally have a shorter life expectancy than women, with the Southwest region having the longest life expectancy for both genders. Urban areas typically have longer life expectancies compared to rural areas due to better access to healthcare, sanitation, and education (Adewale, 2024). Figure 29.2 shows the life expectancy across regions and between genders.

LEADING CAUSES OF MORTALITY

The leading causes of mortality in Nigeria vary but commonly include infectious diseases, noncommunicable diseases (NCDs), and maternal and neonatal conditions. In 2021, neonatal disorders ranked as the primary causes of death in Nigeria. The other leading causes of death in Nigeria during 2021 were malaria, lower respiratory infections, COVID-19, diarrheal diseases, heart disease, stroke, congenital defects, and tuberculosis (Figure 29.3).

INFANT AND MATERNAL MORTALITY

Nigeria lacks comprehensive population-based data on maternal deaths at the national level, and its registration system does not provide reliable estimates. The country relies on statistical models from international agencies, which are often inadequate for evaluating care quality, tracking short-term trends, or setting national health priorities (Oladapo et al., 2015). Nigeria ranks second globally in estimated maternal deaths and has one of the highest neonatal mortality rates in Africa (Nasir et al., 2022). Nigerian women face a one in 22 lifetime risk of dying during pregnancy, childbirth, or postpartum/postabortion, compared to one 1 in 4,900 risk in the most developed countries (World Health Organization [WHO], 2019). In 2020, Nigeria's maternal mortality ratio was 1,047 per 100,000 live births, indicating that maternal deaths account for about a third of all deaths among women of reproductive age (Orjingene et al., 2022). In 2021, Nigeria's infant mortality rate was 57.701 deaths per 1,000 live births, marking a 2.5% decrease from the rate recorded in 2020 (Macrotrends, n.d.).

FIGURE 29.2 Life expectancy in Nigeria according to regions and sex.

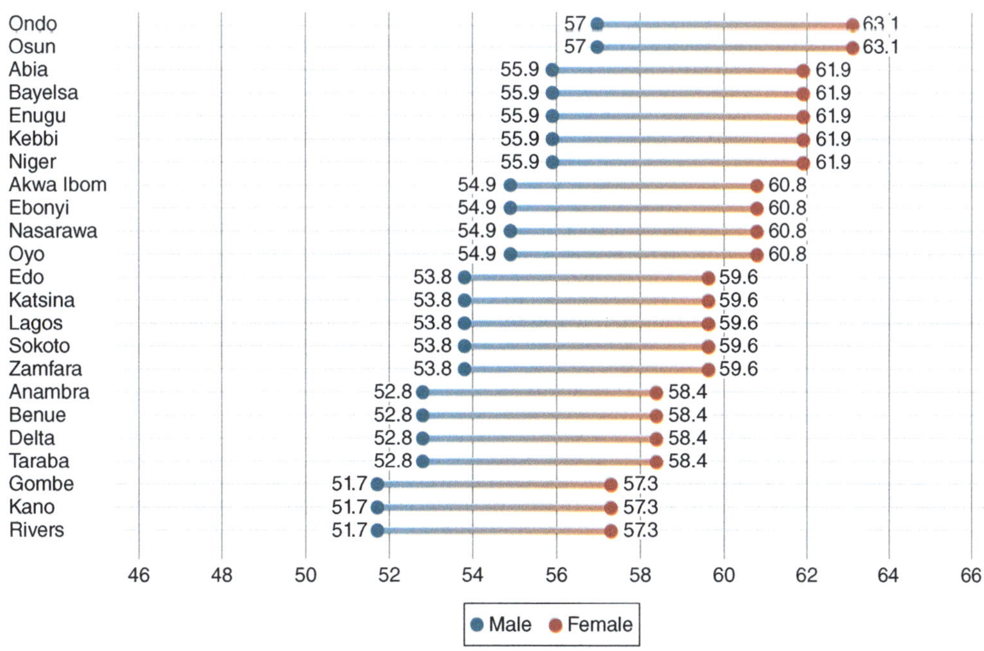

Source: Adewale, Z. (2024). *Data story: What figures tell us about life expectancy across Nigeria.* https://www.premiumtimesng.com/news/headlines/662945-data-story-what-figures-tell-us-about-life-expectancy-across-nigeria.html?tztc=1

FIGURE 29.3 Main causes of death in Nigeria, 2011 and 2021.

Cause	2011 rank	2021 rank	Change in deaths per 100K, 2011–2021
Neonatal disorders	1	1	↓ –42.8
Malaria	2	2	↓ –34.7
Lower respiratory infections	4	3	↓ –50.3
COVID-19	–	4	↑ +56.4
Diarrheal diseases	3	5	↓ –69.9
Ischemic heart disease	8	6	↓ –0.6
HIV/AIDS	5	7	↓ –15.0
Stroke	6	8	↓ –5.3
Congenital defects	10	9	↓ –7.6
Tuberculosis	7	10	↓ –13.7

● Communicable, maternal, neonatal, and nutritional diseases
● Noncommunicable diseases

Source: Institute for Health Metrics and Evaluation. (n.d.). *Health research by location: Country profiles*. https://www.healthdata.org/research-analysis/health-by-location/profiles

COMMUNICABLE DISEASES

In Nigeria, there is a significant burden of both communicable and NCDs (WHO, 2023). In recent times, the country has faced various infectious diseases including yellow fever, meningitis, cholera, Lassa fever, and COVID-19, further challenging its already fragile health system (Idajili et al., 2020; Kassa & Grace, 2020; Omojuyigbe et al., 2023). Other longstanding endemic diseases include malaria, HIV, tuberculosis (TB), and certain neglected tropical diseases (NTDs).

Malaria

Malaria continues to pose a substantial public health challenge in Nigeria, with approximately 65.4 million cases reported in 2021 (equating to an incidence rate of 298.6 cases per 1,000 population) and leading to 193,512 deaths (WHO, 2023). With about 27% of the world's cases of malaria, Nigeria has the largest malaria burden worldwide. There is a year-round danger of transmission across the entire nation. Nonetheless, the country's northeastern and northern regions have the greatest rates of malaria infection (WHO, 2023).

HIV and Tuberculosis

HIV and TB are recognized as the deadliest infectious diseases globally. What's more, these epidemics are closely linked, with TB being the primary cause of death among individuals living with HIV (Centers for Disease Control and Prevention, 2022). Approximately 63,000 Nigerians living with HIV/AIDS contract TB annually, with around 39,000 deaths attributed to the disease (WHO, 2018a). In 2021, the estimated incidence rate of TB cases stood at 229 per 100,000, indicating a persistent burden although showing a declining trend since 2015. The mortality rate for all forms of TB, excluding cases coinfected with HIV, has decreased from 62 to 53 per 100,000 population between 2015 and 2021. Concurrently, the TB mortality rate among individuals with HIV has declined from 23 to 6.2 during the same period (WHO, 2023).

Neglected Tropical Diseases

Nigeria bears approximately 25% of Africa's burden of NTDs, positioning it as one of the world's most endemic nations for these incapacitating conditions. An estimated 100 million individuals in the country face the risk of contracting at least one NTD, with several million cases of coendemicity where individuals are afflicted with multiple NTDs (Nuphi, 2019). Nigeria is considered endemic for four out of the five NTDs that can be controlled through mass drug administration (MDA). These include lymphatic filariasis, schistosomiasis, soil-transmitted helminthiasis, and trachoma (WHO, 2023). Annually, these diseases claim the lives of more than 170,000 individuals globally (The END Fund, 2023), although their mortality rates are lower than that of malaria.

NONCOMMUNICABLE DISEASES

In 2019, NCDs accounted for 27% of deaths in Nigeria (WHO, 2023). In sub-Saharan Africa (SSA), NCDs are pushing the mortality rates higher and higher. In 2021, the age-standardized mortality rate for four major NCDs (cardiovascular disease [CVD], chronic respiratory disease, cancer, and diabetes) was 565 per 100,000 among males and 546 per 100,000 among females (WHO, 2023). Among Nigerians aged 30 to 69 years, there is a 22% risk of premature death from these four NCDs (WHO, 2018b).

Cardiovascular Diseases

Over the past five decades, the predominant manifestations of CVDs were primarily linked to malnutrition and communicable diseases. Among these, rheumatic heart disease (RHD) and cardiomyopathies were the primary CVDs observed during that period (Ike & Onyema, 2020). In 2017, the age-standardized total CVD death rate stood at 7.73%, marking the lowest rate among all African countries analyzed in a study. Among men, approximately 2.5% of disability-adjusted life years (DALYs) were attributed to CVD, while for women, it was 2.8%. The prevalence of atrial fibrillation (AF) and atrial flutter was 0.13%, and that of RHD was 0.75%. Notably, the total mortality rate due to RHD accounted for 0.11% of all deaths recorded (Institute for Health Metrics and Evaluation, 2017).

Cancers

In 2020, Nigeria recorded an estimated 124,815 new cancer cases and 78,899 cancer-related deaths (International Agency for Research on Cancer, 2020). These figures are expected to rise by 85% over the next 15 years (Onah, 2018). Efforts are underway to enhance cancer treatment and improve survival rates in the country. Common types of cancer in Nigeria include breast cancer, prostate cancer, cervical cancer, colorectal cancer, and non-Hodgkin lymphoma (Chidebe et al., 2023). Breast cancer is the most frequent among adults, with a significant mortality rate (Onyeka, 2022). Prostate cancer and cervical cancer are also prevalent, while acute lymphoblastic leukemia (ALL) is the most common form of cancer among children (Onyeka, 2022).

Diabetes

In 2019, an estimated 3.9 million adults in Nigeria were living with diabetes, a figure expected to nearly double to 6.0 million by 2045 (International Diabetes Federation, 2019). Evidence from multiple sources—including a national survey, systematic review and meta-analysis, as well as community-based and other epidemiological studies—indicates a marked rise in diabetes prevalence among Nigerian adults, increasing from approximately 2.2% in 1992 to about 10.5% in 2022 (Adeloye et al., 2017; Ajayi et al., 2023; Uloko et al., 2018).

MENTAL HEALTH

The gap between the existing healthcare services and the demand for mental health services in Nigeria is evident (Wada et al., 2021). A 2019 study conducted by the Africa Polling Institute (API) and EpiAFRIC revealed the low awareness of mental health issues in Nigeria. Most respondents acknowledged having a mental health disorder, often attributing it to drug abuse, spiritual possession, or brain illness. The study also found that a significant number of patients seek spiritual interventions at prayer houses for their mental health concerns. There are fewer than 300 psychiatrists, resulting in a ratio of approximately 700,000 people per psychiatrist. Most of these psychiatrists are based in urban areas. Additionally, due to limited understanding of mental disorders at the primary healthcare level, the responsibility of caring for individuals with mental illness often falls on family members (Ugochukwu et al., 2020).

DETERMINANTS OF HEALTH

SOCIAL AND ECONOMIC FACTORS

The nexus between social and economic determinants and health outcomes in Nigeria is notable. Despite economic growth, health metrics in Nigeria reveal a contrasting picture. Over the last decade, life expectancy in Nigeria increased by 3.4 years, from 50.90 to 54.33 years. However, per-capita income declined 11.3% during the same period, dropping from $2,292.40 to $2,032.70 between 2010 and 2018 (Lawanson & Umar, 2021). Numerous studies have delved into the influence of these determinants on various healthcare facets within the nation. Vincent (2021) highlighted economic disparities, geographic hurdles, instability, education, gender parity, and sociocultural factors as principal socioeconomic determinants affecting maternal and child health in Nigeria.

Poverty

Nigeria has the most extensive gross domestic product (GDP) in Africa. However, its per-capita income of about $2,000 is relatively low, indicating a highly unequal distribution of income, wealth, and, subsequently, health. This presents a paradox of poverty within a wealthy nation, highlighting the disparity in economic prosperity (Abubakar et al., 2022). Approximately 40% of the Nigerian population resides below the global poverty line, with the average Nigerian surviving on $1.90 per day (World Bank Group, 2021). This results in limited financial accessibility to healthcare services, even when such services are available within proximity (Atobatele et al., 2022).

Educational Attainment

Individuals with higher levels of education not only have more significant financial resources to access high-quality healthcare but also possess the skills and knowledge to effectively navigate the healthcare system and seek appropriate care (Atobatele et al., 2022). Numerous studies have established a correlation between a lack of education or lower educational achievement, reduced income, and unfavorable health results (Atobatele et al., 2022). Research has established a correlation between low parental educational and socioeconomic status and inadequate health-seeking behaviors, resulting in elevated childhood mortality rates during emergencies in Nigeria and other SSA nations (Abiodun & Sadoh, 2021). The Nigerian education system has made significant progress in recent decades, but this progress has not been consistent due to a decrease in foreign earnings and policy changes (Atobatele et al., 2022). The average federal government allocation for education between 2009 and 2021, which stands at 7%, is a far cry from global recommendations of 15% to 20% of the total government budget for education following the Incheon Declaration and Framework for Action (FFA) for the Implementation of Sustainable Development Goal-4 (SDG-4; Atobatele et al., 2022).

SOCIAL JUSTICE AND HUMAN RIGHTS ISSUES

Social justice and human rights issues are crucial determinants of health in Nigeria, influencing access to healthcare services, health outcomes, and overall well-being. In Nigeria, achieving social justice necessitates communities to advocate for social accountability, guaranteeing transparency and equity in healthcare provision (Abimbola et al., 2022). As per WHO, health is recognized as a fundamental human right (WHO, 2021). Violations of human rights in Nigeria frequently lead to adverse health effects. For example, the continuing conflict in the northeastern region has caused widespread displacement, leaving more than 2 million internally displaced persons (IDPs) without access to fundamental healthcare services (Amnesty International, 2025).

ENVIRONMENTAL AND CLIMATE CHANGE ISSUES

Nigeria is confronted with many challenges arising from environmental issues, including pollution, climate change, and resource depletion. The nation grapples with heightened health hazards, the proliferation of communicable diseases, and shifts in socioeconomic patterns attributable to climate change–induced factors such as severe weather occurrences, rising temperatures, and precipitation spikes (Monday, 2020). The direct consequences of climate change in Nigeria have been linked to a range of health risks, including cerebrospinal meningitis, cardiovascular and respiratory disorders affecting older adults, skin cancer, malaria, high blood pressure, and increased morbidity rates (Monday, 2020). The incidence of vector-borne diseases is projected to rise due to climate change, which could exacerbate the impact of malaria (estimated to have caused 12% of deaths in 2019) and other diseases that already pose a significant burden on the Nigerian population (Abubakar et al., 2022).

HEALTHCARE BEHAVIORS

Nigeria has taken steps to address NCD progress indicators such as NCD policies and plans, tobacco taxes, bans on tobacco advertising, health warnings on tobacco products, and alcohol taxes. However, progress remains limited in several areas, including smoke-free policies, tobacco media campaigns, salt policies, trans fats policies, marketing of these products to children, and awareness of physical activity (WHO, 2023).

HEALTHCARE SYSTEM

Healthcare access disparities continue to persist in Nigeria, leading to limited availability and affordability of services for many individuals, resulting in out-of-pocket expenses for medical care (Ugochukwu et al., 2020). The healthcare system in Nigeria is grappling with several challenges, including increasing outbound medical tourism, declining medical infrastructure, inadequate government budget allocation, and the emigration of skilled healthcare professionals due to low compensation. In 2021, the federal government allocated only 5% of its budget to healthcare, falling short of the 15% commitment made in the 2001 Abuja Declaration (International Trade Administration [ITA], 2023).

FINANCING AND INSURANCE

Funding a nation's healthcare system is crucial for achieving universal health coverage (UHC), as it directly affects the accessibility and affordability of healthcare services (Uzochukwu et al., 2015). In Nigeria, healthcare funding primarily comes from pooled sources such as budgetary allocations, direct and indirect taxes, and donor contributions (Uzochukwu et al., 2015). Nonpooled sources, which account for over 70% of total health expenditure in Nigeria, mainly consist of out-of-pocket payments (Uzochukwu et al., 2015), which include direct fees paid to healthcare providers during services (about 90%) and purchases of medical goods like bed-nets or condoms (about 10%; Lawanson & Olaniyan, 2013).

To improve healthcare access for all citizens, Nigeria has enacted various laws and policies, including the National Health Insurance Scheme Act of 1999, the National Health Insurance Act of 2014, and the amended National Health Policy of 2016 (Onyedika-Ugoeze, 2023). The National Health Insurance Act, signed into law on May 24, 2022, aims to strengthen health insurance initiatives and boost private sector involvement in healthcare provision (Onyedika-Ugoeze, 2023). This legislation mandates health insurance for all Nigerians and legal residents, standardizes a minimum healthcare package across insurance schemes, and establishes a Vulnerable Group Fund to support vulnerable demographics, ensuring equitable healthcare access (Onyedika-Ugoeze, 2023).

The National Health Insurance Scheme, a government-led social health insurance program, aims to supplement healthcare financing sources and enhance healthcare accessibility for a significant portion of the Nigerian population (Akinyemi, 2023). Despite these efforts, the 2018 Nigeria Demographic and Health Survey indicated that only 3% of individuals age 15 to 49 years have any form of health insurance coverage (National Population Commission, 2019).

DELIVERY

Facilities

Healthcare delivery in Nigeria is diverse, involving both orthodox and traditional providers, with minimal integration and collaboration between the two sectors (Federal Ministry of Health [FMH], 2016). Primary health facilities make up 88% of the total, with secondary and tertiary facilities accounting for 12% and 0.25%, respectively. Government-owned facilities outnumber private ones, constituting 67% compared to 33% (Makinde et al., 2018). There is a higher concentration of public health facilities in the northern regions (Makinde et al., 2018). The healthcare system is structured into three tiers: primary, secondary, and tertiary care (Wada et al., 2021). Primary healthcare services, primarily accessible in rural areas, are overseen by local government authorities in collaboration with state governments and international donors (Wada et al., 2021). Secondary healthcare, managed by state governments, includes comprehensive health centers and general hospitals. Tertiary healthcare, managed by the federal government, comprises federal medical centers, specialist hospitals, and teaching hospitals (Wada et al., 2021). Hospitals are categorized into general wards, offering both outpatient and inpatient care for a fee, and amenity wards, which provide higher-priced services with better aesthetics and therapeutic conditions (Ogunneye et al., 2018). General wards often face overcrowding and long waiting times, with inpatient care sometimes being challenging due to limited direct access to doctors (Ogunneye et al., 2018).

HEALTHCARE PRACTICES

PUBLIC AND PRIVATE HEALTHCARE PRACTICES

The coexistence of public and private healthcare providers characterizes the healthcare system in Nigeria. While public healthcare facilities often struggle with resource constraints and inefficiencies, private healthcare providers are typically more agile and better equipped but may not be accessible to the broader population due to cost factors (Okunade et al., 2023). In Nigeria, public healthcare delivery remains greatly underfunded, significantly contributing to poor health outcomes and notable health disparities. Data from WHO reveal that in 2019 Nigeria allocated only 0.5% of its GDP to healthcare, well below the SSA average of 2%. Furthermore, with just 4.2% of total government expenditure allocated to healthcare in 2020, Nigeria has not met its commitment established in the 2001 **Abuja Declaration** (Chukwuma, 2024).

ALTERNATIVE HEALTHCARE PRACTICES IN NIGERIA

In Nigeria, traditional healthcare practices, including traditional medicine, herbal remedies, and spiritual healing methods, have become increasingly prominent alongside conventional medicine. These practices are deeply rooted in the cultural heritage of diverse ethnic groups in the region. Traditional medicine in Nigeria encompasses the application of native knowledge and methodologies for addressing a variety of health conditions, such as herbal medicines, spiritual healing, and other natural practices (Aka & Balogun, 2022).

Amid the prominent cultural and utilitarian role of herbal medicine, there is a growing concern about the safety, effectiveness, and standardization of these remedies (Chopra et al., 2022). The Nigerian government has committed to establishing the Traditional Medicine Development Division within the Ministry of Health and formulating policies to regulate and standardize herbal medicine practices (Alostad et al., 2020). Despite these efforts, there are still challenges in integrating traditional healing practices with modern healthcare standards, especially regarding safety, efficacy, and regulatory compliance (Jansen et al., 2021).

CONCLUSION

In conclusion, Nigeria's healthcare system embodies a unique blend of traditional and modern practices, reflecting the nation's rich cultural heritage and ongoing development. Addressing current challenges requires a multifaceted approach to improve access, equity, and overall health outcomes for the Nigerian population. By leveraging both public and private healthcare sectors, enhancing healthcare financing, and fostering collaboration among various stakeholders, Nigeria can work toward a more robust and efficient healthcare system. Furthermore, ongoing efforts to address maternal and infant mortality, enhance awareness and utilization of health services, and integrate innovative solutions like telemedicine and health literacy workshops will be crucial in achieving sustainable health improvements across the country.

LEARNING ACTIVITIES

CourseConnect

To access self-assessment questions and interactive, competency-based learning activities for this chapter, visit www.springerpub.com/courseconnect. See inside front cover and tear-out for CourseConnect details.

REFERENCES

Abimbola, S., Drabarek, D., & Molemodile, S. (2022). Self-reliance or social accountability? The raison d'être of community health committees in Nigeria. *The International Journal of Health Planning and Management, 37*(3), 1722–1735. https://doi.org/10.1002/hpm.3438

Abiodun, M. T., & Sadoh, W. E. (2021). Socio-demographic characteristics and pre-hospital care of children with circulatory failure in a children's emergency room in southern Nigeria. *Pan African Medical Journal, 40*, 65. https://doi.org/10.11604/pamj.2021.40.65.30003

Abubakar, I., Dalglish, S. L., Angell, B., Sanuade, O., Abimbola, S., Adamu, A. L., Adetifa, I. M. O., Colbourn, T., Ogunlesi, A. O., Onwujekwe, O., Owoaje, E. T., Okeke, I. N., Adeyemo, A., Aliyu, G., Aliyu, M. H., Aliyu, S. H., Ameh, E. A., Archibong, B., Ezeh, A., . . . Zanna, F. H. (2022). The Lancet Nigeria Commission: Investing in health and the future of the nation. *The Lancet, 399*(10330), 1155–1200. https://doi.org/10.1016/S0140-6736(21)02488-0

Adeloye, D., Ige, J. O., Aderemi, A. V., Adeleye, N., Amoo, E. O., Auta, A., & Oni, G. (2017). Estimating the prevalence, hospitalisation and mortality from type 2 diabetes mellitus in Nigeria: a systematic review and meta-analysis. *BMJ Open, 7*(5), e015424. https://doi.org/10.1136/bmjopen-2016-015424

Adewale, A. (2024). Data story: What figures tell us about life expectancy across Nigeria. *Premium Times Nigeria*. https://www.premiumtimesng.com/news/headlines/662945-data-story-what-figures-tell-us-about-life-expectancy-across-nigeria.html?tztc=1

Ajayi, I. O., Balogun, W. O., Olopade, O. B., Ajani, G. O., Soyoye, D. O., Bolarinwa, O. A., Olamoyegun, M. A., Alatishe-Muhammad, B. W., Odeniyi, I. A., Odukoya, O., Fasanmade, O. A., Diyaolu, F. P., Otrofanowei, E., Akase, I., Agabi, P. O., Adejimi, A., Ajetunmobi, O. A., Durowade, K. A., Gabriel-Alayode, E. O., et al. (2023). Prevalence of haemoglobin A1c based dysglycaemia among adult community dwellers in selected states in Nigeria: a descriptive cross-sectional study. *Frontiers in Endocrinology, 14*. https://doi.org/10.3389/fendo.2023.1192491

Aka, P. C., & Balogun, J. A. (2022). *Healthcare and economic restructuring*. Palgrave Macmillan. https://doi.org/10.1007/978-9 81-16-9543-8_1

Akinyemi, A.I. (2023). *Nigeria's growing population can be an advantage, with better data and a policy focus on young people*. The Conversation. https://theconversation.com/nigerias-growing-population-can-be-an-advantage-with-better-data-and-a-policy-focus-on-young-people-209530#:~:text=The%20country%20has%20the%20largest,of%20food%2C%20lives%20and%20property

Akinyemi O., & Atilola, O. (2012). Nigerian resident doctors on strike: Insights from and policy implications of job satisfaction among resident doctors in a Nigerian teaching hospital. *The International Journal of Health Planning and Management, 28*(1). https://doi.org/10.1002/hpm.2141

Alostad, A. H., Steinke, D. T., & Schafheutle, E. I. (2020). Herbal medicine classification: Policy recommendations. *Frontiers in Medicine, 7*, 31. https://doi.org/10.3389/fmed.2020.00031

Amnesty International. (2025, January). *Nigeria: Boko Haram must end vicious killing spree*. https://www.amnesty.org/en/latest/news/2025/01/nigeria-boko-haram-must-end-vicious-killing-spree/

Angell, B., Sanuade O., Adetifa, I. M. O., Okeke, I. N., Adamu, A. L., Aliyu, M. H., Ameh, E. A., Kyari, F., Gadanya, M. A., Mabayoje, D. A., Yinka-Ogunleye, A., Oni, T., Jalo, R. I., Tsiga-Ahmed, F. I., Dalglish, S. L., Abimbola, S., Colbourn, T., Onwujekwe, O., Owoajeet, E. T., . . . Abubakar, I. (2022). Population health outcomes in Nigeria compared with other West African countries, 1998–2019: A systematic analysis for the Global Burden of Disease Study. *The Lancet, 399*(10330), 1117–1129. https://doi.org/10.1016/S0140-6736(21)02722-7

Atobatele, S., Omeje, O., Ayodeji, O., Oisagbai, F., & Sampson, S. (2022). Situational analysis of access to essential healthcare services in Nigeria: Implication for trans-sectorial policy considerations in addressing health inequities. *Health, 14*(5), 553–575. https://doi.org/10.4236/health.2022.145041

Bala, B., & Tar, U. (2020). The giant of Africa? Explaining the Nigerian governance, security, and development paradox. In K. Omeje (Ed.), *Governance and security in the Sahel* (pp. 315–339). Springer Publishing Company. https://doi.org/10.1007/978-3-030-49348-6_16

Centers for Disease Control and Prevention. (2022). *CDC in Nigeria*. https://www.cdc.gov/globalhealth/countries/nigeria/

Central Intelligence Agency. (n.d.-a). *Nigeria - The world factbook*. https://www.cia.gov/the-world-factbook/countries/nigeria/

Central Intelligence Agency. (n.d.-b). *Country population comparison: The world factbook*. https://web.archive.org/web/20181218221601/https://www.cia.gov/library/publications/the-world-factbook/fields/335rank.html

Chepkemoi, J. (2019). *What languages are spoken in Nigeria*? World Atlas. https://www.worldatlas.com/articles/what-languages-are-spoken-in-nigeria.html

Chidebe, R. C. W., Leibel, L. L., Orjiakor, T. C., Shrestha, A., Agha, A. A., Dindar, D. A., Kisakol, B., Ipiankama, S. C., Okoye, I. J., Mason, M., Auguste, A., Esiaka, D. K. (2023). Promoting cancer prevention through World Cancer Day in Nigeria. *The Lancet Oncology, 24*(4), 319–322. https://doi.org/10.1016/S1470-2045(22)00692-1

Chopra, A. S., Lordan, R., Horbańczuk, O. K., Atanasov, A. G., Chopra, I., Horbańczuk, J. O., Jóźwik, A., Huang, L., Pirgozliev, V., Banach, M., Battino, M., & Arkells, N. (2022). The current use and evolving landscape of nutraceuticals. *Pharmacological Research, 175*, 106001. https://doi.org/10.1016/j.phrs.2021.106001

Chukwuma, J. N. (2024). Implementing health policy in Nigeria: The basic health care provision fund as a catalyst for achieving universal health coverage? *Development and Change, 54*(6), 1480–1503. https://doi.org/10.1111/dech.12808

Commonwealth Governance. (2014). *Countries*. https://commonwealthgovernance.org/countries/africa/nigeria/geography/

Federal Ministry of Health. (2016). *The national strategic health development plan framework (2009–2015)*. UHC2030. https://www.uhc2030.org/fileadmin/uploads/ihp/Documents/Country_Pages/Nigeria/Nigeria

Hemba, E., Trisma, E., & Ikyumbur, T. (2019). Mass concentration and size distribution of atmospheric particulate matter in Plateau State, Nigeria. *International Journal of Environment and Climate Change, 9*(12), 701–707. https://doi.org/10.9734/ijecc/2019/v9i1230151

Idajili, A., Adebayo, T. A., Chijioke, U. W., & Irowa-Omoregie, D. (2020). The impact of global infectious diseases on Nigeria's socioeconomic development. *African Journal of Social Sciences and Humanities*

Research, 3(6), 232–245. https://abjournals.org/ajsshr/papers/volume-3/issue-6/the-impact-of-global-infectious-diseases-on-nigerias-socio-economic-development/

iExplore. (n.d.) *Nigeria holidays and festivals.* https://www.iexplore.com/articles/travel-guides/africa/nigeria/festivals-and-events

Ike, S., & Onyema, C. T. (2020). Cardiovascular diseases in Nigeria: What has happened in the past 20 years? *Nigerian Journal of Cardiology, 17*(1), 21. https://doi.org/10.4103/njc.njc_33_19

Institute for Health Metrics and Evaluation. (2017). *GHDx.* Global Health Data Exchange. https://ghdx.healthdata.org/gbd-2017

International Agency for Research on Cancer. (2020). *Cancer today.* https://gco.iarc.fr/today/home

International Diabetes Federation. (2019). *IDF diabetes atlas* (9th ed.). https://www.diabetesatlas.org

International Trade Administration. (2023). *Nigeria - healthcare.* https://www.trade.gov/country-commercial-guides/nigeria-healthcare

Integral Human Development. (2023). *Nigeria - Migrants & refugees section.* Migrants & Refugees Section. https://migrants-refugees.va/country-profile/nigeria/#:~:text=In%202022%2C%20the%20estimated%20net,and%20current%20database%20on%20migration

Jansen, C., Baker, J. D., Kodaira, E., Ang, L., Bacani, A. J., Aldan, J. T., Shimoda, L. M. N., Salameh, M., Small-Howard, A. L., Stokes, A. J., Turner, H., & Adra, C. N. (2021). Medicine in motion: Opportunities, challenges and data analytics-based solutions for traditional medicine integration into western medical practice. *Journal of Ethnopharmacology, 267*, 113477. https://doi.org/10.1016/j.jep.2020.113477

Kassa, M. D., & Grace, J. M. (2020). Race against death or starvation? COVID-19 and its impact on African populations. *Public Health Rev, 41*(30). https://doi.org/10.1186/s40985-020-00139-0

Kirk-Greene, A. H. M., Falola, T. O., Ajayi, J. A., & Udo, R. K. (2024). *Nigeria | History, Population, flag, Map, Languages, capital, & Facts.* Encyclopedia Britannica. https://www.britannica.com/place/Nigeria

Lawanson A.O., & Olaniyan, O. (2013). Health expenditure and health status in Northern and Southern Nigeria: A comparative analysis using National Health Account Framework. *African Journal of Health Economics, 2*, 31–46.

Lawanson, O. I., & Umar, D. I. (2021). The life expectancy–economic growth nexus in Nigeria: The role of poverty reduction. *SN Business and Economics, 1*, 127. https://doi.org/10.1007/s43546-021-00119-9

Macrotrends. (n.d.). *Nigeria infant mortality rate (1950–2025).* https://www.macrotrends.net/global-metrics/countries/nga/nigeria/infant-mortality-rate

Makinde, O. A., Sule, A., Ayankogbe, O., & Boone, D. (2018). Distribution of health facilities in Nigeria: Implications and options for Universal Health Coverage. *International Journal of Planning and Management, 33*(4), 1179–1192. https://doi.org/10.1002/hpm.2603

Monday, I. (2020). Investigating effects of climate change on health risks in Nigeria. In I. Uher (Ed.), *Environmental factors affecting human health.* IntechOpen. https://doi.org/10.5772/intechopen.86912

Nasir, N., Aderoba, A. K., & Ariana, P. (2022). Scoping review of maternal and newborn health interventions and programmes in Nigeria. *BMJ Open, 12*(2), e054784. https://doi.org/10.1136/bmjopen-2021-054784

National Population Commission. (2019). ICF 2018 Nigeria Demographic and Health Survey. https://www.dhsprogram.com/pubs/pdf/FR359/FR359.pdf

Nuphi, J. Y. (2019). *Using research to reach people at risk of NTDs in Nigeria.* Sightsavers. https://www.sightsavers.org/blogs/2019/03/research-ntds-nigeria/

Okunade, B. A., Adediran, F. E., Balogun, O. D., Maduka, C. P., & Adegoke, A. A. (2023). Capacity building in Nigeria's healthcare sector: A review of skill development and mentorship initiatives. *World Journal of Advanced Research and Reviews, 20*(3), 906–923. https://doi.org/10.30574/wjarr.2023.20.3.2540

Oladapo, O. T., Adetoro, O. O., Ekele, B. A., Chama, C., Etuk, S. J., Aboyeji, A. P., Onah, H. E., Abasiattai, A. M., Adamu, A. N., Adegbola, O., Adeniran, A. S., Aimakhu, C. O., Akinsanya, O., Aliyu, L. D., Ande, A. B., Ashimi, A., Bwala, M., Fabamwo, A., Geidam, A. D., Ikechebelu, J. I., … Nigeria Near-miss and Maternal Death Surveillance Network. (2015). When getting there is not enough: A nationwide cross-sectional study of 998 maternal deaths and 1451 near-misses in public tertiary hospitals in a low-income country. *BJOG, 123*(6), 928–938. https://doi.org/10.1111/1471-0528.13450

Omojuyigbe, J. O., Tikare, O., Oke, A. E., & Hassan, A. (2023). Managing infectious disease outbreaks during an ongoing economic crisis in Nigeria: A call to action, *Health Policy OPEN, 5*(100106), 2590–2296. https://doi.org/10.1016/j.hpopen.2023.100106

O'Neill, A. (2024a). *Age structure in Nigeria 2022.* Statista. https://www.statista.com/statistics/382296/age-structure-in-nigeria/

Ogunneye, Y., Ogunneye, Q., & Kalu, K. (2018). Nigeria. In J. Johnson, C. Stoskopf, & L. Shi (Eds.), *Comparative health systems: Global perspectives.* Jones and Bartlett Publishers.

Onah, J. O. (2018). *New plan will help improve cancer treatment and save lives in Nigeria.* Clinton Health Access Initiative. https://www.clintonhealthaccess.org/blog/new-plan-will-help-improve-cancer-treatment-save-lives-nigeria/

Onyedika-Ugoeze, N. (2023). *NHIA pledges to ensure that all Nigerians have access to affordable, good quality health care.* The Guardian Nigeria News - Nigeria and World News. https://guardian.ng/news/nhia-pledges-to-ensure-that-all-nigerians-have-access-to-affordable-good-quality-health-care/#:~:text=By%20Nkechi%20Onyedika%2DUgoeze%2C%20Abuja&text=The%20National%20Health%20Insurance%20Authority,burden%20of%20paying%20for%20them

Onyeka, T. (2022). *Cancer in my community: Meeting the palliative care needs of people with cancer in Nigeria.* https://www.cancer.net/blog/2022-03/cancer-my-community-meeting-palliative-care-needs-people-with-cancer-nigeria

Orjingene, O., Teryila, O., Baffoe, P., & Ojo, O. (2022). Factors affecting maternal and neonatal mortality in northern Nigeria: A multiple linear regression analysis. *BMJ- Preprint.* https://www.medrxiv.org/content/10.1101/2022.06.30.22276507v1.full.pdf

Sasu, D. D. (2022). Distribution of ethnic groups in Nigeria 2018. Statista. https://www.statista.com/statistics/1203438/distribution-of-ethnic-groups-in-nigeria/

Sasu, D. D. (2023a). *Nigeria: most common languages spoken at home 2022.* Statista. https://www.statista.com/statistics/1268798/main-languages-spoken-at-home-in-nigeria/#:~:text=Main%20languages%20spoken%20at%20home%20in%20Nigeria%202022&text=The%20primary%20languages%20spoken%20at,%2C%20Pidgin%20English%2C%20and%20Ijaw

Sasu, D. D. (2023b). *Immigration in Nigeria.* Statista. https://www.statista.com/topics/7865/immigration-in-nigeria/#topicOverview

Sasu, D. D. (2023c). *Distribution of religions in Nigeria 2018.* https://www.statista.com/statistics/1203455/distribution-of-religions-in-nigeria/

The END Fund. (2023). *The impact of neglected tropical diseases.* https://end.org/ntds-in-focus/#:%7E:text=Neglected%20Tropical%20Diseases%20Statistics,blindness%20results%20in%20social%20isolation

Trading Economics. (n.d.). *Nigeria - Population ages 65 and above (% of total) - 2024 data 2025 forecast 1960-2022 historical.* https://tradingeconomics.com/nigeria/population-ages-65-and-above-percent-of-total-wb-data.html#:~:text=Population%20ages%2065%20and%20above%20(%25%20of%20total%20population)%20in,compiled%20from%20officially%20recognized%20sources

Translators Without Borders. (2022). *Language data for Nigeria.* https://translatorswithoutborders.org/language-data-nigeria

Ugochukwu, O., Mbaezue, N., Lawal, S. A., Azubogu, C., Sheikh, T. L., & Vallières, F. (2020). The time is now: Reforming Nigeria's outdated mental health laws. *The Lancet Global Health, 8*(8), 989–990. https://doi.org/10.1016/S2214-109X(20)30302-8

Uloko, A. E., Musa, B. M., Ramalan, M. A., Gezawa, I. D., Puepet, F. H., Uloko, A. T., Borodo, M. M., & Sada, K. B. (2018). Prevalence and risk factors for diabetes mellitus in Nigeria: A systematic review and meta-analysis. *Diabetes Therapy, 9*(3), 1307–1316. https://doi.org/10.1007/s13300-018-0441-1

UN Data Portal. (n.d.). *UN population division data portal: Interactive access to global demographic indicators.* United Nations. https://population.un.org/dataportal/data/indicators/70,61,54/locations/566/start/1990/end/2025/table/pivotbylocation?df=e93e661b-688e-457e-b31b-3f3c27dad6ec

Uzochukwu, B. S. C., Ughasoro, M. D., Etiaba, E., Okwuosa, C., Envuladu, E., & Onwujekwe, O. E. (2015). Health care financing in Nigeria: Implications for achieving universal health coverage. *Nigerian Journal of Clinical Practice, 18*(4), 437–444. https://doi.org/10.4103/1119-3077.154196

Wada, Y. H., Rajwani, L., Anyam, E., Karikari, E., Njikizana, M., Srour, L., & Khalid, G. M. (2021). Mental health in Nigeria: A neglected issue in public health. *Public Health in Practice, 2*, 100166. https://doi.org/10.1016/j.puhip.2021.100166

World Bank Group. (n.d.). *World Bank open data.* https://data.worldbank.org/indicator/SP.DYN.TFRT.IN?locations=NG

World Bank Group. (2019). *World development indicators: Life expectancy at birth, total (years).* https://data.worldbank.org/indicator/SP.DYN.LE00.IN?locations=NG

World Bank Group. (2021). *Poverty & equity brief, Africa Western & Central, Nigeria.* https://databank.worldbank.org/data/download/poverty/987B9C90-CB9F-4D93-AE8C-750588BF00QA/AM2020/Global_POVEQ_NGA.pdf

World Factbook Glyph. (n.d.). *Nigeria.* https://www.cia.gov/the-world-factbook/countries/nigeria/#people-and-society

World Health Organization. (2018a). *Guideline on management of drug resistance-TB. In WHO Treatment Guidelines for Drug-Resistant Tuberculosis.* https://www.who.int/publications/i/item/9789241550529

World Health Organization. (2018b). *Noncommunicable diseases country profiles 2018.* https://www.who.int/publications/i/item/9789241514620

World Health Organization. (2021). *Constitution of the World Health Organization.* https://www.who.int/about/governance/constitution

World Health Organization. (2023). *Maternal mortality: The urgency of a systemic and multisectoral approach in mitigating maternal deaths in Africa.* WHO African Region. https://files.aho.afro.who.int/afahobckpcontainer/production/files/iAHO_Maternal_Mortality_Regional_Factsheet.pdf

PART VIII: Health and Healthcare in East Africa

CHAPTER 30

OVERVIEW OF EAST AFRICA

Samantha Mason and Thomas Foley

GEOGRAPHY

East Africa is renowned for its stunning and remarkably diverse geography that includes large freshwater lakes such as Lake Victoria, mountainous and volcanic terrain such as Mount Kilimanjaro, the drylands of the eastern Sahara Desert, the extensive East African Rift Valley, vast savanna plains such as the Serengeti, **archipelagos** (island chains) such as Seychelles and Zanzibar, densely populated cities such as Nairobi in Kenya, large peninsulas such as the Horn of Africa, and coastal borders along the Red Sea, Gulf of Aden, and Indian Ocean. East Africa includes the following countries: Eritrea, Djibouti, Ethiopia, Somalia, Kenya, Uganda, Tanzania, Comoros, and Seychelles (Figure 30.1; Berglee, 2016). The countries of East Africa are vulnerable to the effects of climate change, such as drought, flooding, and intense tropical cyclones (Marcus & Low, 2024).

BRIEF HISTORY

East Africa is recognized as the birthplace of early modern humanity, which emerged approximately 200,000 years ago (Liu et al., 2006). Several civilizations, such as the Puntites, Askumites, and Bantu, thrived in East Africa prior to European colonization. Bantu expansion occurred approximately 2,500 years ago and led to the establishment of agriculture in much of East Africa. Other cultures, such as the Arabic, Cushitic, Persian, and Swahili, integrated with the Bantu during this time, creating much of the cultural diversity that exists in present-day East Africa (Vansina, 1995).

The first Europeans to explore the region were the Portuguese, whose colonization of coastal East Africa established a line of spice trade with Asia (Ross, 2002). In the 19th and 20th centuries, European imperialism of Africa was rampant in the event known as the **Scramble for Africa.** The primary perpetrators of East Africa colonization during the Scramble for Africa were England, France, Italy, and Germany. Decolonization of eastern African countries did not begin until the 1960s, and European colonization left a lasting mark on the countries of eastern Africa by furthering ethnic violence, classism, health disparities, educational gaps, and overall political unrest (Gjersø, 2015).

POPULATION

In 2023, the population of East Africa was more than 330 million people. The most populous countries in East Africa during 2023 were Ethiopia (approximately 127 million), Tanzania (approximately 67 million), Kenya (approximately 55 million), and Uganda (approximately 49 million). In 2023, Seychelles was the least populous East Africa nation with a population of 107,660 people (UN Data Portal, n.d.).

Opportunity for agriculture, improved governmental infrastructure, and reduction in infant mortality rates are factors credited for a growing population in East Africa (Alemu, 2020). The growing population in East Africa is exceptionally youthful—the median age during 2023 was approximately 18 years. The crude birth rate in East Africa during 2023 was comparatively high

FIGURE 30.1 Map of East Africa.

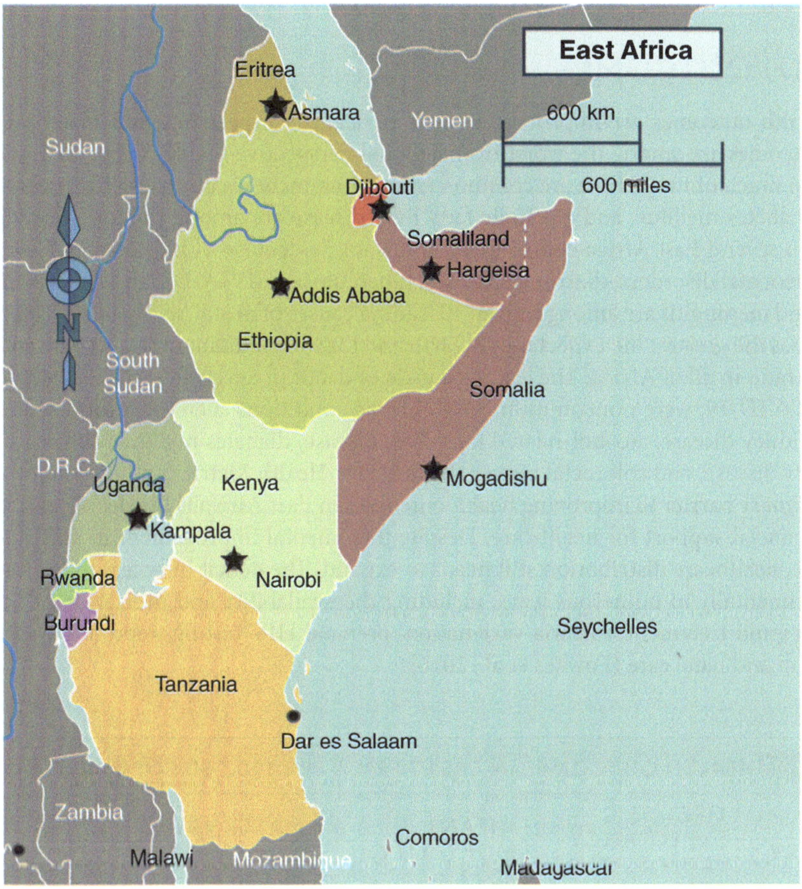

Note: Rwanda and Burundi are considered to be part of both East and Central Africa.

Source: Fitzgerald, P. (2008). *East Africa regions map*. https://commons.wikimedia.org/wiki/File:East_Africa_regions_map.png

with a rate of approximately 33 births per 1,000 people, far exceeding the global birth rate of 16.7 births per 1,000 people. Seychelles is an exception in East Africa as it is experiencing population aging. In Seychelles during 2023, the birth rate was 14.7 and the median age was 33.1 years (UN Data Portal, n.d.).

SOCIOECONOMIC FACTORS

Although East Africa is resource abundant and Ethiopia, Kenya, and Tanzania are leading African economies, the countries of East Africa struggle financially and account for an extremely small percentage of the global gross domestic product (GDP). In 2023, nearly every country in East Africa had a per-capita GDP of less than $4,000, with the per-capita GDP in Somalia as the lowest at approximately $644. Seychelles is the exception, as it has the greatest per-capita GDP in all of Africa. During 2023, the per-capita GDP in Seychelles was approximately $17,880. Educational attainment is an issue in much of East Africa. Again, Seychelles is a notable exception as it has the highest primary and secondary completion rates and literacy rate in all of Africa (World Bank Group, n.d.).

While East Africa struggles with important socioeconomic outcomes, the region is recognized as having an emerging economy and is home to several of the world's fastest-growing economies, including Ethiopia and Tanzania (African Development Bank Group, 2019). This change has contributed to economic and health transitions within East Africa, reducing the number of individuals living in extreme poverty and contributing to positive shifts in related healthcare outcomes.

HEALTH OUTCOMES

While health outcomes are improving in East Africa, life expectancy and maternal and child health outcomes are among the worst from a global perspective (Table 30.1). The leading causes of death in much of East Africa are common among low-income countries. While cardiovascular disease, diabetes mellitus, and alcoholic fatty liver disease are among the top 10 leading causes of death in several East Africa countries, a significant percentage of mortality in East Africa is a result of neonatal disorders, diarrheal diseases, tuberculosis, HIV/AIDS, and malaria. In Somalia, measles and meningitis are among the top 10 leading causes of death. Seychelles is again an exception as it has the greatest life expectancy at birth and the lowest infant mortality rate and maternal mortality ratio in all of Africa. The leading causes of death in Seychelles in 2021, with the exception of COVID-19, were noncommunicable chronic conditions such as cardiovascular diseases, chronic kidney disease, alcohol-related fatty liver disease, diabetes mellitus, chronic obstructive pulmonary disease, and colorectal cancer (Institute for Health Metrics and Evaluation, n.d.).

The primary barrier to improving health outcomes in East Africa is the dearth of access to and lack of financial support for healthcare. Despite incremental improvement in access to modern healthcare, healthcare distribution still needs to expand. The deficit in access to healthcare manifests detrimentally in numerous ways, including the availability and utilization of tuberculosis diagnostics and treatment, malaria vaccination, prenatal HIV testing, reproductive health, and postpartum and natal care (Fowkes et al., 2016).

TABLE 30.1 HEALTH OUTCOMES IN EAST AFRICA PER 100,000 POPULATION

COUNTRY	LIFE EXPECTANCY FROM BIRTH, 2023	INFANT MORTALITY, 2023	MATERNAL MORTALITY, 2020	LEADING CAUSE OF MORTALITY, 2021
Comoros	65.04	43.4	217	COVID-19
Djibouti	63.71	35	234.5	COVID-19
Eritrea	67.32	27.9	321.6	COVID-19
Ethiopia	66.65	29.9	266.7	COVID-19
Kenya	63.34	26	530	COVID-19
Seychelles	75	9.8	3.3	COVID-19
Somalia	57.35	64.3	620.7	COVID-19
Tanzania	67.6	29.5	283.3	COVID-19
Uganda	63.84	29.7	284.1	Malaria

Sources: Adapted from Institute for Health Metrics and Evaluation. (n.d.). *Health research by location: Country profiles*. University of Washington. https://www.healthdata.org/research-analysis/health-by-location/profiles; UN Data Portal. (n.d.). *UN population division data portal*. United Nations. https://population.un.org/dataportal/home/; UN Population Fund. (2024). *Data portal*. United Nations. https://www.unfpa.org/data

LEARNING ACTIVITIES

CourseConnect

To access self-assessment questions and interactive, competency-based learning activities for this chapter, visit www.springerpub.com/courseconnect. See inside front cover and tear-out for CourseConnect details.

REFERENCES

African Development Bank Group. (2019). *East Africa regional overview*. www.afdb.org/en/countries/east-africa/east-africa-overview

Alemu, K. (2020). The relationship between population growth and economic growth in Ethiopia. *Journal of Economic and Sustainable Development, 11*(15), 52–65.

Berglee, R. (2016). *World regional geography*. University of Minnesota Libraries Publishing.

Fowkes, F. J. I., Draper, B. L., Hellard, M., & Stoové, M. (2016). Achieving development goals for HIV, tuberculosis and malaria in sb-Saharan Africa through integrated antenatal care: Barriers and challenges. *BMC Medicine, 14*(1), 202. https://doi.org/10.1186/s12916-016-0753-9

Gjersø, J. F. (2015). The scramble for East Africa: British motives reconsidered, 1884–95. *The Journal of Imperial and Commonwealth History, 43*(5), 831–860. https://doi.org/10.1080/03086534.2015.1026131

Institute for Health Metrics and Evaluation. (n.d.). *Health research by location: Country profiles*. University of Washington. https://www.healthdata.org/research-analysis/health-by-location/profiles

Liu, H., Prugnolle, F., Manica, A., & Balloux, F. (2006). A geographically explicit genetic model of worldwide human-settlement history. *American Journal of Human Genetics, 79*(2), 230–237. https://doi.org/10.1086/505436

Marcus, H. G., & Low, D. A. (2024). *Eastern Africa*. Britannica. https://www.britannica.com/place/eastern-Africa

Ross, A. E. (2002). *Heilbrunn timeline of art history: The Portuguese in Africa, 1415–1600*. Metropolitan Museum of Art. www.metmuseum.org/toah/hd/agex/hd_agex.htm

UN Data Portal. (n.d.). *UN population division data portal*. United Nations. https://population.un.org/dataportal/home/

Vansina, J. (1995). New linguistic evidence and "the Bantu expansion." *The Journal of African History, 36*(2), 173–195.

World Bank Group. (n.d.). *The World Bank open data*. https://data.worldbank.org/

CHAPTER 31

ETHIOPIA

Adugnaw Berhane

GEOGRAPHY AND DEMOGRAPHICS

GEOGRAPHIC FEATURES

The Federal Democratic Republic of Ethiopia, located in the Horn of Africa, covers 1,112,000 square kilometers (69,000 square miles) and is Africa's 10th largest country. It has 12 regional states and two chartered cities (Figure 31.1). The capital city, Addis Ababa, is centrally located in Ethiopia and is home to the headquarters of the **African Union**, which stands as a pivotal center for African diplomacy, shaping the continent's political landscape and fostering cooperation among nations. Only 12% of the land in Ethiopia is arable, and agriculture and animal husbandry are crucial for subsistence. The country's topography, characterized by a massive highland complex divided by the Great Rift Valley, influences regional variations in climate, vegetation, soil, and settlement patterns.

FIGURE 31.1 Map of Ethiopia.

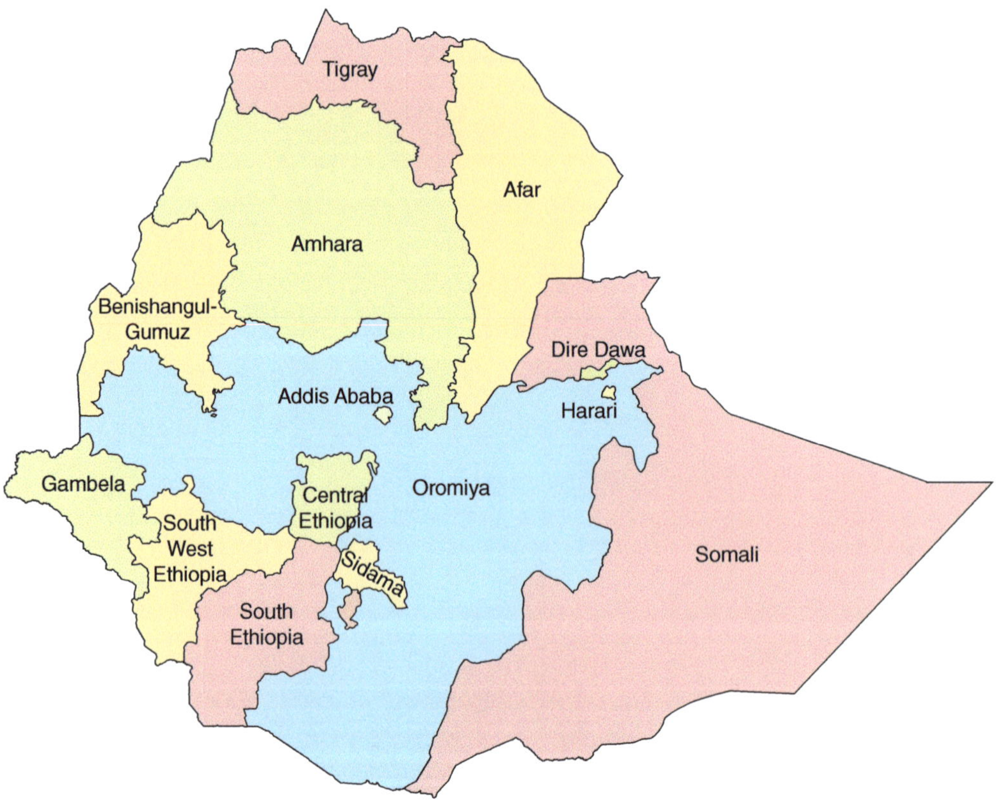

Source: Jfblanc. (2020). *Regions of Ethiopia*. https://en.wikipedia.org/wiki/Regions_of_Ethiopia

The five major topographic classifications of Ethiopia are the Western Highlands, the Western Lowlands, the Eastern Highlands, the Eastern Lowlands, and the Rift Valley. The Western Highlands are the most extensive and rugged topographic component of Ethiopia (Britannica, 2024).

POPULATION CHARACTERISTICS

Ethiopia is the second most populated country in Africa next to Nigeria and the 11th most populous country in the world. Ethiopia's 2023 population was approximately 128.7 million. The population density in Ethiopia during 2023 was 129 people per square kilometer, which was more than double the global average of 62 people per square kilometer. In 2023, 46.21% of Ethiopia's population was younger than 18 years, while only 3.17% of the population was 65 years or older. Life expectancy at birth in 2023 was 67.32 years—64.08 years for males and 70.73 years for females. The median age was 18.7 years, well below the global 2023 average of 30.4 years. The birth rate in Ethiopia during 2023 was 31.9 births per 1,000 people, which was nearly double the global birth rate (UN Data Portal, n.d.). Ethiopia is a predominantly rural-living country, concentrated in densely populated highland settlements. However, the rural population in Ethiopia steadily decreased from 94% in 1964 to 77% in 2023 (World Bank Group, n.d.).

From 2015 to 2020, more than 839,000 Ethiopians, mostly young adults, migrated out of Ethiopia seeking jobs in other countries. The United States, Canada, Europe, the Middle East, and neighboring African countries were popular destinations. Many migrants face perilous journeys and risks. More than 51,000 were missing during that time period, and many are feared to have died (International Organization for Migration [IOM], 2021). Ethiopia is also a major refugee-hosting country in Africa, with most refugees coming from neighboring nations such as South Sudan, Somalia, Djibouti, Eritrea, Uganda, Rwanda, and Burundi. The Gambelia, Somali, and Tigray regions host the majority of these refugees. Ethiopia's net migration rate in 2023 was an estimated –0.19 migrant(s)/1,000 population.

CULTURE

Ethiopia is a diverse country with numerous ethnic groups. According to the Ethiopian census, there are more than 80 different ethnic groups in the country, each with its own unique cultural, linguistic, and historical characteristics. The **Oromo** are the largest ethnic group in Ethiopia, making up approximately 34% of the population. The **Amhara** are the second-largest group, accounting for about 27% of the total population. Other ethnic groups in Ethiopia include the Somali, Tigray, Sidama, Gurage, Wolayita, Afar, Hadiya, and Gamo (Central Statistical Agency, 2008).

There are more than 80 languages in Ethiopia that can be categorized into four main groups: Semitic, Cushitic, Omotic, and Nilotic. The majority of languages belong to the Semitic, Cushitic, or Omotic groups, which are all part of the Afro-Asiatic language family. A smaller number of languages are Nilotic, belonging to the Nilo-Saharan language family. Although Ethiopia has many languages, **Amharic** is the working language of the federal government; however, Oromo is widely spoken. In 2020, the government made Afan Oromo, Afar, Somali, and Tigrigna official languages at the federal level (Osoblivaia, 2023).

Ethiopia is a land of important ancient history and religious diversity. Christianity, introduced in the fourth century, is the dominant religion. Islam, arriving in the seventh century, is prevalent in eastern regions. Small minorities adhere to traditional African religions or Judaism. Efforts have been made to promote religious tolerance and equality (Corsini, 2018). Ethiopians value respect for human life, social etiquette, and wisdom. Religion, especially the Ethiopian Orthodox Church, shapes morality and social interactions. Hospitality and respect for older adults are highly valued. The Ethiopian Orthodox Church has influenced national culture, with holidays like Easter, Christmas, Meskel, and Timket widely celebrated.

Ethiopian culture is deeply rooted in its rich heritage, encompassing religion, language, and family. The country has cultural institutions like the National Museum and the Museum of the Institute of Ethiopian Studies. Ethiopia's cultural history is evident in sites like Lalibela and Fasil

Ghebbi (Figure 31.2), which are both recognized as World Heritage Sites. The government also invests in tourism projects, including transforming Addis Ababa into a tourist destination.

POLITICAL SYSTEM

Ethiopia has experienced significant political shifts. Since the overthrow of the Derg regime in 1991, the country has transitioned to a federal republic. The ruling Prosperity Party, formed in 2019, succeeded the Ethiopian People's Revolutionary Democratic Front. The government is led by a powerful prime minister and a titular president. The legislature is **bicameral** (having two branches), with members elected at federal and regional levels, and the constitution guarantees an independent judiciary (Britannica, 2024).

HEALTH OUTCOMES

LEADING CAUSES OF DEATH

In Ethiopia, infectious diseases continue to be a significant health challenge. Respiratory infections, diarrheal diseases, HIV/AIDS, tuberculosis (TB), and malaria are among the most common causes of death. However, noncommunicable diseases (NCDs), such as cardiovascular diseases, cancer, diabetes, chronic renal disease, cirrhosis of the liver, and chronic respiratory diseases, are also making a substantial impact on mortality rates (Institute of Health Metrics and Evaluation [IHME], n.d.).

Maternal and child health is also a major concern as neonatal disorders are a leading cause of mortality in Ethiopia (IHME, n.d.) Acute respiratory tract infections (ARTI) are the primary cause of death among children younger than 5 years in Ethiopia, accounting for 18% of mortality. Other significant contributors to mortality include diarrhea (13%), prematurity (12%), newborn infections

FIGURE 31.2 Fasil Ghebbi in Ethiopia's Gondar region.

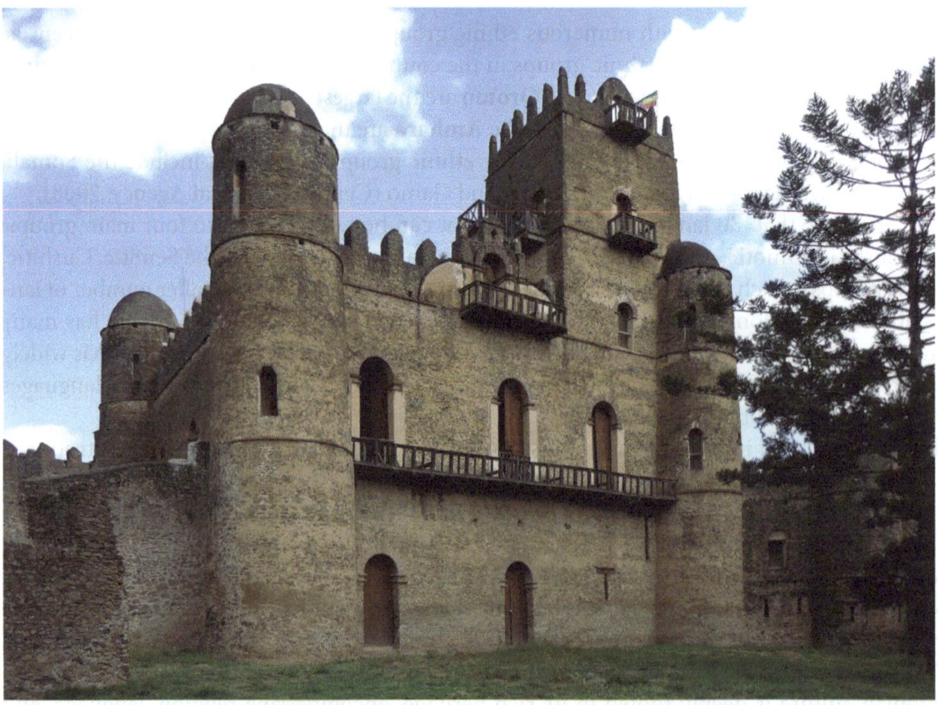

Source: Gagnon, B. (2012). *Fasilides Palace in the Fasil Ghebbi, Gondar, Ethiopia*. https://commons.wikimedia.org/wiki/File:Fasilides_Palace_01.jpg

(10%), asphyxia (9%), meningitis (6%), injuries (6%), measles (4%), malaria (2%), TB (3%), congenital anomalies (2%), HIV (2%), pertussis (1%), and other causes (17%). Malnutrition is a significant underlying factor, contributing to nearly 50% of deaths among children younger than 5 years in Ethiopia (World Health Organization [WHO], 2024). However, it is important to note that Ethiopia has made significant strides in improving maternal and child health. Maternal mortality ratios have declined dramatically from 871 maternal deaths per 100,000 live births in 2000, to 267 maternal deaths per 100,000 live births in 2020. Additionally, child deaths have been reduced by two thirds since 1990. Similarly, Ethiopia made significant strides in improving child nutrition. The prevalence of stunting among children younger than 5 years decreased from 51% to 37%, underweight from 33% to 21%, and wasting from 12% to 7%. Despite these advancements, certain health indicators, such as stunting rates and neonatal mortality, continue to lag behind. These areas require further attention to ensure that Ethiopia's health progress is sustained and equitable (World Bank Group, n.d.).

INFECTIOUS DISEASES

Ethiopia is currently grappling with a triple burden of diseases: communicable diseases, NCDs, and injuries. This burden disproportionately affects children and women of reproductive age. In 2019, 58% of disability-adjusted life years (DALYs) were attributed to maternal and neonatal conditions, communicable diseases, and malnutrition. NCDs accounted for 35% of total DALYs and injuries accounted for 7%. Over the past two decades, the share of NCDs has increased from 17% to 35% (Federal Ministry of Health [FMoH], 2024). Infectious diseases continue to be a major public health concern in Ethiopia, contributing to both morbidity and mortality. Malaria, TB, HIV/AIDS, and other **neglected tropical diseases** (NTDs) are some of the most prevalent infectious diseases in the country.

While significant progress has been made in reducing malaria morbidity and mortality in Ethiopia, the disease remains a public health concern. Between 2016 and 2019, confirmed malaria cases decreased by 47%, and malaria-attributed deaths declined by 58%. However, recent years have seen a resurgence in malaria cases due to factors such as the COVID-19 pandemic, armed conflict, and displacement. Between 2021 and 2022, confirmed malaria cases increased by 32.5%. In 2023, compared to the same periods in 2021 and 2022, reported malaria cases have increased by 150% and 120%, respectively (WHO, 2024).

Ethiopia has a high burden of TB and TB/HIV coinfection. In 2021, there were an estimated 143,000 TB cases with an annual incidence of 119 per 100,000 population. Ethiopia has achieved significant progress in reducing TB incidence and mortality rates, successfully transitioning out of the global list of high-risk countries for rifampicin-resistant/multidrug-resistant TB. However, ongoing drought, conflict, and large population movements pose significant risks for TB transmission and require urgent attention. Ethiopia's national HIV prevalence is 0.9%, but the epidemic varies significantly across different regions, sexes, and population groups. The Gambella region and Addis Ababa have the highest HIV prevalence rates at 4.8% and 3.4%, respectively (Qanche et al., 2021).

Ethiopia is endemic for all five NTDs that can be treated through mass drug administration (MDA): lymphatic filariasis, onchocerciasis, soil-transmitted helminthiasis, schistosomiasis, and trachoma. In 2021, more than 31 million people were targeted for MDA, and nearly 25 million received treatment for at least one NTD. In addition to these NTDs, Ethiopia also remains endemic for dracunculiasis (Guinea worm disease), leishmaniasis (cutaneous and visceral), dengue, chikungunya, scabies, leprosy, and rabies (WHO, 2024).

COVID-19 and acute respiratory infections (ARIs) remain significant public health threats in Ethiopia. ARIs, particularly among children younger than 5 years, continue to be a leading cause of morbidity and mortality. In Ethiopia, these infections place a substantial burden on the healthcare system. As of February 25, 2024, Ethiopia had conducted more than 5.5 million COVID-19 tests, resulting in 501,373 confirmed cases and 7,574 deaths, with a case fatality rate (CFR) of 1.5%. The positivity rate (PR) was calculated to be 9%. Despite these figures, only 38% of the population has completed the primary COVID-19 vaccination series, highlighting the ongoing challenges in achieving widespread immunization (Ethiopian Public Health Institute [EPHI], 2024b).

NONCOMMUNICABLE DISEASES

NCDs are a growing public health concern in Ethiopia. The high burden of NCDs is compounded by limited access to essential medications, particularly for diabetes and hypertension. In 2021, the age-standardized mortality rate for four major NCDs (cardiovascular disease, chronic respiratory disease, cancer, and diabetes) was significantly higher for men (631 per 100,000) than for women (549 per 100,000; Awedew et al., 2023). The study by Awedew et al. (2023) highlights the need for increased investment in NCD prevention and treatment in Ethiopia. Between 2010 and 2019, the burden of NCDs in Ethiopia increased significantly. Death counts rose by 21%, incidence cases by 25%, and DALYs by 17%. Heart disease, stroke, chronic kidney disease, and liver cirrhosis were leading causes of death in Ethiopia during 2021 (IHME, n.d.). Modifiable risk factors contributed to 52% of all NCD-related deaths in 2019, highlighting the potential for prevention and intervention.

Despite these challenges, Ethiopia has taken steps to address NCDs. The government developed NCD policies, treatment guidelines, and physical activity recommendations. They implemented tobacco control measures and regularly revise alcohol taxes. However, policies regarding trans fats, salt reduction, and marketing to children require further development. As the population ages, NCDs become more prevalent, and conflicts continue, the need for rehabilitation services will likely increase.

MENTAL HEALTH

Mental health disorders are significant contributors to the burden of disease in Ethiopia, accounting for approximately 15% of mortality. People with mental health disorders often face stigmatization and discrimination. The most common mental health disorders in Ethiopia are depressive disorders (4.65%), anxiety disorders (3.46%), bipolar disorders (0.63%), and schizophrenia (0.5%). From 1990 to 2019, the prevalence of these disorders remained relatively consistent across different regions. Addis Ababa had the highest DALYs due to mental health conditions; the Somali region had the lowest (Ababi et al., 2023).

QUALITY OF LIFE

Ethiopia ranks 175 out of 191 countries on the Human Development Index (HDI), a composite index measuring life expectancy, education, and income. While Ethiopia's HDI score has been improving, it still faces significant health, education, and income challenges (UN Data Portal, 2022). Additionally, Ethiopia ranks 118 out of 121 countries on the 2023 **Digital Quality of Life Index (DQL)**, which assesses internet affordability, quality, infrastructure, security, and e-government.

DETERMINANTS OF HEALTH

HEALTH BEHAVIORS

Ethiopian health practices encompass a wide range of activities that contribute to overall well-being and disease prevention. These include regular exercise, proper nutrition, adequate sleep, avoiding harmful substances, seeking timely medical care, practicing good hygiene, and adhering to vaccination schedules.

Promoting positive health behaviors is crucial for improving quality of life and reducing the burden of preventable diseases in Ethiopia. Government initiatives, community programs, and educational campaigns can play a significant role in raising awareness and encouraging healthy habits. By emphasizing preventive care and empowering individuals to take control of their health, Ethiopia can improve health outcomes and reduce healthcare costs that result from risky behaviors such as unsafe sex, alcohol use, and poor diet, which were among Ethiopia's leading mortality risk factors in 2021 (IHME, n.d.).

SOCIOECONOMIC FACTORS

Ethiopia's economy expanded by 7.1% in 2022/2023, surpassing the previous year's growth rate of 6.4%. The services sector, which accounts for 40% of Ethiopia's gross domestic product (GDP), led the growth at 7.9%. Industry (28% of GDP) grew by 6.9%, and agriculture (32% of GDP) expanded by 6.3%. Despite its economic growth, Ethiopia's per-capita GDP of $1,293.80 in 2023 (World Bank Group, n.d.) places it firmly in the low-income category. Poverty rates have declined from 31.1% in 2016 to 27% in 2019; however, unemployment remains a concern, estimated at 8% in 2020/2022. Approximately 2.5 million new jobs are needed annually to absorb new entrants into the workforce. Additionally, approximately 31.4 million people require humanitarian support due to conflict and climate-related shocks (African Development Bank, 2025). Education is a key driver of economic success; however, Ethiopia faces several challenges in this area, including limited access to education, inadequate educational infrastructure, and a shortage of qualified teachers. According to the UN Educational, Scientific, and Cultural Organization (UNESCO) Institute for Statistics, approximately 48.93% of Ethiopian adults were literate in 2022 (UNESCO Institute for Statistics, 2022).

SOCIAL JUSTICE AND HUMAN RIGHTS

Ethiopia faces significant challenges in the areas of social justice, human rights, and the well-being of marginalized populations. Women, children, people living with disabilities, and ethnic minorities are particularly affected by health inequities and disparities (Lemu, 2019). Social justice issues in Ethiopia include poverty, inequality, and discrimination. Despite progress in poverty reduction, a significant portion of the population still lives in extreme poverty, exacerbating social inequalities and limiting access to basic services. Women and girls often experience gender-based violence, limited education, and economic marginalization. Children, especially in rural areas, may lack access to quality healthcare and education, making them vulnerable to poverty and exploitation. People living with disabilities face barriers to employment, education, and social inclusion. Ethnic minorities encounter discrimination, marginalization, and conflicts, hindering their development and well-being (EPHI, 2024a).

ENVIRONMENTAL AND CLIMATE CHANGE

Human activities, primarily through greenhouse gas emissions, have unequivocally caused global warming. This has led to widespread adverse impacts on food and water security, human health, economies, and society, disproportionately affecting vulnerable communities. Ethiopia is facing significant environmental and climate change challenges, including deforestation, soil erosion, loss of biodiversity, droughts, floods, and unpredictable weather patterns. These issues pose serious threats to Ethiopia's ecosystems, agriculture, and overall sustainability (World Bank Group, n.d.).

HEALTHCARE SYSTEM

BRIEF HISTORY OF HEALTHCARE IN ETHIOPIA

The history of Western medicine in Ethiopia dates back to 1521 when Emperor Lebne Dingil requested physicians and surgeons from the Portuguese king. While Western medicine was initially limited to royal palaces, its influence grew over time as subsequent emperors embraced healthcare advancements (Torrey, 1967). Allopathic medicine was first adopted in Ethiopia during the 16th century, but initial adoption was slow due to limited information and infrastructure.

A turning point came in 1896 with the establishment of a Russian Red Cross Hospital in Addis Ababa. Allopathic healthcare practices continued to expand throughout the 19th century with the construction of additional hospitals. By 1936, Ethiopia had 11 hospitals and a serological facility for vaccine production. However, the war between Ethiopia and Italy from 1936 to 1941 disrupted the expansion of modern medical services. Nevertheless, "hospitals and clinics were gradually added and the country was able to strengthen its overall infrastructure" following the war (Torrey, 1967, p. 278).

Efforts to improve access to modern healthcare in Ethiopia include the establishment of the Public Health Laboratory and Research Institute in 1946, the Ministry of Public Health in 1948, and the Public Health College and Training Center in Gondar in 1954. However, significant challenges remain. Notably, "modern healthcare is very limited, and in many rural areas it is virtually nonexistent," and "only major cities have hospitals with full-time physicians, most of which are in Addis Ababa" (Crummey et al., 2024). Furthermore, the growing demand for healthcare services continues to outpace the number of trained specialists and general practitioners, and a lack of medical equipment and medication further restricts access to modern healthcare in Ethiopia. The Health Sector Development Program has sought to address these shortcomings and improve healthcare coverage and access in 21st-century Ethiopia (WHO, 2024).

HEALTHCARE FINANCING

Ethiopia's healthcare financing has historically been characterized by low government spending and limited private sector participation. Government spending on healthcare has fluctuated over time, influenced by political changes. Per-capita spending has remained below the sub-Saharan African average. According to the Third National Health Accounts (NHA), the government and other public enterprises provide approximately 31% of healthcare financing; donors and non-governmental organizations (NGOs) provide 37%; households provide 31%; and other private employers and funds account for about 2% of healthcare financing. The share of government and household financing has decreased since 1999/2000, while foreign financing and NGOs have grown. To address limitations in the healthcare financing system, the Ethiopian government has implemented various reforms. These include the development of a healthcare financing strategy in 1998 and a health insurance strategy in 2008. The government established **social health insurance (SHI)** for formal sector employees (i.e., workers in government-registered businesses registered with benefits such as social security and medical insurance) and **community-based health insurance (CBHI)** for the agricultural and informal sectors. While there have been implementation and enrollment issues, there is a growing demand for both schemes (FMoH, 2024).

HEALTHCARE TRAINING AND EDUCATION

Ethiopia's medical education landscape has evolved significantly over time. The country's unique political history has shaped its specific trajectory. The Imperial Period (1900–1974) witnessed initial steps toward formal medical training, primarily through missionary hospitals and government-established programs. The establishment of the Gondar Public Health College and the subsequent founding of the Faculty of Medicine at Haile Selassie University marked significant milestones (Woldeyes, 1990). The Socialist Period (1974–1990) presented challenges, including the temporary closure of the medical school and disruptions to training programs. Despite these setbacks, the medical schools in Addis Ababa and Gondar continued to expand, relying heavily on foreign faculty to fill the gaps (Woldemariam & Assefa, 1990). The Developmental Democracy Period (1990–present) ushered in a new era of growth and expansion. Increased medical student intake, staff development, and the opening of new medical schools were key developments. The **New Innovative Medical Education Initiative (NIMEI)** aimed to accelerate the production of healthcare professionals through a shorter medical program.

HEALTHCARE COST, ACCESS, AND QUALITY

Healthcare costs in Ethiopia vary based on facility type, location, and specific services. While healthcare is generally more affordable than in more developed countries, there are still access issues. The Healthcare Access Quality (HAQ) Index measures personal healthcare access and quality based on risk-standardized mortality rates. Ethiopia's HAQ Index improved from 10.6 in 1990 to 28.1 in 2016, with an average annual improvement of 4.4% from 2000 to 2016. In 2019, Ethiopia's national HAQ Index was 33 out of 100, with Addis Ababa performing the best at 45 (National Data Management Center for Health, 2019).

TRADITIONAL MEDICINE

Ethiopia's rich plant life has been a cornerstone of traditional medicine for centuries. These practices, passed down through generations, remain a vital source of healthcare for many Ethiopians, particularly in rural areas. Despite the introduction of modern medicine, an estimated 80% of the population still relies primarily on traditional healing methods. Moreover, over 95% of traditional medical preparations are derived from plants, highlighting the enduring importance of Ethiopia's botanical heritage (EPHI, 2024).

CONCLUSION

Ethiopia, a dynamic nation with a youthful population, faces a "triple burden" of communicable, NCDs, and injuries. Despite advancements in maternal and child health, the country grapples with a rising burden of NCDs, alongside persistent infectious diseases. To ensure sustained progress, Ethiopia must prioritize investments in healthcare, especially for NCDs, and address the multifaceted health needs of its diverse population.

REFERENCES

Ababi Z., Tadesse, S., Taju, A., Berheto, T. M., Agachew, M., Arja, A., Bitew, S., Tollera, G., Dheresa, M., Naghavi, M., & Misganaw, A. (2023). The burden of mental disorders in Ethiopia, from 1990 to 2019: A systematic analysis of the Global Burden of Diseases Study 2019. *Ethiopian Journal of Health Development*, *37*(2), 1–6. https://www.ajol.info/index.php/ejhd/article/view/257583/243297

Awedew, A. F., Berheto, T. M., Dheresa, M., Tadesse, S., Hailemariam, A., Tollera, G., Mohammed, S., Acham, Y., Walker, A., Worku, A., Abebe, B., & Misganaw, A. (2023). The burden of non-communicable diseases and its implications for sustainable development goals across regions in Ethiopia. *Ethiopian Journal of Health Development, 37*(2). https://www.ajol.info/index.php/ejhd/article/view/257585

African Development Bank. (2025). *Homepage*. https://www.afdb.org/en

Britannica. (2024, September 5). *Ethiopia—mountains, plateaus, valleys*. https://www.britannica.com/place/Ethiopia

Central Statistical Agency. (2008). *Summary and statistical report of the 2007 population and housing census results*. Addis Ababa, Ethiopia. https://www.ethiopianreview.com/pdf/001/Cen2007_firstdraft(1).pdf

Corsini, A. (2018). *Operation Solomon: From Ethiopian Jews to Ethiopian Israelis—The Jewish Museum London*. The Jewish Museum London. https://jewishmuseum.org.uk/2018/10/24/operation-solomon-from-ethiopian-jews-to ethiopian-israelis/

Crummey, D. E., Marcus, H. G., & Mehretu, A. (2024, August 26). *Ethiopia*. Encyclopedia Britannica. https://www.britannica.com/place/Ethiopia/Economy

Ethiopian Public Health Institute. (2024a). *Traditional and modern medicine*. Ethiopian Public Health Institute. https://ephi.gov.et/research/traditional-modern-medicine/

Ethiopian Public Health Institute. (2024b). *Public Health Emergency Operations Center and its functions*. https://ephi.gov.et/public-health-emergency/public-health-emergency-management-center-and-its-functions/

Federal Ministry of Health. (2024). *Homepage*. https://www.moh.gov.et/en/node/35?language_content_entity=en.

Institute of Health Metrics and Evaluation. (n.d.). *Ethiopia*. https://www.healthdata.org/research-analysis/health-by-location/profiles/ethiopia

International Organization for Migration. (2021). *More than 800,000 Ethiopians migrated abroad over the past five years*. IOM Regional Office for East and Horn of Africa. https://eastandhornofafrica.iom.int/news/more-800000-ethiopians-migrated-abroad-over-past-five-years

Lemu, A. (2019, September). *Ethnic politics vs. citizenship politics in Ethiopia*. Aiga Forum. https://aigaforum.com/article2019/Citizenship-Politics-Vs-Ethinic-Politics-in-Ethiopia.htm

National Data Management Center for Health. (2019). *Healthcare access and quality profile, 2019*. https://ndmc.ephi.gov.et/ethiopia-healthcare-access-and-quality-profile-2019/

Osoblivaia, T. (2023). *Official and national languages of Ethiopia*. PoliLingua. https://www.polilingua.com/blog/post/official-and-national-languages-of-ethiopia.htm

Qanche, Q., Wondimu, W., Asefa, A., Yosef, T., Midaksa, G., & Nigussie, T. (2021). Factors contributing to high HIV prevalence in Majang Zone, southwest Ethiopia: What lies beneath the tip of the iceberg? *Journal of Multidisciplinary Healthcare, 14*, 3273–3283. https://doi.org/10.2147 jmdh s331708 ON jmulti.org

Torrey, E. F. (1967). Health services in Ethiopia. *The Milbank Memorial Fund Quarterly, 45*(3), 275–285.

UN Data Portal. (n.d.). *UN population division data portal*. United Nations. https://population.un.org/dataportal/home/

UNESCO Institute for Statistics. (2022). *Ethiopia*. https://uis.unesco.org/en/country/et

Woldemariam, T., & Assefa, M. (1990). Historical perspective of Jimma Institute of Health Sciences. *Bulletin of Jimma Institute of Health and Science, 1*(2), 11–19.

Woldeyes, A. (1990). The postliberation period (1941–1973). In R. Pankhurst (Ed.), *An introduction to the medical history of Ethiopia* (pp. 241–264). Red Sea Press.

World Bank Group. (n.d.). *The World Bank open data*. https://data.worldbank.org/

World Health Organization. (2024). *The world health data hub*. https://data.who.int/

CHAPTER 32

UGANDA

Joshua Ojodale Aruwa

INTRODUCTION

The healthcare system in the Republic of Uganda is a multifaceted and decentralized structure that includes various providers and governance levels (Uganda's Ministry of Health [MoH], n.d.). The majority of not-for-profit providers are religiously based, with prominent organizations like the Uganda Catholic Medical Bureau, the Uganda Protestant Medical Bureau, and the Uganda Muslim Medical Bureau. For-profit providers consist of clinics and informal drugstores, while formal providers include medical and dental practitioners, nurses, midwives, pharmacies, and allied health professionals. Traditional providers encompass herbalists, spiritual healers, and traditional birth attendants. Uganda's health system operates on national and district levels, delivering the national minimum healthcare package through a decentralized system. The lowest level comprises **Village Health Teams (VHTs)**, followed by Health Centers II, III, and IV, which provide increasingly comprehensive services. Uganda's MoH coordinates planning, budgeting, policy formulation, and regulation, implementing the Health Sector Strategic and Investment Plan. Governance at the district level is managed by **District Health Management Teams (DHMTs)**, ensuring alignment with national policies and supported by **Health Unit Management Committees (HUMCs)** for community involvement. When considering Uganda's health system, it is important to reflect on how decentralization and diverse provider types impact healthcare delivery and what can be learned from Uganda's approach to addressing healthcare challenges.

GEOGRAPHIC FEATURES

Uganda is a landlocked country in East Africa with a total surface area of approximately 241,038 square kilometers (approximately 150,000 square miles; World Bank Group, n.d.). It is bordered by Kenya to the east, South Sudan to the north, the Democratic Republic of the Congo to the west, Rwanda to the southwest, and Tanzania to the south. The country's diverse geography includes several notable features:

- *Mountain ranges*: Uganda is home to the Rwenzori Mountains, also known as the "Mountains of the Moon," which contain the third highest peak in Africa, Margherita Peak.
- *Lakes and rivers*: The country has extensive freshwater resources, including Lake Victoria, the largest lake in Africa and the source of the Nile River. Other significant lakes include Lake Albert, Lake Edward, and Lake Kyoga.
- *Savannahs and national parks*: Uganda's savannah regions are rich in wildlife, with notable national parks such as Murchison Falls, Queen Elizabeth, and Kidepo Valley, which are vital for conservation and tourism.
- *Forests*: The country has lush tropical forests, including the Bwindi Impenetrable Forest, a UNESCO World Heritage Site known for its population of mountain gorillas.
- *Urban and rural areas*: Kampala, the capital city, is densely populated and serves as the economic and political hub. In contrast, much of the country consists of sparsely populated rural areas where agriculture is the primary livelihood (Uganda Bureau of Statistics, n.d.).

DEMOGRAPHIC FEATURES

Uganda has a rapidly growing and youthful population. At the start of the 21st century, Uganda's population was approximately 24 million; in 2023, it was more than 48.6 million. The median age in 2023 was 16.5 years, and approximately 56% of the population was younger than 20 years. Adults 65 years and older accounted for only an approximate 2% of the total population. Uganda's high birth rate contributes to the youthful demographic, with a birth rate of 35.2 live births per 1,000 people in 2023. It is important to note that while the birth rate in Uganda is high, it has decreased since the start of the 21st century, when the birth rate was 48.2 live births per 1,000 people (UN Data Portal, n.d.).

Uganda's young, rapidly growing population is also ethnically diverse. There are more than 56 recognized ethnic groups in Uganda. The largest ethnic groups include the Baganda, Banyankole, Basoga, Bakiga, and Iteso. Ethnic diversity influences cultural practices, languages, and social structures. Uganda is a multilingual country with more than 40 languages spoken. English is the official language, while Swahili is also widely spoken and recognized as a second official language. **Luganda**, widely spoken in the central region, is one of the most commonly used local languages (Uganda Bureau of Statistics, n.d.). Gender roles and dynamics are deeply influenced by cultural and traditional norms, although there are ongoing efforts toward gender equality. Data on sexual orientation in Uganda are limited due to societal and legal challenges. However, there are emerging discussions and advocacy efforts for the rights of LGBTQ+ individuals despite significant cultural and legal hurdles.

BRIEF COUNTRY HISTORY

The land that makes up present-day Uganda has been inhabited for thousands of years. Early human settlements were established by various Indigenous groups, with significant kingdoms such as Buganda, Bunyoro, Toro, and Ankole emerging in the region. These kingdoms had well-organized political systems and engaged in trade, agriculture, and ironworking long before the arrival of Europeans.

European explorers first arrived in Uganda in the mid-19th century, with the British establishing their influence in the region by the late 19th century. The British declared Uganda a protectorate in 1894, leading to the imposition of colonial rule. This period included the introduction of cash crops like cotton and coffee and the construction of infrastructure such as railways and roads to support colonial economic interests (Kiwanuka, 1968). The impact of British colonial rule on Uganda was far-reaching and devastating, resulting in significant changes to the social, economic, and political fabric of the region. Colonial policies often disrupted traditional governance structures and prioritized the interests of the colonial administration over those of the Indigenous populations. This led to economic inequalities and social tensions that persisted even after independence (Mutibwa, 1992).

Uganda gained independence from British rule on October 9, 1962, with Milton Obote becoming the first prime minister. However, the postindependence period was marked by political instability and conflict. In 1971, General Idi Amin seized power through a military coup, leading to a brutal regime characterized by human rights abuses and economic decline. Amin's rule ended in 1979 when he was overthrown by a coalition of Ugandan exiles and Tanzanian forces (Jørgensen, 1981). Following Amin's ousting, Uganda experienced further political turmoil, with several short-lived governments until Yoweri Museveni's National Resistance Army (NRA) took power in 1986. Museveni's government implemented various reforms aimed at stabilizing the country and promoting economic recovery. Despite these efforts, Uganda has faced ongoing challenges, including political repression, corruption, and regional conflicts (Mutibwa, 1992).

Uganda's recent history centers on economic development and social progress. The country has made significant strides in areas such as healthcare, education, and infrastructure development. However, challenges remain, including poverty, human rights issues, and the need for political reforms to ensure greater democratic governance (World Bank Group, n.d.).

HEALTH OUTCOMES

LIFE EXPECTANCY AT BIRTH

Life expectancy in Uganda has improved significantly over the past several decades. In 2023, life expectancy at birth in Uganda was 68.25 years (Bamba et al., 2024), an increase by more than 20 years from 2000 when life expectancy at birth was 49.64 years (UN Data Portal, n.d.). Despite these gains, Uganda still ranks lower in life expectancy than many other countries. Contributing factors include high rates of infectious diseases, maternal and child mortality, and limited access to healthcare services.

LEADING CAUSES OF MORBIDITY AND MORTALITY

In Uganda, the leading causes of morbidity and mortality include neonatal disorders and several communicable diseases. Figure 32.1 shows the leading causes of mortality in Uganda during 2011 and 2021 (Institute for Health Metrics and Evaluation [IHME], n.d.). While there has been a decrease in mortality from neonatal disorders and communicable diseases from 2011 to 2021, neonatal concerns and infectious diseases remain significant public health challenges in Uganda. In 2021, the major causes of death included neonatal disorders, HIV/AIDS, lower respiratory infections, COVID-19, malaria, tuberculosis, and diarrheal diseases. An estimated 1.4 million people were living with HIV in 2021 (IHME, n.d.). Malaria continues to be a major health issue, particularly among children younger than 5 years, accounting for a high number of hospital admissions and deaths (MoH, n.d.).

While improvements in healthcare have reduced morbidity and mortality from neonatal conditions and some infectious diseases, noncommunicable diseases (NCDs) like cardiovascular diseases, cancer, and diabetes are on the rise (Owachi, 2024). Lifestyle changes, urbanization, and increased life expectancy have contributed to the rise in NCDs. In 2021, NCDs accounted for approximately 27% of total deaths in Uganda (WHO, n.d.), with strokes and heart diseases both the top 10 leading causes of mortality (IHME, n.d.).

FIGURE 32.1 Top 10 leading causes of mortality in Uganda per 100,000 population in 2021 and rate change 2011–2021, all ages combined.

Cause	2011 rank	2021 rank	Change in deaths per 100K, 2011–2021
Malaria	3	1	↑ +3.3
COVID-19	–	2	↑ +95.9
Neonatal disorders	2	3	↓ −42.1
HIV/AIDS	1	4	↓ −80.6
Lower respiratory infections	4	5	↓ −17.8
Stroke	7	6	↓ −1.0
Tuberculosis	5	7	↓ −11.4
Diarrheal diseases	6	8	↓ −17.5
Ischemic heart disease	9	9	↑ +0.4
Congenital defects	8	10	↓ −7.8

● Communicable, maternal, neonatal, and nutritional diseases ● Noncommunicable diseases

Source: Institute for Health Metrics and Evaluation. (n.d.) *Uganda*. https://www.healthdata.org/research-analysis/health-by-location/profiles/uganda

MATERNAL AND INFANT MORTALITY

Maternal and infant mortality rates in Uganda are high but have shown improvement over the years. The maternal mortality ratio was approximately 336 maternal deaths per 100,000 live births in 2021, down from 438 per 100,000 in 2010 (MoH, n.d.). Factors contributing to maternal mortality include inadequate access to skilled birth attendants, poor healthcare infrastructure, and high rates of teenage pregnancies. The infant mortality rate was about 28.3 infant deaths per 1,000 live births in 2023, a significant improvement when compared to 89.2 infant deaths per 1,000 live births in 2000 (UN Data Portal, n.d.). Disparities exist, however, based on geographic location and socioeconomic status (Uganda Bureau of Statistics, n.d.).

MENTAL HEALTH

Mental health issues in Uganda are often underreported and inadequately addressed due to stigma and limited resources. Common mental health conditions include depression, anxiety, and post-traumatic stress disorder, particularly among populations affected by conflict and displacement. Mental health services are scarce, with only a few specialized facilities and a shortage of trained professionals (Kaggwa et al., 2022).

DETERMINANTS OF HEALTH

HEALTH BEHAVIORS

In Uganda, risky behaviors, such as unsafe sex, tobacco use, poor dietary intake, physical inactivity, and alcohol use, significantly impact the prevalence of diseases and overall health outcomes. Adopting healthy behaviors is critical for preventing communicable diseases and NCDs.

Tobacco use remains a significant public health issue in Uganda. According to the Global Adult Tobacco Survey (GATS), about 7.9% of Ugandan adults use tobacco products (GATS, 2013). Smoking and the use of other tobacco products contribute to the rising burden of NCDs, including heart disease, cancer, and respiratory illnesses (Ogbodo & Onyekwum, 2024). Efforts to reduce tobacco use include public awareness campaigns and legislation to control tobacco sales and consumption.

Dietary habits in Uganda are influenced by socioeconomic factors, cultural practices, and food availability. Many Ugandans do not meet the dietary intake recommendations for fruits, vegetables, and whole grains. Instead, the diet is often high in starchy foods, such as maize and plantains, with low intake of protein-rich foods and micronutrients. Malnutrition, including undernutrition and micronutrient deficiencies, remains prevalent, particularly among children younger than 5 years (Amegbor et al., 2020).

Physical inactivity is an emerging concern in Uganda, particularly in urban areas where sedentary lifestyles are becoming more common. WHO recommends at least 150 minutes of moderate-intensity physical activity per week for adults, but many Ugandans, especially those in urban centers, do not meet this guideline (WHO, n.d.). Physical inactivity contributes to the rise in NCDs such as hypertension and diabetes.

Alcohol use in Uganda is widespread, with significant social and health impacts. A study by the MoH indicated that about 10% of Ugandan adults have an alcohol use disorder (MoH, n.d.). Alcohol use disorder is associated with an increased risk of liver disease, accidents, and mental health issues. Community-based interventions and public health campaigns are being implemented to address alcohol use and its consequences.

SOCIAL AND ECONOMIC FACTORS

In Uganda, social and economic determinants, including income, education, and employment, profoundly influence health outcomes with education a critical socioeconomic determinant of health. Higher educational attainment is associated with better health outcomes, improved access to healthcare, and healthier behaviors. However, disparities in educational attainment persist, with rural areas and marginalized groups having lower access to quality education. According to the Uganda Bureau of Statistics, about 70% of Ugandans age 15 years and older are literate, with significant gender and regional disparities (Uganda Bureau of Statistics, n.d.).

Poverty also remains a significant barrier to health in Uganda. World Bank Group (n.d.) reports that about 21.4% of Ugandans lived below the national poverty line in 2021. Poverty limits access to healthcare, nutritious food, clean water, and sanitation. Rural areas are disproportionately affected by poverty, which exacerbates health disparities. Efforts to reduce poverty through economic development and social protection programs are critical to improving health outcomes.

ENVIRONMENTAL FACTORS

Environmental determinants, including access to clean water, sanitation, and living conditions, play a crucial role in health outcomes in Uganda. Access to clean water and adequate sanitation is essential for preventing waterborne diseases and promoting overall health. In 2021, about 72% of Ugandans had access to basic drinking water services, and only 19% had access to basic sanitation services (UNICEF Uganda, n.d.). Lack of access to clean water and sanitation contributes to the prevalence of diarrheal diseases and other health issues, particularly in rural areas. Living conditions, including housing quality and overcrowding, affect health outcomes in Uganda. Poor housing conditions are associated with a higher risk of respiratory infections, vector-borne diseases, and mental health issues. Government and nongovernmental organizations are working to improve living conditions through housing programs and infrastructure development.

HEALTHCARE SYSTEM

FINANCING AND INSURANCE

Uganda's healthcare system is a multipayer model funded by public sources, private contributions, and international aid. Unlike centralized healthcare systems in many wealthy nations that are primarily financed through the government, Uganda relies on a mix of public funding, private payments, and out-of-pocket expenses. The public sector is predominant, especially in rural areas, while private and faith-based organizations significantly contribute to service delivery. Public healthcare financing in Uganda is primarily sourced from government allocations, donor funding, and international aid, accounting for about 50% of healthcare expenditures (World Bank Group, n.d.). The government funds essential health services through initiatives like the Health Sector Development Plan and the Uganda National Minimum Health Care Package (UNMHCP), which provide free services at public facilities. Private healthcare financing includes out-of-pocket payments by patients and contributions from private health insurance schemes. However, private health insurance coverage remains low, covering less than 1% of the population (MoH, n.d.). Most private healthcare costs are paid directly by patients, posing significant access barriers for low-income households.

HEALTHCARE DELIVERY

Healthcare facilities in Uganda are categorized into national referral hospitals, regional referral hospitals, district hospitals, and health centers (HCs) at levels II, III, and IV. There are also private and faith-based hospitals that complement public healthcare services (MoH, n.d.). The following are descriptions of the common healthcare facilities in Uganda:

- ***National referral hospitals*:** Mulago National Referral Hospital and Butabika National Referral Hospital provide specialized care.
- ***Regional referral hospitals*:** Fourteen regional hospitals offer tertiary care across regions.

- *District hospitals and HCs*: Each district has a hospital, with HCs serving at different levels. HC II provides basic outpatient services; HC III offers inpatient and maternity services; and HC IV provides emergency surgical care and blood transfusions.
- ***Community health centers** (CHCs)*: These centers are crucial for delivering primary healthcare services, particularly in rural and underserved areas. CHCs provide essential services like immunizations, maternal and child health, and treatment of common illnesses.
- *Long-term care facilities*: In Uganda, these facilities are limited, with most long-term care provided informally by family members. Institutionalized long-term care facilities, such as nursing homes and hospices, are scarce.

Uganda's healthcare workforce comprises physicians, nurses, midwives, clinical officers, and allied health professionals. The country faces a significant shortage of healthcare workers, especially in rural areas. The doctor-to-population ratio is approximately 1:25,000, far below the WHO's recommended ratio of 1:1,000 (WHO, 2024). Physicians in Uganda undergo rigorous training, including medical school and internships. Efforts to increase the number of physicians include training programs and incentives for working in rural areas. Nurses and midwives are essential for maternal and child health services; they are trained at nursing schools and provide primary and specialized care. Allied health professionals in Uganda include clinical officers, laboratory technicians, pharmacists, and other specialized health workers who support healthcare delivery in Uganda.

TRADITIONAL AND COMPLEMENTARY CARE

Traditional medicine remains an integral part of Uganda's healthcare system. Many Ugandans rely on traditional healers for primary healthcare, especially in rural areas. Traditional healers use herbal medicines, spiritual healing, and other practices passed down through generations. The government recognizes traditional medicine's importance and has established the **National Council for Traditional Healers and Herbalists Associations** to regulate and integrate traditional practices in modern healthcare.

ACCESS, QUALITY, AND COST

Uganda's healthcare system faces significant challenges related to access, quality, and cost (MoH, n.d.). Although public healthcare services are intended to be free, many patients incur out-of-pocket expenses for drugs, diagnostics, and informal payments to healthcare workers. These costs can be prohibitive for low-income households, limiting access to essential services. Out-of-pocket expenditures account for a large portion of healthcare spending, and financial barriers prevent many from seeking timely care. The government and international partners are working to improve healthcare financing mechanisms, such as expanding health insurance coverage and increasing funding for public health programs. The quality of healthcare services varies widely, with significant disparities between urban and rural areas. Urban centers typically have better-equipped facilities and more healthcare workers, while rural areas struggle with shortages of staff, equipment, and supplies.

CONCLUSION

Uganda's healthcare system is characterized by a multipayer model supported by public funding, private contributions, and international aid. While the system has made significant strides in improving healthcare access and outcomes, it continues to face substantial challenges. Challenges include a shortage of healthcare workers, particularly in rural areas, and significant disparities in healthcare quality and access between urban and rural populations. Public healthcare financing covers a substantial portion of healthcare expenditures, but out-of-pocket costs remain a barrier for many low-income households. Efforts to address these challenges include expanding public health programs, increasing healthcare funding, and integrating traditional medicine with modern healthcare practices.

The history of Uganda's healthcare system reflects its journey from rudimentary beginnings to a more structured and scientifically informed approach, with recent reforms focusing on improving access, quality, and cost-efficiency. Continued investment in healthcare infrastructure, workforce training, and health insurance coverage is crucial for enhancing Uganda's healthcare system. By addressing these key areas, Uganda can work toward achieving better health outcomes for its population, ensuring that healthcare services are accessible, affordable, and of high quality for all Ugandans.

REFERENCES

Amegbor, P. M., Yankey, O., & Sabel, C. E. (2020). Examining the effect of geographic region of residence on childhood malnutrition in Uganda. *Journal of Tropical Pediatrics, 66*(6), 598–611. https://doi.org/10.1093/TROPEJ/FMAA019

Bamba, G., abboud, J. A., Olal, E., & Kitara, D. L. (2024). Comparative analysis of the evolution of life expectancy in the United Republic of Tanzania, Uganda, and Kenya in 61 years (1960–2021): A secondary data analysis of the World Population Prospects (WPPs) on the three East African countries. *MedRxiv*. https://doi.org/10.1101/2024.04.12.24305722

Global Adult Tobacco Survey. (2013). *2013 GATS country report Uganda*. WHO. https://www.who.int/publications/m/item/2013-gats-country-report-ugand

Institute for Health Metrics and Evaluation. (n.d.). *Uganda*. https://www.healthdata.org

Jorgensen, J. J. (1981). *Uganda: A modern history*. Routledge.

Kaggwa, M. M., Harms, S., & Mamun, M. A. (2022). Mental health care in Uganda. *The Lancet Psychiatry, 9*(10), 766–767. https://doi.org/10.1016/S2215-0366(22)00305-4

Kiwanuka, M. S. M. (1968). Bunyoro and the British: A reappraisal of the causes for the decline and fall of an African kingdom. *The Journal of African History, 9*(4), 603–619. https://doi.org/10.1017/S0021853700009063

Mutibwa, P. (1992). *Uganda since independence: A story of unfulfilled hopes*. Africa World Press.

Ogbodo, S. C., & Onyekwum, C. A. (2024). Social determinants of health, religiosity, and tobacco use in sub-Saharan Africa: Evidence from the global adult tobacco surveys in seven countries. *Journal of Public Health, 32*(6), 895–908. https://doi.org/10.1007/s10389-023-01882-9

Owachi, D. (2024). *Open access BMC infectious diseases*. https://doi.org/10.1186/s12879-024-09112-7

Uganda Bureau of Statistics. (n.d.). *Explore statistics: Public health*. https://www.ubos.org/explore-statistics/25/#

Uganda's Ministry of Health. (n.d.). *Ministry of health: Republic of Uganda*. https://www.health.go.ug/

UN Data Portal. (n.d.). *UN Population division data portal: Interactive access to global demographic indicators*. United Nations. https://population.un.org/dataportal/home

UNICEF Uganda. (n.d.). *Water, sanitation and hygiene (WASH)*. https://www.unicef.org/uganda/what-we-do/wash

World Bank Group. (n.d.). *The World Bank open data*. https://data.worldbank.org/

World Health Organization. (2024). *Uganda*. https://data.who.int/countries/800

CHAPTER 33

TANZANIA

Kathleen Visovatti Weaver and Thomas Foley

GEOGRAPHY

Tanzania, officially the United Republic of Tanzania, is the 13th largest country in all of Africa and the second largest in Eastern Africa. Tanzania's total surface area is 947,300 square kilometers (588,624 square miles) of which 885,800 square kilometers (550,410 square miles) cover land (World Bank Group, n.d.). Tanzania is on the eastern side of Africa with Kenya and Uganda to its north, Mozambique to its south, Zambia to its southwest, and the Indian Ocean on its eastern border. Zanzibar, an archipelago with more than 50 islands and islets, is a semiautonomous zone of Tanzania located in the Indian Ocean. Tanzania also includes Mount Kilimanjaro (Figure 33.1), which is the highest African mountain. Remarkable geographic features such as Mount Kilimanjaro and Zanzibar help make Tanzania a popular tourist and safari destination.

THE ECONOMY

Tanzania is resource abundant with one of Africa's leading and rapidly developing economies. The major contributors to Tanzania's economic power are manufacturing, tourism, and agriculture. Agriculture is the leading employment industry (Mascarenhas et al., 2020). Tanzania's 2023 unemployment rate was only 2.6%. However, Tanzania, along with most other East African countries, has low per capita gross national product (GDP). In 2023, the per-capita GDP in Tanzania was approximately $1,225. The poverty rate in Tanzania, which has been decreasing during the 21st century, is about 26% (World Bank Group, n.d.).

HUMAN RIGHTS

There are several noted human right concerns in Tanzania (U.S. Department of State [DoS], 2022). These human right concerns include

- government restricted access to the internet,
- arresting and prosecuting the media for language against the government,
- restricting peaceful assembly,
- domestic violence against women is not protected by law,
- female genital mutilation is still allowed on women over the age of 18 years,
- reproductive health services are limited by environmental barriers and negative actions by service providers,
- corporal punishment by teachers in schools is allowed, and
- although there are laws about what age someone can marry, girls as young as 7 years old can be arranged in a forced marriage where a dowry is paid to the bride's parents.

ENVIRONMENTAL CLIMATE CHANGE ISSUES

Severe drought conditions make water scarcity a major environmental concern in Tanzania and affect farming crops and livestock. Forests in Tanzania, especially in rural areas, are a part of the ongoing water cycle. In the rural areas, however, Tanzanians use trees for firewood, causing

FIGURE 33.1 Mount Kilimanjaro.

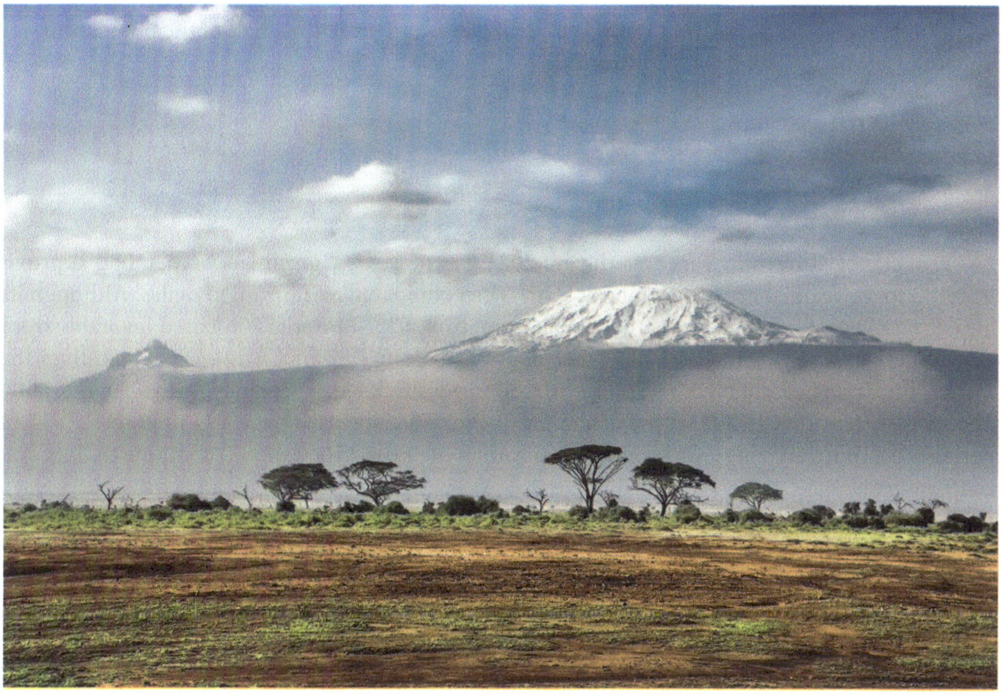

Source: Pesterev, S. (2012). *View of Kilimanjaro from Amboseli National Park, Kenya*. https://commons.wikimedia.org/wiki/File:Kilimanjaro_from_Amboseli.jpg

deforestation that contributes to drought conditions. In order to combat the inability to farm due to droughts, the rural populations have resorted to other means to improve their income such as beekeeping and sewing (UN Environment Programme, 2024).

BRIEF HISTORY

Archeologists have designated Tanzania as a "Cradle of Mankind." Some of the oldest human fossils, estimated at 3.6 million years old, were located in the area, making it a "birthplace of humanity, and the oldest known footprints" (Embassy of the United Republic of Tanzania, n.d.). The Indigenous populations were basic hunter–gatherers. Migration into the area brought agriculture, cattle farming, food production, and political organization. As the country grew, it became a trading location for gold, ivory, and other goods along with being the center for the Arab slave trade (Embassy of the United Republic of Tanzania, n.d.). Via colonization, several countries influenced culture and society in Tanzania, including Portugal, Persia, Britain, Oman, Germany, and France.

Prior to 1964, modern day Tanzania was two separate countries: Tanganyika, which was on the mainland of Africa; and the Zanzibar islands. In 1964, Tanganyika and Zanzibar unified into one country, becoming the United Republic of Tanzania. Prior to unification, both Tanganyika and Zanzibar were under British rule—Tanganyika as a British colony and Zanzibar as a British protectorate. After 40 years of being ruled as a colony of Britain, Tanganyika gained its independence in 1961. As well, after more than 70 years of being a protectorate, Zanzibar gained its independence from Britain in October of 1963 (Embassy of the United Republic of Tanzania, n.d.).

POPULATION

The population in Tanzania during 2023 was approximately 66.6 million people, making Tanzania the second most populous country in Eastern Africa and the fifth most populous country in all of

Africa. The population of Tanzania is predominately rural as only approximately one third lives in urban areas. Tanzania's population is also young; the median age of Tanzanians in 2023 was 17.2 years. Only 3% of the population was 65 years or older, and more than half of the population was under the age of 20 (UN Data Portal, n.d.).

HEALTH OUTCOMES

LIFE EXPECTANCY

Life expectancy at birth in Tanzania during 2023 was 67 years. Tanzanian women had approximately 5 more years of life expectancy at birth when compared to Tanzanian males. Although its life expectancy at birth was below the global average in 2023, Tanzania compared favorably from a regional perspective. The 2023 life expectancy at birth in Tanzania was greater than then the average life expectancy at birth in Eastern Africa. In addition, life expectancy from birth is rapidly improving. From 2000 to 2023, life expectancy in Tanzania increased by nearly 14 years (UN Data Portal, n.d.). With an emerging economy, Tanzanian life expectancy should continue to improve.

INFANT AND MATERNAL MORTALITY

While Tanzania has high infant and maternal mortality, there are indicators of recent success in the prevention of such deaths. In 2023, the infant mortality rate in Tanzania was 28.9 infant deaths per 1,000 live births, which was near the global rate and well below the Eastern Africa regional rate. In addition, infant mortality has drastically decreased in Tanzania during the 21st century; in 2000, the infant mortality rate in Tanzania was 83.2 infant deaths per 1,000 live births. The maternal mortality ratio in Tanzania during 2021was 283.3 maternal deaths per 100,000 live births, which was also similar to the global ratio and well below the regional ratio (UN Population Fund, n.d.).

LEADING CAUSES OF MORTALITY

Tanzania experiences significant mortality from preventable infectious diseases and maternal–child health issues, as is the case in most African countries. In 2021, the leading causes of death in Tanzania were COVID-19, HIV/AIDS, neonatal disorders, lower respiratory tract infections, stroke, ischemic heart disease, diarrheal diseases, malaria, tuberculosis, and congenital defects (Figure 33.2). With the exception of deaths due to heart disease, the mortality rates for these leading causes have been decreasing (Institute for Health Metrics and Evaluation [IHME], n.d.). As Tanzania's economy continues to improve, it will be imperative to stress the importance of preventing an increase in noncommunicable diseases such as heart disease.

LEADING MORBIDITY AND MORTALITY RISK FACTORS

The leading morbidity and mortality risk factors in Tanzania during 2021 were malnutrition, air pollution, unsafe sex, water/sanitation/hygiene (WaSH), hypertension, dietary risks, tobacco use, obesity, hyperglycemia, and occupational hazards (Figure 33.3). The morbidity and mortality attributed to malnutrition, air pollution, unsafe sex, WaSH, tobacco use, and occupational hazards have declined since 2011. However, the impact on disease and death from hypertension, dietary risks, obesity, and hyperglycemia has increased, which is reflected in the increase in mortality from heart disease (IHME, n.d.). Promoting health education about heart-healthy lifestyles and diabetes prevention are needed in Tanzania as it develops economically.

CULTURE

Tanzania is a culturally diverse area with approximately 120 ethnic groups and more than 100 spoken languages. Swahili is the official language; however, most Tanzanians speak both English and

FIGURE 33.2 Leading causes of death in Tanzania in 2011 and 2021.

Cause	2011 rank	2021 rank	Change in deaths per 100K, 2011–2021
COVID-19	–	1	↑ +109.6
HIV/AIDS	1	2	↓ −89.1
Neonatal disorders	2	3	↓ −32.3
Lower respiratory infection	3	4	↓ −29.2
Stroke	5	5	↓ −2.8
Ischemic heart disease	8	6	↑ +3.4
Diarrheal diseases	4	7	↓ −28.0
Malaria	7	8	↓ −6.9
Tuberculosis	6	9	↓ −13.1
Congenital defects	9	10	↓ −11.3

Communicable, maternal, neonatal, and nutritional diseases
Noncommunicable diseases

Source: Institute of Health Metrics and Evaluation. (n.d.). *United Republic of Tanzania*. https://www.healthdata.org/research-analysis/health-by-location/profiles/tanzania

FIGURE 33.3 Leading morbidity and mortality risk factors in Tanzania in 2011 and 2021.

Risk	2011 rank	2021 rank	Change in DALYs per 100K, 2011–2021
Malnutrition	1	1	↓ −6,679.4
Air pollution	3	2	↓ −1,963.4
Unsafe sex	2	3	↓ −3,858.3
WaSH	4	4	↓ −2,523.5
High blood pressure	5	5	↑ +35.2
Dietary risks	7	6	↑ +15.1
Tobacco	6	7	↓ −245.1
High body-mass index	11	8	↑ +143.4
High fasting plasma glucose	10	9	↑ +74.7
Occupational risks	8	10	↓ −103.2

Behavioral risks Metabolic risks
Environmental/occupational risks

DALY, disability-adjusted life year; WaSH, water/sanitation/hygiene.

Source: Institute of Health Metrics and Evaluation. (n.d.). *United Republic of Tanzania*. https://www.healthdata.org/research-analysis/health-by-location/profiles/tanzania

Swahili. Religion and religious practices are an integral part of the Tanzanian culture. Christianity and Islam are the most common religions with a smaller percent of the population practicing traditional Indigenous religions, Hinduism, and Buddhism. Zanzibar, however, is predominately Muslim (DoS, 2022).

POLITICAL SYSTEM

Tanzania, which officially unified as a country in 1964 after gaining independence from British rule, enacted its Constitution in 1977. Tanzania added a Bill of Rights in 1984. The President of the United Republic is the head of the country and commander of the armed forces. The President rules with an advisory Cabinet. The government is unicameral, having only one national legislative body (Mascarenhas et al., 2020). The unicameral structure of its legislative body is unlike that of the United States, which has a bicameral Congress with the Senate and House of Representatives, and the United Kingdom's Parliament, which has the House of Commons and the House of Lords.

EDUCATION SYSTEM

The education system in Tanzania is based on the British system, which includes 7 years of primary education, 6 years of secondary and advanced education, and, after passing the Advanced Certificate Exam, the opportunity to attend college. University programs are 3 years. The education system supports two levels of higher education: the University level, which focuses on diplomas and degrees for professional qualifications, and the Higher Education level, which offers Bachelor degree programs. Approximately 335,000 students are enrolled in higher education, seeking professional and Bachelor degrees. The three top fields of study are education, business, and medicine and health sciences (Tanzania Commission for Universities, 2023).

Approximately 1.2 million Tanzanian children have never attended school and only 27% of children attend secondary schooling (UNICEF, n.d.). There are efforts to encourage more girls to attend school. The healthcare system finds it difficult to expand and meet the healthcare needs of the populations, making the dearth of students pursuing degrees in medicine and the health sciences especially problematic.

HEALTH CARE SYSTEM

HEALTH INSURANCE AND FINANCING

Tanzania is progressing toward universal healthcare coverage. Major healthcare schemes in Tanzania include the National Health Insurance Fund (NHIF), which it started in 1999, and the Community Health Fund (CHF), which started in 2000. While the NHIF is mandatory for employers and employees, participation in the CHF is voluntary. These schemes help to reduce out-of-pocket expenses and to improve the quality of care due to improved reimbursement. Participation in any health insurance scheme in Tanzania, however, is low, often because Tanzanians find it difficult to pay insurance premiums on a regular basis. Out-of-pocket expenses are problematic in Tanzania, accounting for about 22% of healthcare expenditures (Mori, 2023).

HEALTH SERVICES

Healthcare facilities are more available in urban areas. Approximately 60% of healthcare facilities are operated by the government and 40% are operated by faith-based or private entities (Ministry of Health [MoH], 2024). Hospitals are arranged within the 26 regions of the country. Some regions have several hospitals while others only have one hospital. In total, there is less than one bed per 1,000 population. In 2018, there were approximately 2,600 physicians and 20,800 nurses in Tanzania (Cowling, 2024), which equated to less than one physician or nurse per 1,000 population. Pharmacies are connected to hospitals in large urban areas, but very limited in rural areas (MoH, 2024).

Tanzania has a Mental Health Association, two mental health hospitals, five mental health service centers located in general hospitals, and four mental health residential facilities. The mental health workforce of physicians, nurses, social workers, psychologists, and occupational therapists does not meet the needs of the population (Ambikile & Isesselo, 2023). The limited infrastructure of mental health services impacts the quality of mental health care in Tanzania.

TRADITIONAL HEALTHCARE

Because there are limited biomedical resources in Tanzania, traditional medicine is practiced throughout the country. Approximately 80% of the population seeks care and treatment from traditional healers, shamans, and plants and herbs.

CONCLUSION

Tanzania is a country of remarkable beauty and economic promise. Its large, youthful population, abundant resources, popular tourist locations, and diverse cultural makeup should place Tanzania in a good position to promote health equity. However, Tanzania needs to develop its biomedical healthcare system with more inland healthcare services in the rural areas to complement traditional healing practices. Doing so should result in continued decreases in incidences of preventable infectious diseases and maternal and infant deaths. In addition, Tanzania needs to bolster primary and secondary prevention of noncommunicable diseases such as heart disease and diabetes to mitigate their increasing prevalence.

LEARNING ACTIVITIES

CourseConnect

To access self-assessment questions and interactive, competency-based learning activities for this chapter, visit www.springerpub.com/courseconnect. See inside front cover and tear-out for CourseConnect details.

REFERENCES

Ambikile, J.S., & Iseselo, M.K. (2023). Challenges to the provision of home care and support for people with severe mental illness: Experiences and perspectives of patients, cargivers, and healthcare providers in Dar es Salaam, Tanzania, *PLOS Global Public Health, 3*(1), e0001518. https://doi.org/10.1371/journal.pgph.0001518

Cowling, N. (2024). *Medical staff in Tanzania 2018, by category*. Statista. https://www.statista.com/statistics/1249293/number-of-medical-personnel-in-tanzania-by-category

Embassy of the United Republic of Tanzania. (n.d.). *Brief history*. https://www.de.tzembassy.go.tz/tanzania/category/history

Institute of Health Metrics and Evaluation. (n.d.). *Health research by location: Country profiles*. University of Washington. https://www.healthdata.org/research-analysis/health-by-location/profiles

Mascarenhas, A.C., Bryceson, D.F., Ingham, K., & Chiteji, F.M. (2020). *Tanzania*. Britannica. https://www.britannica.com/place/Tanzania

Ministry of Health. (2024). *Health facility registry*. https://hfrs.moh.go.tz/web/index.php

Mori, A.T. (2023). Mandatory health insurance for the informal sector in Tanzania—Has it worked anywhere? *Frontiers in Health Services*, 3, 1247301. https://doi.org/10.3389/frhs.2023.1247301

Tanzania Commission for Universities. (2023). *VitalStats on university education in Tanzania 2023*. https://www.tcu.go.tz/publications/higher-education-statistics

UN Data Portal. (n.d.). *UN population division data portal: Interactive access to global demographic indicators*. United Nations. https://population.un.org/dataportal/home

UN Environment Programme. (2024). *On front lines of climate change, Tanzanian communities search for answers to deepening drought*. https://www.unep.org/news-and-stories/story/front-lines-climate-change-tanzanian-communities-search-answers-deepening

UNICEF. (n.d.). *Maternal and child health*. https://www.unicef.org/tanzania/media/711/file/UNICEF-Tanzania-2017-MCH-fact-sheet.pdf

UN Population Fund. (2024). *Data portal*. United Nations. https://www.unfpa.org/data

U.S. Department of State. (2022). *2022 country reports on human rights practices: Tanzania*. https://www.state.gov/reports/2022-country-reports-on-human-rights-practices/tanzania/

World Bank Group. (n.d.). *The World Bank open data*. https://data.worldbank.org/

PART IX. Health and Healthcare in Middle and Southern Africa

CHAPTER 34

OVERVIEW OF MIDDLE AND SOUTHERN AFRICA

Anna Foucek Tresidder

INTRODUCTION

Middle and Southern Africa are diverse and dynamic subregions of Africa. They are characterized by varied geographic, socioeconomic, and cultural landscapes. The health systems of countries such as South Africa, Botswana, Zimbabwe, Rwanda, Namibia, and Eswatini face unique challenges due to historical legacies, high disease burdens, and resource constraints. Health outcomes in the region reflect persistent inequities, with marginalized groups disproportionately affected by preventable diseases and limited access to care. Despite these challenges, there have been notable strides in combating major public health issues, such as HIV/AIDS and maternal mortality.

GEOGRAPHY

Middle and Southern Africa span diverse terrains, from Namibia and Botswana's arid deserts to Mozambique and Zimbabwe's subtropical climates (Figure 34.1). These variations profoundly influence health systems, particularly regarding healthcare access and disease prevalence. Rural areas, constituting about 60% of the population in many countries, face logistical challenges in accessing healthcare due to long distances and lack of roads and transportation to facilities (World Bank Group, 2022); for example, Namibia's vast desert regions necessitate **mobile clinics** to reach isolated communities. Malaria is endemic in wetter areas such as Mozambique, contributing to more than 5,000 deaths annually (World Health Organization [WHO], 2022). Conversely, arid areas report higher respiratory disease rates, exacerbated by dust and limited ventilation.

HISTORY

Colonial histories left indelible marks on political and health systems in Middle and Southern Africa, creating inequitable structures for Indigenous populations. For example, in the country of South Africa, apartheid-era policies established a tiered healthcare system, favoring urban and White populations while marginalizing rural and Indigenous Black communities. Although postapartheid reforms increased healthcare access, disparities persist, with only 20% of the population receiving private healthcare (National Department of Health, South Africa, 2021). Zimbabwe achieved early successes in immunization, with coverage exceeding 80% by the late 1980s, but economic instability has reversed these gains, leaving maternal mortality at 458 deaths per 100,000 live births. Botswana, leveraging diamond revenues, built one of the most robust healthcare systems in the region, with **antiretroviral therapy (ART)** coverage exceeding 90% for HIV-positive individuals (UNAIDS, 2022).

FIGURE 34.1 Map of Southern Africa.

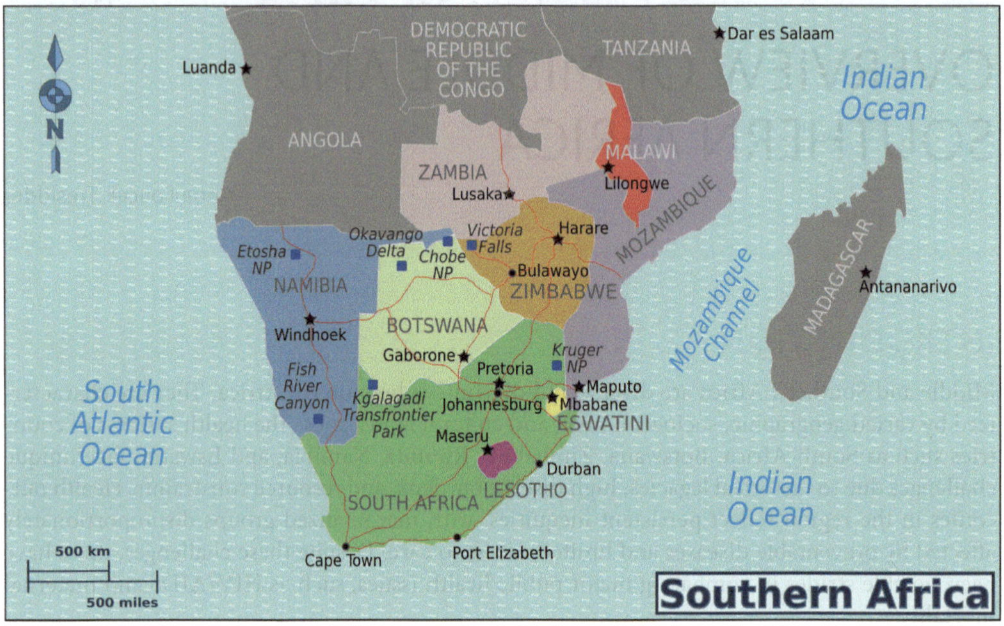

Source: Burmesedays. (2010). *Southern Africa new map*. https://commons.wikimedia.org/wiki/File:Southern_Africa_new_map.png

POPULATION

The populations of Middle and Southern Africa are predominantly young, with over 60% under 25 years (World Bank Group, 2022). This creates significant demand for maternal and child health services in many countries. Eswatini, with an HIV prevalence rate of 27%, has seen substantial reductions in mortality due to ART programs, yet 58% of orphans in the country are AIDS-related (UNAIDS, 2022). Urbanization, increasing at 4% annually in the region, transforms health needs—for example, in informal settlements where overcrowding and poor sanitation drive outbreaks of diseases like cholera in Mozambique and South Africa.

SOCIOECONOMIC FACTORS

Health outcomes in Middle and Southern Africa are deeply tied to socioeconomic disparities. South Africa, with a Gini coefficient of 0.63, exemplifies stark inequality: While private hospitals provide world-class care, public hospitals suffer from underfunding and workforce and resource shortages (World Bank Group, 2022). Zimbabwe's economic instability has contributed to a "**brain drain**," with 60% of trained healthcare workers migrating abroad for better opportunities. Educational attainment varies: Botswana's investment in universal primary education correlates with high health literacy, while Mozambique's literacy rate of 60% hinders health understanding (UNESCO, 2022). Food insecurity compounds health challenges. Malnutrition affects 33% of children younger than 5 years in Malawi and Zambia, while rates of obesity exceed 25% in South Africa, highlighting the region's wide-ranging burden of disease (UNICEF, 2023).

HEALTH OUTCOMES

Middle and Southern Africa bear a dual disease burden (Table 34.1), with infectious diseases coexisting alongside rising noncommunicable diseases (NCDs). HIV/AIDS remains the leading health challenge, with Botswana, Lesotho, and Eswatini reporting adult prevalence rates exceeding 20% (UNAIDS, 2022). ART has dramatically improved survival, reducing HIV-related mortality by 60% since 2010. Maternal and neonatal health varies widely: Namibia reports a maternal mortality ratio of 195 deaths per 100,000 live births due to skilled birth attendance, while Mozambique exceeds 289 deaths per 100,000 due to healthcare access barriers (WHO, 2022). NCDs, such as diabetes and cardiovascular diseases, are surging. South Africa reports a diabetes prevalence of 12% among adults (International Diabetes Federation, 2022). Mental health remains underaddressed, with limited facilities and underreporting due to pervasive stigma.

CONCLUSION

The health systems of Middle and Southern African countries reflect the interplay of geography, history, and socioeconomic determinants. While the region has made significant progress in combating infectious diseases and expanding healthcare access, challenges remain, particularly in addressing disparities and the rising burden of NCDs. Strengthening health systems requires investment in infrastructure, human resources, and equitable financing. Regional collaboration and international partnerships will be pivotal in addressing shared challenges and advancing the goal of universal health coverage.

TABLE 34.1 LIFE EXPECTANCY AND MORTALITY RATES IN MIDDLE AND SOUTHERN AFRICA, 2022–2023

COUNTRY	LIFE EXPECTANCY AT BIRTH (YEARS)	INFANT MORTALITY RATE (PER 1,000 LIVE BIRTHS)	MATERNAL MORTALITY RATIO (PER 100,000 LIVE BIRTHS)	LEADING CAUSE OF DEATH
Angola	61.1	72	241	Malaria
Botswana	66.8	31	144	HIV/AIDS
Eswatini	59.8	43	437	HIV/AIDS
Lesotho	55.3	59	544	HIV/AIDS
Madagascar	67.2	35	335	Lower respiratory infections
Malawi	65.4	37	349	HIV/AIDS
Mozambique	60.7	65	289	Malaria
Namibia	63.1	35	195	HIV/AIDS
Nigeria	55.0	72	917	Lower respiratory infections
Rwanda	69.4	29	203	Neonatal conditions
South Africa	64.5	25	119	HIV/AIDS
Zambia	64.4	45	213	HIV/AIDS
Zimbabwe	65.5	37	458	HIV/AIDS

Note: Leading causes of death are based on WHO Global Health Estimates, considering the predominance of diseases like HIV/AIDS in Southern Africa and malaria in Middle Africa.

Sources: World Health Organization. (2022). *Global health observatory data repository: Southern Africa*. https://www.who.int; World Bank Group. (2022). *World development indicators database*. https://data.worldbank.org.

LEARNING ACTIVITIES

CourseConnect

To access self-assessment questions and interactive, competency-based learning activities for this chapter, visit www.springerpub.com/courseconnect. See inside front cover and tear-out for CourseConnect details.

REFERENCES

International Diabetes Federation. (2022). *IDF diabetes atlas* (10th ed.). https://diabetesatlas.org

National Department of Health, South Africa. (2021). *Annual health statistics report 2021.* https://www.unaids.org/en/resources/fact-sheet

UNAIDS. (2022). *Global HIV and AIDS statistics—Fact sheet.* https://www.unaids.org

UNESCO. (2022). *Global education monitoring report: Southern Africa focus.* https://www.unesco.org

UNICEF. (2023). *The state of the world's children 2023: Food security and nutrition.* https://www.unicef.org

World Bank Group. (2022). *World development indicators database.* https://databank.worldbank.org/source/world-development-indicators

World Health Organization. (2022). *Global health observatory data repository: Southern Africa.* https://www.who.int

CHAPTER 35

RWANDA

Victor Bassey Archibong, Abdullahi Abiodun Mohammed,
Samson Ehindero Olorunnado, Mathias Ruhosha,
Jean Paul Rugambwa, and Olivier Kubwimana

GEOGRAPHY, SIZE, AND DEMOGRAPHICS

Rwanda's western and north-central regions are dominated by mountains and foothills of the Congo–Nile Divide, the Virunga Volcano range, and the northern highlands. Events have influenced Rwanda's development in the Great Lakes region of Banyarwanda, which includes the neighboring countries of eastern Zaire (Congo), Uganda, northwestern Tanzania, and Burundi. The Banyarwanda region is populated by people who speak the Kinyarwanda language and share a common heritage throughout modern history (Sellstrom et al., 1996).

IMPORTANT GEOGRAPHIC FEATURES AND DIVISIONS

Rwanda is a small, landlocked country in east-central Africa (Rwanda Basic Education Board [REB], 2023). It is located south of the Equator between 104' and 2051' south latitude and 28063' and 30054' east longitude. Due to its mountainous terrain, Rwanda is known as the Land of a Thousand Hills (Institut National de la Statistique du Rwanda and ORC Macro, 2006).

POPULATION

Based on the general population census of August 2022, the population of Rwanda has increased from 12,089,720 in 2018 (Rurangwa & Whittaker, 2020) to 13,246,394 in 2022. The life expectancy at birth is now 69.6 years, increasing from 51.2 years in 2002 to 64.5 years in 2012 (National Institute of Statistics of Rwanda [NISR], 2023). The population breakdown of Rwanda shows that females make up the majority at 6,817,068 (51.5%), while males are the minority (48.5%) at 6,429,326 (NISR, 2023). There are no data on the transgender population in Rwanda.

URBAN/RURAL AND AGE DISTRIBUTION

About 83% of the Rwandan population live in rural areas, with one in every two persons younger than 19 years. People age 65 years and older constitute 3% of the resident population (NISR, Ministry of Finance and Economic Planning [MINECOFIN], 2012). Administratively, Rwanda is divided into five provinces according to their geographic positioning. The provinces are Kigali City, Northern Province, Eastern Province, Southern Province, and Western Province (NISR, MINECOFIN, 2012).

RACIAL AND ETHNIC GROUPS

Rwanda is made up of three main ethnic groups: Hutus (85%), Tutsi (14%), and Twa (1%; Europa Publications Staff, 1998; Rwanda Assessment, 2000). Historians believe that the Twa were the original inhabitants of Rwanda from as early as 2000 BCE. However, around 1000 CE, the Hutus displaced the Twa and became the dominant group in the region. Between the 11th and 15th centuries, the Tutsi immigrated to the area and established the geographic entity of present-day Rwanda (Sellstrom et al., 1996).

CULTURAL BELIEFS

RELIGIONS

The two predominant religions in Rwanda are Christianity and Islam. Roman Catholicism remains the religion of choice for over two fifths of Rwandans, followed by Adventism, with over one tenth of the population. About 38% of the country's population identifies as Protestant (Britannica n.d.). Traditional African beliefs also persist and often blend with Christianity (Schliesser, 2018; Simonsson, 2019).

LANGUAGES

While Kinyarwanda is the official language, French and English also hold official status, reflecting the country's complex colonial past. However, there has been a recent shift toward English as the primary language for education and government functions (Government of Rwanda, n.d.).

POLITICAL SYSTEM

The president of Rwanda is both the head of state and head of government. The political climate is characterized by a commitment to national unity, reconciliation, and socioeconomic development (Government of Rwanda, n.d.). Rwanda is a constitutional republic with a multiparty political system. Like other democracies, it has three distinct branches—the executive, legislature, and judiciary—that operate independently while complementing each other.

IMPORTANT TRADITIONS, PRACTICES, EVENTS, AND LEISURE PURSUITS

In Rwanda, oral tradition holds a powerful presence, with a great emphasis on storytelling and poetry. Celebrating harvests and showing gratitude is a revered practice in the form of the Umuganura Festival. The rich cultural heritage of Rwanda is showcased through traditional dances like the Intore dance (Dahlmanns, 2015; Grayson, 2017; Kingston, 2015). Additionally, the regular community work day, known as *umuganda,* reminds Rwandans of the vital role collective participation plays in nation building (Britannica, n.d.; Dahlmanns, 2015).

HISTORICAL CONSIDERATIONS

The aftermath of the 1994 genocide has undeniably shaped Rwanda's journey toward reconciliation, unity, and rebuilding. President Paul Kagame's Rwandan government has prioritized initiatives aimed at national healing, economic growth, and social harmony. One notable example is the implementation of the Gacaca courts, which have played a crucial role in promoting accountability and fostering reconciliation in the aftermath of the genocide. The nation's commitment to unity and progress is a testament to the transformative power of reconciliation and collective efforts in overcoming adversity (Grayson, 2017; Kingston, 2015).

HEALTH OUTCOMES

TOP 10 CAUSES OF DEATH

The healthcare system in Rwanda has gone through significant changes over the years. However, despite the improvements, the causes of mortality remain a concern. The most common causes of mortality in Rwanda include: (a) prematurity and low birth weight, (b) birth asphyxia and birth trauma, (c) nephritis and nephrosis, (d) cerebrovascular disease, (e) HIV/AIDS, (f) road traffic accidents, (g) diabetes mellitus, (h) lower respiratory infections, (i) endocrine disorders, and (j) tuberculosis (TB; World Health Organization [WHO], 2022b).

MENTAL HEALTH

According to a survey conducted in 2018, mental health disorders were found to be more common among women (23.2%) than men (16.6%). The most prevalent disorders noted were major depressive episodes (12%), panic disorders (8.1%), and posttraumatic stress disorder or PTSD (3.6%; Kayiteshonga et al., 2022). Among genocide survivors, more women (53.3%) were affected by mental health disorders than men (48.8%). The most common disorders found were major depressive episodes (35%), PTSD (27.9%), and panic disorders (26.8%; Kayiteshonga et al., 2022).

Epilepsy is generally the primary cause of mental health consultation, accounting for 52% of cases. However, most of these cases can be managed at district hospitals since the Ministry of Health (MoH) has decentralized their treatment (MoH, 2011).

INFECTIOUS DISEASES

Malaria is a common disease in Rwanda. However, the country has implemented adequate measures to reduce the mortality and hospitalization rates associated with the disease. HIV/AIDS and HIV-TB coinfection are also present in Rwanda. Still, the country has strengthened its TB control measures, leading to a reduction in HIV-TB coinfection cases. According to WHO's 2018 report, the prevalence of TB in Rwanda was 85 per 100,000 people, with a mortality rate of 81% (National Institute of Allergy and Infectious Diseases, 2024; WHO, 2022b). Rwanda was also affected by the COVID-19 pandemic, but the situation was controlled through public awareness, vaccination, and preventive measures, as reported by Rwanda Biomedical Center (RBC, 2023a).

NONCOMMUNICABLE DISEASES

Noncommunicable diseases (NCDs) have been responsible for 50% of deaths in Rwanda, according to WHO in 2023. Rwanda's four significant NCD burdens are cardiovascular diseases (CVD), chronic respiratory disease, cancer, and diabetes. These four NCDs led to 695 deaths per 100,000 and 609 deaths per 100,000 mortality in males and females, respectively, as reported by WHO in 2023. CVD is on the rise in Rwanda and has caused numerous deaths (Taghian et al., 2024). To manage NCDs, Rwanda has introduced a bimonthly Car Free Day for physical exercise, health screening, and public awareness on NCDs (RBC, 2023b).

INFANT AND MATERNAL MORTALITY AND LIFE EXPECTANCY

In 2014 to 2015, the infant mortality rate per 1,000 live births was 20, while maternal mortality per 100,000 live births was 210, according to the the Demographic Health Survey (MOH, 2024). Rwanda's life expectancy at birth is 69.6 years (NISR, 2022b).

DETERMINANTS OF HEALTH

NATIONAL AND PER-CAPITA GROSS DOMESTIC PRODUCT AND POVERTY RATES

Rwanda plans to gain Middle Income Country status by 2035 and High-Income Country status by 2050 through a series of 7-year National Strategies for Transformation (NST1), underpinned by sectoral strategies focused on meeting the United Nation's Sustainable Development Goals (SDGs; World Bank Group, 2024). Growth averaged 7.2% annually over the decade to 2019, while per-capita gross domestic product (GDP) grew at 5%.

EDUCATION AND LITERACY RATES

The adult literacy rate of Rwanda increased from 38.2% in 1978 to 75.9% in 2021. The education sector has 31 General Higher Education Institutions and 5,076 adult literacy centers (Ministry of Education [MOE], 2023).

UNEMPLOYMENT RATES

In February 2022 (Q1), the unemployment rate declined to 16.5% compared to 23.8% in November 2021 (Q4). The unemployment rate is higher among youths age 16 to 30 years (21.5%) compared to adults older than 31 years (13.1%), with females (18.2%) more affected than males (15%; NISR, 2022a).

FOOD/NUTRITION

The agriculture industry contributes to Rwanda's economy, accounting for 39% of the country's GDP, 80% of employment opportunities, and 63% of foreign exchange earnings while also fulfilling 90% of food requirements. However, challenges such as topography, high population density, inadequate water management, and limited sector commercialization have resulted in low agricultural productivity (World Bank Group, 2013). Alarming statistics reveal that 38% of children younger than 5 years experience stunted growth, with 2% suffering from acute malnutrition. It is essential to note that stunting is more prevalent among children in rural areas (41%) than in urban centers (24%). Additionally, a clear correlation exists between a mother's education level and wealth quintile and the prevalence of stunting, as revealed by the NISR's 2016 report.

SOCIAL JUSTICE INCLUDING HUMAN RIGHTS ISSUES AND VULNERABLE AND UNDERSERVED POPULATIONS

Since Rwanda emerged from the devastating 1994 genocide against the Tutsi, significant efforts have been made to ensure the realization of fundamental human rights. The Constitution of the Republic of Rwanda (Rwanda Bar Association, 2015) recognizes the right to **social protection** as a fundamental right (Ministry of Local Government, 2020).

ENVIRONMENTAL AND CLIMATE CHANGE ISSUES

The Rwanda National Environment and Climate Change Policy goal is for "Rwanda to have a clean and healthy environment resilient to climate variability and change that supports a high quality of life for its society" (Ministry of Environment, 2019).

HISTORICAL/THEORETICAL BACKGROUND OF HEALTHCARE

HEALTHCARE DELIVERY, FINANCE, INSURANCE, AND PAYMENT

Healthcare insurance is accessible to every citizen in Rwanda for only $2 a year, while the actual cost ranges between $14 and $20 per citizen. The government provides half of this cost, while international donors contribute to the other half. Rwanda achieves over 93% vaccination coverage, and more than 90% of mothers give birth at health centers (WHO, 2019). There are four main health insurance schemes in Rwanda: (a) Rwandaise d'Assurance Maladie, which provides medical insurance to civil servants and state-owned enterprise employees; (b) military medical insurance, offering basic insurance coverage to military personnel; (c) community-based health insurance schemes or Mutuelles de Santé, which cater to both formal and informal sector members; and (d) private insurance products (International Labour Office [ILO], 2016).

HEALTHCARE TRAINING AND EDUCATION

Healthcare training and education in Rwanda involve one public medical school under the University of Rwanda, with a preclinical campus in Butare and a clinical campus in Kigali. Two private medical schools, namely the Adventist School of Medicine of East-Central Africa in Kigali, and the University of Global Health Equity in Butaro, were established in 2019. The Rwandan MOH, in collaboration with the University of Rwanda and other key stakeholders, recently launched new medical training programs, including fellowships, to sustain the quality of teaching for students at both undergraduate and postgraduate levels (RBC, 2022).

HEALTHCARE COST, QUALITY, AND ACCESS

Rwanda operates a **community-based health insurance (CBHI) program** known as Mutuelles de Santé. This program makes healthcare delivery accessible through donations from foreign charities, the Rwandan government, and international organizations such as the Global Fund to Fight AIDS, Tuberculosis, and Malaria. As a result of these efforts, in 2020 more than 90% of Rwanda's population had some form of health insurance (Rwanda Voluntary National Review, 2023).

GAPS IN CARE OR HEALTHCARE SHORTAGE AREAS

Access to healthcare facilities remains a challenge, particularly in rural areas of Rwanda. The government is taking active measures to create more health posts to reduce accessibility barriers. These health posts bridge community health workers and health centers, providing essential primary care services (WHO, 2022a). However, training medical professionals and healthcare workers remains a significant challenge for Rwanda (National Academies of Sciences, Engineering, and Medicine, Health and Medicine Division, Board on Global Health, & Committee on the Evaluation of Strengthening Human Resources for Health Capacity in the Republic of Rwanda Under the President's Emergency Plan for AIDS Relief, 2020).

HEALTHCARE PRACTICES

Allopathic, Traditional, Complementary, and Alternative Medicine Practices

In Rwanda, several recognized complementary and alternative medicine practices exist, including acupuncture, therapeutic reflexology, traditional Chinese medicine, naturopathy, and homeopathy (MOH, 2017). However, traditional medicine is not subject to official legislation or regulatory documents, and there are no protocols for endorsing traditional medical treatments and procedures. Despite this, traditional medicine is often more accessible and affordable, and it is well-liked by local people, making it a potential tool for achieving universal health coverage (Muganga et al., 2019).

CONCLUSION

Rwanda aims to achieve middle-income status by 2035, but accessibility to healthcare posts and availability of healthcare professionals are significant challenges. The government is actively working to resolve these issues.

LEARNING ACTIVITIES

CourseConnect

To access self-assessment questions and interactive, competency-based learning activities for this chapter, visit www.springerpub.com/courseconnect. See inside front cover and tear-out for CourseConnect details.

REFERENCES

Britannica. (n.d.). *Rwanda—Ethnicity, unity, democracy.* https://www.britannica.com/place/Rwanda/Government-and-society

Dahlmanns, E. (2015). New community, old tradition: The Intore warrior as a symbol of the new man. Rwanda's itorero-policy of societal recreation. *Modern Africa: Politics, History and Society, 3*(1), Article 1. https://doi.org/10.13140/RG.2.2.13168.12806

Europa Publications Staff. (1998). *Africa: South of the Sahara 2000*. Taylor and Francis Group.

Government of Rwanda.(n.d.). *Governance and home grown solutions.* https://www.gov.rw/highlights/governance

Grayson, H. (2017). A place for individuals: Positive growth in Rwanda. *Eastern African Literary and Cultural Studies, 3*(2–4), 107–130. https://doi.org/10.1080/23277408.2017.1374052

International Labour Office. (2016). *Rwanda: Progress towards universal health coverage*. https://www.socialprotection.org/gimi/gess/Media.action;jsessionid=NW8Ns9QzWXol08oL5rq1beTy2xXWP51NnfrlW1JIkW2hMTpxNajY!1945465934?id=15435

Institut National de la Statistique du Rwanda and ORC Macro. (2006). *Rwanda demographic and health survey 2005.* INSR and ORC Macro.

Kayiteshonga, Y., Sezibera, V., Mugabo, L., & Iyamuremye, J. D. (2022). Prevalence of mental disorders, associated co-morbidities, health care knowledge and service utilization in Rwanda—Towards a blueprint for promoting mental health care services in low- and middle-income countries?. *BMC Public Health, 22*(1), 1858. https://doi.org/10.1186/s12889-022-14165-x

Kingston, L. (2015). The destruction of identity: Cultural genocide and Indigenous peoples. *Journal of Human Rights, 14*(1), 63–83. https://doi.org/10.1080/14754835.2014.886951

Ministry of Education. (2023). *The Rwanda education statistical yearbook for 2021–2022 report*. https://www.scribd.com/document/735401003/Education-Statistical-Yearbook-2021-22

Ministry of Environment. (2019). *National environment and climate change policy*. https://faolex.fao.org/docs/pdf/rwa195923.pdf

Ministry of Health. (2011). *National mental health policy in Rwanda, Kigali*. Ministry of Health. https://www.rbc.gov.rw/fileadmin/user_upload/mental/men/4.%20National-Mental-health-Policy.pdf

Ministry of Health. (2017). Rwanda: National policy of traditional, complementary, and alternative medicine. http://www.moh.gov.rw/fileadmin/user_upload/Publication/Traditional_2cC_A_Medicine_National0001.pdf

Ministry of Health. (2024). *Key health indicators*. https://www.moh.gov.rw/publications/key-health-indicators

Ministry of Local Government. (2020). *National social protection policy*. https://www.minaloc.gov.rw/fileadmin/user_upload/Minaloc/Publications/Policies/Social_Protection_Policy_Adopted__1_.pdf

Muganga, O., Kasilo, J., Wambebe, C., Nikiema, J., & Nabyonga-orem, J. (2019). Towards universal health coverage: Advancing the development and use of traditional medicines in Africa. *BMJ Global Health, 4*(Suppl 9), e001517. https://doi.org/10.1136/bmjgh-2019-001517

National Academies of Sciences, Engineering, and Medicine, Health and Medicine Division, Board on Global Health, & Committee on the Evaluation of Strengthening Human Resources for Health Capacity in the Republic of Rwanda Under the President's Emergency Plan for AIDS Relief. (2020). *Evaluation of PEPFAR's contribution (2012–2017) to Rwanda's Human Resources for Health Program*. National Academies Press. https://www.ncbi.nlm.nih.gov/books/NBK558442/

National Institute of Allergy and Infectious Diseases. (2024). *Global research in Rwanda*. https://www.niaid.nih.gov/research/niaid-research-rwanda

National Institute of Statistics of Rwanda. (2016). *Comprehensive food security and vulnerability analysis report—2015*. https://e-ihuriro.rcsprwanda.org/wp-content/uploads/2023/05/CFSVA-Report_Final.pdf

National Institute of Statistics of Rwanda. (2022a). *Labor force survey trends—February 2022*. https://www.statistics.gov.rw/data-sources/surveys/Labour-Force-Survey/labour-force-survey-2022/labour-force-survey-february-2022-q1#:~:text=In%20February%202022%20(Q1)%2C,labour%20force%20(4%2C293%2C305%20persons)

National Institute of Statistics of Rwanda. (2022b). *Life expectancy at birth*. https://statistics.gov.rw/publication/life-expectancy-birth

National Institute of Statistics of Rwanda. (2023). *Rwanda's population reaches 13,2 million in 2022*. https://www.statistics.gov.rw/publication/Rwanda_population_2022

National Institute of Statistics of Rwanda, Ministry of Finance and Economic Planning. (2012). *Rwanda fourth population and housing census—2012. Thematic report: Population size, structure and distribution*. NISR. https://dataspace.princeton.edu/handle/88435/dsp01qb98mh92m
Rurangwa, M. L., & Whittaker, R. J. (2020). Making space for birds: Sourcing solutions from the mountain gorilla conservation model in Rwanda. *Journal for Nature Conservation, 54*, 125797. https://doi.org/10.1016/j.jnc.2020.125797
Rwanda Bar Association. (2015). *Constitution of the Republic of Rwanda (as revised in 2015)*. https://www.rwandabar.org.rw/attached_pdf/Constitution%20of%20the%20Republic%20of%20Rwanda-1608275353.pdf
Rwanda Assessment. (2000, October). *Country information and policy unit*. http://www.homeoffice.gov.uk/ind/asylum/asylum_contents02.html
Rwanda Basic Education Board. (2023). *Geography*. https://elearning.reb.rw/course/view.php?id=484&section=3
Rwanda Biomedical Center. (2022). *The Ministry of Health launches 13 medical training programs*. https://rbc.gov.rw/index.php?id=100&tx_news_pi1%5Bnews%5D=640&tx_news_pi1%5Bday%5D=20&tx_news_pi1%5Bmonth%5D=5&tx_news_pi1%5Byear%5D=2022&cHash=d322466b34896dae2bcf0fd5f7545d85#:~:text=Kigali%20May%204%2C%202022.,at%20undergraduate%20and%20postgraduate%20levels
Rwanda Biomedical Center. (2023a). *Coronavirus disease (COVID-19)*. https://rbc.gov.rw/index.php?id=707
Rwanda Biomedical Center. (2023b). *Noncommunicable diseases*. https://rbc.gov.rw/index.php?id=677
Schliesser, C. (2018). From "a theology of genocide" to a "theology of reconciliation"? On the role of Christian churches in the nexus of religion and genocide in Rwanda. *Religions, 9*(2), Article 2. https://doi.org/10.3390/rel9020034
Sellstrom, T., Wohlgemuth, L., & Dupont, P. (1996). *The international response to conflict and genocide: Lessons from the Rwanda experience: Synthesis report*. Steering Committee of the Joint Evaluation of Emergency Assistance to Rwanda. https://www.oecd.org/content/dam/oecd/en/toolkits/derec/evaluation-reports/derec/unitedstates/50189764.pdf
Simonsson, O. (2019). *God rests in Rwanda: The role of religion in the 1994 genocide in Rwanda*. https://urn.kb.se/resolve?urn=urn:nbn:se:uu:diva-380153
Taghian, G., Fisher, S., Chiles, T. C., Binagwaho, A., & Landrigan, P. J. (2024). The burden of cardiovascular disease from air pollution in Rwanda. *Annals of Global Health, 90*(1), 2. https://doi.org/10.5334/aogh.4322
World Bank Group. (2013). *Agricultural development in Rwanda*. https://www.worldbank.org/en/results/2013/01/23/agricultural-development-in-rwanda
World Bank Group. (2024). *The World Bank in Rwanda*. https://www.worldbank.org/en/country/rwanda/overview#:~:text=Rwanda%20aspires%20to%20become%20a,Sustainable%20Development%20Goals%20(SDGs)
World Health Organization. (2019). *Rwanda: The beacon of universal health coverage in Africa*. https://www.afro.who.int/news/rwanda-beacon-universal-health-coverage-africa
World Health Organization. (2022a). *Rwanda's primary health care strategy improves access to essential and life-saving health services*. http://apps.who.int/gho/data/node.cco%0Ahttp://apps.who.int/gho/data/node.cco%0Ahttp://apps.who.int/iris/bitstream/handle/10665/136986/ccsbrief_rwa_en.pdf?sequence=1
World Health Organization. (2022b). *Rwanda vital statistics report 2021*. https://data.who.int/countries/646
World Health Organization. (2023). *Country disease outlook*. https://www.afro.who.int/sites/default/files/2023-08/Rwanda.pdf

CHAPTER 36

BOTSWANA

Sunil K. Khanna, Megan MacDonald, Courtney Jost,
and Benjamin Roberts

GEOGRAPHY, SIZE, DEMOGRAPHICS

Botswana (Figure 36.1), officially known as the Republic of Botswana, is a landlocked country in Southern Africa, bordered by Namibia, Zimbabwe, Zambia, and South Africa. It is renowned for its stable democracy, robust economic growth, and commitment to wildlife conservation. Botswana covers an area of approximately 362,102 square kilometers (225,000 square miles), making it the 48th largest country in the world and slightly larger than France. Botswana's geography is predominantly flat, with up to 70% of its territory being the Kalahari Desert. Despite its arid environment, Botswana has diverse ecosystems, including savannas, grasslands, and the Okavango Delta.

Botswana has several administrative districts, including 10 main districts and six town councils. These include the Central District, Ngamiland District, Chobe District, Ghanzi District, Kgalagadi District, Kweneng District, Southern District, North-East District, South-East District, and Kgatleng District. These districts play an important role in local administration, handling governance and infrastructure locally.

POPULATION SIZE

As of the latest estimates, Botswana has approximately 2.4 million people, making it one of the least densely populated countries in the world. The average population density in Botswana is about nine people per square mile (World Population Review, 2022). The country has experienced steady population growth over the past few decades, driven by a combination of natural increase and, to a lesser extent, migration. The majority of the population resides in the eastern part of the country, and the largest ethnic group is the Tswana, with Setswana and English as the official languages. The capital city is Gaborone.

AGE DISTRIBUTION

Botswana has a young population, with a significant proportion of its citizens younger than 30 years. The age distribution is shown in Table 36.1.

MEDIAN AGE AND BIRTH RATE

In 2020, the median age in Botswana was approximately 23.3 years. This relatively young median age reflects the high proportion of children and young adults. The birth rate in Botswana is estimated to be approximately 22 births per 1,000 people per year. This birth rate has gradually declined due to increased access to family planning and reproductive health services, education, and improved economic conditions (The World Factbook, 2024).

IN-AND-OUT MIGRATION

Botswana has historically attracted labor migrants from neighboring countries, particularly Zimbabwe, Zambia, and Namibia. Many migrants come to Botswana seeking better economic opportunities, as the country has one of the more stable economies in the region. Sectors such

FIGURE 36.1 Map of Botswana.

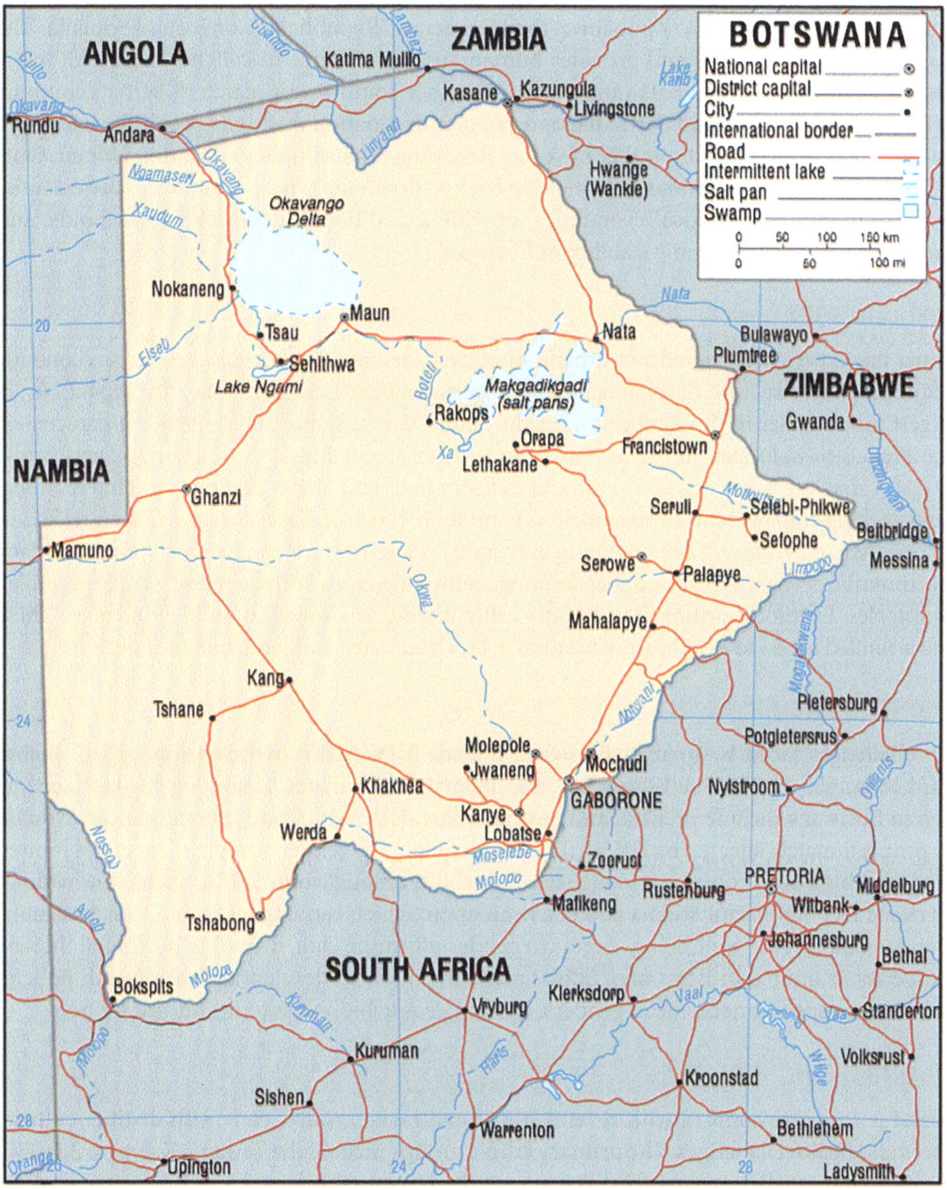

Source: University of Texas Libraries, The University of Texas at Austin. (n.d.). *Botswana*. https://maps.lib.utexas.edu/maps/africa/botswana-pol-2005.png

TABLE 36.1 AGE DISTRIBUTION IN BOTSWANA, 2024

AGE RANGE (YEARS)	POPULATION DISTRIBUTION (%)
0–14	28.7
15–64	65.2
65+	6.1

Source: The World Factbook. (2024). *Botswana*. https://www.cia.gov/the-world-factbook/countries/botswana/#:~:text=Age%20structure%20*%200%2D14%20years:%2028.7%%20(male,6.1%%20(2024%20est.)%20(%20male%2059%2C513/female%2089%2C747)

as mining, agriculture, and construction are significant employers of foreign labor. Botswana has also been a destination for refugees and asylum seekers from countries experiencing political instability and conflict, such as Zimbabwe, the Democratic Republic of Congo, and Somalia. The country hosts refugee camps and provides humanitarian assistance in collaboration with international organizations. Some Batswana migrate to other countries in search of better economic opportunities. South Africa, in particular, is a popular destination due to its proximity and more robust economy. A significant number of young Batswana pursue higher education abroad. Outmigration often results in remittance being sent back to Botswana. These remittances are essential in supporting families and local economies, providing additional income for households, and contributing to overall economic stability in Botswana.

RURAL–URBAN

Botswana has experienced significant urbanization over the past few decades, driven by economic opportunities, infrastructure development, and government policies. Gaborone, the capital city, is the largest urban center in the southeast, near the South African border. Other major urban centers include Francistown, located in the northeast, and Maun, situated near the Okavango Delta in the northwest. Urban areas serve as economic and industry hubs and attract domestic and international migrants seeking employment. Despite rapid urbanization, much of Botswana's population resides in rural areas, where livelihoods are predominantly based on agriculture and livestock farming. Many rural communities engage in subsistence farming, cultivating crops such as maize, sorghum, millet, and vegetables. Livestock farming, particularly cattle rearing, is also common in rural areas. These areas face limited access to healthcare, education, jobs, clean water, and sanitation facilities.

SEX AND GENDER

Health challenges faced by men in Botswana include HIV/AIDS, hypertension, type 2 diabetes, cardiovascular diseases, substance use, and mental health issues. Health challenges faced by women in Botswana include prenatal and postnatal care, HIV/AIDS, and cervical cancer. Women are disproportionately affected by HIV/AIDS. Gender inequity, gender-based violence, and limited decision-making power contribute to higher vulnerability among women. Transgender individuals in Botswana face significant stigma and discrimination, which can impact their access to healthcare services and overall well-being. Access to gender-affirming care, including hormonal therapy and surgeries, is limited in Botswana. Efforts are being made to develop inclusive health policies that address the specific needs of all genders, ensuring equitable access to healthcare services.

RACIAL/ETHNIC GROUPS

Botswana is a diverse country with several ethnic and racial groups, each with distinct cultural practices and health challenges. The primary ethnic groups include the Tswana, Kalanga, Basarwa (San), and other smaller groups. The Tswana are the largest ethnic group in Botswana, making up approximately 79% of the population. Their health status and challenges are representative of national trends. These include high rates of HIV/AIDS and noncommunicable diseases (NCDs) and limited access to maternal and child health services. The Kalanga are the second largest ethnic group, constituting about 11% of the population. The Basarwa (San) are an Indigenous minority group and face significant health disparities, including high rates of malnutrition and infectious diseases and limited access to healthcare services. Their traditional nomadic lifestyle and marginalization contribute to these challenges. Botswana also has small populations of White and Indian communities, primarily involved in business and professional sectors. These groups have better access to healthcare services due to their socioeconomic status.

Botswana faces significant health challenges and has made substantial efforts to improve its healthcare system. One of Botswana's most pressing health issues has been the HIV/AIDS epidemic. The country has one of the highest HIV prevalence rates in the world, with approximately

20% of the adult population living with the virus. In collaboration with international organizations, the Botswana government has implemented comprehensive strategies to combat the epidemic, including widespread antiretroviral therapy (ART), significantly improving life expectancy and quality of life for those affected.

HISTORICAL BACKGROUND OF HEALTHCARE

Before Botswana gained independence from the United Kingdom in 1966, the country's healthcare system was fragmented, primarily provided by missionaries and colonial authorities. Healthcare services were limited, with few facilities and trained health professionals available to serve the population, especially in rural areas. Following independence, Botswana's government prioritized healthcare as a critical component of national development. The Ministry of Health was established to oversee expanding and improving healthcare services. The government focused on building healthcare infrastructure, training medical personnel, and increasing access to health services. Since the early 1990s, Botswana has been confronting a severe HIV/AIDS epidemic. The Botswana government has taken decisive actions to address the HIV/AIDS epidemic, becoming one of the first African countries to provide free ART to all citizens in need, significantly reducing HIV-related mortality and improving the quality of life for people living with HIV.

The historical and theoretical background of healthcare in Botswana reflects a commitment to expanding access to health services, addressing significant health challenges, and building a robust and resilient healthcare system. Guided by the principles of primary healthcare, health system strengthening, and universal health coverage, Botswana continues to make significant strides in improving the health and well-being of its population.

CULTURAL BELIEFS

Cultural beliefs significantly shape Botswana's health behaviors, healthcare practices, and attitudes toward illness and treatment. The interplay between cultural beliefs and Western medical practices creates a unique healthcare landscape in Botswana. Developed within the Tswana culture in Southern Africa, Tswana medicine has several culturally specific characteristics and plays a prominent role in social control in the Indigenous society in Botswana. In traditional Tswana thought, illness, death, and misfortune are not regarded as natural events but are often attributed to the supernatural interventions of an external agent. The *Badimo*, or ancestors, are considered the guardians of community morality and can punish any transgression against the moral code or one's failure to show proper veneration with illness or misfortune. Similar punishment can be meted out by *modimo*—the supreme being and creator of the universe, who controlled rainfall and could inflict punishment by sending thunder, lightning, drought, or death (Dennis, 1978).

HEALTH OUTCOMES

Botswana has significantly improved health outcomes over the past few decades but faces many significant health challenges. The country's healthcare system has improved dramatically, especially in areas such as HIV/AIDS treatment, maternal health, and child survival. However, NCDs, health inequities, and healthcare access in rural areas remain concerns.

LIFE EXPECTANCY AT BIRTH

Life expectancy at birth has improved by 15.6 years, from 45.6 years in 2000 to 61.2 years in 2021 (Figure 36.2). Botswana has experienced declines in mortality and fertility levels since the 1980s. From the mid-1990s, the country experienced an increase in mortality, mainly due to the increased number of deaths associated with the HIV/AIDS epidemic. However, as a result of the introduction of free ARTs, mortality has declined since 2001.

FIGURE 36.2 Life expectancy at birth in Botswana.

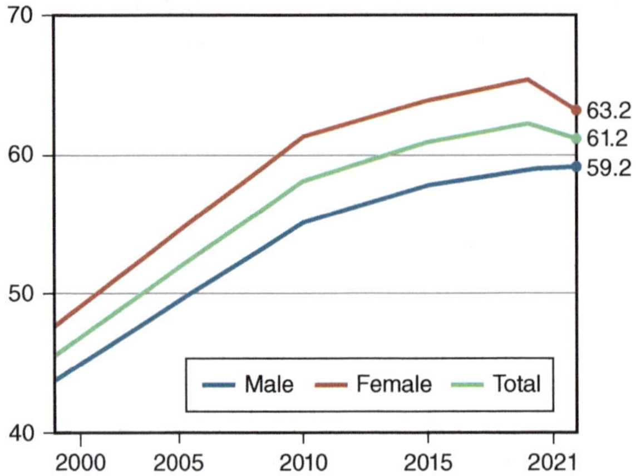

Source: World Health Organization. (n.d.). *Botswana*. https://data.who.int/countries/072

LEADING CAUSES OF MORTALITY

The leading causes of death in Botswana (Figure 36.3) include both communicable and NCDs. These include HIV/AIDS, lower respiratory infections, cardiovascular diseases, diabetes, neonatal infections, tuberculosis, and road injury (World Health Organization [WHO], 2023). The leading causes of death in Botswana have shifted significantly over time due to various social, economic, and healthcare developments. Before Botswana's independence in 1966, the country faced limited healthcare infrastructure, with most medical services concentrated in urban areas. Rural populations primarily relied on traditional healers. The leading causes of death during this period were predominantly infectious diseases and conditions related to poverty, poor sanitation, and limited access to healthcare. Malaria, tuberculosis, pneumonia, and gastrointestinal infections (diarrhea and dysentery) were the leading causes of mortality (Jamison et al., 2006).

Following independence, Botswana began to build its healthcare infrastructure, improving access to hospitals, clinics, and vaccination programs. However, infectious diseases still dominated mortality statistics during this period. Tuberculosis, malaria, diarrheal diseases, and pneumonia remained the leading causes of mortality, particularly among children.

HIV/AIDS

In the early 1990s, Botswana faced a devastating HIV/AIDS epidemic that dramatically altered the country's mortality patterns. By the mid-1990s, HIV/AIDS became the leading cause of death in Botswana. The epidemic overwhelmed the healthcare system, leading to high mortality rates among young adults, who were the most affected demographic. Opportunistic infections such as tuberculosis and pneumonia surged due to weakened immune systems in HIV-positive individuals, further increasing mortality. During this period, Botswana's life expectancy plummeted from approximately 65 years in the early 1990s to below 40 years in the early 2000s due to the HIV/AIDS crisis (Gona et al., 2020). Despite its relatively small population, Botswana has been impacted by the HIV/AIDS epidemic, posing substantial health, social, and economic challenges. Ranked among the top four countries in the world most affected by HIV/AIDS, Botswana has one of the highest HIV/AIDS prevalence rates in the world. However, HIV/AIDS death rates continued to decline due to comprehensive ART programs.

In the early 2000s, Botswana made remarkable progress in controlling the HIV/AIDS epidemic, but the country began to face the dual burden of infectious diseases and emerging NCDs. HIV/AIDS remained a leading cause of mortality, but mortality rates declined sharply as ART coverage expanded to over 90% of people living with HIV. Mother-to-child transmission of HIV also dropped due to the success of prevention programs. As Botswana's economy grew, lifestyle changes

FIGURE 36.3 Leading causes of death (2019) in Botswana.

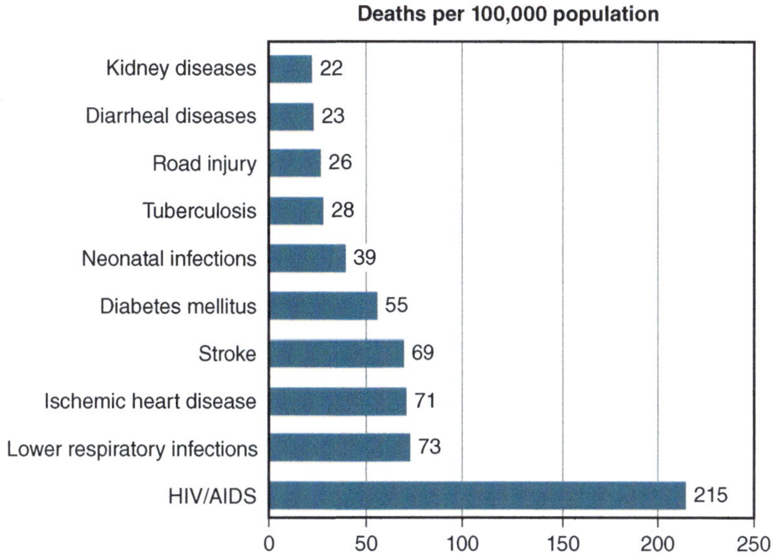

Source: Adapted from World Health Organization. (2023). *What are the leading causes of death in the African region?* https://files.aho.afro.who.int/afahobckpcontainer/production/files/iAHO_Mortality_Regional-Factsheet.pdf

led to the rise of NCDs, such as diabetes, hypertension, and cardiovascular diseases. These became significant causes of mortality, particularly in urban areas where dietary and lifestyle changes were more pronounced. Cervical and prostate cancer emerged as significant causes of mortality among adults, with cervical cancer being linked to HIV prevalence. Tuberculosis, particularly in coinfection with HIV, also emerged as a significant cause of death. While the ART helped reduce tuberculosis mortality, the emergence of multidrug-resistant tuberculosis (MDR-TB) posed new challenges. Although maternal and child mortality rates declined during these years, this decline was primarily in urban areas. Communities in rural Botswana continued to record high levels of maternal and child mortality due to limited access to government-sponsored healthcare services.

In the last decade, Botswana has made significant progress in reducing deaths from infectious diseases while facing a rising burden of NCDs and other health challenges. The prevalence of HIV in the 15 to 49 age group in Botswana has dropped from 25.3% in 2000 to 16.4% in 2022 (UNAIDS, 2022; Figure 36.4). Currently, the leading causes of mortality in Botswana reflect a combination of infectious diseases, NCDs, and conditions related to maternal and child health.

NONCOMMUNICABLE DISEASES

Recent epidemiological data suggest that prevalence rates of NCDs, including heart disease, stroke, diabetes, and cancer, are rising in Botswana (Haacker et al., 2019). As Botswana's population ages and lifestyles shift, NCDs are placing increasing strain on Botswana's healthcare system. Cervical cancer remains the most common cancer-related cause of death among women. In 2015, the Botswana government rolled out a nationwide human papillomavirus (HPV) vaccination program for 9- to 13-year-old girls to reduce future cases. Botswana plans to expand these efforts by launching a National Cervical Cancer Prevention Program (Masisi & Briceno, 2024). In addition, road traffic collisions have recently emerged as a leading cause of death, particularly among young adults in Botswana.

ALCOHOL USE

Alcohol use disorder is a persistent and growing concern in Botswana, with rates of alcohol use disorder (7.1%) and alcohol dependence (2.5%) significantly exceeding the WHO African Region

FIGURE 36.4 HIV/AIDS-related deaths in Botswana, 2010–2022.

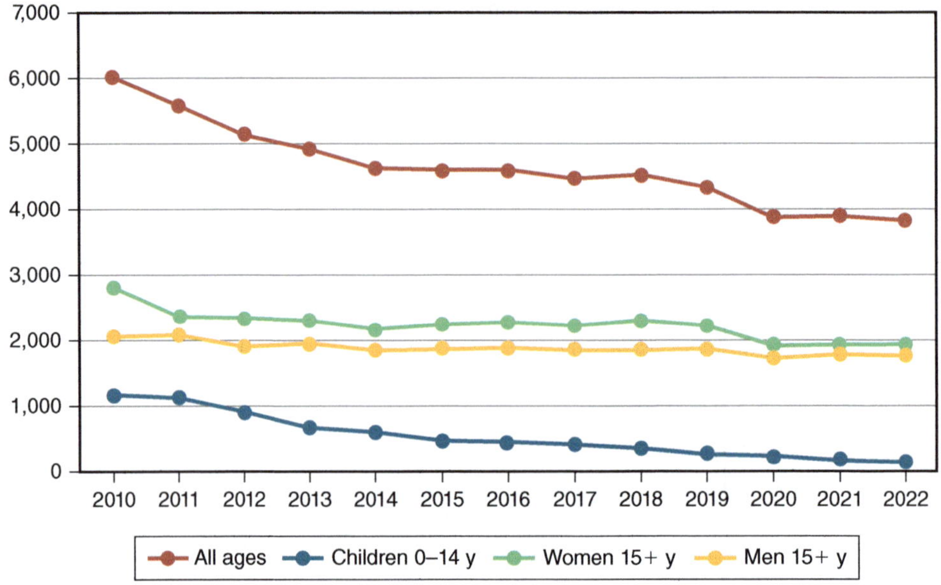

Source: UNAIDS. (2022). *UNAIDS data 2022.* Joint United Nations Program on HIV/AIDS. https://www.unaids.org/sites/default/files/media_asset/data-book-2022_en.pdf

averages of 3.7% and 1.3%, respectively (WHO, 2018). Heavy episodic drinking (HED), or binge drinking, is also widespread, affecting 19% of the population aged 15 years and older (WHO, 2018). The direct health impact of alcohol use in Botswana is alarming. Age-adjusted alcohol-related death rates per 100,000 males are notably high: 23.2% for liver cirrhosis, 27.9% for traffic injuries, and 138.5% for cancer (WHO, 2018). These figures reflect the severe consequences of excessive alcohol consumption in the country. Beyond these direct health effects, alcohol use contributes to a range of broader social and health issues, including increased rates of gender-based violence, risky sexual behavior, and a high susceptibility to HIV/AIDS.

ROAD TRAFFIC COLLISIONS

Road traffic collisions in Botswana have become a growing public health problem, contributing to injury, disability, and death. Botswana has experienced rapid economic growth, leading to increased vehicles on the road. Equivalent improvements in road infrastructure and safety measures have not matched this growth. Speeding, drunk driving, and poor road conditions contribute to the high traffic collision rates. Botswana has one of the highest road traffic death rates in the sub-Saharan region (Motsumi et al., 2021). Beyond fatalities, road traffic accidents result in a high number of injuries, leading to long-term disabilities and increasing the burden on the healthcare system.

DISABILITY

Approximately 4.2% of Botswana's population lives with a disability (Statistics Botswana, 2018). Significant disparity exists between the Botswana National Census and modeled estimates of disability prevalence (approximately 15% of the world's population has a disability), indicating that the prevalence of disability in Botswana could be much higher than estimated (Oyaro, 2015). Disability in Botswana profoundly impacts health status, quality of life, and access to healthcare and social services for affected individuals. The interplay between disability and health outcomes in Botswana is shaped by a variety of factors, including access to medical care, social and economic marginalization, and lack of supportive infrastructure. Individuals with disabilities have limited access to healthcare services, making them more vulnerable to increased physical and mental health risks.

They also face increased social marginalization and barriers to education and health promotion. Although Botswana has made efforts to address disability through its National Policy on Care for People with Disabilities, the implementation of this policy remains inconsistent, and there is an urgent need for more robust systems to ensure that healthcare services are accessible to all.

SOCIAL DETERMINANTS OF HEALTH

Botswana's health policy recognizes the importance of the social determinants of health and their influence on health equities/inequities (WHO, 2013). The social determinants of health in Botswana play a critical role in shaping the health outcomes of its population. Several factors, including socioeconomic status, education, employment, access to healthcare, housing, and environmental conditions, profoundly influence people's health in the country. Botswana has many good policies and strategies to promote positive change in social determinants of health. However, implementation is weak, and societal structural attributes make achieving health equity difficult. These relate to high poverty levels, uneven infrastructural development, and highly skewed income distribution.

INCOME/POVERTY

Botswana has a relatively high gross domestic product (GDP) per capita for Africa, but income disparity remains a significant challenge. Poverty levels, especially in rural areas, contribute to health disparities. While the country's economy has grown due to diamond mining, unemployment remains high, particularly among youth. The income gap limits access to quality healthcare, nutritious food, and health-promoting environments, contributing to poor health outcomes for low-income communities.

Botswana's economic growth and welfare improvements have slowed over the last decade. The share of the population living below the International Poverty Line ($2.15 per person per day) declined from 29.1% in 2002/2003 to 17.7% in 2009/2010, and more slowly to 15.4% in 2015/2016 (World Bank Group, 2023). Broad-based employment increases contributed to the fast pace of poverty reduction earlier. In contrast, the lack of employment generation in the more recent period, combined with a deep drought in 2015, resulted in poverty reversals, particularly among rural households. Botswana has faced structural challenges and slow growth since 2015 and is vulnerable to external shocks, particularly because it mainly depends on a single commodity, diamonds. The unemployment rate increased from 17.6% in 2015 to 22.5% by 2021, disproportionately affecting women and youth in rural communities (World Bank Group, 2023).

LITERACY

Botswana's education system includes early childhood, primary, junior, and senior secondary education. Botswana has made progress in increasing literacy rates, but disparities remain between urban and rural areas. Recognizing the importance of education for its citizens, Botswana has articulated in its Vision 2036 that education and skill-building are critical to human resource development (UNICEF, 2024). However, more access to quality education for many rural communities is needed to improve health knowledge and overall health outcomes. Only 43% of children between 4 and 5 years access early learning opportunities; approximately one third of children taking the Primary School examination do not pass; and approximately two thirds of children taking the Junior Certificate examinations do not pass. To address these challenges, the government of Botswana is collaborating with **UNICEF** to develop national remediation and enrollment interventions to enhance learning outcomes (UNICEF, 2024).

INFANT MORTALITY

Botswana's infant mortality rate (IMR) has significantly declined from approximately 40 to 50 deaths per 1,000 live births in the 1990s to around 27.7 deaths per 1,000 live births in 2023. This improvement is attributable mainly to the government's efforts to strengthen healthcare infrastructure, expand access to maternal and child health services, and address the country's HIV/AIDS epidemic.

Botswana was one of the first African countries to implement a national **Prevention of Mother-to-Child Transmission (PMTCT) program**, and this has dramatically reduced the transmission of HIV from mothers to their infants. In addition, Botswana has a robust immunization program, which has decreased deaths from vaccine-preventable diseases like measles, diphtheria, and polio. Finally, the government promotes exclusive breastfeeding for the first 6 months of life and runs nutrition programs to improve maternal and infant nutrition. Despite these advancements, Botswana's IMR is still higher than in many high-income countries, and it is considered relatively high for a country with Botswana's economic standing. Shortages of skilled healthcare professionals, inadequate medical equipment, and long travel distances to healthcare facilities contribute to higher IMRs in rural Botswana.

POPULATION CHANGE (AGING)

Aging in Botswana is an emerging issue as the country experiences a demographic shift due to improved healthcare and reduced mortality rates from communicable diseases like HIV/AIDS. Life expectancy has risen significantly to 69 years, partly due to the success of HIV/AIDS treatment programs. The proportion of older persons has increased from 5% in 2001 to 8.5% in 2021, and is projected to rise to 20% in 2051 (WHO, 2022). Although Botswana has made significant advances in healthcare delivery, these efforts have not fully translated into access to quality healthcare services for older adults. Botswana's healthcare delivery system is not well aligned with the emerging health needs of older adults, especially those related to NCDs and comorbidities associated with living with HIV/AIDS. Botswana's Ministry of Health has recently adopted WHO's Integrated Care for Older Adults (ICOPE) plan to better serve older adults in the country (WHO, 2022).

HEALTHCARE SYSTEM

OVERVIEW

Botswana's commitment to universal health coverage is central to its healthcare policy. Botswana's healthcare system is heavily funded by the government, with over 80% of healthcare services being publicly provided. The government spends a substantial portion of its budget on health, ensuring widespread access to medical services and reducing health disparities. Although the healthcare system is accessible to a majority of the population, achieving universal health coverage remains challenging. People living in rural areas often need to travel long distances to reach healthcare facilities, and staffing shortages can limit the availability of services.

HUMAN RESOURCES AND INFRASTRUCTURE

The healthcare infrastructure in Botswana is structured into primary, secondary, and tertiary care facilities, forming a three-tiered system designed to serve rural and urban areas.

- *Primary care facilities*: Primary healthcare services are delivered through a network of health posts, clinics, and health centers. Botswana has 17 primary hospitals, 311 clinics, 351 health posts, and 931 mobile stops (Nkomazana et al., 2014). Extensive primary healthcare is the cornerstone of Botswana's delivery system. These facilities provide essential services such as immunization, maternal and child healthcare, family planning, HIV testing and ARV delivery, and treatment for common illnesses.
- *Secondary care facilities*: Botswana's 15 district hospitals represent the secondary tier of healthcare. Each country's 27 districts have a district hospital providing more advanced

care than clinics and primary health centers. These hospitals offer diagnostic services, surgical procedures, emergency care, and the treatment of more complex health problems.

- *Tertiary care facilities*: Tertiary care is provided at referral hospitals equipped to handle specialized medical cases. Botswana has three fully operational tertiary care hospitals. These hospitals offer advanced treatments, including specialized surgeries, oncology services, and comprehensive care for HIV/AIDS and tuberculosis.

Botswana's health sector has been dominated by nurses, who comprise over 70% of the health workforce (Tapela et al., 2019). Other healthcare professionals, such as physicians, pharmacists, lab technicians, lay counselors, and healthcare auxiliaries, comprise the remaining 30% of Botswana's healthcare workforce. Despite advancements in healthcare infrastructure, Botswana faces several challenges related to rural–urban disparities in healthcare access, human resource shortages, and limited availability of specialized care (Oleribe et al., 2019). Botswana needs help in maintaining a sufficient and well-trained workforce. The country has struggled with shortages of healthcare professionals, particularly doctors and specialists, leading to a reliance on expatriate staff in many healthcare facilities. The distribution of healthcare workers is uneven, with rural areas being particularly underserved. To address these challenges, Botswana has invested in training healthcare professionals locally through the University of Botswana's medical school and nursing programs. Additionally, the government has strengthened partnerships with international organizations to provide continuous medical education and training.

HEALTHCARE PRACTICES: TRADITIONAL, COMPLEMENTARY, AND ALTERNATIVE MEDICINE

Traditional and complementary healthcare practices are integral to the healthcare system in Botswana, particularly in rural and semi-urban areas. These practices involve a wide range of healing traditions passed down through generations. Traditional healers (*dingaka* or *ngaka*) are respected figures in Botswana. They play a significant role in providing care, especially in areas with limited access to biomedical healthcare. Specifically, Botswana has two major groups of traditional healers: the *dingaka Isa Dichochwa,* or **herbalists**, and the *dingaka Isa Tanaka,* or **divine healers**. Their healing roles are broad, addressing physical and spiritual symptoms and a few veterinary treatments (Ulin, 1975). Dingakas are highly respected individuals in the community. They can treat a range of physical, psychologic, and spiritual ailments. Their methods often involve herbal remedies, spiritual rituals, and divination.

Witchcraft is commonly believed to cause illness, misfortune, and death. Many Batswana (people of Botswana) attribute certain illnesses or misfortunes to curses or witchcraft, especially if the cause of the illness is unclear. Many people in Botswana view health holistically, encompassing physical, mental, and spiritual well-being. The harmony between individuals and their ancestors is essential for maintaining good health. The use of herbal medicine is widespread in Botswana. People use various plant-based remedies to treat illnesses like colds, fevers, and digestive issues. These remedies are often passed down through generations and are seen as complementing biomedicinal remedies. Ancestor worship plays a central role in health beliefs. Finally, traditional birth attendants are actively involved in childbirth, especially when access to biomedical healthcare facilities is limited. Family members and the community often play active roles in healing, offering physical and emotional support.

While **biomedicine** is widely practiced in Botswana, many integrate their cultural beliefs and practices with biomedicine, sometimes using both simultaneously. Botswana recognizes traditional healers and has taken steps to promote their work. Botswana's Ministry of Health, the apex government body regulating healthcare services in the country, has a policy that recognizes traditional healers and fosters collaboration with biomedical practices. Many in Botswana consult dingaka for health issues, especially for conditions believed to have spiritual or supernatural causes.

CONCLUSION

Botswana, a landlocked country in Southern Africa, is known for its stable democracy, economic growth, and wildlife conservation. With a population of approximately 2.4 million, Botswana is one of the least densely populated nations. Most people reside in the east, and the Tswana ethnic group is the largest. Gaborone is the capital city. The country's population is young, with 28.7% age 0 to 14 years and a median age of 23.3 years. Health challenges are prominent in Botswana, mainly due to HIV/AIDS, which affects around 20% of the country's adult population. Men face additional health risks associated with NCDs, while women are vulnerable to maternal health issues and gender-based violence.

In the early 1990s, Botswana was hit hard by the HIV/AIDS epidemic, becoming one of the countries most affected by the virus. By the mid-1990s, HIV/AIDS was the leading cause of death, with a significant impact on young adults. Life expectancy dropped from 65 years in the early 1990s to below 40 years in the early 2000s. However, Botswana's response, including widespread ART, helped reduce mortality rates and improve life expectancy. By 2022, the prevalence of HIV in the 15- to 19-years age group has significantly decreased.

Despite progress in combating HIV, Botswana now faces a double burden of infectious diseases and NCDs, such as diabetes, hypertension, and cancers like cervical and prostate cancer. Coinfection of tuberculosis with HIV remains a challenge, particularly with the rise of multidrug-resistant tuberculosis (MDR-TB).

In addition to the HIV/AIDS crisis, other health challenges have surfaced. Alcohol use is a significant issue, with rates of alcohol use disorder and heavy episodic drinking above regional averages. Alcohol-related issues contribute to high death rates from liver cirrhosis, traffic injuries, and cancer while also exacerbating social issues like gender-based violence and risky sexual behavior, which fuel HIV transmission.

Road traffic collisions have also become a leading cause of death, especially among young adults, due to increased vehicle numbers, poor infrastructure, and reckless driving. Disability rates in Botswana are underreported, and those with disabilities face barriers in accessing healthcare and social services.

Botswana is committed to universal health coverage, with over 80% of healthcare services publicly provided and primarily funded by the government. The healthcare system is designed in three tiers—primary, secondary, and tertiary care—ensuring services for rural and urban populations. Primary care is the foundation, offering essential services such as immunizations, maternal care, and HIV testing across 17 primary hospitals, 311 clinics, and hundreds of health posts and mobile stops. Secondary care is delivered through 15 district hospitals, while tertiary care, including specialized treatments, is provided at three referral hospitals.

Despite significant investments, Botswana needs help in achieving universal health coverage. Rural areas are particularly underserved, with patients often traveling long distances to access healthcare. Staffing shortages, especially doctors and specialists, have led to a reliance on expatriate healthcare professionals. Nurses form over 70% of the health workforce, but the overall distribution of healthcare workers is uneven. Botswana invests in local medical and nursing training to address these gaps and partners with international organizations for continuous education and training.

LEARNING ACTIVITIES

CourseConnect

To access self-assessment questions and interactive, competency-based learning activities for this chapter, visit www.springerpub.com/courseconnect. See inside front cover and tear-out for CourseConnect details.

REFERENCES

Dennis, C. (1978). The role of "Dingaka Tsa Setswana" from the 19th century to the present. *Botswana Notes and Records, 10*, 53–66. http://www.jstor.org/stable/40979537

Gona, P. N., Gona, C. M., Ballout, S., Rao, R. S., Kimokoti, R., Mapoma, C. C., & Mokdad, A. H. (2020). Burden and changes in HIV/AIDS morbidity and mortality in Southern Africa development community countries, 1990–2017. *BMC Public Health, 20*(1), 867. https://doi.org/10.1186/s12889-020-08988-9

Haacker, M., Barnighausen, T., & Atun, R. (2019). HIV and the growing burden of noncommunicable diseases in Botswana: Modeling study. *Journal of Global Health, 9*(1), 010482. https://doi.org/10.7189/jogh.09.010428

Jamison, D. T., Feachem, R. G., Makgoba, M. W., Bos, E. R., Baingana, F. K., Hofman, K. J., & Khama, Rogo O. (Eds.). (2006). *Disease and mortality in sub-Saharan Africa*. (2nd ed.). World Bank.

Masisi, N., & Briceno, R. (2024). *Decisive action is needed to stop cervical cancer deaths*. Johns Hopkins Bloomberg School of Public Health. https://globalhealthnow.org/2024-03/eliminating-cervical-cancer#:~:text=Botswana%20rolled%20out%20a%20national,but%20it%20is%20not%20enough

Motsumi, M., Ayane, G., Morapedi, K., Panzirah-Mabake, K., & Walsh, M. (2021). Preventable deaths following road traffic collisions in Botswana: A retrospective review. *Injury, 52*(9), 2665–2671. https://doi.org/10.1016/j.injury.2021.04.020

Nkomazana, O., Phaladze, N., Peersman, W., Willcox, M., & Mash, R. (2014). Human resources for health in Botswana: The results of in-country database and reports analysis. *African Journal of Primary Health Care & Family Medicine, 6*(1), 1–8. https://doi.org/10.4102/phcfm.v6i1.716

Oleribe, O., Momoh, J., Uzochukwu, B., Mbofana, F., Adebiyi, A., Barbera, B., Williams, R., & Taylor-Robinson, S. (2019). Identifying key challenges facing healthcare systems in Africa and potential solutions. *International Journal of General Medicine, 12*, 395–403. https://doi.org/10.2147/ijgm.s223882

Oyaro, L. (2015). Africa at crossroads: The United Nations convention on the rights of persons with disabilities. *American University of Law Review, 30*(2), 347–377.

Statistics Botswana. (2018). *Botswana demographic survey report 2017*. Statistics Botswana.

Tapela, N., Tshisimogo, G., Shatera, B. P., Letsatsi, V., Gaborone, M., Madidimalo, T., Ovberedjo, M., Jibril, H. B., Tsima, B., Nkomazana, O., Dryden-Peterson, S., Lockman, S., Masupe, T., Hirschhorn., L. R., & El Halabi, S. (2019). Integrating noncommunicable disease services into primary health care, Botswana. *Bulletin of the World Health Organization, 97*(2), 142. https://doi.org/10.2471/blt.18.221424

Ulin, P. (1975). The traditional healer of Botswana in a changing society. *Botswana Notes and Records, 7*, 95–102.

UNAIDS. (2022). *UNAIDS data 2022*. Joint United Nations Program on HIV/AIDS. https://www.unaids.org/sites/default/files/media_asset/data-book-2022_en.pdf

UNICEF. (2024). *Education: Every child has a right to accessible quality education*. https://www.unicef.org/botswana/education

World Bank Group. (2023). *Poverty and equity brief: Africa Eastern & Southern, Botswana*. https://databankfiles.worldbank.org/public/ddpext_download/poverty/987B9C90-CB9F-4D93-AE8C-750588BF00QA/current/Global_POVEQ_BWA.pdf

The World Factbook. (2024). *Botswana*. https://www.cia.gov/the-world-factbook/countries/botswana/#:~:text=Age%20structure%20*%200%2D14%20years:%2028.7%%20(male,6.1%%20(2024%20est.)%20(%20male%2059%2C513/female%2089%2C747)

World Health Organization. (2013). *Integrating social determinants of health in all public policies: The case of health development in Botswana*. https://www.afro.who.int/sites/default/files/2018-02/Botswana%20case%20study.pdf

World Health Organization. (2018). *Global status report on alcohol and health*. https://www.who.int/substance_abuse/publications/global_alcohol_report/en/

World Health Organization. (2022). *Health data overview for the republic of Botswana*. https://data.who.int/countries/072

World Health Organization. (2023). *What are the leading causes of death in the African region?* https://files.aho.afro.who.int/afahobckpcontainer/production/files/iAHO_Mortality_Regional-Factsheet.pdf

World Population Review. (2022). *Botswana population 2024*. https://worldpopulationreview.com/countries/botswana-population

CHAPTER 37

ZIMBABWE

Paul Ndebele and Florence Mandebvu

INTRODUCTION

Zimbabwe, a low-income country in Southern Africa, is characterized by several health threats and challenges, including HIV, tuberculosis (TB), and malaria. Zimbabwe is one of the countries that was significantly affected by the HIV/AIDS epidemic, and the number of cases is still significant despite the global drop in new infections. Zimbabwe is one of the 22 countries with a substantial burden of TB, and the incidence has been rising over the past decade for various reasons, including poor housing conditions. More than 8 million Zimbabweans are at risk of **malaria**, and malaria is one of the significant health problems that contribute to more than 40% of deaths. These three diseases contribute significantly to maternal and childhood illnesses and deaths. Other diseases that are on the rise and are affecting Zimbabweans include cancers, diabetes, lower respiratory infections, hypertension, cardiovascular conditions, and mental health conditions. Zimbabwe's decades-old economic crisis has severely impacted the health delivery system in many ways and has led to a mass exodus of healthcare workers, weakened disease prevention efforts, and underdiagnosis and undertreatment of both communicable and noncommunicable diseases (NCDs; Mugwagwa et al., 2017).

GEOGRAPHY AND POPULATION

Zimbabwe, officially referred to as the Republic of Zimbabwe, is a landlocked country in Southern Africa and lies between the Zambezi River to the north and the Limpopo River to the South. Zimbabwe is bordered by South Africa to the south, Botswana to the southwest, Zambia to the north, and Mozambique to the east and is a member of the United Nations, the **Southern African Development Community**, the African Union, and the Common Market for Eastern and Southern Africa. The capital and largest city is Harare, followed by Bulawayo. Most of the country is elevated, consisting of a central plateau (the high veld) stretching from the southwest northward with altitudes between 1,000 and 1,600 meters (3,280 and 5,250 feet). The country's extreme east is mountainous and is referred to as the Eastern Highlands. Mount Nyangani, situated in the Eastern Highlands, is the highest point at 2,592 meters (8,504 feet). The country's total size is 390,757 square kilometers (242,805 square miles), consisting of 386,847 square kilometers (386,847 square miles) of land and 3,910 square kilometers (2,429 square miles) of water (Britannica, 2024).

Zimbabwe has a subtropical climate with many local variations. The southern areas are known for their heat and aridity, while parts of the central plateau receive frost in winter. The Zambezi valley between Zimbabwe and Zambia is known for its extreme heat, and the Eastern Highlands, famous for agriculture production, usually experience lower temperatures and the highest rainfall in the country.

The country's rainy season generally runs from late October to March, and the hot climate is moderated by increasing altitude. Zimbabwe is faced with recurring droughts, which have been worsening during the past two decades due to the effects of climate change and El Nino.

The Republic of Zimbabwe is divided into 10 administrative provinces, which are divided into 64 districts and 1,970 wards. The administrative provinces are Bulawayo, Harare, Manicaland, Mashonaland Central, Mashonaland East, Mashonaland West, Masvingo, Matabeleland North, Matabeleland South, and Midlands (Figure 37.1).

FIGURE 37.1 Map showing Zimbabwe's 10 provinces.

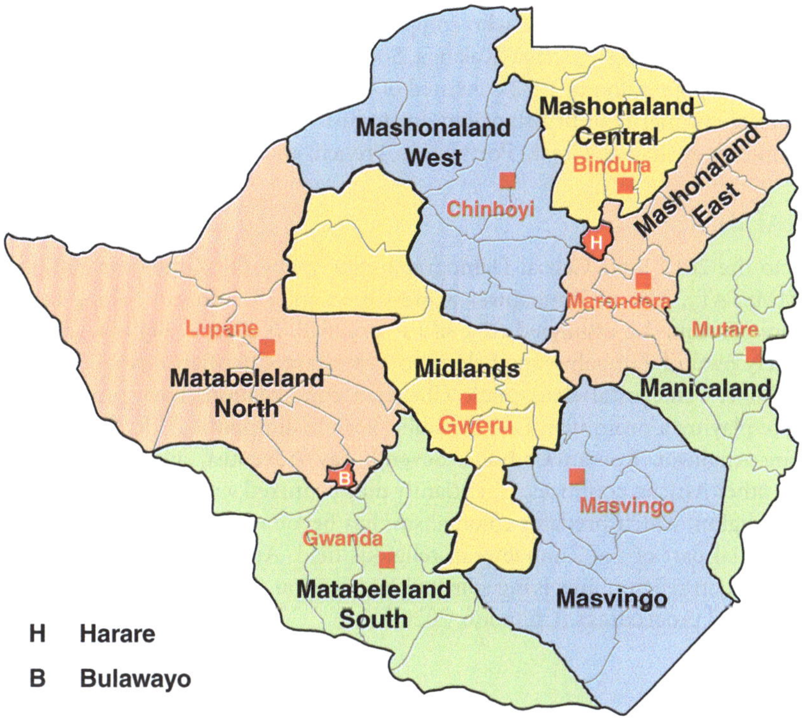

Source: Mangwanani. (2008). *A map showing the administrative divisions of Zimbabwe*. https://commons.wikimedia.org/wiki/File:Administrative_Divisions_of_Zimbabwe.svg

POPULATION SIZE

Zimbabwe has a population of around 17,150,352 people and an estimated annual population growth rate of 1.91%. The total population consists of 8,343,790 males and 8,806,562 females. The population is relatively young in 2023, there were 40% of people age 0 to 14 years in 2023, 56% age 15 to 64 years, and 4.2% older than 65 years. The age breakdown of Zimbabwe's population is as follows: 0 to 4 years, 13.9%; 5 to 12 years, 21.2%; 13 to 17 years, 11.6%; 18 to 24 years, 14.3%; 25 to 34 years, 14.3%; 35 to 44 years, 11.7%; 45 to 54 years, 6.6%; 55 to 64 years, 3.2%; and 65 years and older, 3.3%. The population pyramid for Zimbabwe is expansive with a wide base and narrow top, indicating high birth and fertility rates, high death rates, and lower life expectancies. As of 2023, the median age of Zimbabwe's population was 18.4 years. This marked an increase from 17.9 years in 2020. The birth rate for Zimbabwe in 2023 was 27.689 births per 1,000 people, a 2.23% decline from 2022. Zimbabwe's net migration rate has been declining since 2021, with a –3.405 per 1,000 people in 2024, a 13.99% decrease from 2023. The 2022 Population and Housing Census found that 84% of the approximately 908,000 emigrants left the country for employment, while 5% left for education or training. Other reasons for migration include economic hardship. Most emigration has been to the United Kingdom, South Africa, Botswana, Zambia, Mozambique, Canada, Australia, and New Zealand. The World Bank reported that 67.4% of Zimbabweans lived in rural areas in 2022 (CIA, 2021; World Population Review, 2024).

ETHNICITY AND RACE

Zimbabwe's population is made up of many ethnic and racial groups. According to the 2012 census report, 99.7% of the population is of African origin (Central Intelligence Agency [CIA],

2021). The majority of the Zimbabwean population are the Shona people, who comprise 82% of the Zimbabwean population, while Ndebele people make up 14% (CIA, 2021). Minority ethnic groups include White Zimbabweans, who comprise less than 1% of the population. Other ethnic groups include Venda, Tonga, Tsonga, Kalanga, Sotho, Ndau, Nambya, Tswana, Xhosa, and Lozi. About 0.4% of the population in 2022 consisted of White, Asiatic, and mixed-race groups. White Zimbabweans are primarily of British origin due to historical ties through colonialism, but there are also significant Afrikaner, Greek, Portuguese, French, and Dutch communities (CIA, 2021).

CULTURAL BELIEFS

According to the 2017 Inter Censal Demography Survey by the Zimbabwe National Statistics Agency (ZIMSTAT), 84% of Zimbabweans are Christian, 10% do not belong to any religion, and 0.7% are Muslim. An estimated 62% of the population attend religious services regularly. Approximately 69% of Zimbabweans belong to Protestant Christian formations, while 8% are Roman Catholic. Pentecostal-charismatic Christian congregations have proliferated in recent years and are playing a prominent role in public, social, and political life. The largest Christian churches are Anglican, Roman Catholic, Seventh-day Adventist, and Methodist (ZIMSTAT, 2017). As in other African countries, Christianity may be mixed with enduring traditional beliefs. Indigenous religion, which predates colonialism, has become relatively marginal but continues to be an essential part of the Zimbabwean religious field. Ancestral worship is the most practiced non-Christian religion, involving spiritual intercession. The *mbira* instrument is important during ceremonial proceedings (Chitando, 2020).

LANGUAGES AND FOOD

Zimbabwe has 16 official languages, and English is the primary language used in the education, commerce, and judicial systems. The Bantu languages, Shona and Ndebele, are the principal Indigenous languages of Zimbabwe. Shona is spoken by 78% of the population, Ndebele by 20%. Other minority Bantu languages include Venda, Tsonga, Shangaan, Kalanga, Sotho, Ndau, and Nambya. Less than 2.5%, mainly consisting of White and mixed-race minorities, consider English their native language (CIA, 2021). English is primarily spoken in the cities but less so in rural areas. Radio and television news are mainly broadcast in Shona, Ndebele, and English, although there are slots for the other official minority languages.

Sadza is the most common dish in Zimbabwe. It is a stiff maize meal like a thickened porridge. It can be rolled into a ball and dipped into meat, sauce, gravy, sour milk, or stewed vegetables.

SYSTEM OF GOVERNMENT

Zimbabwe is a republic with a presidential system of government. In 1987, Zimbabwe revised the constitution, abolishing the ceremonial presidency and the prime ministerial posts to form an executive president—a presidential system. The semipresidential system was abolished with the adoption of a new constitution after a referendum in 2013. Under the constitutional changes in 2005, an upper chamber, the Senate, was introduced (CIA, 2021). The House of Assembly is the lower chamber of Parliament. The Senate consists of 80 seats: 60 members are directly elected in multiseat constituencies—6 seats in each of the 10 provinces—by proportional representation vote; 16 seats are indirectly elected by the regional governing councils; 18 seats are reserved for the National Council Chiefs; and two seats are reserved for members with disabilities. Members of the Senate serve 5-year terms. The National Assembly consists of 280 seats: 210 members directly elected in single-seat constituencies by simple majority vote and 60 seats reserved for women directly elected by proportional representation vote; 10 additional seats are reserved for candidates between ages 21 and 35 years directly elected by proportional representation. Members of the National Assembly also serve 5-year terms (CIA, 2021).

BRIEF HISTORY OF ZIMBABWE

In 1880, Zimbabwe became a British colony, called Rhodesia, in honor of Cecil John Rhodes, who led the colonizing party. The colony status lasted until 1965, when the White minority declared independence from Britain to avoid having majority rule. Precolonial Zimbabwe societies were mainly farming communities that adopted iron tools to modernize their agriculture and cultivate more extensively than their Stone Age predecessors (Mlambo, 2014). They also practiced pastoralism and heavily depended on their livestock for milk and protein. The livestock also played an important role in facilitating marriage as they were used as *lobola* (dowry). Zimbabwe achieved majority rule and internationally recognized independence in April 1980 following a long period of colonial rule and 15 years of White-dominated minority rule, instituted after the minority regime's so-called Unilateral Declaration of Independence (UDI) in 1965. UN sanctions and an uprising led to free elections in 1979 and the creation of the independent country of Zimbabwe in 1980 (Mlambo, 2014). Prior to its recognized independence as Zimbabwe in 1980, the nation had been known by several names: Rhodesia, Southern Rhodesia, and Zimbabwe Rhodesia.

One of the earliest known Zimbabwe traditions is the use of totems. These totems, known as *mitupo*, are used by the various tribal groups to identify the different clans that made up the ancient civilizations of the dynasties. The symbols are usually associated with animal names and provide the social identity of the clan. Zimbabwe is renowned for numerous internationally acclaimed tourist destinations that offer sightseeing, game and bird viewing, game hunting, camping, rafting, elephant rides, walking with lions, and bungee jumping. Many Zimbabweans celebrate the Christian holidays, including Good Friday, Easter, Christmas Day, and Boxing Day. Other major holidays are New Year's Day (January 1), Independence Day (April 18), International Workers' Day (May 1), Africa Day (May 25), and National Unity Day (December 22). Natural resources include coal, chromium ore, asbestos, gold, nickel, copper, iron ore, vanadium, lithium, tin, and platinum group metals. Agricultural products include sugarcane, maize, beef, milk, cassava, wheat, bananas, vegetables, tobacco, and cotton. Primary industries include mining (coal, gold, platinum, copper, nickel, tin, diamonds, clay, numerous metallic and nonmetallic ores), steel, wood products, cement, chemicals, fertilizer, clothing and footwear, food, and beverages.

HEALTH OUTCOMES

Despite some improvements in key healthcare indicators, Zimbabwe's healthcare system still faces significant challenges as the life expectancy from birth is still low. In the past few years (2020–2021), life expectancy slowed down globally due to death rates from COVID-19 (population.un.org), and Zimbabwe is no exception. Between 2000 and 2021, Zimbabweans' life expectancy at birth increased by about 11.9 years, from 46.6 years to 58.5 years, and reached 60.7 years in 2019 before the pandemic (World Health Organization [WHO], 2023). In comparison, life expectancy for Africa as a whole for the same period (2000–2021) increased by 10.9 years, from 52.7 years to 63.6 years (WHO, 2023). Additionally, the infant mortality rate has steadily declined significantly due to public health measures the Zimbabwean government supports and enforces. Overall, infant mortality dropped from 103.31 deaths per 1,000 live births in 1954, to 53.47 in 2010, to 34.64 in 2022 (United Nations, 2024). The rate of HIV/AIDS is among the highest in the world despite a decrease from a rate of 29% to 15% since 1997 (CIA, 2021). The number one leading cause of death in Zimbabwe is HIV/AIDS, followed by respiratory infections, neonatal conditions, ischemic heart diseases, road injuries, cardiovascular events, diarrheal diseases, diabetes mellitus, protein-energy malnutrition, and congenital anomalies. For children younger than 5 years, the leading cause of mortality is also HIV/AIDS (WHO, 2023). Despite the high mortality rate from HIV, progress is being made, as 96% of people living with HIV are aware of their status and are receiving treatment with viral suppression in 93% of the affected people (WHO, 2023).

Malaria continues to be a significant health problem, with approximately 342,543 cases and 876 deaths in 2021. Tuberculosis also continues to be a challenging health problem, with an incidence rate of 181.3 cases per 10,000 people in 2020 (WHO, 2023). Neglected tropical diseases (NTD) that are endemic to Zimbabwe include trachoma, schistosomiasis (bilharzia), lymphatic filariasis, soil-transmitted helminthiasis, human Africa trypanosomiasis, leprosy, among others (WHO, 2023). As for the cause of death by broad categories, death due to communicable diseases and conditions related to maternal, perinatal, and nutritional issues is 47.6%. In comparison, 39.3% are due to NCDs, and 13.1% of deaths are related to injuries (WHO, 2023). Zimbabwe depends on local and external funding to combat some common disease outbreaks. WHO (2022) assists with testing, treatment, and vaccination efforts against infectious diseases such as tuberculosis and malaria and disease outbreaks of diarrheal diseases such as cholera. In 2021, there was also an outbreak of measles and rubella; both are preventable, yet approximately 66,300 children were under-mmunized, and an additional 33,150 children received no vaccinations.

Through coordinated efforts by the U.S. Agency for International Development (USAID) and the **Global Fund** to combat three major diseases (HIV, tuberculosis, and malaria), Zimbabwe was able to significantly and positiively impact maternal and childhood health by decreasing disease burden and reducing preventable deaths among women and children younger than 5 years (USAID, n.d.). Malaria is endemic to sub-Saharan Africa, including Zimbabwe, and significantly impacts public health in this region as it is one of the highest contributors to premature death and disability, especially among children younger than 5 years (Gunda et al., 2016). Although infant mortality has decreased (Figure 37.2), it is still above that of most countries.

Recently, Zimbabwe experienced cholera outbreaks in some regions of the country, and this required coordinated efforts to contain the spread of the disease using conventional cholera prevention methods (WHO, 2023). The measures to combat cholera are still relevant and enforced. At the same time, with external funding resources, Zimbabwe was able to launch a cholera

FIGURE 37.2 Neonatal, infant, and child mortality rates in Zimbabwe.

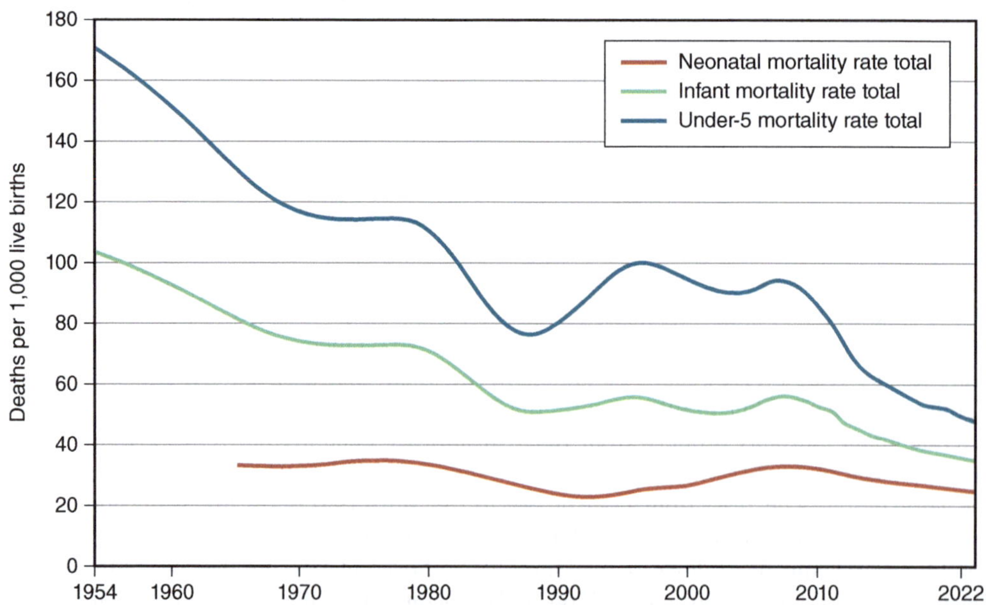

Source: United Nations. (2024). *Inter-agency group mortality estimation (IGME) all-cause mortality.* https://childmortality.org/all-cause-mortality/data?refArea=ZWE&indicator=MRY0&sex=_T

vaccination campaign with the target of vaccinating 2.3 million people in the regions impacted the most (WHO, 2024).

Mental Health

Like most countries, Zimbabwe also faces an increase in mental health conditions and a severe shortage of mental health providers. This often overlooked and severely underfunded component of health and well-being is now drawing more attention from the health industry, policymakers, and government officials. WHO estimates there is one psychiatrist for every 1 million people in Zimbabwe. Several mental health conditions affect a significant portion of the population in Zimbabwe, with WHO estimating that about 4% of the population suffers from depressive disorders and 2.8% suffer from anxiety disorders (WHO, 2022). Additionally, the prevalence of alcohol use is 6.4%, and dependency disorder is 2.2%—rates higher than the African region (WHO, 2022). Higher rates of depression are also noted among those living with HIV/AIDS (WHO, 2022).

DETERMINANTS OF HEALTH

Poverty is a significant social determinant of health. As of 2022, the national gross national product (GDP) for Zimbabwe was $27.37 billion; the GDP per capita is $1,676.8. The GDP annual growth is 6.5%, and inflation is 104.7%, while the unemployment rate in 2023 was at 9.1% (World Bank Group, 2024). The overall average literacy rate for Zimbabwe is approximately 90% for age 15 years to adult, a higher average rate than that of the sub-Saharan region (68%) and the world average of 87% (World Bank Group, 2024).

Zimbabwe is already experiencing the impact of climate change with more recurrent droughts and unpredictable rainfall patterns, which threaten food and water security and worsen the economy, which is dependent on the agriculture industry (UNDP Climate Change Adaptation, 2024). Vector-borne diseases such as malaria and bilharzia (schistosomiasis) also worsen with climate change. With support from different organizations, Zimbabwe is building climate resilience for vulnerable agricultural livelihoods in high risk areas (UN Development Programme, 2024; Gavi, 2024). In March of 2019, Zimbabwe was impacted by Cyclone Idai, which left 340 people dead, many casualties, and 51,000 people displaced. This experience was something to learn from in terms of preparedness, timely response, and mitigation of negative consequences on health outcomes (Ray et al., 2022).

According to UNICEF (2024), fewer than one in 10 children consume food per the recommended daily diet of five or more food groups, and it is estimated that over one-half million (25%) children in Zimbabwe are malnourished on a chronic basis, leading to stunted growth and other poor outcomes. Since the COVID-19 pandemic, acute malnutrition is worse, with 15,000 children with severe wasting and requiring treatment (UNICEF, 2024). Drought conditions due to El Nino could worsen food insecurity. UNICEF, other organizations, and the local government are supporting mitigating interventions such as community-based nutrition programs that provide nutrition-dense and affordable foods. Integrated along with the nutrition programs are HIV and tuberculosis services for children younger than 5 years, and, to improve nutrition for older children, there are school-based feeding programs.

In addition to concerns about children's health and the long-standing diseases common in the region, Zimbabweans now face a growing threat of conditions that some developed nations grapple with. These conditions that require health behavior change include diabetes, heart disease, strokes, hypertension, and associated obesity. In their cross-sectional study, Tozivepi et al. (2021) identified low adherence to recommended health lifestyle behavior changes in patients diagnosed with hypertension. They defined nonadherence as poor diet, low physical activity, smoking, drinking, and not taking prescribed medications.

HISTORICAL/THEORETICAL BACKGROUND OF HEALTHCARE

When Southern Rhodesia (present-day Zimbabwe) became a British colony in 1890, the healthcare system was dominantly rudimentary and organized by enclaves; it primarily served the medical needs of the minority population consisting of White colonialists and their African employees through private practitioners who arrived with the settlers (Woelk, 1994). However, in the aftermath of a landmark transition to a self-governed colony from imperial Britain in the early 1920s, there was mounting pressure to improve the health services available to Africans and create a buffer between the African populations that were considered to be "diseased" and the European community (Woelk, 1994). By the early 1930s, rural health facility expansion was prioritized by the new colonial administration due to transcolonial learning, the emergence of a colonial regime sympathetic to natives' affairs, and pressure to prove the colony's capacity for self-governance. In this regard, the development of medical services in Southern Rhodesia was directed by the central colonial administration with the assistance of churches that established mission hospitals (Mhazo et al., 2023).

Zimbabwe's healthcare system is mainly divided into the public and private sectors. The government owns around 70% of the country's healthcare facilities, while the private sector owns the remaining 30%. The public health system consists of central hospitals that serve as national referral centers, provincial hospitals, district hospitals, and central government and local government clinics. It is complemented by mission hospitals and healthcare delivered by nongovernmental organizations (NGOs).

Finance and Insurance

The health system in Zimbabwe is mainly financed through a mix of public and private sources. Public funds are sourced by the Ministry of Finance and the municipalities. Private funding sources include corporations, households, nonprofit organizations, and donors. Financing sources as a percentage of total health expenditure in 2018 were as follows: government 44.1%; corporations 15.8%; households 13.43%; and the rest of the world 26.7% (Mhazo et al., 2023). Central general revenue, obtained by the central government from taxes and nontaxable revenue, remains the primary funding source for government through fiscal allocation. However, most of this money is directed toward salaries and other employee-related costs (30%), with low capital investment (1% in 2017 and 4% in 2018). As a result, service availability and quality is severely hampered at public health facilities, and the user-fee policy is strictly enforced for consultation, and for inpatient and outpatient services to cover the deficits. The private healthcare sector in Zimbabwe, which initially catered to upmarket clients, is now open to low-income urban populace. With the number of trained medical personnel on the rise, even people living in "high-density" suburbs can seek treatment privately. The Medical Aid Societies are responsible for the growing number of private healthcare centers in Zimbabwe (Mhazo et al., 2023).

Zimbabwe has one of the highest rates in the world of private health insurance (PHI) expenditures as a share of total health expenditures. Zimbabwe's current PHI coverage is segmented along socioeconomic lines due to a long history of elitist and exclusionary politics in coverage patterns. While PHI was considered to perform relatively well up to the mid-1990s, the economic crisis of the 2000s eroded trust among insurers, providers, and patients. That culminated in agency problems that severely lessened PHI coverage quality with concurrent deterioration in efficiency and equity-related performance dimensions. Both the urban and the semiurban populations depend on polyclinics managed by local government authorities or city councils. They can access private medical facilities in their localities through medical insurance coverage. Sometimes, due to disagreements between clinics and insurance companies, medical insurance holders still end up paying out of pocket. Most of the working population in the country cannot afford private medical centers and clinics, and depend on the more affordable state and mission hospitals and clinics. Zimbabwe has more than 30 medical aid societies, 10 of which are restricted to respective industries or employees (Mhazo et al., 2023).

Training of Healthcare Workers

Traditionally, training of healthcare personnel in Zimbabwe has been the responsibility of the government. However, competing priorities and socioeconomic and political uncertainties in the past two decades have greatly reduced government funding of both training institutions and government-run health facilities. Prior to the year 2000, government funding of public health institutions and training institutions was adequate. Zimbabwe had a single medical school at the University of Zimbabwe in Harare training doctors and several schools that trained nurses, dentists, and other healthcare cadres. During this period, hospitals were well equipped and staff adequately remunerated, and patients could afford services offered by the public health system. The training was of an adequate standard and was able to meet the needs of the communities and the nation at large. High-end medical procedures like open-heart surgery, cochlear implants, and separation of conjoined twins by locally trained pediatric surgeons all attest to the high standard of training prior to the "brain drain" and the decline in patients treated in public institutions. The overall output of healthcare training was a well-trained medical practitioner. Furthermore, retention of trained healthcare workers always met the needs of the population (Chidziva & Soko, 2021).

After the economic and political upheaval at the start of the millennium, a new reality set in affecting both healthcare provision and training institutions. The net effect of the deteriorating economic climate was a reduction in government investment in public health institutions and state universities. Consequently, retention of academic faculty began to decline as academics left public institutions, usually in pursuit of better remuneration and working conditions. Deteriorating economic conditions reduced remuneration of healthcare practitioners. A natural "brain drain" followed with the majority of practitioners migrating to better resourced countries while those that remained entered private practice. Currently, health practitioners in state institutions dedicate more time to private practice where working conditions, infrastructure, and remuneration are higher. Cycles of hyperinflation have eroded disposable income in the general population, and public institutions have seen a decline in patient numbers. Patients who could afford to do so chose private healthcare over public health systems. Dwindling patient numbers at public institutions reduced clinical exposure for trainees at both undergraduate and postgraduate levels and for faculty. This has been compounded by outdated and dilapidated infrastructure and ill-equipped training to meet the standard of quality training required at both undergraduate and postgraduate levels (Chidziva & Soko, 2021).

However, despite deterioration in public health systems, private health systems in Zimbabwe tell a different story. Private healthcare in Zimbabwe is a robust industry. There is significant investment in infrastructure and remuneration of personnel and much higher staff retention than the public health system. Accountability and transparency are higher in the private healthcare systems; hence, investors find it to be a lucrative investment opportunity. Activities in the private sector have therefore remained steady and robust. However, private healthcare has benefited tremendously from the health training provided by the public health system and state training institutions but has put very little back into the training system. It is the authors' view that it is time for private–public synergies to be actively pursued to ensure the survival and resuscitation of quality training of health personnel in Zimbabwe (Chidziva & Soko, 2021).

Access to Healthcare

In Zimbabwe, access to healthcare services is influenced by long distances and travel times to health facilities, the availability of financial resources to travel or pay for care, and the availability of medical drugs as well as competent healthcare workers. For example, in Zimbabwe, people in rural areas often have to walk between 10 and 50 kilometers (6 to 31 miles) to access the nearest health facility. Access can be further impeded by a lack of infrastructure, such as roads that are not maintained, resulting in poor road conditions and potholes that create barriers to transport. In Zimbabwe, because of economic challenges, bridges that have collapsed because of rain are not repaired, hindering traveling of patients during critical times and negatively affecting the timely delivery of drugs and medical supplies to rural health centers (Chidziva & Soko, 2021).

Gaps in Care or Healthcare Shortage Areas

Even where healthcare services are available and affordable, access to medical drugs is limited. There is often a shortage in the supply of medical drugs, especially in the rural parts of Zimbabwe. It is evident that the economic crisis in Zimbabwe has also led to a shortage of medical supplies and equipment in public health facilities, leaving professional nurses with limited options to provide treatment. The economic crisis has caused community outreach programs to be closed, as they were likely to place a further burden on the few nurses available. The family planning distribution program has crumbled, as family planning drugs are not available, and thus the birth rate has increased. There were challenges with access to antiretroviral drugs for people living with HIV in the rural areas because of shortages, transportation challenges, and nurses' attitudes at designated rural health facilities (Mangundu et al., 2020).

Zimbabwe has also failed to meet the minimum 15% annual health budget allocation as indicated in the Abuja Declaration of 2001, where African leaders agreed to allocate 15% of their countries' total annual budget to the health sector. Although some efforts were made by Zimbabwe's government in 2010 to reverse the significant declines in the health allocation of the annual budget (12.3% of the total allocated annual budget), the increase was reversed in subsequent years to 7% in 2012, 8.2% in 2013, 7.3% in 2015, and 8.3% in 2016 (Mangundu et al., 2020). The country's once-efficient medical system has been deteriorating over the years and is facing shortages of medical facilities, supplies, and staff. The country is abundant with natural resources but faces challenges related to healthcare and its economy (Chidziva & Soko, 2021).

HEALTHCARE PRACTICES

Zimbabwe's healthcare system uses a combination of conventional medicine (allopathic) and nonconventional (traditional/Indigenous, alternative, complementary) approaches to deliver healthcare to the population. The most commonly used approach is the allopathic or conventional approach, whereby trained healthcare professionals such as physicians, nurses, pharmacists, psychologists, and others provide healthcare services. Conventional medicine is well established and regulated but underfunded, and there is a severe shortage of healthcare professionals, as highlighted previously. Despite the well-established conventional healthcare system, Zimbabweans also rely heavily on traditional methods they have used since ancient times, which incorporate herbalists and *n'angas* (medicine men/women or traditional healers). Zimbabweans also rely on Eastern methods of healing as well as spiritual healing through their places of worship. Some religious sects do not use conventional or traditional methods of healing and strictly abide by their religious teachings, relying on spiritual healing alone. In general, Zimbabweans understand illness as a physical phenomenon but also perceive it through traditional and religious lenses, hence, the use of a combined approach to healthcare. Traditional practices and different Christian faiths support current knowledge that religion and tradition play a critical role in health-seeking behaviors that facilitate adherence to treatment regimens (Wüthrich-Grossenbacher et al., 2023). Conceptions about HIV, risk-taking, and health-seeking behaviors were significantly influenced by religious beliefs that moralized HIV infections, and were associated with higher viral loads of HIV, higher treatment failure, and high risk for opportunistic infections along with high rates of rejecting screenings for preventing cancers such as cervical cancer (Wüthrich-Grossenbacher et al., 2023).

Overall, traditional or Indigenous health practices are a significant part of healthcare for many African countries with an estimated 80% of Africans using the Indigenous treatments for their primary healthcare (Oseni & Shannon, 2020). Much of traditional health practices are unregulated, despite many Africans relying on Indigenous healthcare. The challenge of unregulated care is the threat to public health that can result from unregistered and unsafe treatments (Usai et al., 2021) or unsafe combinations of treatments from both traditional (Indigenous) and allopathic systems. Zimbabwe has an Indigenous health system with two regulatory bodies for registration and control of the sale of traditional medicines; however, the system needs improvement (Usai et al., 2021). There are many concerns about unregulated medicinal products, which can range from contaminants such as heavy metals (mercury, lead, arsenic, chromium); microorganisms (bacteria, parasites, fungi); and improper, inadequate, or lacking labeling (Usai et al., 2021). Another challenge is the lack of established standards to identify competent traditional practitioners in diagnosing and treating conditions, thereby protecting the public as well as rooting out imposter traditional practitioners (Mwaka et al., 2023). Many traditional health practitioners believe healing powers are inherited from their family line, bestowed upon them by senior healers through dreams and visions that provide the how-to instructions, or during spiritual activities (Mwaka et al., 2023). Additionally, there are several perceived causes of illness among traditional practitioners, including natural causes, infections, poor hygiene, fate, curses, witchcraft, evil actions, and heredity/generational curses (Mwaka et al., 2023). Traditional health practitioners' diagnostic approaches include consulting with the spirits, diagnostic ritual performances, use of artifacts such as animal bones and more, observations of patterns of recurrent events, evaluation of known signs and symptoms of disease, and use of health facilities' biomedical laboratory testing (Mwaka et al., 2023).

RECENT OR IN-DEVELOPMENT HEALTHCARE INNOVATIONS

While the right to healthcare is enshrined in the 2013 Constitution of Zimbabwe, financing healthcare continues to be challenging. However, several initiatives have been implemented to help alleviate some of Zimbabwe's healthcare challenges. In 2021, with the help of external financial support, Zimbabwe launched the Health Resilience Fund (HRF) and strategic frameworks to help make Universal Health Coverage (UHC) a reality for all people with a special focus on ending preventable maternal, newborn, child, and adolescent deaths; improve health security; and strengthen health systems (Chimbwanda, 2023).

The WHO Regional Office also launched an initiative to improve access for services for early detection and treatment of breast and cervical cancers (World Health Organization Regional Office for Africa, 2023). Additionally, WHO's mhGAP program is used in Zimbabwe to train non–mental health specialist healthcare workers. The FRIENDZ project is also part of the Zimbabwe Special Initiative for Mental Health that was implemented in partnership with WHO and Friendship Bench. This 2023 initiative is financially supported by the Grand Challenges Canada and will run until 2025 (WHO, 2022). Lastly, the Global Fund and other interagency groups continue to finance HIV/AIDS screening, prevention, and treatment programs in Zimbabwe (WHO, 2022).

CONCLUSION

The health challenges affecting Zimbabwe can be resolved if health and healthcare are prioritized in the national budget. Zimbabwe's decades-old economic crisis continues to severely impact the health delivery system in many ways, including creating a shortage of medical supplies and equipment and the mass exodus of healthcare workers. All these challenges have weakened disease prevention efforts and led to underdiagnosis and undertreatment of both communicable and NCDs. Efforts by the government of Zimbabwe to improve access to healthcare after attaining political independence in 1980 need to be revived. Revival of these efforts will ensure that Zimbabwe is better placed to address health burdens that include HIV, malaria, tuberculosis, cancers, diabetes, lower respiratory infections, mental health conditions, hypertension, and other cardiovascular conditions.

RECOMMENDATIONS TO IMPROVE HEALTH AND HEALTHCARE

- More sustainable funding is required to support the healthcare delivery system. Such funding would support various areas including workforce development and procurement of equipment, drugs, and supplies.
- Public education should remain a priority and should focus on both communicable disease and NCD prevention strategies.
- The government of Zimbabwe should prioritize research by providing funding to support research that addresses the needs of the country.
- The Ministry of Health should prioritize the training of mental health specialists and should ensure that psychiatry is included in the general nursing curriculum.
- The government and Ministry of Health should employ strategies to ensure rural areas can attract qualified staff.
- Advanced practice nurse training should be prioritized as an option in addressing the shortage of medical doctors in rural areas. Universities around the country along with the relevant ministries should also rethink the role of the nurse practitioner in Zimbabwe to alleviate the chronic provider shortage. Lessons can be learned from several examples of developed nations as well as the robust literature supporting this role, including the Robert Woods Johnson Foundation's *Future of Nursing Report* at the former Institute of Medicine (2010) now the National Academies of Sciences, Engineering and Medicine.
- More resources should be devoted to mobile clinics that can play a significant role in reaching isolated and underserved communities.

LEARNING ACTIVITIES

CourseConnect >

To access self-assessment questions and interactive, competency-based learning activities for this chapter, visit www.springerpub.com/courseconnect. See inside front cover and tear-out for CourseConnect details.

REFERENCES

Britannica. (2024). *Zimbabwe*. https://www.britannica.com/place/Zimbabwe

Central Intelligence Agency. (2021). *The world factbook 2021*. https://www.cia.gov/the-world-factbook/countries/zimbabwe/

Chidziva, C, & Soko, N. D. (2021). Training and capacity development in healthcare: What role can the private sector play? A case of Zimbabwe. *East and Central Africa Journal of Otolaryngology, Head and Neck Surgery, 5*, 45–46. https://kenyaentsociety.or.ke/wp-content/uploads/2021/10/ENT-July-2021-full-Journal.pdf

Chimbwanda, T. A. (2023). *Zimbabwe launches health resilience fund and strategic framework to bolster universal health coverage*. https://www.afro.who.int/countries/zimbabwe/news/zimbabwe-launches-health-resilience-fund-and-strategic-frameworks-bolster-universal-health-coverage

Chitando, E. (2020). *Politics and religion in Zimbabwe: The deification of Robert Mugabe*. Routledge.
Gavi, the Vaccine Alliance. (2024). *Zimbabwe's battle to control a skin-burrowing worm faces a new challenge: Climate change*. https://www.gavi.org/vaccineswork/zimbabwes-battle-control-skin-burrowing-worm-faces-new-challenge-climate-change
Gunda, R., Chimbari, M., & Mukaratirwa, S. (2016). Assessment of burden of malaria in Gwanda District, Zimbabwe, using the disability adjusted life years. *International Journal of Environmental Research and Public Health, 13*(2), 244. https://doi.org/10.3390/ijerph13020244
Institute of Medicine. (2010). *A summary of the February 2010 forum on the future of nursing: Education*. The National Academies Press. https://doi.org/10.17226/12894
Mangundu, M., Roets L., & Janse van Rensberg, E. (2020). Accessibility of healthcare in rural Zimbabwe: The perspective of nurses and healthcare users. *African Journal of Primary Health Care & Family Medicine, 12*(1), 2071–2936. https://doi.org/10.4102/phcfm.v12i1.2245
Mhazo, A. T., Maponga, C. C., & Mossialos, E. (2023). Inequality and private health insurance in Zimbabwe: History, politics and performance. *International Journal for Equity in Health, 22*(54). https://doi.org/10.1186/s12939-023-01868-9
Mlambo, A. S. (2014). *A history of Zimbabwe*. Cambridge University Press.
Mugwagwa, J. T., Chinyadza, J. K., & Banda, G. (2017). Private sector participation in health care in Zimbabwe: What's the value-added? *Journal of Healthcare Communications, 2*(2), 10. https://doi.org/10.4172/2472-1654.100050
Mwaka, A. D., Achan, J., & Orach, C. G. (2023). Traditional health practices: A qualitative inquiry among traditional health practitioners in northern Uganda on becoming a healer, perceived causes of illnesses, and diagnostic approaches. *PLoS One, 18*(4), e0282491. https://doi.org/10.1371/journal.pone.0282491
Oseni, Z., & Shannon, G. (2020). The relationship between Indigenous and allopathic health practitioners in Africa and its implications for collaboration: A qualitative synthesis. *Global Health Action, 13*(1), 1838241. https://doi.org/10.1080/16549716.2020.1838241
Ray, S., Goronga, T., Chigiya, P. T., & Madzimbamuto, F. D. (2022). Climate change, disaster management and primary health care in Zimbabwe. *African Journal of Primary Health Care & Family Medicine, 14*(1), e1–e3. https://doi.org/10.4102/phcfm.v14i1.3684
Tozivepi, S. N., Takawira, S., Chikaka, E., Mundagowa, P., Chadambuka, E. M., Mukora-Mutseyekwa, F. (2021). The nexus between adherence to recommended lifestyle behaviors and blood pressure control in hypertensive patients at Mutare Provincial Hospital, Zimbabwe: A cross-sectional study. *Journal of Patient Prefer Adherence, 15*, 1027–1037. https://doi.org/10.2147/PPA.S306885
UNDP Climate Change Adaptation. (2024). *Zimbabwe: Africa*. https://www.adaptation-undp.org/explore/africa/zimbabwe
UNICEF. (2024). *Child food poverty*. https://www.unicef.org/media/157661/file/Child-food-poverty-2024.pdf
UN Agency International Development. (n.d.). *Global health: Zimbabwe*. https://www.usaid.gov/zimbabwe/global-health
Usai, J., Ekeocha, Z., Byrn, S. R., & Clase, K. L. (2021). Herbal medicines registration process for Zimbabwe: Overview of the process. *BIRS Africa Technical Report Papers*. Paper 8. http://doi.org/10.5703/1288284317434
Woelk, G. B. (1994). Primary health care in Zimbabwe: can it survive? An exploration of the political and historical developments affecting the implementation of PHC. *Social Science & Medicine, 39*(8), 1027–1035. https://doi.org/10.1016/0277-9536(94)90374-3
World Bank Group. (2024). *Zimbabwe*. https://data.worldbank.org/country/zimbabwe
World Health Organization. (2022). *Prevention and management of mental health conditions in Zimbabwe: The case for investment*. MHIC Report. https://www.afro.who.int/sites/default/files/2023-04/1.-zimbabwe-mental-health_investment_case_report_2022_%20%281%29_0.pdf
World Health Organization. (2023). *Zimbabwe*. https://data.who.int/countries/716
World Health Organization Regional Office for Africa. (2023). *Ending disease in Africa: Responding to communicable and noncommunicable diseases 2023*. https://www.afro.who.int/sites/default/files/2024-04/UCN%20Cluster%20Report_2023.pdf
World Population Review. (2024). *Zimbabwe population*. https://worldpopulationreview.com/countries/zimbabwe-population

Wüthrich-Grossenbacher, U., Midzi, N., Mutsaka-Makuvaza, M. J., & Mutsinze, A. (2023). Religious and traditional beliefs and practices as predictors of mental and physical health outcomes and the role of religious affiliation in health outcomes and risk taking. *BMC Public Health, 23*(1), 2170. https://doi.org/10.1186/s12889-023-17030-7

Zimbabwe National Statistics Agency. (2017). *Inter-censal demographic survey, 2017 report.* https://www.zimstat.co.zw/wp-content/uploads/publications/Population/population/ICDS_2017.pdf

PART X. Health and Healthcare in West and Central Asia

CHAPTER 38

OVERVIEW OF WEST AND CENTRAL ASIA

James Giallella, Sheena Malla, and Thomas Foley

GEOGRAPHY

Central and West Asia are recognized as climate change–vulnerable regions that are susceptible to intense heat waves, drought, and water scarcity (Intergovernmental Panel on Climate Change [IPCC], 2025). **Central Asia,** the least-populated Asian subregion, comprises five countries: Tajikistan, Uzbekistan, Kazakhstan, Turkmenistan, and Kyrgyzstan. Major geographic features in Central Asia include Kazakhstan's grassy steppes, the Aral Sea drainage basin, vast deserts with sparse fertile land along the Amu Darya River and Syr Darya River systems, and bordering mountain ranges such as the Tian Shan. While Central Asia contains urban centers such as Uzbekistan's capital Tashkent, the geography of the land has led to uneven population distribution (Britannica, 2025). Figure 38.1 is a map of Central Asia. **West Asia**, often referred to as the Middle East, is the second least-populated Asian subregion (UN Data Portal, n.d). West Asia is a geographically complicated region that includes Syria, Lebanon, Israel, Palestine, Jordan, Iraq, Iran, Kuwait, Bahrain, Qatar, Saudi Arabia, United Arab Emirates (UAE), Oman, and Yemen. It also includes several transcontinental countries—Asian–European nations that are considered to be part of West Asia

FIGURE 38.1 Map of Central Asia.

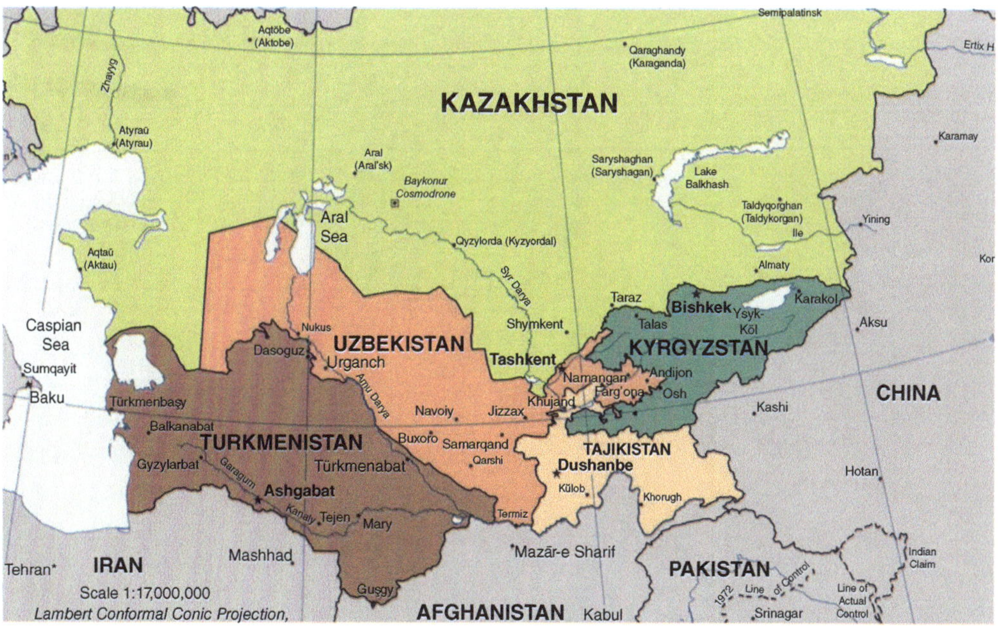

Source: U.S. Embassy in Uzbekistan. (n.d.). *United States strategy for Central Asia 2019-2025: Advancing sovereignty and economic prosperity.* https://uz.usembassy.gov/united-states-strategy-for-central-asia-2019-2025-advancing-sovereignty-and-economic-prosperity/

but have stronger geopolitical associations with Europe, including Georgia, Armenia, Azerbaijan, Turkey, and Cyprus. Egypt is a North African–West Asian nation that is primarily located in North Africa. Arid deserts cover large portions of West Asia; however, there are points of access to large bodies of water such as the Arabian Sea, Black Sea, Caspian Sea, Red Sea, Persian Gulf, Gulf of Aiden, and the Tigris–Euphrates River. In addition, there are cool mountainous regions such as the Pontiac Mountains in the Asian region of Turkey (Asia Society, 2025). Major cities in West Asia include Istanbul (located in both Europe and Asia Turkey), Baghdad (Iraq), Tehran (Iran), and Dubai (UAE). Figure 38.2 is a map of West Asia.

BRIEF HISTORY

West Asia is historically rich as it contains cradles of civilizations arising in the **Fertile Crescent** region, such as the Sumerians of Mesopotamia (4100–1750 BCE). Landmark developments that emerged in the Fertile Crescent include agriculture, farming, the use of irrigation, and writing. The region would become an area of imperial strife from antiquity through the early modern period among the Roman, Sassanid, Seljuk, Mongol, and Ottoman Empires (HistoryWorld, 2012). During the 17th century, the vast Ottoman Empire began to weaken due to European

FIGURE 38.2 Map of West Asia.

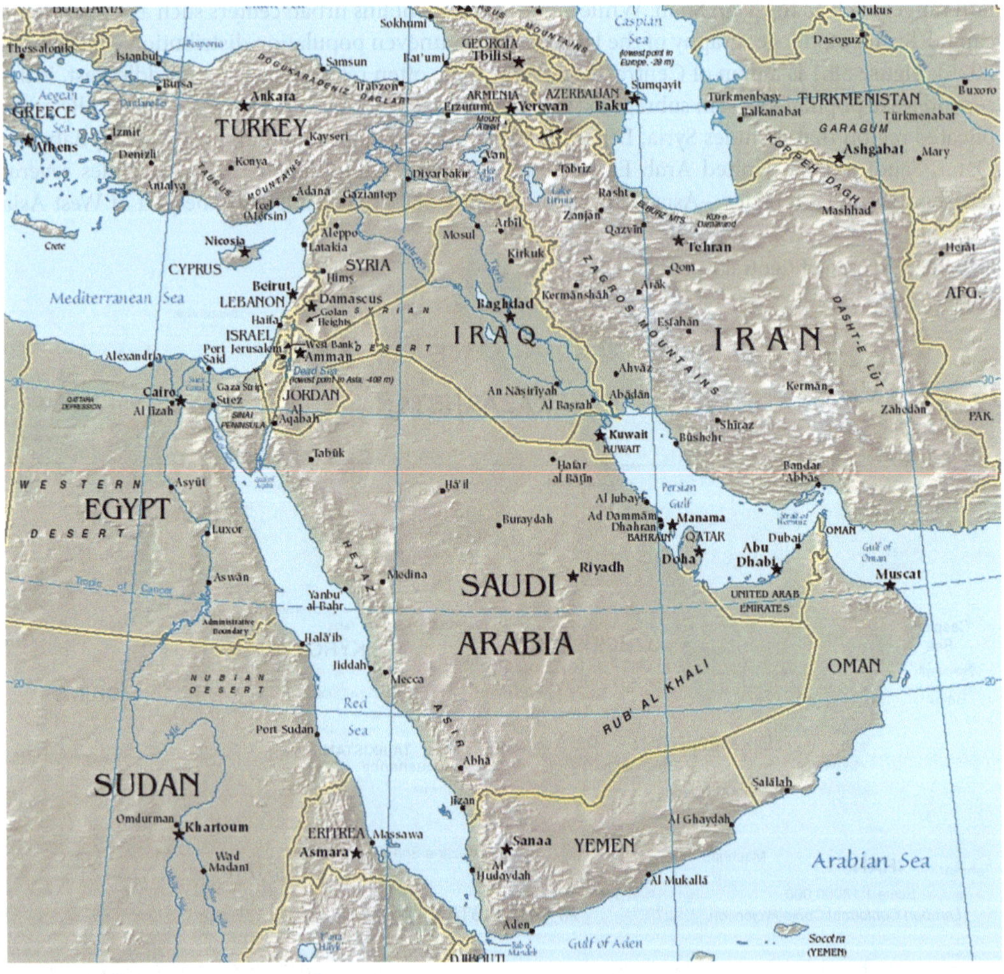

Source: Central Intelligence Agency. (n.d.). *Middle east.* https://en.wikipedia.org/wiki/Middle_Easthttps://en.wikipedia.org/wiki/Middle_East

expansion. It completely collapsed following World War I as it had sided with the losing German Empire. The defeated Ottoman Empire was partitioned into several new separate nations that included diverse people and territories with conflicting views. The **Partitioning of the Ottoman Empire** by the British and French created tension that persists in the modern Arab world. The end of World War II brought decolonization to West Asian nations. However, colonial interference was quickly replaced by the competing interest of the United States and Soviet Union. The growth of the region's oil industry along with the Iranian Revolution, U.S. and Russian interference, the rise of terrorist organizations such as Al-Qaeda and the Islamic State, the War on Terror, and Israel–Palestine conflicts have greatly shaped modern-day West Asia (Flynn, 2024).

Central Asia's history can be traced back to early nomadic groups such as the Cimmerians and Scythians in the first millennium BCE. The ethnic character of the region was influenced by the dominance of various Turkish peoples during the Iron Age and Middle Ages, such as the Xionghu, Uyghur, Khitan, and Karakhanids. The Mongols took control of Central Asia in the 13th century, opening up the area to allow trade between Europe and China. The collapse of the Mongol Empire diminished trade between European nations and China, leaving Central Asia isolated and impoverished. During the 17th century, Russia expanded their interests into Central Asia to trade with China. By the late 19th century, Russia controlled most of Central Asia. After the Russian Revolution of 1917, Soviet rule replaced Russian tsars, and the region was integrated into the Soviet system. In the 20th century, the Soviet system created five Soviet socialist republics in Central Asia. When the Soviet Union collapsed, these republics obtained their independence in 1991, becoming the five sovereign nations that now constitute the Central Asian region (Britannica, 2025).

POPULATION AND SOCIOECONOMIC FACTORS

Central Asia is a lower-income, majority-rural, and sparsely populated region. There were only 21 people per square kilometer (0.6 square miles) in Central Asia during 2023. The total population of Central Asia in 2023 was 80.81 million, making it one of the least populated regions in the world. Central Asia is also a young region with a low median age and high birth rate. Tajikistan had the lowest median age (21.9 years) among Central Asian countries in 2023. Uzbekistan had the highest birth rate (26.5 births per 1,000 people) among Central Asian countries in 2023 (UN Data Portal, n.d.).

The population of West Asia during 2023 was 303.97 million. Population statistics between West Asian countries vary drastically. The most populated country in West Asia during 2023 was Iran (90.61 million), while the least populated was Cyprus (1.34 million). Yemen had the lowest median age (18.2 years) during 2023, while Cyprus had the highest (37.8 years). The UAE and Qatar had the lowest West Asian birth rates in 2023, 9.8 and 9.9 births per 1,000 people, respectively. Yemen had the highest birth rate (35.2 births per 1,000 people) in West Asia (UN Data Portal, n.d.). With the exception of Yemen, West Asia is predominantly urban. West Asia is also a region of extreme economic inequities. It is home to some of the world's wealthiest and poorest countries. For example, the per-capita gross domestic product (GDP) in Qatar during 2023 was $80,196, while the per-capita GDP in Yemen was less than $500 (World Bank Group, n.d.).

HEALTH OUTCOMES

The leading causes of death in Central and West Asia during 2021 were COVID-19 and ischemic heart disease (Institute for Health Metrics and Evaluation, 2024). With the exceptions of the infant mortality rates (IMR) in Turkmenistan (31.77 infant deaths per 1,000 live births) and Tajikistan (24.50 infant deaths per 1,000 live births), the countries of Central Asia have relatively low IMRs and maternal mortality ratios (MMR). In addition, life expectancy at birth does not vary much among Central Asian countries. In 2023, life expectancy at birth for Central Asia was 72.65 years, which was near the global life expectancy at birth. In contrast to Central Asia, health outcomes in West Asian countries widely vary, resulting in intraregional disparities. For example, life expectancy at birth for Israel (82.41 years), IMR (2.78), and MMR (2.8) were significantly healthier than Yemen's life expectancy at birth (69.30), IMR (32.27), and MMR (183.40) (UN Data Portal, n.d.; UN Population Fund, n.d.). Addressing income inequities between West Asian nations is essential to ameliorating the health disparities that exist between its countries. See Table 38.1 for a list of health outcomes in Central and West Asia.

TABLE 38.1 CENTRAL AND WESTERN ASIA HEALTH DATA, 2020, 2021, AND 2023

REGION/ COUNTRY	LIFE EXPECTANCY AT BIRTH (2023)	INFANT MORTALITY RATE (2023)	MATERNAL MORTALITY RATIO (2020)	LEADING CAUSE OF MORTALITY (2021)
Central Asia	72.65	14.33	24.9	
Kazakhstan	74.40	8.12	13.4	COVID-19
Kyrgyzstan	71.68	14.26	50.4	Heart disease
Tajikistan	71.79	24.50	16.6	COVID-19
Turkmenistan	70.07	31.77	5.1	Heart disease
Uzbekistan	72.39	11.14	30.2	Heart disease
Western Asia	75.41	17.01	62.9	
Azerbaijan	74.43	14.95	40.8	Heart disease
Armenia	75.68	8.66	27.2	Heart disease
Bahrain	81.28	5.33	15.9	COVID-19
Cyprus	81.65	3.12	68.4	Heart disease
Georgia	74.50	8.14	27.6	COVID-19
Iraq	72.32	19.02	76.1	Heart disease
Iran	77.65	9.9	22	COVID-19
Israel	82.41	2.78	2.8	COVID-19
Jordan	77.81	11.75	41.3	COVID-19
Kuwait	80.40	7.25	7.2	Heart disease
Lebanon	77.82	15.72	20.6	COVID-19
Oman	80.03	8.56	17	COVID-19
Qatar	82.37	4.18	7.6	COVID-19
Saudi Arabia	78.73	5.06	16.2	Heart disease
State of Palestine	65.17	14.18	20.4	Heart disease
Syrian Arab Republic	72.12	16.74	29.9	Heart disease
Turkey	77.16	9.16	17.3	Heart disease
United Arab Emirates	82.91	4.86	9.3	COVID-19
Yemen	69.30	32.27	183.4	Heart disease

Sources: Adapted from Institute for Health Metrics and Evaluation. (2024). *Health research by location: Country profiles*. University of Washington. https://www.healthdata.org/research-analysis/health-by location/profiles; UN Data Portal. (n.d.). *UN population division data portal*. United Nations. https://population.un.org/dataportal/home/; UN Population Fund. (n.d.). *Data portal*. United Nations. https://www.unfpa.org/data

LEARNING ACTIVITIES

CourseConnect

To access self-assessment questions and interactive, competency-based learning activities for this chapter, visit www.springerpub.com/courseconnect. See inside front cover and tear-out for CourseConnect details.

REFERENCES

Asia Society. (2025). *West Asia*. https://asiasociety.org/countries-regions/west-asia

Britannica. (2025). *Central Asia*. https://www.britannica.com/place/Central-Asia

Flynn, R. J. (2024). *A history of the Middle East*. Portland Community College.

HistoryWorld. (2012). *Timeline: West Asia*. Oxford Reference.

Institute for Health Metrics and Evaluation. (2024). *Health research by location: Country profiles*. University of Washington. https://www.healthdata.org/research-analysis/health-by-location/profiles

Intergovernmental Panel on Climate Change. (2025). *Intergovernmental panel on climate change*. United Nations.

UN Data Portal. (n.d.). *UN population division data portal*. United Nations. https://population.un.org/dataportal/home/

UN Population Fund. (n.d.). *Data portal*. United Nations. https://www.unfpa.org/data

World Bank Group. (n.d.). *World Bank open data*. The World Bank Group. https://data.worldbank.org

CHAPTER 39

IRAN

Parisa Broomandkhoshbacht

INTRODUCTION

The Islamic Republic of Iran (also known as Persia or Iran, henceforth referred to as Iran) is a country located in West Asia that is rich with history, culture, and diversity. Iran (*ee-RAHN*) has a robust primary healthcare system with a strong focus on prevention. While Iran has seen significant improvement in recent decades in health outcomes with expansion of care, medical innovations, and improvement of socioeconomic conditions, inequities persist.

GEOGRAPHY AND POPULATION

GEOGRAPHIC FEATURES

Iran is located in the southwestern region of Asia, east of the Mediterranean Sea. It is bordered by Afghanistan, Armenia, Azerbaijan, Iraq, Pakistan, Turkey, and Turkmenistan. It shares coastlines with the Caspian Sea in the north and with the Persian Gulf and the Gulf of Oman in the south. With a total land surface area of 1,630,848 square kilometers (1,013,362 square miles), Iran is the second largest country in West Asia and the sixth largest country on the Asian continent (UN Statistics Division, 2023). Iran contains a diversity of landscapes, including mountains, plains, deserts, forests, wetlands, and glaciers. Mountainous land and plains make up about 52% of the territory, whereas deserts and forests constitute about 22% and 7%, respectively (Lumsden, 2018; World Bank Group, n.d.). As Iran's geography is diverse, so too is its population.

DEMOGRAPHIC FEATURES

Approximately 88,551,000 people live in Iran, about 9,013,700 of whom live in its capital city of Tehran (UN Statistics Division, 2023). Iran's population is shifting to be older, more urban, and more equal in number between sexes.

Age

The pyramid-shaped age distribution in Iran is relatively symmetric between the male and female populations with a median age of approximately 33 years old (UN Population Division, 2022; World Health Organization [WHO], 2024). The total fertility rate has seen a steep decline since the early 1980s, with the median total fertility rate at 6.6 births per woman in 1982 and 1.7 births per woman in 2022 (UN Population Division, 2022). Meanwhile, life expectancy in Iran has steadily increased over the past several decades, with a current life expectancy at birth of 75 years. This combination of increasing life expectancy and decreasing fertility rates is shifting Iran's population toward aging and is projected to result in a more pillar-shaped age distribution by the year 2050 (WHO, 2024).

Urban and Rural Populations

As of 2019, Iran's urban population constitutes about 75.4% of the total population while the remaining 24.6% live in rural areas (UN Statistics Division, 2023). Rural Iranians face notable health disparities compared to their urban counterparts due to challenges of access to medical and other resources; for instance, 87.7% of Iran's rural population has access to safe drinking water, compared to 96.2% of Iran's urban population (Danaei et al., 2019; UN Statistics Division, 2023). These disparities are improving as Iran implements measures to address health equity.

Sex and Gender

Iran has a sex ratio of 102 males per 100 females (Statistical Center of Iran, 2016; UN Statistics Division, 2023). This ratio may vary across different provinces; for instance, Iran's 2016 census revealed the Bushehr, Yazd, Ardebil, and Kerman provinces had sex ratios of greater than 105 males per 100 females (Statistical Center of Iran, 2016). Respective to gender equality, some progress on women's rights has been made, yet gender gaps persist in social, economic, and political sectors of Iran (World Bank Group, 2024). Regarding gender-diverse individuals, there are an estimated 1.46 transgender individuals per 100,000 Iranians with a transwoman/transman ratio of 1:2 (Talaei et al., 2022). Iranian law permits legal recognition of transgender individuals' gender identity so long as they are diagnosed with gender dysphoria, fit under a binary identity (thereby excluding nonbinary individuals), and have completed a long process of legal and medical gender transition. Iranian law fails to recognize the gender identity of transgender individuals who do not meet these criteria.

Ethnicity

While Persians make up Iran's largest ethnic group, numerous ethnic groups contribute to Iran's demographic diversity. Aside from Persians, the most populous ethnic and national groups living in Iran include Turks, Kurds, Baluchis, Arabs, Turkmans, and Lurs (Iran Chamber Society, n.d.). Iran also has a large but diminishing nomadic population, comprised of around 1 million nomads (96 tribes and 547 independent clans) of various ethnic origins who migrate throughout the provinces.

CULTURE

Iran's rich cultural fabric is colored by various religions, languages, and traditions in the context of its societal and political structures. Its culture may be defined by its elasticity—despite enduring numerous conquests and empires, Iran maintained a strong cultural identity that absorbed each new ruling power (Koutlaki, 2010).

RELIGION

Iran has been shaped by a diversity of faiths throughout its history. It is the birthplace of Zoroastrianism, one of the world's oldest organized religions. Iran today is an Islamic republic with a predominantly (over 99%) Muslim population, most of whom follow Shia Islam (Danaei et al., 2019). Religious minorities recognized by the Iranian constitution include Zoroastrians, Christians, and Jews. Other religious minorities, such as Baha'is or Yarsanis, are not recognized.

LANGUAGE

Persian (Farsi) is the official language of Iran and is spoken by most Iranians (Moradi, 2019). In descending order of the estimated number of speakers of languages other than Persian are Azeri, Kurdish, Gilaki, Mazandarani, Luri, Arabic, Balochi, Turkmen, Qashqai, Taleshi, Baadi, and numerous other local languages. Iran's language geography is further diversified by various dialects and subbranches of different languages.

POLITICAL SYSTEM

Iran established the Islamic Republic in 1979 after the Iranian Revolution abolished the institution of the monarchy (Koutlaki, 2010). Power is divided among different political bodies to deter anyone from seizing absolute power. All Iranians over the age of 18 years are entitled to vote and elect the president, the Parliament, local government, and the Assembly of Experts. The Assembly of Experts elect and advise the Supreme Leader, who must approve the president-elect before they can take office. Furthermore, the Supreme Leader appoints the head of the judiciary as well as six of 12 jurists on the Guardian Council, the most powerful body. Remaining jurists are proposed by the judiciary and must be approved by Parliament. The unelected Expediency Council advises the Supreme Leader and has the final say when Parliament and the Guardian Council disagree.

IMPORTANT TRADITIONS AND LEISURE PURSUITS

Iran follows the Persian Calendar, which is a solar calendar that begins in the vernal equinox and has the same starting point as the lunar Islamic calendar (Koutlaki, 2010). Major public holidays observed in Iran include Zoroastrian, Islamic, and international holidays as well as observances of major historical events. The festival of Nowruz, or Persian New Year, is perhaps the most widely celebrated holiday in Iran and in the diaspora. This holiday, marked by the spring equinox, symbolizes new beginnings and is celebrated by Iranians of all religious backgrounds. Iranians also enjoy various leisure pursuits including traveling, picnicking, watching television, eating out, and entertaining guests (which often entails serving tea).

HISTORICAL CONSIDERATIONS FOR CONTEXT

Iran is home to one of the world's oldest continuous civilizations, with evidence of settlements dating back over 5,000 years (Danaei et al., 2019). Much of its history is defined by various empires, dynasties, and conquests. In more recent history, the Islamic Republic of Iran was established in 1979 after the Iranian Revolution resulted in the collapse of the Pahlavi dynasty. The birth of this republic was shortly followed by prolonged military conflict with the Iran–Iraq War (1980–1988). Since its inception, the Islamic Republic of Iran has faced repeated economic sanctions by prominent Western powers, especially the United States. These sanctions place heavy economic burden on the Iranian people, especially among vulnerable populations (Sahraian et al., 2021). Such sanctions have resulted in shortages and increased costs of medical resources, including medications and medical equipment.

HEALTH OUTCOMES

LEADING CAUSES OF DEATH

Per 2024 WHO data, the top 10 causes of death in Iran include the following (in descending order): ischemic heart disease, stroke, road injury, hypertensive heart disease, diabetes mellitus, kidney diseases, chronic obstructive pulmonary disease, lower respiratory infections, Alzheimer disease and other dementias, and neonatal conditions (Figure 39.1). Noncommunicable diseases (NCDs) as a group have emerged as the leading cause of mortality in Iran.

NONCOMMUNICABLE DISEASES

As Iran's population ages and disease risk factors change, NCDs have replaced communicable diseases as the country's leading cause of death and disease burden (Danaei et al., 2019). NCDs—such as cardiovascular diseases (CVDs), hypertension, diabetes, mental and psychiatric disorders, substance use disorder, and road injuries—cause 81.3% of the deaths in Iran (WHO, 2024). In efforts to reduce mortality and disease burden of NCDs, the Iranian Non-Communicable Diseases Committee (INCDC) was formed in 2015, with a stated target of reducing premature NCD-related deaths by 25% by 2025 by engaging in multisectoral collaboration (Peykari et al., 2017).

Cardiovascular Disease

CVD is the leading cause of death in Iran, with an age-standardized rate in 2019 of 241.2 deaths per 100,000 population for both males and females (WHO, 2020). CVD disproportionately affects

FIGURE 39.1 Top 10 causes of death in Iran per 100,000 population.

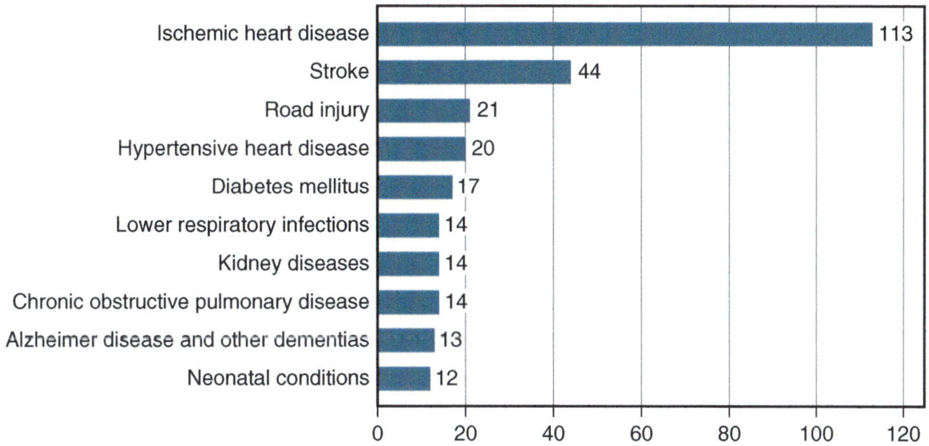

Source: Adapted from World Health Organization. (2020). *Global health estimates: Leading causes of death*. https://www.who.int/data/gho/data/themes/mortality-and-global-health-estimates/ghe-leading-causes-of-death

Iranian men; the age-standardized rate for CVD-related deaths in the male population of Iran is about 15% greater than that of the female population. Ischemic heart disease causes both the most deaths and disability adjusted life years (DALYs), followed by stroke (Farzadfar et al., 2022; WHO, 2020).

Road Injury

Road injuries are the third leading cause of death and second leading cause of DALYs (Farzadfar et al., 2022; WHO, 2020). Better policies to control road traffic injuries are needed in Iran, as evidenced by the low prevalence of seatbelt (around 75%) and helmet use (about 14%) in the Iranian population—both major contributors to road traffic injuries (Farzadfar et al., 2022). Low-quality domestic vehicles and poor driving behaviors also contribute to this problem, despite recent improvements in road infrastructure. In efforts to reduce this burden, the INCDC set a target for a 20% relative reduction in mortality rate due to road traffic injuries (Peykari et al., 2017).

Mental Health and Substance Use

Mental and behavioral disorders are the second group of diseases (behind CVDs) causing the highest DALYs and the first group of diseases causing years of life with disability (YLDs) in Iran (Danaei et al., 2019). According to the most recent national mental health survey data, nearly one in four Iranians in the 15 to 64 years age range has had at least one psychiatric disorder in a 12-month period; women have greater odds (1.47:1, adjusted for multiple factors) compared to men of meeting criteria for any psychiatric disorder (Sharifi et al., 2015). Anxiety disorders are most prevalent, followed by mood disorders. Nearly two thirds of those with a psychiatric disorder have a serious- or moderate-level disorder. Furthermore, 2.8% of respondents (5.2% of male respondents, 0.4% of female respondents) reported having any substance use disorder; however, these may be underestimated figures given the self-report nature of the survey and the strict legal punishments for use and possession of alcohol and other substances.

INFECTIOUS DISEASES

While NCDs have largely replaced communicable (infectious) diseases in terms of mortality rates and disease burden, infectious diseases—such as HIV/AIDS, tuberculosis, viral hepatitis, respiratory infections, and zoonoses—continue to be a priority area (WHO Regional Office for the Eastern Mediterranean, n.d.). Lower respiratory infections are the eighth leading cause of death in Iran, and the leading cause of mortality in children under 5 (WHO, 2020). Iran has also experienced a high number of COVID-19 deaths compared to other countries globally, as well as increased disabilities and socioeconomic disparities since the start of the pandemic (Rezaei et al., 2022).

INFANT AND MATERNAL MORTALITY

The infant mortality rate has steeply declined in past decades, dropping from 209 infant deaths per 1,000 live births in 1950 to 10 deaths per 1,000 live births in 2022 (UN Population Division, 2022). Similarly, maternal mortality has been halved between 2000 (44 deaths per 100,000 live births) and 2020 (22 deaths per 100,000 live births) and is lower than the regional average (World Bank Group, 2024).

LIFE EXPECTANCY AND QUALITY OF LIFE

Life expectancy in Iran has been steadily increasing over the past several decades as socioeconomic conditions and healthcare infrastructure improve; the most recent data estimate life expectancy at birth is 75 years (UN Population Division, 2022). Healthy life expectancy at birth has also improved from 62.6 years in 2000 to 64 years in 2019 (WHO, 2020). Overall disease burden has shown improvement in the past few decades; between 2000 and 2019, DALYs decreased from 1,200 years to 685.5 years per 100,000 population.

DETERMINANTS OF HEALTH

SOCIAL AND ECONOMIC FACTORS

Economic Factors

Iran has a national gross domestic product (GDP) of $594.9 billion (approximately 25 quadrillion Iranian rial [IRR]), with a per-capita GDP of $6,766.0 (approximately 284.8 million IRR) and an annual GDP growth of 4.7% (UN Statistics Division, 2023). In 2022, approximately 20% of the population were living below the societal poverty line, representing a 12-point decrease since 1986 (World Bank Group, n.d.). Poverty trends higher in eastern provinces, where life expectancy trends lower (Rezaei et al., 2022).

Unemployment and Education

Per most recent estimates, 16.1% of women and 69.3% of men in Iran participate in the labor force, while about 11.1% of the total labor force are unemployed (UN Statistics Division, 2023). Unemployment, in addition to informal jobs, dangerous working conditions, poverty, child labor, and lack of socioeconomic protections negatively affect health (Rezaei et al., 2022). Tangential to employment is education. Literacy rates among youth age 15 to 24 years have increased in recent decades from 87% in 1991 to 99% in 2022. Though gender- and location-based inequities in employment and education persist, they are progressively decreasing (Rezaei et al., 2022, World Banl, n.d.).

Nutrition

Iran has seen rapid urbanization and changing dietary patterns in recent decades, with a shift from traditional diets to diets higher in red and processed meats, refined grains, and fried foods (Damari et al., 2018). Increased food expenses in the last decade resulted in decreased caloric intake in rural areas (especially among lower-income households) and increased caloric intake among high-income urban households, leading to both under- and overnutrition. Notably, prevalence of undernourishment and adult obesity in Iran increased from 5.0% and 15.3% in 2001 to 6.1% and 23.9% in 2021, respectively (World Bank Group, n.d.; WHO, 2024).

HEALTH BEHAVIORS

Risk Factors

Prominent modifiable risk factors for NCDs in Iran include hypertension (26.2% prevalence), obesity (24.3% prevalence), and tobacco use (10% prevalence; Danaei et al., 2019; WHO, 2024). Major drivers of these modifiable risk factors include poor diet and physical inactivity. Air pollution, unsafe water, and unsafe sanitation are among major environmental risk factors in Iran with strong impacts on health status (Farzadfar et al., 2022). In 2019, air pollution was the fifth leading contributor to death and disability in Tehran and is estimated to have contributed to deaths from CVD, diabetes and kidney diseases, and chronic respiratory diseases.

SOCIAL JUSTICE AND HUMAN RIGHTS ISSUES

Numerous rights abuses and accounts of discrimination and persecution in Iran have been reported, with recent escalation of security forces' crackdowns on protestors following Mahsa Jina Amini's 2022 death while in custody of the morality police and the subsequent "Woman, Life, Freedom" protests (Human Rights Watch, 2024). Other human rights abuses include arbitrary detention and unfair trials; excessive and lethal force, torture, and sexual assault from security forces; executions of individuals convicted of crimes committed as children or vaguely worded offenses; restricted freedoms of assembly and expression; discrimination and violence against women and girls; punishment of same-sex conduct by flogging and (for men) the death penalty; and persecution of ethnic and religious minorities, especially Baha'is. Furthermore, Iran has been criticized for failure to adequately address its environmental crisis and substantial contributions to climate change (Elmore, 2021; Human Rights Watch, 2024).

ENVIRONMENTAL AND CLIMATE CHANGE ISSUES

Iran, like many countries, is adversely affected by climate change and related environmental issues and is seeing a worsening water crisis and increasing desertification (Elmore, 2021; Lumsden, 2018). Deforestation, overgrazing, and water overexploitation accelerate these crises and threaten Iran's diverse landscapes (Lumsden, 2018). Iran is also a sizable contributor to climate change—it is the largest greenhouse gas emitter in West Asia and the eighth-largest emitter in the world, with emissions primarily related to its petroleum industry (Elmore, 2021). Health and quality of life in Iran have worsened due to climate change and will continue to worsen without appropriate action and global collaboration.

HEALTHCARE SYSTEM

HEALTHCARE SYSTEM AND SERVICE DELIVERY

Iran's healthcare system is predominantly comprised of public healthcare providers that include government-funded hospitals, clinics, and health centers, with the private sector contributing to a lesser extent (Aboutorabi et al., 2023). Much of the population is covered by a national health insurance system called the Islamic Republic of Iran Health Insurance Organization, which provides coverage for services including hospitalization, outpatient care, and prescription medications. Iran emphasizes primary healthcare with prioritization of universal access, equity, and community involvement. Services are delivered through a referral system, starting from the first level and moving to higher levels based on degree of specialization required. Urban and rural health centers provide less specialized services, while hospitals, polyclinics, and academic hospitals offer specialized and super-specialized services.

HEALTHCARE EDUCATION AND TRAINING

Medical education is well-established in Iran, with over 50 publicly funded medical schools and numerous private ones since significant expansion in the 1980s (Danaei et al., 2019). These reputable institutions educate and train physicians, nurses, dentists, pharmacists, and allied health workers including **community health** workers.

HEALTHCARE COSTS

Since 1910, all Iranian citizens are entitled to primary healthcare services free of charge (Danaei et al., 2019). As of 2021, healthcare expenditures in Iran were 5.8% of the GDP, with a health expenditure per capita of $392.54 (WHO, 2024). The proportion of out-of-pocket expenditures, as a percentage of current health expenditure, was 34.5% in Iran in 2021 (World Bank Group, n.d.). This figure has decreased over time but remains higher than the global average. Healthcare expenditures are primarily spent via hospitals, outpatient providers, and pharmacies or other retailers of medical products (Danaei et al., 2019). For hospital services, households pay 52% of the costs while public health insurance pays 21%.

HEALTHCARE SHORTAGE AREAS

Despite investments in expansion of care, Iran struggles with shortages of healthcare professionals, with greater shortages in rural areas (Danaei et al., 2019). In Iran, the density of healthcare professionals has steadily improved in the past two decades but remains below the world average for most professional types except for dentists (WHO, 2024; Figure 39.2).

FIGURE 39.2 Healthcare professional density by profession and region.

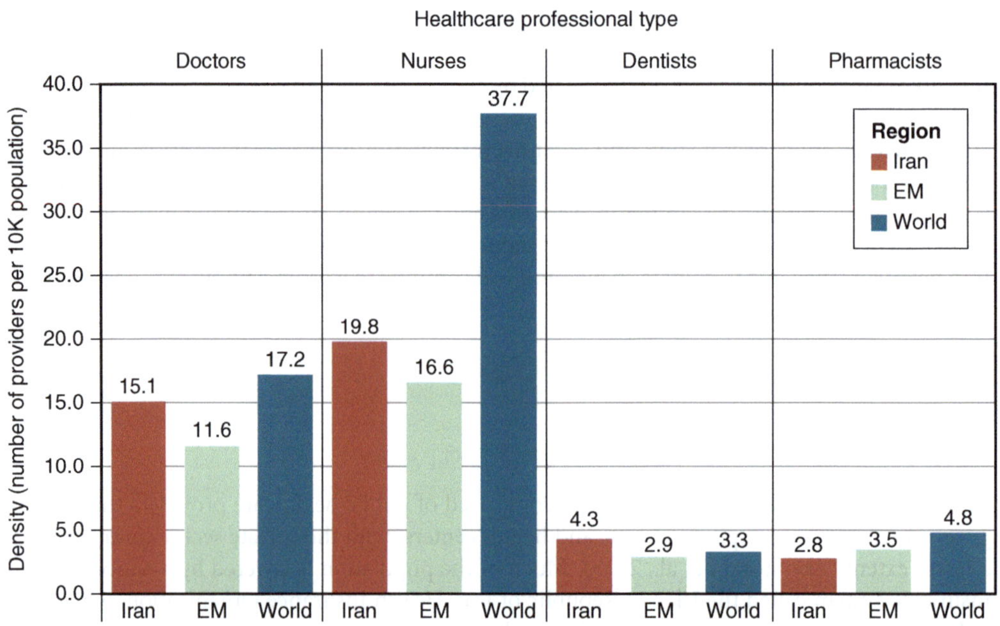

Note: Side-by-side regional densities (count per 10,000 population) of different healthcare professionals.

EM, Eastern Mediterranean.

Source: Adapted from World Health Organization. (2024). *Iran (Islamic Republic of) data*. WHO Data. https://data.who.int/ countries/364

HEALTHCARE PRACTICES

ALLOPATHIC MEDICINE

Modern allopathic medicine, sometimes referred to as "conventional" medicine, has existed in Iran since at least the mid-19th century with the establishment of modern medical institutions (Danaei et al., 2019). However, Iran's relationship to allopathic medicine dates back millennia. Historical Iranian medical scholars and scientists, such as Rhazes and Avicenna from the 10th and 11th centuries, introduced several foundational principles of allopathic medicine. Today, allopathic physicians (MDs) are trusted medical authorities in Iran who often integrate allopathic medicine with traditional medicine.

TRADITIONAL MEDICINE

Iranian traditional medicine (ITM) is a holistic practice of medicine with roots dating back to 8,000 BCE (Rezaeizadeh et al., 2009). ITM encompasses the sum of all the diagnostic, preventive, and treatment-related knowledge and practices used in Iran from ancient to present times. Ingrained in Iranian culture, ITM continues to be practiced and is integrated into the overall healthcare system (Aboutorabi et al., 2023). ITM emphasizes prevention and health maintenance based on six essential factors (*Setteh-e-Zarurieah)*: air, food and drink, sleep and wakefulness, evacuation and retention, body movement and repose, and mental movement and repose (Rezaeizadeh et al., 2009). Diagnosis and treatment processes center on identifying imbalances of different "temperaments"—hot, cold, wet, and dry—and correcting those imbalances. Modes of treatment for ITM include lifestyle modifications, diet therapy, pharmacotherapy (such as use of medicinal herbs and plant extracts), and hands-on physical manipulation.

CONCLUSION

Iran is a country enriched by a long history, a strong cultural identity, and a diverse population that parallels the diversity of its geography. The tradition of medicine in Iran dates to ancient times and has contributed many scientific and medical advancements throughout history. In the past century, Iran increased healthcare accessibility, improved control of infectious diseases, and decreased mortality rates. Iran has made significant progress in implementing and expanding a robust primary healthcare network in both urban and rural areas, delivering a wide range of community-based health interventions, and integrating Iranian traditional medicine within its healthcare system. Due to these advancements, as well as sociodemographic changes, NCDs have replaced communicable diseases as the leading cause of death and disability in Iran. Health disparities are broadly improving but persist based on income level, geography, gender, and other factors. Furthermore, the health and overall welfare of Iranians is threatened by climate change, economic sanctions, human rights abuses, and systematic discrimination against women and minority groups. Potential actions to address existing and emerging health issues include engaging in multisectoral collaboration to control NCDs and risk factors; increasing investments in healthcare infrastructure, including education and training; implementing policies to help identify, monitor, and remedy health disparities; and prioritizing steps to address environmental crises and climate change.

LEARNING ACTIVITIES

CourseConnect

To access self-assessment questions and interactive, competency-based learning activities for this chapter, visit www.springerpub.com/courseconnect. See inside front cover and tear-out for CourseConnect details.

REFERENCES

Aboutorabi, A., Darvishi Teli, B., Rezapoor, A., Ehsanzadeh, S. J., Martini, M., & Behzadifar, M. (2023). History of primary health care in Iran. *Journal of Preventive Medicine and Hygiene, 64*(3), E367–E374. https://doi.org/10.15167/2421-4248/jpmh2023.64.3.3081

Damari, B., Abdollahi, Z., Hajifaraji, M., & Rezazadeh, A. (2018). Nutrition and food security policy in the Islamic Republic of Iran: Situation analysis and roadmap towards 2021. *Eastern Mediterranean Health Journal, 24*(2), 177–188. https://doi.org/10.26719/2018.24.2.177

Danaei, G., Farzadfar, F., Kelishadi, R., Rashidian, A., Rouhani, O. M., Ahmadnia, S., Ahmadvand, A., Arabi, M., Ardalan, A., Arhami, M., Azizi, M. H., Bahadori, M., Baumgartner, J., Beheshtian, A., Djalalinia, S., Doshmangir, L., Haghdoost, A. A., Haghshenas, R., Hosseinpoor, A. R., & Islami, F. (2019). Iran in transition. *The Lancet, 393*(10184), 1984–2005. https://doi.org/10.1016/s0140-6736(18)33197-0

Elmore, L. (2021, July 27). *The implications of climate change in Iran*. American Iranian Council. https://www.us-iran.org/news/2021/7/2/covid-19-in-iran-r6by5

Farzadfar, F., Naghavi, M., Sepanlou, S. G., Moghaddam, S. S., Dangel, W. J., Weaver, N. D., Aminorroaya, A., Azadnajafabad, S., Koolaji, S., Mohammadi, E., Rezaei, N., Abbas, J., Abbasi, B., Abbasifard, M., Abbasi-Kangevari, M., Abbasi-Kangevari, Z., Abbastabar, H., Abdoli, A., Abdollahi, M., . . . Larijani, B. (2022). Health system performance in Iran: A systematic analysis for the Global Burden of Disease Study 2019. *The Lancet, 399*(10335), 1625–1645. https://doi.org/10.1016/S0140-6736(21)02751-3

Human Rights Watch. (2024). *World report 2024* (pp. 310–317). https://www.hrw.org/world-report/2024/

Iran Chamber Society. (n.d.). *People of Iran: Iranian ethnic groups*. https://www.iranchamber.com/people/articles/iranian_ethnic_groups.php

Koutlaki, S. A. (2010). *Among the Iranians: A guide to Iran's culture and customs*. Nicholas Brealey.

Lumsden, A. (2018, November 10). *Myth vs. fact: Geography of Iran*. American Iranian Council. https://www.us-iran.org/resources/2018/11/10/myth-vs-fact-geography-of-iran

Moradi, S. (2019). Languages of Iran: Overview and critical assessment. In S. D. Brunn & R. Kehrein (Eds.), *Handbook of the changing world language map* (pp. 1–32). Springer International Publishing. https://doi.org/10.1007/978-3-319-73400-2_137-1

Peykari, N., Hashemi, H., Dinarvand, R., Haji-Aghajani, M., Malekzadeh, R., Sadrolsadat, A., Sayyari, A. A., Asadi-lari, M., Delavari, A., Farzadfar, F., Haghdoost, A., Heshmat, R., Jamshidi, H., Kalantari, N., Koosha, A., Takian, A., & Larijani, B. (2017). National action plan for non-communicable diseases prevention and control in Iran; A response to emerging epidemic. *Journal of Diabetes & Metabolic Disorders, 16*(1). https://doi.org/10.1186/s40200-017-0288-4

Rezaei, N., Moghaddam, S. S., Farzadfar, F., & Larijani, B. (2022). Social determinants of health inequity in Iran: A narrative review. *Journal of Diabetes & Metabolic Disorders, 22*(1), 5–12. https://doi.org/10.1007/s40200-022-01141-w

Rezaeizadeh, H., Alizadeh, M., Naseri, M., & Shams Ardakani, M. R. (2009). The Traditional Iranian Medicine point of view on health and disease. *Iranian Journal of Public Health, 38*(Suppl 1), 169–172.

Sahraian, M. A., Moghadas, A. N., & Eskandarieh, S. (2021). Economic sanctions against Iran as an important factor in threatening the health of patients with multiple sclerosis. *Current Journal of Neurology, 20*(1), 15–22. https://doi.org/10.18502/cjn.v20i1.6375

Sharifi, V., Amin-Esmaeili, M., Hajebi, A., Motevalian, A., Radgoodarzi, R., Hefazi, M., & Rahimi-Movaghar, A. (2015). Twelve-month prevalence and correlates of psychiatric disorders in Iran: The Iranian Mental Health Survey, 2011. *Archives of Iranian Medicine, 18*(2), 76–84.

Statistical Center of Iran. (2016). *Selected results of the 2016 national population and housing census*. https://irandataportal.syr.edu/census/census-2016

Talaei, A., Hedjazi, A., Moosavi, B., Dadgarmoghaddam, M., Lotfinejad, N., & Khorashad, B. S. (2022). The epidemiology of gender dysphoria in Iran: The first nationwide study. *Archives of Sexual Behavior, 51*(4), 1881–1889. https://doi.org/10.1007/s10508-021-02250-y

UN Population Divison. (2022). *UN population division data portal*. United Nations. https://population.un.org/dataportal/

UN Statistics Division. (2023). *World statistics pocketbook 2023* (p. 133). United Nations. https://unstats.un.org/unsd/publications/pocketbook/files/world-stats-pocketbook-2023.pdf

World Bank Group. (n.d.). *Country profile: Iran, Islamic Republic.* World Development Indicators. https://databank.worldbank.org/views/reports/reportwidget.aspx?Report_Name=CountryProfile&Id=b450fd57&tbar=y&dd=y&inf=n&zm=n&country=IRN

World Bank Group. (2024). *Iran, Islamic Republic.* World Bank Gender Data Portal. https://genderdata.worldbank.org/en/economies/iran-islamic-rep

World Health Organization. (2020). *Global health estimates: Leading causes of death.* World Health Organization. https://www.who.int/data/gho/data/themes/mortality-and-global-health-estimates/ghe-leading-causes-of-death

World Health Organization. (2024). *Iran (Islamic Republic of) data.* WHO Data. https://data.who.int/countries/364

World Health Organization Regional Office for the Eastern Mediterranean. (n.d.). *Communicable diseases.* https://www.emro.who.int/iran/priority-areas/communicable-diseases.html

CHAPTER 40

TURKEY

Serdar Atav

INTRODUCTION

Straddling Europe and Asia, Turkey is a transcontinental country reflecting characteristics of both regions geographically and culturally. With a rich history spanning centuries, Turkey has been a bridge between Eastern and Western civilizations, blending influences from various empires and cultures. As a long-time member of NATO and the only fully secular and democratic country with a large Muslim-majority population, Turkey's alliances and aspirations have historically been aligned with the West. Despite its unique position at the crossroads of continents, Turkey has faced challenges in balancing its diverse identities and forging a distinct path. The transformation of its healthcare system into a solid universal health system since the early 2000s coincided with an unprecedented period of economic growth, wealth creation, and deep integration with global markets and institutions.

GEOGRAPHY AND GOVERNANCE

Turkey's unique geographic position spanning Europe and Asia has profoundly shaped its history, culture, and governance. Its landmass extends across the Anatolian peninsula in Western Asia and a small portion in the Balkan region of Southeast Europe, known as East Thrace (Figure 40.1). This intersection of continents has enabled Turkey to absorb and synthesize influences from various empires and cultures over centuries.

Governance in Turkey has evolved from its Ottoman imperial past to a modern republic established in 1923 under the leadership of Mustafa Kemal Atatürk. Following a constitutional referendum in 2018, the country is now a unitary presidential republic, with the president serving as both the head of state and head of government. President Recep Tayyip Erdoğan, who previously served as Prime Minister from 2003 to 2014, has been the head of state and government since the system change in 2018.

Turkey has a unitary system of provincial governance, with each of the 81 provinces headed by a governor appointed by the central government. These provincial governors represent the national government at the provincial level and serve as the highest civilian authority in the provinces. While provinces have elected provincial assemblies, the provincial governor chairs the executive body of the special provincial administration, reflecting the centralized nature of Turkey's governance despite some devolution of powers to local administrations.

While Turkey is constitutionally a secular state, the role and influence of religion in Turkish society and politics remain subjects of ongoing debate, reflected by the policies of the Erdoğan administration, which has aimed to increase the role of religion in public life.

Turkey's strategic location and governance have played a crucial role in shaping its international relations and alliances. With NATO membership and accession negotiations with the European Union, Turkey has historically aligned itself culturally, militarily, and economically with Western institutions and values, while also maintaining strong cultural and economic ties with the Middle East and Central Asia. This unique position combined with membership in the **Group of Twenty (G20)**, a group of 20 of the world's largest economies, allowed Turkey to act as a nexus, influencing its approach to various policy areas, including healthcare, by drawing from its diverse cultural and geopolitical connections.

FIGURE 40.1 Map of Turkey.

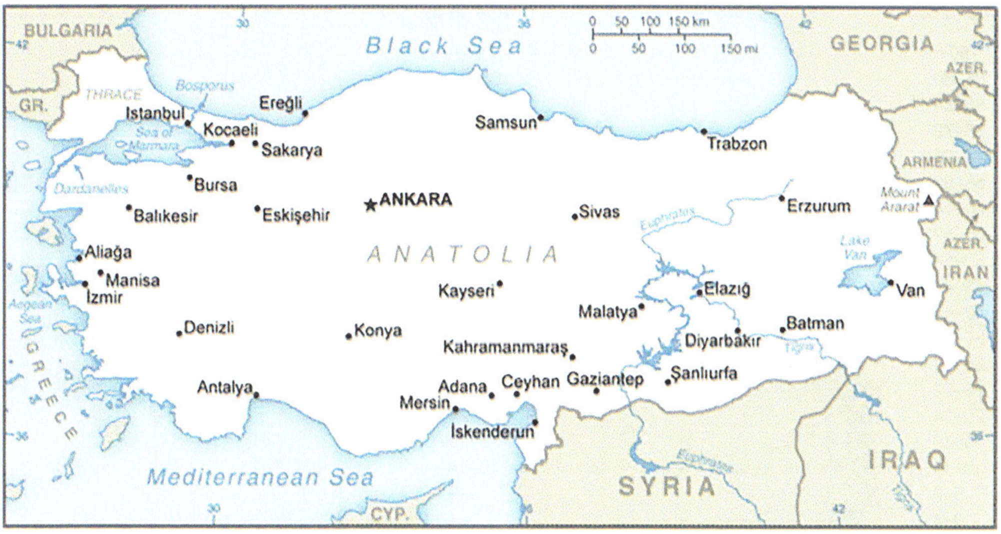

Source: Central Intelligence Agency. (n.d.). *The world factbook*. https://www.cia.gov/the-world-factbook/countries/turkey-turkiye/map/

TURKEY'S POPULATION DYNAMICS

Turkey's population in 2024 is just under 86 million, up from 85 million in 2022. Despite this increase, Turkey's population growth rate continues to decline, from 1.4% in 2019 to 0.9% in 2022. In 2024, the growth rate is expected to go down to a historic low of 0.7% (World Bank Group, 2024). According to the Turkish Statistics Institute (TUIK, 2024a), the primary characteristics of Turkey's growing population are:

- *Aging demographics*: In 2023, 21.4% of the population was younger than 15 years, a large drop from 27.4% in 2007 (Figure 40.2). The population 65 years and older grew to 10.2% from 7.1% in 2007. These trends indicate a rapid continuing growth in middle-aged and older groups, similar to the population trends of other developed economies of the world. Turkey's projected median age in 2024 was 34 years.
- *Urbanization*: More than 75% of the Turkish population live in urban areas, with an urbanization rate of 1.11% annually. Sixty-five percent of people in Turkey live in 19 cities with more than 1 million people, including Istanbul (16 million), the capital Ankara (5.8 million), and Izmir (4.5 million). Istanbul is one of the most populous metropolitan areas in the world. It straddles Europe and Asia and serves as the economic, cultural, and historic powerhouse of the country.
- *Immigration*: Turkey has a long history of immigration, particularly from the Balkans, Caucasus, and other parts of the former Ottoman Empire following its dissolution. Waves of Muslim immigrants, including Turks, Albanians, Bosniaks, Circassians, and others, resettled in modern-day Turkey and shaped its demographic makeup.

In recent years, Turkey has experienced a major influx of refugees and migrants (Ministry of Interior, 2024):

- Turkey hosts the largest refugee population in the world, estimated at around 4 million.
- In addition to Syrians (3.1 million in 2024, with a slight decrease from 3.5 million in 2022), Turkey also hosts refugees from Afghanistan, Africa, and other conflict zones.

FIGURE 40.2 Age pyramid of Turkey, 2007 and 2023.

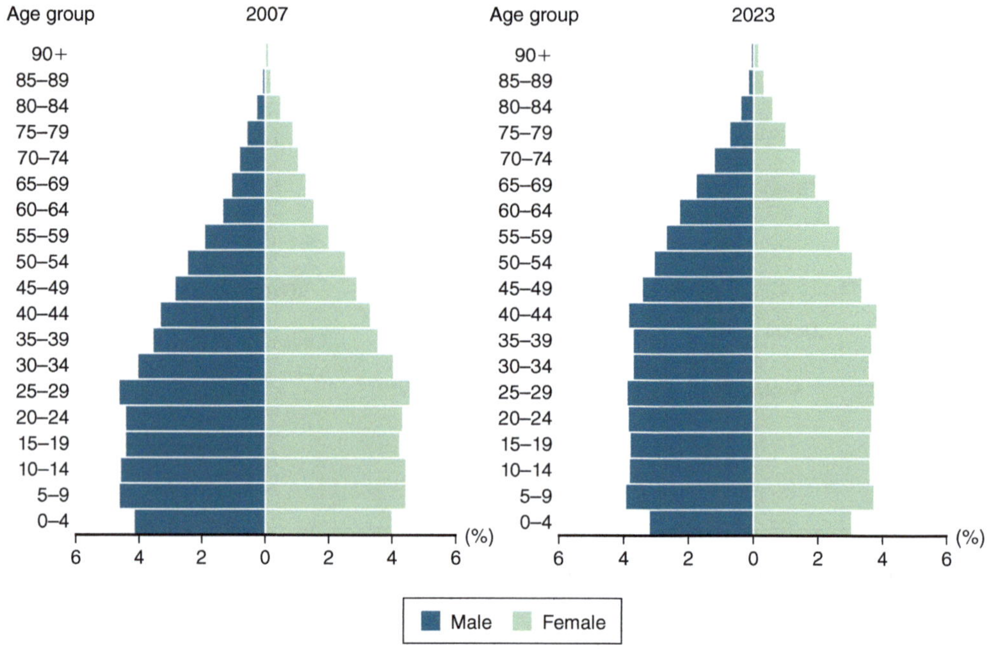

Source: Turkish Statistics Institute. (2024). *Address-based population registration system results, 2023*. https://data.tuik.gov.tr/Bulten/Index?p=Adrese-Dayali-Nufus-Kayit-Sistemi-Sonuclari-2023-49684

- Around 96,000 Ukrainians sought refuge in Turkey as of May 2023 following the Russian invasion.
- In 2022, nearly 100,000 Russian citizens migrated to Turkey, the highest number of foreign migrants that year.

ETHNIC AND LINGUISTIC DIVERSITY

Turkey exhibits considerable ethnic, linguistic, and cultural heterogeneity, despite being perceived as a largely Turkish and Muslim nation. While ethnic Turks and Turkish speakers constitute the majority at around 70% to 75% of the population, there are several significant minority groups (Joshua Project, 2024), as discussed in the following sections.

KURDISH MINORITY

Kurds are the largest ethnic minority in Turkey, comprising an estimated 15% to 20% of the population. Kurdish languages like Kurmanji and Zazaki have millions of native speakers. The Kurdish minority in Turkey faces multifaceted challenges such as cultural suppression, political marginalization, economic discrimination, and conflict arising from the Kurdish separatist movement. International human rights groups have consistently criticized Turkey's policies toward its Kurdish population.

ARAB MINORITY

Arabs form another sizable minority concentrated in southeastern Turkey near the Syrian border. Arabic is spoken by this community as well as the large Syrian refugee population. The Syrian refugees are ethnically diverse, including Arabs (80%), Kurds (10%–15%), Syrian Turkmen (10%–15%), and minority groups like Assyrian Christians and Circassians. In addition to Arabic, they speak Kurdish, Turkmen, and other minority languages, adding to Turkey's linguistic diversity.

OTHER MINORITIES

Smaller ethnic minorities include Circassians, Laz, Roma, Jews, Armenians, Greeks, Georgians, and Caucasian groups like Abkhaz and Ossetians. Minority languages spoken include Laz, Romani, Armenian, Greek, Georgian, Circassian, and Caucasian languages (Tomedes, 2024).

FERTILITY AND MORTALITY

According to TUIK (2024a), Turkey's total fertility rate declined for the eighth consecutive year in 2023, reaching 1.51 live births per woman (Figure 40.3). This is below the 2.1 children per woman needed to sustain population levels. An aging population, costs associated with raising children, urbanization, increasing age of marriage and childbearing, rising educational levels, and empowerment of women have contributed to the drastic drops in fertility rates in Turkey (BBC, 2024).

The infant mortality rate was 9.2 per 1,000 live births in 2022 (TUIK, 2023a), while life expectancy at birth was 77.5 years (74.8 years for males and 80.3 for females; TUIK, 2023b). These numbers are lower than in 2020, reflecting the impact of COVID-19. Life expectancy at age 65 years is also higher for women (15.3 years for males and 18.8 for females).

SEX, GENDER, AND SEXUAL ORIENTATION

WOMEN'S RIGHTS AND GENDER EQUALITY

Despite being a secular republic and an early adopter of women's suffrage in 1934, Turkey continues to face significant challenges in upholding women's rights and achieving gender equality. Gender-based violence remains one of the foremost women's rights issues in Turkey. Approximately four out of 10 Turkish women experience sexual and/or physical violence at some point in their lives. In 2022 alone, at least 392 women were murdered by men, highlighting the serious problem of femicides and violence against women (Stockholm Center for Freedom [SCF], 2023).

Turkey ranked a low 130th out of 153 countries in the World Economic Forum's **2020 Global Gender Gap Index** (2019) on economic participation and political empowerment. Women

FIGURE 40.3 Fertility rates in Turkey by year.

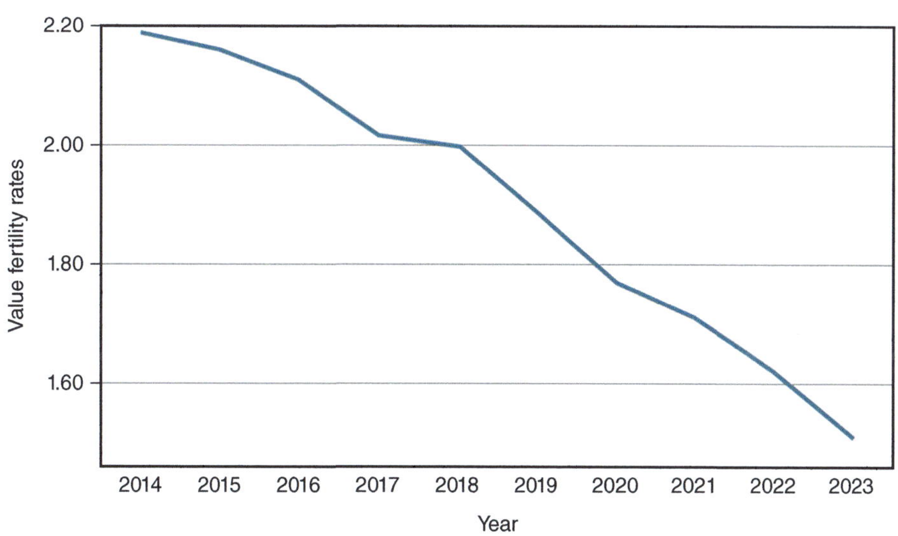

Source: Adapted from Turkish Statistics Institute. (2024a, May 15). *Doğum istatistikleri, 2024* [Birth statistics, 2024]. https://data.tuik.gov.tr/Bulten/Index?p=Birth-Statistics-2024-54196&dil=2

encounter obstacles in areas like employment, political representation, and access to financial resources and opportunities.

In a controversial move in 2022, Turkey's top court ruled that President Erdoğan had the right to unilaterally withdraw from the Council of Europe Convention on Preventing Violence Against Women (Istanbul Convention). This decision was criticized by opposition parties and women's rights groups as a major setback in combating domestic violence. Under President Erdoğan's AKP government, there has been a conservative religious pushback against women's rights and gender equality. This includes promoting traditional gender roles, restricting reproductive rights, and opposing career-oriented women. Despite a vibrant women's movement, gender equality efforts in Turkey face headwinds from violence, regressive policies, lack of legal safeguards, and socio-cultural resistance rooted in patriarchal norms and religious conservatism. Local women's groups are working to advance rights through grassroots initiatives, data collection, and transnational solidarity networks to counter setbacks and advocate for substantive reforms (Arat, 2020).

Homosexuality was decriminalized in Turkey during the Ottoman period in 1858 and has remained legal to date. However, there are no specific legal protections for LGBTQ+ individuals in the country. This lack of codified rights, combined with prevailing social attitudes, creates challenges for Turkey's sexual minority population. Public opinion surveys reveal widespread disapproval and rejection of homosexuality in Turkish society.

According to a 2020 study by Kadir Has University, 45% of respondents believed that LGBTQ+ individuals should have equal rights and should be accepted by society (Kadir Has University, 2020). This represented a marginal increase from previous years when acceptance levels were lower. A 2019 survey by the same university showed that 46.5% of respondents would not want a homosexual person as a neighbor, down from 55.3% in 2018. While the level of disapproval has decreased, the data indicate that a significant portion of the Turkish public still holds negative views toward homosexuality and nonheterosexual orientations.

LEADING CAUSES OF MORTALITY

Leading causes of mortality in Turkey reflect a transition toward noncommunicable diseases (NCDs), except for COVID-19. In 2022, the top causes of death were categorized as follows (TUIK, 2023b):

- cardiovascular diseases (35.4%)
- cancer (15.2%)
- chronic respiratory diseases (13.4%)
- endocrinologic diseases (4.5%)
- COVID-19 (4.4%)
- neurologic disorders (3.6%)
- unintended injuries (3.3%)

As with most countries, in 2021 COVID-19 was one of the leading causes of death at 11.5% (ranked fourth). Lifestyle behaviors like tobacco use, unhealthy diets, and physical inactivity remain significant risk factors contributing to the prevalence of NCDs like cancer, cardiovascular diseases, and chronic respiratory diseases in Turkey.

The leading causes of death in Turkey highlight the necessity to implement public health interventions—first and foremost, to reduce tobacco use. According to the most recent statistics, 28.3% of Turks older than 15 years use tobacco daily. The gender gap is significant in this number as 41.3% of males and only 15.5% of females reported daily smoking (TUIK, 2023c).

QUALITY OF LIFE

Turkey ranks 32nd in quality of life, trailing the United States, which placed 23rd. However, on safety, climate, healthcare, and cost of living, Turkey ranks better than or similar to most other European and North American countries (U.S. News & World Report, 2024).

TURKISH HEALTHCARE SYSTEM

Prior to 2003, Turkey's healthcare system faced numerous challenges, including

- poor population health indicators and outcomes;
- disparities in access between rural/urban populations and income groups;
- major inefficiencies in healthcare delivery;
- excessive fragmentation across insurance schemes;
- incomplete health insurance coverage for the population;
- duplication of services and low productivity;
- high out-of-pocket costs burdening patients;
- shortages of facilities and personnel, especially in eastern/southeastern regions;
- increasing pressures from an aging population; and
- rising NCDs and chronic diseases.

THE HEALTH TRANSFORMATION PROGRAM (2003 TO PRESENT)

To address these systemic issues, the Health Transformation Program (HTP) was launched in 2003 as an ambitious reform agenda by Erdoğan's AK Party government. The overall objectives were to improve governance, efficiency, user/provider satisfaction, and long-term financial sustainability of the healthcare system (Akdag, 2011). The HTP's initial planning was financed by a World Bank loan. Its underlying principles consisted of

- strengthening of the Ministry of Health's stewardship capacity,
- provision of universal health insurance,
- reorganization of healthcare service delivery,
- human resource development in the health sector, and
- establishment of a national health information system.

Adopting a neoliberal approach, the Ministry of Health transitioned from being a service provider to a policymaker and regulator through decentralization and public–private partnerships. While the public sector serves most of the population, the private sector serves those with private insurance or ability to pay out of pocket.

UNIVERSAL HEALTH INSURANCE

A key reform was the establishment of a single health insurance fund by consolidating four existing schemes. For salaried workers, premiums are automatically deducted from wages. For others, premiums are determined on a sliding income-based scale. The economically disadvantaged have premiums paid by the government. By 2012, 98% of Turkish citizens had gained access to health insurance under this new system.

SERVICE DELIVERY REORGANIZATION

The delivery system adopted a primary care focus, new patient referral pathways, and greater autonomy for hospitals. This aimed to improve care coordination, efficiency, and responsiveness to patient needs. Family physicians are paid per capita for up to 3,500 patients in their assigned neighborhoods. Hospitals were modernized, and many new hospitals were built across the country.

HUMAN RESOURCE DEVELOPMENT

Healthcare personnel education was revamped with a focus on allied health professionals and the training of family physicians. The work schedules of physicians were restructured so that only full-time work in the public sector was allowed. Salaries of all public healthcare personnel were adjusted. However, the exodus of public-sector physicians to the private sector and to other countries could not be prevented. The government's overly centralized policy to healthcare personnel was criticized by many for ignoring input from key stakeholders.

NATIONAL HEALTH INFORMATION SYSTEM

All stakeholders agree that the establishment and implementation of an infrastructure for information flow among various components of the healthcare system were necessary. The new national health database and its ease of access by all stakeholders are a success. More recently, the Ministry of Health revised the appointment system nationally and established a single system of appointments in the public sector for primary care providers and specialists. The new appointment system is also perceived favorably by providers and the public alike.

Through an ambitious slate of reforms financed by loans and premised on principles like decentralization and public–private partnerships, Turkey achieved unprecedented public satisfaction and improved health outcomes, such as lower infant/maternal mortality ratios and improved longevity. In addition, Turkey became one of the top destinations in the world for medical tourism. However, long-term financial sustainability, retention of public providers, and addressing socioeconomic inequalities impacting health remain key challenges.

DETERMINANTS OF HEALTH

SOCIOECONOMIC STATUS AND INEQUALITY

Turkey has the world's 17th largest economy, with a gross domestic product (GPD) per capita based on purchasing power parity (PPP) of $33,149. Nominally, GDP per capita is projected to be $12,765 in 2024. The ambitious reforms under the Erdoğan governments in the last 20 years have put Turkey at the higher end of the upper middle–income status and reduced poverty, doubling the country's GDP. However, economic inequality persists, as indicated by 14.4% of the population under the national poverty line. Job losses due to the COVID-19 pandemic and the huge earthquake that hit southeast Turkey in 2023 have contributed to the level of poverty. The southeast region of Turkey contains 39% of the country's poor, and its poverty level is twice the national average (World Bank Group, 2023).

EDUCATION

Access to education is a constitutional right with 12 years of schooling compulsory for all citizens. Primary and secondary education is offered free in all public schools. Along with the public system, there is a private system that offers primary, secondary, and higher education. Even though the public university system is not free, the tuition and fees in public universities are very low.

The education system is highly centralized under the Ministry of National Education. The primary and secondary education system in the public sector suffers from frequent policy changes, a memorization focus, an exam-oriented curriculum, an oppressive disciplinary environment, and a rural–urban divide. For Kurdish students, these challenges are exacerbated by the restrictions on the Kurdish minorities' linguistic, cultural, and educational rights and needs (Pardo, 2022). Furthermore, the inclusion of the children of the millions of Syrian refugees in the education system is still facing challenges.

The literacy rate in Turkey is around 98%. In 2023, 24.6% of individuals held higher education degrees; in 2008, this number was 9.8%. The expansion of primary, secondary, and higher educational facilities in both the public and private domains explains the rapid increase in secondary and higher education graduates (TUIK, 2024b).

EMPLOYMENT AND INCOME SUPPORT

The unemployment rate in Turkey in 2025 is projected to be 8.6% (Strategy and Budget, 2025), with significant variations across regions. Unemployment benefits pay up to 30% of salary for a maximum of 10 months. However, the rules are strict, and individuals in the informal job sector do not qualify for any benefits. There are also separate cash payouts for food and nutrition, but only the poorest of the poor qualify for them.

HEALTH BEHAVIORS

The most prevalent health risk behaviors in Turkey are tobacco use, unhealthy eating, inactivity, and stress and anger issues (TUIK, 2023b). While tobacco use is clearly a major cause of morbidity and mortality, according to a Gallup study Turks are among the top five in the world for experiencing stress and lacking enjoyment (Gallup, 2022).

HUMAN RIGHTS AND SOCIAL JUSTICE

Turkey does not have a stellar human rights record. The oppression of minorities like the Kurds, the Alawites, and the LGBTQ+ community, severe limitations on freedom of expression and assembly, and the fading separation of powers due to Erdoğan's authoritarian regime are only some of the concerns voiced by Amnesty International (2020).

Economic inequalities and the uneven distribution of economic development are major contributors to social justice challenges in Turkey. The lack of any comprehensive social justice policy perpetuates the economic, political, cultural, and educational disparities experienced by the Kurds.

ENVIRONMENTAL ISSUES

Turkey experiences air and water pollution, biodiversity loss, water scarcity, and gaps in environmental infrastructure as major challenges. However, the government does not consistently enforce concrete policies to address such challenges. Much stronger implementation of laws and strategies is needed to address Turkey's environmental issues.

CONCLUSION

Through the ambitious, two-decade HTP reforms premised on principles like decentralization, universal health coverage, and public–private partnerships, Turkey achieved remarkable progress in improving healthcare access, quality, and outcomes. The establishment of a consolidated national health insurance system, reorganization of service delivery with a primary care focus, modernization of facilities, and development of health information systems contributed to unprecedented public satisfaction. However, challenges persist in ensuring long-term financial sustainability of the reformed healthcare model, retaining skilled professionals in the public sector, and addressing socioeconomic inequalities that perpetuate disparities in health determinants and outcomes. As Turkey's population continues to age and the burden of NCDs grows, the nation must build on the HTP's successes while prioritizing equitable access, preventive interventions targeting risk factors like tobacco use, and evidence-based policies tailored to the needs of diverse populations, including ethnic minorities. Robust implementation of a comprehensive, multisectoral approach to public health will be crucial for Turkey to fully realize the potential of its healthcare transformation.

LEARNING ACTIVITIES

CourseConnect

To access self-assessment questions and interactive, competency-based learning activities for this chapter, visit www.springerpub.com/courseconnect. See inside front cover and tear-out for CourseConnect details.

REFERENCES

Akdag, R. (2011). *Turkey health transformation program evaluation report 2003–2010*. Ministry of Health. https://www.sesric.org/imgs/news/image/729-doc-Turkey-Health-Transformation-Programme.pdf

Amnesty International. (2020, May 18). *Human rights in Turkey*. https://www.amnesty.org.uk/human-rights-turkey

Arat, Z. (2020, December 31). *Women's struggle in Turkey and a new transnational declaration*. Wilson Center. https://www.wilsoncenter.org/blog-post/womens-struggle-turkey-and-new-transnational-declaration

BBC. (2024, May 16). *Dogum oranlari rekor seviyeye dustu* [Birth rates hit record low]. https://www.bbc.com/turkce/articles/c1ejenpdllko

Gallup. (2022). *What is the world's emotional temperature?* https://news.gallup.com/interactives/248240/global-emotions.aspx

Ministry of Interior. (2024, April 30). *Temporary protection*. https://en.goc.gov.tr/temporary-protection27

Joshua Project. (2024). *Türkiye*. https://joshuaproject.net/countries/TU

Kadir Has University. (2020). *The perception of gender and women in Turkey 2020*. https://gender.khas.edu.tr/en/survey-public-perceptions-gender-roles-and-status-women-turkey

Pardo, E. (2022, January 13). *Kurdish education in Turkey: A joint responsibility. Modern Diplomacy*. https://moderndiplomacy.eu/2022/01/13/kurdish-education-in-turkey-a-joint-responsibility/

Stockholm Center for Freedom. (2023, March 8). *Women's rights in Turkey: 2022 in review*. https://stockholmcf.org/womens-rights-in-turkey-2022-in-review/

Strategy and Budget. (2025). *İstihdam* [Employment]. https://www.sbb.gov.tr/istihdam/

Tomedes. (2024, March 4). *Which languages are spoken in Turkey*? https://www.tomedes.com/translator-hub/language-spoken-in-turkey

Turkish Statistics Institute. (2023a, September 18). *Hayat tabloları, 2020–2022* [Life tables, 2020–2022]. https://data.tuik.gov.tr/Bulten/Index?p=Life-Tables-2020-2022-49726

Turkish Statistics Institute. (2023b, June 22). *Ölüm ve ölüm nedenleri, 2022* [Deaths and causes of death, 2022]. https://data.tuik.gov.tr/Bulten/Index?p=Death-and-Causes-of-Death-Statistics-2022-49679

Turkish Statistics Institute. (2023c, June 2023). *Türkiye sağlık araştırması, 2022* [Turkey health survey, 2022]. https://data.tuik.gov.tr/Bulten/Index?p=Turkiye-Saglik-Arastirmasi-2022-49747

Turkish Statistics Institute. (2024a, May 15). *Doğum istatistikleri, 2024* [Birth statistics, 2024]. https://data.tuik.gov.tr/Bulten/Index?p=Dogum-Istatistikleri-2023-53708

Turkish Statistics Institute. (2024b, May 30). *Ulusal eğitim istatistikleri, 2023* [National education statistics, 2023]. https://data.tuik.gov.tr/Bulten/Index?p=Ulusal-Egitim-Istatistikleri-2023-53444

U.S. News & World Report. (2024). *Quality of life*. https://www.usnews.com/news/best-countries/rankings/quality-of-life

World Bank Group. (2023, April). *Poverty and equity brief: Türkiye*. https://databankfiles.worldbank.org/public/ddpext_download/poverty/987B9C90-CB9F-4D93-AE8C-750588BF00QA/current/Global_POVEQ_TUR.pdf

World Bank Group. (2024). *Population growth (annual %)—Türkiye*. https://data.worldbank.org/indicator/SP.POP.GROW?locations=TR

World Economic Forum. (2019, December 16). *Global gender gap report 2020*. https://www.weforum.org/publications/gender-gap-2020-report-100-years-pay-equality/

CHAPTER 41

KAZAKHSTAN

Ardak Nurbakyt, Maksut Kulzhanov, Lyazzat Kosherbayeva, Maiya Zhakupova,
Dinara Sukenova, Laila Nazarova, Nazerke Narymbayeva,
Sharapat Moiynbayeva, Nadira Aitambayeva, and Shnara Svetlanova

INTRODUCTION

The Republic of Kazakhstan (Kazakhstan) is a vast nation in Central Asia, renowned for its diverse landscapes—from sweeping steppes to towering mountains. As one of the world's largest countries, it hosts a multifaceted population with a rich mix of ethnicities, languages, and cultures. Its strategic location at the crossroads of Europe and Asia adds to its historical and cultural complexity, making its geographic and demographic diversity a key part of its national identity and global significance.

IMPORTANT GEOGRAPHIC FEATURES AND DIVISIONS

As of July 2022, Kazakhstan is divided into 20 first-level administrative units: 17 regions and three cities of republican significance (Almaty, Astana, and Shymkent; Figure 41.1). It also includes 224 second-level units, such as 170 districts and 38 cities of regional significance, and 2,352 third-level units, including 48 akimats (local administration or local government) of cities and 2,179 rural district akimats. Kazakhstan has 89 cities, 29 settlements, and 6,293 villages. Russia leases 95,727 square kilometers (59,500 square miles) for the Baikonur Cosmodrome and military testing grounds. In 2022, three new regions were created: Abai, Zhetysu, and Ulytau (Classifier of Administrative-Territorial Objects, 2018).

POPULATION SIZE AND AGE DISTRIBUTION

As of January 1, 2024, Kazakhstan's population reached 20,033,546, with 12.45 million urban residents (up 1.9%) and 7.58 million rural residents (up 0.3%). In 2023, 387,900 children were born, with the highest birth rates in Mangystau, Turkestan, and Shymkent. The overall **birth rate** was 19.5 live births per 1,000 people, while the mortality rate was 6.56 deaths per 1,000 people, with 130,600 deaths overall. Infant mortality decreased from 8.1 infant deaths per 1,000 people in 2023 to 6.7 infant deaths per 1,000 live births in 2024. The marriage rate dropped by 5.9%, with 120,000 marriages registered, and divorces fell by 5.3%, totaling 16,700.

In absolute numbers, there were

- 4,279,888 people under 15 years (males: 2,186,488; females: 2,093,400);
- 14,101,618 people over 14 and under 65 years (men: 6,871,281; women: 7,230,337); and
- 1,466,789 people over 64 years (men: 502,162; women: 964,627; Countrymeters, n.d.).

MEDIAN AGE AND BIRTH RATES

In 2023, Kazakhstan's median age was approximately 31.3 years, reflecting a relatively young population. The birth rate in 2022 was 21.4 live births per 1,000 people, higher than in many European countries but showing a gradual decline (as evidenced by the 2024 birth rate mentioned previously) due to urbanization, economic factors, and lifestyle changes. Fertility is influenced by economic conditions, government family support policies, and cultural traditions, with higher birth rates in rural areas. Despite a declining birth rate, the young population presents opportunities for economic growth,

FIGURE 41.1 Administrative division map of Kazakhstan.

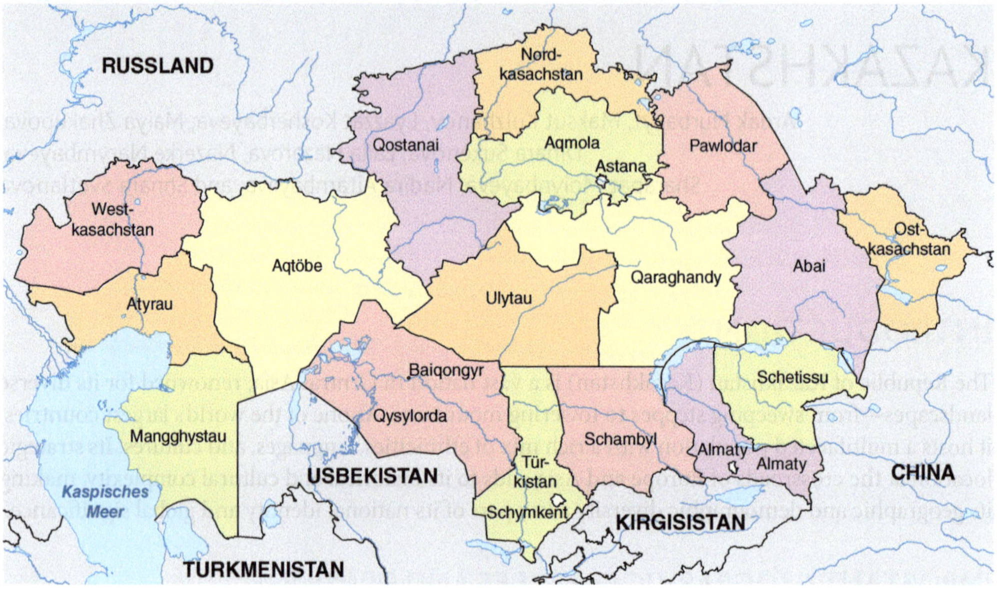

Source: TUBS. (2012). *Kazakhstan, administrative divisions*. https://commons.wikimedia.org/wiki/File:Kazakhstan,_administrative_divisions_-_de_-_colored.svg

provided that education and employment policies are effectively implemented (Bureau of National Statistics, 2023a).

IN- AND- OUT-MIGRATION

The number of people moving into Kazakhstan in the first quarter of 2024 compared to the same period last year increased 2.2-fold (158,600 people). In terms of external migration, in the first 3 months of 2024, the number of arrivals in the country totalled 7,471 people, a decrease of 2.7% compared to 2023. Those who left the Republic of Kazakhstan increased by more than 40%. At the same time, the main migration exchange is with the Commonwealth of Independent States (CIS)—the share of both arrivals (5,651 people) and departures (2,828 people) to the CIS countries fluctuates around 75% (AqZhaiyq, 2023).

URBAN/RURAL

During 2024, about 60% of Kazakhstan's population lived in cities, driven by urbanization, economic growth, and improved living standards. Major cities like Astana, Almaty, and Shymkent serve as centers of economic, educational, and cultural activity. Meanwhile, 40% of the population resides in rural areas, where agriculture and animal husbandry dominate, but access to quality services remains a challenge. To address this, the government has implemented programs like Auyl – El Besigi to modernize infrastructure, the agro-industrial development program to boost agriculture, and the Digital Kazakhstan program to improve digital access (Government of Kazakhstan, 2025). These initiatives aim to enhance rural living conditions, reduce migration to cities, and support sustainable economic growth across all regions (Satubaldina, 2022).

GENDER

Kazakhstan's gender issues reflect its traditionally patriarchal society, with men often in more influential roles and women facing expectations related to family duties. While efforts to promote gender equality are ongoing, especially in urban areas, gaps remain in political representation and economic opportunities. The Constitution guarantees equal rights, but challenges persist in practice. Transgender individuals can legally change their gender following medical certification but face significant social stigma and discrimination. Activists and LGBTQ+ organizations work to improve transgender rights, though they encounter resistance. Gender-based violence and discrimination remain serious issues, with government initiatives lagging behind public awareness efforts.

RACIAL/ETHNIC GROUPS

As of early 2024, Kazakhs make up 70.98% of Kazakhstan's population, exceeding 14 million people for the first time and their proportion more than doubling since independence in 1991. In five regions, Kazakhs account for over 80% of the population, with the highest concentrations in Kyzylorda, Atyrau, and Mangystau. Russians remain the second-largest ethnic group, comprising 14.89% of the population, though their numbers are declining. Uzbeks, the third-largest group, now constitute 3.3%, followed by Ukrainians (1.88%), Uighurs (1.51%), and other ethnic groups like Germans, Tatars, and Koreans, all representing smaller shares of the population (Vlast, 2023).

BRIEF HISTORY

The Kazakh people, descendants of various Turkic tribes, historically led a nomadic lifestyle. The region's first state, the Turkic Kaganate, was established in the sixth century CE, followed by Mongol rule in the 13th century. By the mid-15th century, Kazakhs formed three hordes, later unified by Abylai Khan in the 18th century. Despite establishing ties with Russia and China, Kazakhstan was eventually conquered by Russia. In 1917, Kazakh nationalists briefly formed the Alash Orda before Soviet control. Kazakhstan became a Soviet republic in 1936, enduring Stalin's devastating collectivization policies. After declaring independence in 1991, Kazakhstan transitioned to a parliamentary republic under Nursultan Nazarbayev, experiencing rapid urbanization and demographic shifts (Academy of Preventive Medicine [Kazakhstan] & Macro International Inc., 1999).

RELIGIONS

According to the Constitution, Kazakhstan claims to be a secular state and provides for freedom of religion and belief, as well as freedom to renounce religious affiliation (Constitution of the Republic of Kazakhstan, 1995). In 2021, Kazakhstan's population was estimated at 19.2 million, with 92.8% identifying as religious. Muslims made up approximately 70% of the population, primarily adhering to Sunni Islam, while Christians, mostly Orthodox, accounted for 17.19%. Other religious groups in Kazakhstan include Jews, Buddhists, Baha'is, and smaller Christian denominations (U.S. Mission Kazakhstan, 2022). According to a 2019 study by the government, nonbelievers or atheists accounted for 18.8% of the population.

LANGUAGES

Kazakhstan is a multinational state, with representatives of over 124 nationalities (Panchenko, 2019). The country's state policy emphasizes tolerance, and its constitution designates Kazakh as the official language, while Russian is used in state organizations alongside Kazakh and English is the language of international communication (Language Act of Kazakhstan, 1997). As of 2017, 83.1% of the population had mastered Kazakh, and 92% of document circulation in government bodies was conducted in the state language. Media in Kazakhstan is available in 11 languages, including Ukrainian, German, and Korean, with 170 Sunday language centers across the country (Skaley, 2019).

THE POLITICAL SYSTEM

Kazakhstan is a unitary state with a presidential form of government, declaring itself a democratic, secular, and social state that prioritizes human rights and freedoms. Gaining independence on December 16, 1991, Kazakhstan's capital is Astana and the currency is the tenge. The president is the head of state, guiding domestic and foreign policy, while the government manages executive functions. Legislative power is held by a bicameral Parliament, consisting of the Senate and the Mazhilis. The Senate includes appointed and elected deputies, while the Mazhilis comprises deputies elected through a mixed electoral system. Kazakhstan's administrative structure includes 17 regions and three cities of national importance (Akorda, n.d.).

IMPORTANT TRADITIONS, CUSTOMS, ACTIVITIES, OR LEISURE ACTIVITIES

Kazakhs, originally nomadic, have transitioned to a settled lifestyle while preserving their ancient traditions based on trust, openness, tolerance, and cultural heritage. Hospitality is a cornerstone of Kazakh culture, with guests honored and given the best place in the yurt, and special customs like the *shapan* robe still practiced. Weddings are significant events with numerous rituals, including matchmaking and the *kalym* payment (monies given by the groom to the bride's parents). Family life is central, with traditions like *zheti ata, which* emphasizing knowledge of seven ancestral generations. Daily life includes a range of customs, from household traditions to sports and games. Modern leisure activities are diverse, supported by the state, and include concerts, fitness centers, and creative courses (Advantour, n.d.).

Kazakhstanis have a diverse range of leisure activities, including attending concerts and movies, frequenting fitness centers and swimming pools, and participating in creative courses and master classes. The state supports this variety in leisure options, with spending on sports, recreation, and entertainment reaching 334.9 billion tenge ($670 million) in the first half of 2023, a 31.5% increase from the previous year (Sputnik Kazakhstan, 2023).

HEALTH OUTCOMES

Noncommunicable diseases (NCDs), particularly cardiovascular diseases, are the leading cause of mortality in Kazakhstan. However, preventative efforts are having a positive effect. Mortality rates for circulatory system diseases have dropped by 25.6%, with urban areas seeing a 30.5% decrease due to reductions in coronary heart disease and stroke; rural areas experienced a 20.4% reduction. Advances in oncology services and screening programs for cancer have also contributed to a decrease in preventable cancer deaths.

In 2022, the number of people newly diagnosed with mental and behavioral disorders (MBD) in Kazakhstan increased to 11,461, up from 9,924 in 2021. The primary incidence rate was 59.9 per 100,000 population, with the highest rates in Astana, Karaganda, and East Kazakhstan, and the lowest in Almaty, Atyrau, and West Kazakhstan. For children and adolescents, the rate was 89.9 per 100,000, but higher in Pavlodar, Kostanay, and Karaganda.

Infectious diseases saw notable increases from 2022 to 2023. Acute upper respiratory infections rose to 14,581.23 per 100,000 population, with the highest rates in Astana and West Kazakhstan. Acute intestinal infections were at 69.35 per 100,000, with peaks in Kyzylorda and Zhetisu. Incidence rates for viral hepatitis, pediculosis, and measles also surged, with significant outbreaks reported in Astana and Shymkent (Kazakhstan Pharm Reviews, 2023).

NONCOMMUNICABLE DISEASES

According to World Health Organization (WHO), NCDs accounted for 87% of deaths in Kazakhstan during 2019, with cardiovascular diseases being the leading cause at 47%, followed by cancer at 17%, chronic respiratory diseases at 7%, and diabetes at 2%. Contributing factors included high rates of obesity (21%), sedentary lifestyle (18%), excessive alcohol consumption (5 liters per person per year), and smoking (24%), with the Zhambyl region having the highest smoking rates (Medicine MCFER —Kazakhstan, 2022). It is important to note that COVID-19, a communicable disease, was the leading cause of death in Kazakhstan during 2021 (WHO, 2024).

INFANT AND MATERNAL DISEASES

The primary causes of infant and maternal disease in Kazakhstan, according to the structure of morbidity and mortality, are extragenital infections at 77%, then gestosis at 6.1%, obstetric hemorrhage at 5.5%, and uterine rupture at 3.5%, as well as other causes.

Considering the mortality rate of children under 5 years of age, the highest rates for Kazakhstan were from 2008 to 2019. The trend has been decreasing since 2017, not counting the fact that 2021 shows a slightly higher coefficient.

LIFE EXPECTANCY

In 2022, life expectancy in Kazakhstan rose significantly for both sexes, with women's life expectancy at birth reaching a notable 78.41 years. This figure reflects the average number of years a newborn is expected to live, assuming current mortality rates persist (O'Neill, 2024).

In March 2023, 41.8% of Kazakhs were satisfied with their lives, with higher satisfaction in rural areas (46.5%) than in cities (39.6%), and with men (45.4%) more satisfied than women (39.5%). This is a slight increase from 2022 but significantly lower than the 2021 level of 61.3%. Satisfaction with health rose to 47.6%, though it decreased with age, and financial satisfaction improved to 34%. Most respondents (72.2%) felt their material security was average, with low wages and pensions being major concerns impacting household income (Bureau of National statistics, 2023b).

DETERMINANTS OF HEALTH

SOCIOECONOMIC FACTORS

In the first quarter of 2024, Kazakhstan's per-capita GDP was $2,514.21. The poverty rate, defined as the percentage of the population with incomes below the subsistence level, was 4.6%. The depth and severity of poverty were 0.6% and 0.2%, respectively. The highest poverty rate was in the Turkestan region (7.9%), while the lowest was in Karaganda and Astana (2.4% each).

Kazakhstan ranks 15th in youth literacy and ninth in youth education globally. Its education system, overseen by the Ministry of Education and the Ministry of Science and Higher Education, spans from preschool to postgraduate levels. In the first quarter of 2024, the unemployment rate was 4.7%, with 76.2% of the employed in hired positions and 23.8% self-employed (Law of the Republic of Kazakhstan on Education, 2007). The employment rate for those age 15 and older was 64.8%, and youth unemployment was 3.1%. As of April 2024, 315,600 people were registered as unemployed, making up 3.3% of the labor force.

FOOD/NUTRITION

Kazakh cuisine, rooted in a nomadic lifestyle, traditionally centered on hearty meat and dairy dishes suited to harsh conditions. Over time, as Kazakhs transitioned to a sedentary life and interacted with other cultures, their diet expanded to include legumes, fruits, vegetables, fish, and sweets (Advantour, n.d.). Between 2016 and 2020, there was a notable shift toward high-calorie foods like meat, chicken, eggs, and ultraprocessed items, driven by urbanization, rising incomes, and changing lifestyles (Figures 41.2 and 41.3). This shift highlights the need for updated food security and nutrition policies in Kazakhstan.

FIGURE 41.2 Changes in per-capita food consumption between 2016 and 2020 (kg/person/year).

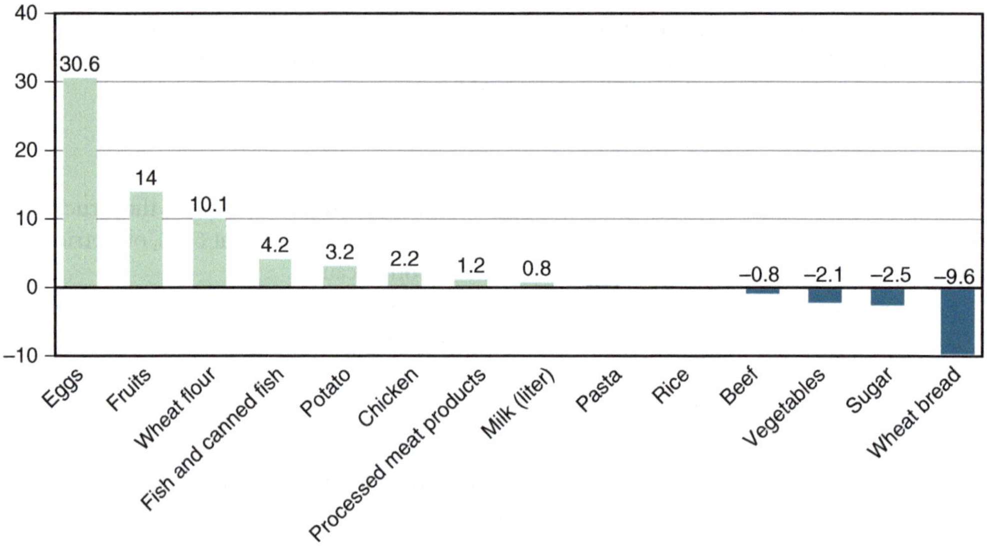

FIGURE 41.3 Retail value of ultraprocessed food sales per capita.

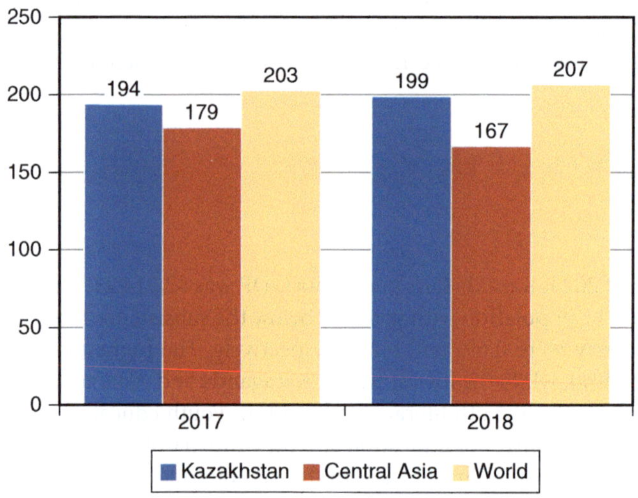

TOP MORTALITY RISK FACTORS

In Kazakhstan, NCDs, especially circulatory system disorders like coronary heart disease and stroke, are the leading causes of mortality. Despite a recent decrease in mortality rates from these diseases, the COVID-19 pandemic caused an increase in 2020 and 2021. Respiratory disease mortality also rose during the pandemic but has since decreased. While mortality rates from cancers and accidents have improved, premature mortality from major NCDs has seen minimal reduction. Key risk factors include high blood pressure, tobacco use, poor nutrition, and a sedentary lifestyle, with nearly 31% of deaths linked to high systolic blood pressure (Government of the Republic of Kazakhstan, 2022; Figure 41.4).

FIGURE 41.4 Top 10 risk factors as a share of all deaths.

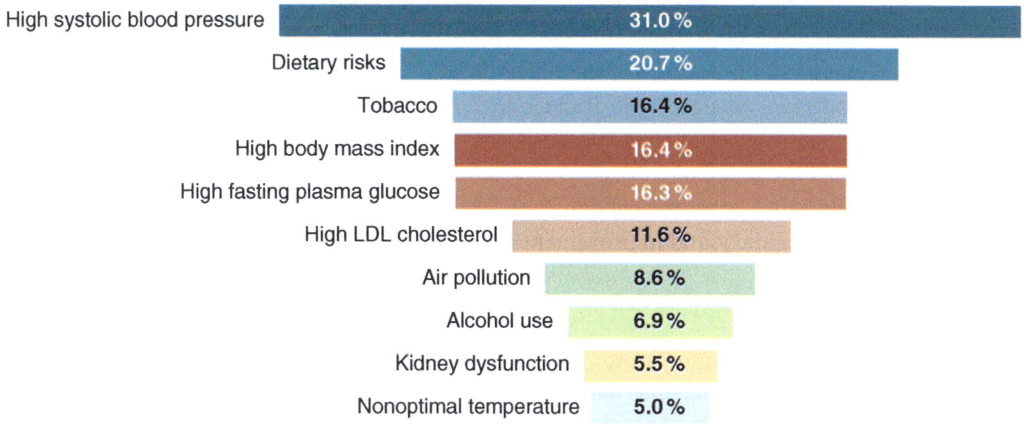

LDL, low-density lipoprotein.

Source: Adapted from European Observatory on Health Systems and Policies & World Health Organization Regional Office for Europe. (2022). *Health systems in action: Kazakhstan: 2022 edition*.https://iris.who.int/handle/10665/362324

ENVIRONMENTAL AND CLIMATE CHANGE ISSUES

Kazakhstan faces significant challenges from global climate change, including desertification, increased forest and steppe fires, melting glaciers, and degraded water systems. Direct impacts include more frequent natural disasters such as floods and fires, worsening drinking water quality due to natural and consumption-related factors, rising temperatures linked to increased cardiovascular and mental health issues, and deteriorating air quality leading to respiratory and other diseases. Additionally, climate warming may increase the prevalence of infectious diseases such as cholera, hepatitis A, and malaria (UN Development Programme Kazakhstan, 2022).

The above-mentioned negative consequences of climate change affect different social groups differently. The most vulnerable categories are women, children, elderly people, large families, disabled people and low-income families (UN Development Programme Kazakhstan, 2022).

HISTORICAL/THEORETICAL BACKGROUND OF HEALTHCARE

Since gaining independence in 1991, Kazakhstan has evolved its Soviet-era, centrally planned healthcare system. Initial reforms in the mid-1990s included decentralizing power, introducing compulsory health insurance, and restructuring primary care, though not all planned changes were fully implemented. By 2004, the service delivery structure was outlined, with the Ministry of Health developing national policy and regional administrations managing healthcare provision and financing (Katsaga et al., 2012). Health financing is regulated by the Ministry of Economics and Budget Planning and the Ministry of Finance, while healthcare providers, trade unions, associations, and nongovernmental organizations also play key roles. Strategic planning is conducted at the ministerial level, guided by the Code on People's Health and the Health Care System (President of Kazakhstan, 2009).

Policymaking in Kazakhstan is highly centralized in an executive-type government headed by the president. The Ministry of Health is responsible for developing national health policy. Strategic planning is outlined in the Ministry of Health's strategic development plans (Katsaga et al., 2012). The latest plan—National Project "Healthy Nation" for 2020–2025—is designed to achieve the following results (Government of the Republic of Kazakhstan, 2022):

- introduction and improvement of the compulsory health insurance system
- development of the concept of the "State Program for Improving Public Health for 2020–2025," and a new version of the draft Code "On the Health of the People and the Healthcare System"
- adoption of the new Code
- large-scale fight against the pandemic of coronavirus infections
- further development and improvement of the country's healthcare system

MEDICAL EDUCATION IN KAZAKHSTAN

Kazakhstan's medical education sector has advanced with modern teaching methods, improved research facilities, and greater international collaboration. Universities are accredited by global bodies like WHO and the World Federation for Medical Education (WFME), ensuring worldwide recognition of their degrees.

Medical education in Kazakhstan follows international standards with these key stages (Figure 41.5):

- *Undergraduate education:* 5 to 6 years covering basic sciences and clinical training
- *Internship:* 1-year, hands-on training period in clinical settings
- *Residency:* 2 to 5 years of specialized training in a chosen field
- *Continuing medical education (CME):* ongoing education through workshops and courses to maintain licensure and stay updated

GAPS IN CURRENT HEALTHCARE SYSTEM

Historically, Kazakhstan's healthcare system emphasized infectious diseases over chronic conditions like diabetes and cancer (Organisation for Economic Co-operation and Development [OECD], 2018). Recently, the government expanded primary care services to address rising chronic disease mortality and aims to transition to a universal healthcare system with better cost transparency and quality of life. The Compulsory Social and Health Insurance (CSHI) program, effective January 2020, seeks to create a single-payer system to reduce out-of-pocket costs and regulate care quality

FIGURE 41.5 Structural overview of healthcare education in Kazakhstan.

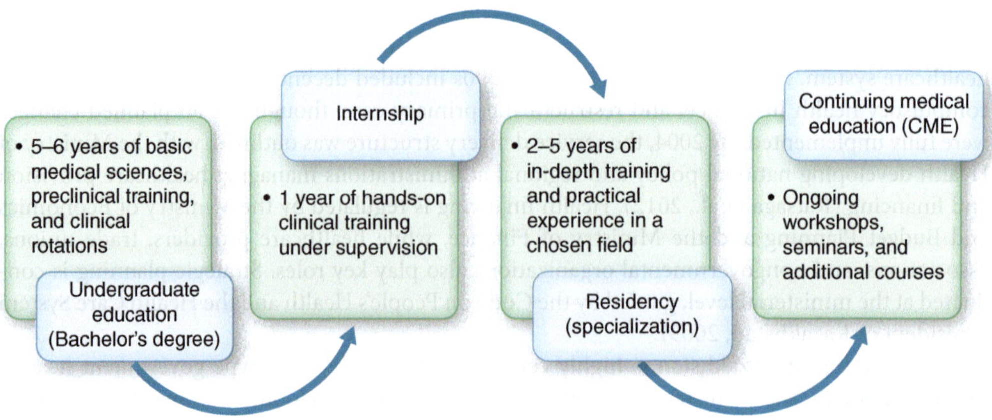

(Altynsarina, 2019). Despite increased funding, healthcare expenditure remains low at 3.1% of the gross domestic product (GDP), compared to the global average of 9.89% (The Borgen Project, 2020).

ALTERNATIVE/COMPLEMENTARY MEDICINE

Recognized as a specialty in the USSR in 1977, alternative medicine gained popularity in Kazakhstan postindependence due to economic conditions and a deteriorating public health system (Penkala-Gawecka, 2002). Despite being removed from the official list of health professions, it is still practiced through certification by government authorities and registered in the National Register of Healers (Katsaga et al., 2012).

RECENT HEALTHCARE INNOVATIONS

Kazakhstan's National Healthy Nation Project 2021–2025 focuses on universal health coverage. It is supported by WHO through initiatives in evidence-based policy, health worker capacity building, and various health programs (WHO Regional Office for Europe, 2022). The COVID-19 pandemic prompted efforts to enhance emergency response, infection control, and essential health services (WHO Regional Office for Europe, 2022).

RECOMMENDATIONS TO IMPROVE HEALTH AND HEALTHCARE IN KAZAKHSTAN

After analyzing the current healthcare system in Kazakhstan, the following recommendations are suggested:

- *Increase healthcare funding:* Align funding with the global average (9.89% of GDP) to improve service quality and accessibility.
- *Focus on NCDs:* Shift emphasis from infectious diseases to chronic conditions like diabetes and cancer. Expand primary care services to manage these effectively.
- *Strengthen public health insurance:* Ensure the CSHI program's effective rollout to reduce out-of-pocket costs and improve access.
- *Promote alternative medicine:* Integrate evidence-based complementary treatments within mainstream care while ensuring proper certification and regulation.
- *Enhance health worker training:* Invest in training for health workers in key areas such as maternal and child health, HIV, and tuberculosis, with support from international organizations like WHO.
- *Improve infrastructure and emergency response:* Strengthen health infrastructure and emergency systems to better handle public health crises and ensure continuous essential services.
- *Adopt a health-in-all-policies approach:* Incorporate health considerations into all policies to address social determinants of health and promote healthy living environments.

CONCLUSION

This chapter discussed the current state of health and healthcare in Kazakhstan, highlighting both achievements and challenges. Kazakhstan has made significant strides in improving health outcomes, such as having a relatively high life expectancy and low maternal and infant mortality rates compared to its Central Asian neighbors. However, it still lags behind WHO European Region and the EU in these health indicators. Economically, Kazakhstan's per-capita GDP is higher than the Central Asia average but lower than that of WHO European Region and the EU. The country's poverty rate is significantly lower compared to Central Asia, WHO European Region, and the EU.

LEARNING ACTIVITIES

CourseConnect

To access self-assessment questions and interactive, competency-based learning activities for this chapter, visit www.springerpub.com/courseconnect. See inside front cover and tear-out for CourseConnect details.

REFERENCES

Academy of Preventive Medicine [Kazakhstan] and Macro International Inc. (1999). *Kazakhstan Demographic and Health Survey.* Calverton, Maryland: Academy of Preventive Medicine and Macro International Inc.

Advantour. (n.d.). *Kazakhstan travel.* https://www.advantour.com/kazakhstan/

Akorda. (n.d.). *The Republic of Kazakhstan.* https://akorda.kz/en/republic_of_kazakhstan/kazakhstan

Altynsarina, E. (2019, November). *Kazakhstan to launch compulsory health insurance 10 years in the making. Astana Times.* https://astanatimes.com/2019/09/kazakhstan-to-launch-compulsory-health-insurance-10-years-in-the-making

AqZhaiyq. (2023). *News of Kazakhstan.* https://azh.kz/ru/news/view/101784

The Borgen Project. (2020, August 17). *Healthcare in Kazakhstan: Problems and solutions.* The Borgen Project. https://borgenproject.org/healthcare-in-kazakhstan/

Bureau of National Statistics. (2023a). *On the birth rate in 2022.* https://stat.gov.kz/ru/news/o-rozhdaemosti-v-2022-godu/

Bureau of National Statistics. (2023b). *Quality of life of the population.* Bureau of National Statistics. https://stat.gov.kz/en/industries/labor-and-income/stat-life/publications/71526/?sphrase_id=427477

Classifier of Administrative-Territorial Objects. (2018, September). *Zakon* [Law]. https://online.zakon.kz/Document/?doc_id=30438024

Constitution of the Republic of Kazakhstan. (1995, August 30). *Constitution of the Republic of Kazakhstan.* https://www.akorda.kz/en/constitution-of-the-republic-of-kazakhstan-50912

Countrymeters. (n.d.). *Distribution of population by age groups.* https://countrymeters.info/ru/Kazakhstan

Government of Kazakhstan. (2025). *About Kazakhstan.* https://www.gov.kz/?lang=en

Government of the Republic of Kazakhstan. (2022, November 24). *Decree on approval of the concept of healthcare development of the Republic of Kazakhstan until 2026.* Adilet.zan.kz - Information and legal system of normative legal acts of the Republic of Kazakhstan. https://adilet.zan.kz/rus/docs/P2200000945#z38

Katsaga, A., Kulzhanov, M., Karanikolos, M., & Rechel, B. (2012). Kazakhstan: Health system review. *Health Systems in Transition, 14*(4), 1–154. PMID: 22894852.

Kazakhstan Pharm Reviews. (2023). *Pharm reviews.* https://pharmreviews.kz/

Language Act of Kazakhstan. (1997, July 11). *Legislation.* Al-Farabi Kazakh National University. https://www.kaznu.kz/ru/1969

Law of the Republic of Kazakhstan on Education. (2007, July 27). *Legal acts.* https://www.gov.kz/legalacts/details/Z070000319_?lang=ru

Medicine MCFER — Kazakhstan. (2022, November 1). *The cause of 87% of deaths in Kazakhstan is non-communicable diseases.* Medicine—Information support portal for healthcare managers. https://med.mcfr.kz/news/3639-prichina-87-smertey-v-kazahstane-neinfektsionnye-zabolevaniya

Organisation for Economic Co-operation and Development. (2018). *OECD reviews of health systems: Kazakhstan 2018.* OECD-ilibrary. https://doi.org/10.1787/9789264289062-en

O'Neill, A. (2024). *Kazakhstan: Life expectancy at birth from 2012 to 2022, by gender.* Statista. https://www.statista.com/statistics/970802/life-expectancy-at-birth-in-kazakhstan-by-gender/

Panchenko, T. (2019, March 28). *How many languages are needed in Kazakhstan?* Forbes Kazakhstan. https://forbes.kz/articles/skolko_yazyikov_nujnyi_v_kazahstane

Penkala-Gawecka, D. (2002). Korean medicine in Kazakhstan: Ideas, practices and patients. *Anthropology & Medicine,* 9(3), 315–336. https://doi.org/10.1080/13648470216338

President of Kazakhstan. (2009, September). *Code on people's health and the health care system.* https://adilet.zan.kz/eng/docs/K090000193_.

Satubaldina, A. (2022). *Building a digital Kazakhstan: Kazakhstan seeks to provide 100 percent of population with internet by 2025.* https://astanatimes.com/2022/08/building-a-digital-kazakhstan-kazakhstan-seeks-to-provide-100-percent-of-popul

Skaley, Y. (2019, April 17). *How many languages are spoken in Kazakhstan?* https://365info.kz/2019/04/na-skolkih-yazykah-govoryat-v-kazahstane

Sputnik Kazakhstan. (2023, October 21). *What types of leisure activities do Kazakhstanis choose?* https://ru.sputnik.kz/20231021/kakie-vidy-dosuga-vybirayut-kazakhstantsy-39545946.html

U.S. Mission Kazakhstan. (2022, June 3). *2021 Report on international religious freedom: Kazakhstan.* U.S. Embassy & Consulate. https://kz.usembassy.gov/2021-report-on-international-religious-freedom-kazakhstan/

UN Development Programme Kazakhstan. (2022, July 2022). *How climate change affects the health of the population of Kazakhstan?* https://www.undp.org/kazakhstan/stories/how-climate-change-affects-health-population-kazakhstan

Vlast. (2023). *The share of Kazakhs in the ethnic composition of Kazakhstan approached 71%.* https://vlast.kz/novosti/59876-dola-kazahov-v-etniceskom-sostave-kazahstana-priblizilas-k-71.html

World Health Organization. (2024). *Kazakhstan.* https://data.who.int/countries/398

World Health Organization Regional Office for Europe. (2022). *Health systems in action: Kazakhstan: 2022 edition.* IRIS. https://iris.who.int/handle/10665/362324

CHAPTER 42

IRAQ

Sarah Al-Aubaidy and Thomas Foley

GEOGRAPHIC AND DEMOGRAPHIC FEATURES

The Republic of Iraq (Iraq) is located in the central region of Western Asia and holds a total surface area of approximately 435,050 square kilometers (270,327 square miles; World Bank Group, 2024). The country is fully bordered by Turkey to the north, Iran to the east, Syria and Jordan to the west, and Saudi Arabia and Kuwait to the south. It is divided into 18 governorates, each composed of 120 districts and further subdistricts. **Baghdad** is considered the smallest governorate and spans only 673 square kilometers (418 square miles); yet it is the capital and most populated region with around 7.2 million inhabitants. Najaf, Karbala, Erbil, Mosul, Basra, and Kirkuk are other major and densely occupied urban cities that are fundamental to the nation's culture and commerce. Iraq has a widely diverse geography with characteristics segregated into various topographic regions: the central and southeastern alluvial plains crucial for agriculture; the northern Al-Jazeera region that constitutes the many mountains of Iraq and is found between the Tigris–Euphrates Rivers; the western and southern deserts exhibited in more than 40% of the total land; and the northern highlands (Iraq Embassy, 2024). The **Tigris–Euphrates** rivers flow through parts of Turkey, Syria, and Iraq and provide irrigation which has allowed for the early growth of civilization in those exceptionally dry areas.

In 2023, approximately 45 million people lived in Iraq, making it the third most populated country in Western Asia after Iran and Turkey. Iraq has a young populace with a median age of 20 years and a birth rate of 25.6 births per 1,000 people, contributing to its rapidly growing population (UN Data Portal, n.d.). Despite its major Arab population (approximately 78%), the country holds an abundance of diversity, as it is home to various ethnic groups including Kurds, Turkmen, Assyrians, Armenians, Shabaks, Chaldeans, and Romani. The Kurds are the second largest ethnic group (approximately 17%) and primarily reside in northern Iraq within the **Kurdistan** region (UN High Commissioner for Refugees [UNHCR], 2023). With Iraq's diverse backgrounds also comes a need for a robust healthcare system that effectively addresses the challenges of its youthful population and enhances healthcare access in its communities. Table 42.1 displays an overview of Iraq's demographic information.

CULTURAL BELIEFS

Iraq's culture has been profoundly influenced by its ancient history, traditions, and practices, allowing it to emerge as a nation of prominent civilization. The country's prevalent religion is Islam with the majority of the population being **Shiite (Shia)** Muslims. There is also, however, a considerable number of **Sunni** Muslims in Iraq. Shia and Sunni are different sects of Islam, in which the groups share many of the same core values but differ in their leaders, hierarchies, and religious interpretations. While Shia is the predominant sect of Islam in Iraq, Sunni Muslims constitute approximately 85% of the global Muslim population. There are also minority religious groups such as Christians and Yezidis, among others, all partly responsible for the country's intricate cultural traditions and customs. Approximately 60% of the Muslim population in Iraq is Shia, a sect of Islam that practices various religious observances such as the annual remembrance of **Ashura**, which has been commemorated for more than 1,000 years

TABLE 42.1 ESTIMATES OF KEY IRAQ DEMOGRAPHIC INFORMATION, 2023	
Median age	20.3 years
Total population	45,074,049
Percent of population by age	0–19 years: 47.4% 20–64 years: 49.2% 65+ years: 3.4%
Fertility rate	3.25 children per woman
Birth rate	77.2 live births per 1,000 people
Death rate	12.4 per 1,000 people
Life expectancy	Males: 70.43 Females: 74.05
Percent of population by ethnicity/ race	Arabs: 75%–80% Kurds: 15%–20% Other: Assyrian, Turkmen, Armenians, etc. (<5%)
Religious composition	Shiite (Shia) Muslims: 60% Sunni Muslims: 35% Christians: 3% Other: <1%
Languages	Arabic: 77.2% Kurdish: 18.0% Others: Azerbaijani, Turkmen, Assyrian, Persian, etc. (<5%)
Education levels	Basic education: 78.4% Secondary education: 48.6% Higher education: 50.2%
Female-to-male ratio	1.5 females per 1.6 males
Urban population	72% of the population
Migration rate	–5,710

Sources: Adapted from UN Data Portal. (n.d.). *UN population division data portal.* United Nations. https://population.un.org/dataportal/home/; UN High Commissioner for Refugees. (2023). *Web archive.* https://webarchive.archive.unhcr.org/; U.S. Department of State. (2023). *U.S. Department of State home page.* https://www.state.gov/; World Bank Group. (2024). *The World Bank open data.* https://data.worldbank.org/; UNESCO. (2024). *UNESCO home page.* https://www.unesco.org/en

and maintains a prominent occurrence in Iraq (U.S. Department of State, 2023). Ashura signifies a time of mourning for the martyrdom of Prophet Muhammad's grandson Hussein ibn Ali. Furthermore, Iraq's culture has been deeply enriched by its diverse traditions, ethnicities, and practices. The primary languages spoken are Arabic (77%) and Kurdish (18%), with a small minority (5%) speaking Azerbaijani, Persian, Assyrian, and Turkish (Central Intelligence Agency [CIA], 2024).

BRIEF MODERN HISTORY

Originally part of the Ottoman Empire, Iraq was colonized by Britain and placed under a mandate in 1920 following World War I. This was largely due to Iraq's rich natural resources, particularly oil, which has made it the country with the fifth largest petroleum reserves in the world. Iraq gained its independence from Britain in 1932 and declared itself a republic in 1958. Following a revolution in 1968, Saddam Hussein gained control of the government and Iraq transitioned under his dictatorship between 1979 and 2003. During this time period, Iraq experienced numerous wars, including jurisdictional conflicts with Iran leading to the **Iran–Iraq War** from 1980 until 1988. This was preceded by the **Gulf War** in 1990, triggered by Saddam Hussein's invasion of Kuwait. In 2003, the **Iraq War** began due to Iraq's noncompliance with UN resolutions and the U.S. administration's goal of ending Saddam Hussein's presidency based on beliefs that Iraq possessed weapons of mass destruction (WMDs) and had links to terrorism. This invasion was later deemed unjustifiable due to the unreliable evidence of WMDs. However, U.S. interference in Iraq officially ended Hussein's rule, creating a federal parliamentary-republic government with multiple political parties as well as an additional independent government in the Kurdistan region of Iraq. Despite the end of a 23-year dictatorship, the nation continued to suffer from persistent instability in governance and occupancy and attacks by an armed extremist organization, ISIS, from 2014 to 2017. Iraq was able to retrieve much of its ISIS-controlled territory, officially proclaiming victory in 2017, as well as regaining disputed land in the Kurdistan region (CIA, 2024).

Iraq has had a unique history that has greatly transformed its political system over time from the excessive fluctuation of political disruptions and key events such as the 2003 U.S. invasion. The invasion led to the transition from a dictatorship to a republic, introducing a new political structure with a president, prime minister, parliament, and political parties that reflect the country's diverse ethnic groups. Regardless, Iraq is significantly affected by sectarianism from previous conflicts between Arabs and Kurds as well as the Shiite and Sunni Islamic sects. Iraq is working to address problems regarding safety, misconduct, and renovation inside its reconciled borders.

Iraq is home to one of the world's original civilizations—the **Sumer** in the Mesopotamia region of the Fertile Crescent. Sumerians are credited with some of the earliest developments in written language, mathematics, astronomy, time keeping, architecture, and urban planning; all of which have a primary effect on the nation's modern identity (Chambers & Kennedy, 2024).

HEALTH OUTCOMES

MENTAL HEALTH

With the enduring consequences of war, instability, and expulsion, mental health is an amplifying concern in Iraq. The emotional burden of coping with wars and terrorist movements has led to an emergent need for mental health professionals and services in Iraq. However, there is a shortage of skilled mental health professionals and a widespread misunderstanding about mental health disorders. As a result, approximately 20% of the population, or more than 9 million people, have reported experiencing mental health disorders, with many more silently struggling (Saied et al., 2023). Approximately 67% of displaced children exposed to violence suffer from PTSD. Depression is also widespread, affecting almost 70% of students and 50% of children. Additionally, 58% of older individuals report anxiety symptoms and about 10% of adolescents exhibit signs of separation anxiety, specific phobias, and learning disorders (Ahmed, 2022).

In 2021, Iraq reported more than 700 suicides. According to the Iraq Ministry of Interior (MOI), 36.6% of these suicides involved individuals under 20 years old and more than 50% were from individuals aged 29 years or younger. Males were more likely than females to commit suicide, 56% and 44%, respectively. In a country where a notable percentage of suicides includes youths and young adults, there is an evident link with social and economic insecurity (Younis & John, 2023). Nevertheless, many cases go unreported due to the stigma around mental illness, discouraging people from seeking help. Raising awareness about mental health is crucial to ensure people receive necessary care, especially among youths and young adults.

INFANT AND MATERNAL MORTALITY AND LIFE EXPECTANCY

Regionally, Iraq has high infant and maternal mortality and low life expectancy. The maternal mortality ratio in Iraq during 2020 was 76 maternal deaths per 100,000 live births (UN Population Fund, 2024). While maternal mortality continues to be a major concern in Iraq, its maternal mortality ratio decreased from 117 in 2006 to 76 in 2020 (World Bank Group, 2024). In 2023, Iraq's infant mortality rate was 19 infant deaths per 1,000 live births. At the start of the 21st century, however, the infant mortality rate in Iraq was 36.2 infant deaths per 1,000 live births. While infant mortality in Iraq is higher than in most other West Asian nations, it is important to recognize Iraq's improvements in the prevention of infant deaths. Iraq has also experienced significant gains in life expectancy at birth over the past several decades. In 1960, life expectancy at birth in Iraq was 57 years; in 2023, it was 72.3 years. Although a great improvement, this remains low when compared to other West Asian nations, with the exception of Yemen (UN Data Portal, n.d.).

LEADING CAUSES OF MORTALITY

Noncommunicable diseases (NCDs) account for a significant percentage of mortality in Iraq. Diseases of the heart, stroke, diabetes mellitus, chronic kidney diseases, and lung cancer were among the top 10 leading causes of death in Iraq during 2021. Cardiovascular disease (CVD) is the leading cause of death in Iraq, and deaths from CVD has steadily increased in Iraq over the past decade. Metabolic risks such as hypertension, hyperglycemia, obesity, and hypercholesterolemia in addition to poor diets and tobacco use are driving the NCD epidemic in Iraq (Institute for Health Metrics and Evaluation [IHME], 2021).

While infectious diseases, neonatal complications, and injuries account for a smaller percentage of mortality in Iraq, they persist as leading causes of death. Communicable diseases in Iraq are intensified by restricted access to nonpolluted communities, clean water, and adequate sanitation. Iraq also has a relatively low vaccination rate of 17.7% and a vaccine hesitancy rate of around 61.4%, indicating a growing apprehension of vaccines making the population more vulnerable to avoidable deaths caused by communicable diseases (Alatrany et al., 2023). In 2021, COVID-19 was the second leading cause of death in Iraq. In addition, road injuries ranked as the eighth leading cause of death due to insufficient traffic safety laws, poor road infrastructure, limited emergency services, unenforced vehicle inspections, and a significant deficiency in law enforcement. Consequently, individuals in Iraq are four times more likely to die from road accident-related injuries than acts of terrorism (World Health Organization [WHO], 2024). Figure 42.1 lists the leading causes of death in Iraq during 2011 and 2021 (IHME, 2021).

FIGURE 42.1 Leading causes of mortality in Iraq during 2011 and 2021.

Cause	2011 rank	2021 rank	Change in deaths per 100K, 2011–2021
Ischemic heart disease	1	1	↑ +20.9
COVID-19	–	2	↑ +88.0
Stroke	2	3	↑ +9.9
Diabetes	6	4	↑ +6.1
Chronic kidney disease	8	5	↑ +4.5
Neonatal disorders	3	6	↓ −22.8
Hypertensive heart disease	12	7	↑ +1.7
Road injuries	7	8	↓ −3.7
Lung cancer	14	9	↑ +2.6
Interpersonal violence	11	10	↓ −2.2

Communicable, maternal, neonatal, and nutritional diseases
Noncommunicable diseases   Injuries

Source: Institute for Health Metrics and Evaluation. (2021). *Country profiles: Iraq*. https://www.healthdata.org/research-analysis/health-by-location/profiles/iraq

DETERMINANTS OF HEALTH

SOCIAL AND ECONOMIC FACTORS

In 2023, Iraq's gross domestic product (GDP) was approximately $251 billion, representing 0.25% of the world's GDP. This is largely due to the abundant natural resources, especially oil. The country's per-capita GDP, however, was only $5,565, which was well below the international average of $12,688 (World Bank Group, 2024). Despite being rich in resources, Iraq struggles to achieve widespread economic growth due to prolonged criminality, war, and instability. Iraq, subsequently, has a low Human Development Index (HDI) score of 0.673 (UN Development Programme, 2024). Iraq's low HDI score is based on insufficient access to proper healthcare, education, and essential living services.

Unemployment and inflation have driven the country's poverty rate from 20% in 2018 to nearly 30% post-COVID pandemic, with adolescents particularly affected. The number of children living in poverty nearly doubled to 37.9% and almost 50% of children were susceptible to experiencing deprivation in different areas such as education and living conditions. Many Iraqis have lack of access to healthcare, shelter, education, and financial stability, leading to a decline in quality of life (UNICEF, n.d.). In 2022, approximately 1 million internally displaced people (IDPs) required humanitarian aid. A multitude of IDPs live in rural overcrowded areas or camps, where there is limited aid and inadequate resources. IDPs are vulnerable to poverty due to restricted financial prospects and the absence of housing, aid, and security. Poverty rates among IDPs are 50%, which is substantially higher than the national average. IDPs struggle to attain fundamental requirements such as food, clean water, and sanitation (UN Development Programme, 2024). These factors sustain social and economic barriers and poor health outcomes, further complicating Iraq's overall growth. Figure 42.2 portrays a substantial change in Iraq's social rankings between 2007 and 2020, as the country's upper class lowered from 16% to 10% of the population, the middle class declined from 61% to 30%, and the lower class rose from 23% to 60% (Dagher, 2020).

FIGURE 42.2 Percentage of the population change in social class distribution in Iraq—2007, 2014, and 2020.

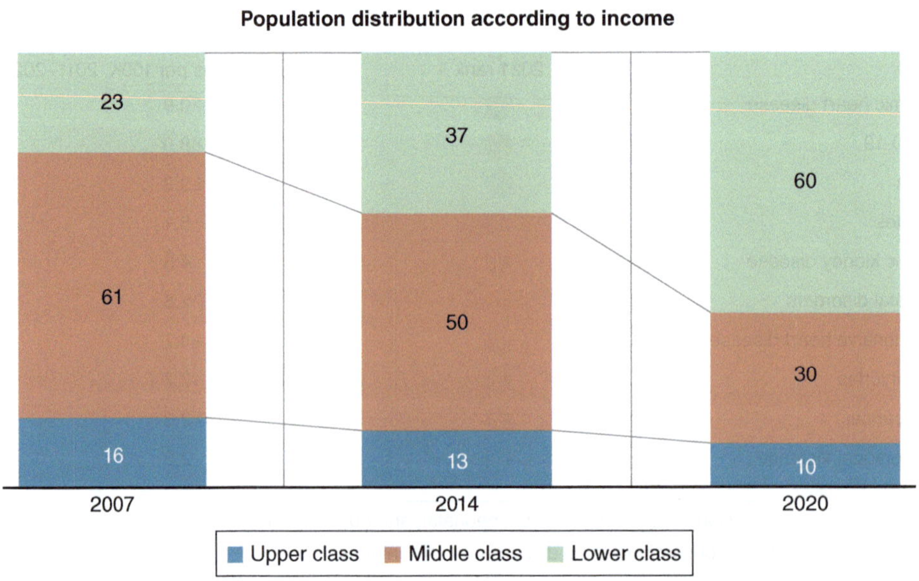

Source: Dagher, M. (2020). *Iraqi stability and its free-falling mddle class.* https://www.csis.org/analysis/iraqi-stability-and-its-free-falling-middle-class

EDUCATION AND UNEMPLOYMENT RATES

In Iraq, where most of the population is young and opportunities are scarce, there is a need for well-resourced education and employment options to drive the nation's development. In 2023, the completion rate for primary education was 78.4%. About 48.6% of the population had completed their lower secondary education and nearly 50% had completed an upper secondary education, which is equivalent to a high school diploma (UNESCO, 2024). These relatively low education rates are tied to Iraq's economic inequality. The unemployment rate in 2023 was approximately 15.5%, which equated to an approximate 7 million unemployed. Women encounter increased challenges to employment and education in comparison to men. By 2021, only 11.4% of females were employed, relative to 72.1% of males. The literacy rate among women age 15 and older was nearly 80%, compared to 91% for men (World Bank Group, 2024).

ENVIRONMENTAL AND CLIMATE FACTORS

Iraq has been intensely impacted by the long-lasting effects of climate change as it experiences nearly year-long dry conditions that cause the country to be progressively vulnerable to environmental challenges. Iraq is the fifth ranked country most vulnerable to climate change worldwide and the most vulnerable among all Middle Eastern and North African (MENA) countries. Experts estimate that Iraq will have the warmest average annual temperatures by 2050, surpassing an annual average of 36°C (96.8°F). The combination of severe heat and scarce rainfall reduces work efficiency, particularly in areas of farming and construction, where 35% of employees endure temperatures above 50°C (122°F). The absence of clean water is also a primary issue, disturbing agriculture and, therefore, the country's food supply. Due to the climate crisis, **desertification** damaged 70% of the land in 2023, further affecting crops, the populations who reside in those arable regions, and the number of IDPs in the country (The New Arab, 2023). Iraq also experiences severe weather occurrences, as heatwaves and sandstorms occur multiple times annually. These uncontrollable environmental strains jeopardize agriculture, general health, and water sources, making adjusting to climate changes and proper resource control vital for Iraq's future.

The nation's carbon intensity is exceptionally high, with yearly carbon dioxide emissions escalating from 61 million tons in 2007 to 185 million tons in 2021. To manage these climate issues, World Bank Group suggests three areas of crucial priority in Iraq:

- adaptations that address the scarcity of water and agriculture
- mitigation regarding the reduction of carbon emissions
- a shift to a low-carbon economy

This plan requires an estimated investment of $233 billion by 2040. Consequently, Iraq ratified the **Paris Agreement**, an internationally enforced treaty designed to address climate change and global warming, and the **ZEF Agreement**, which includes a pledge to stop gas flaring by 2030 (Atlantic Council, 2024).

Iraq is also considered to be one of the most polluted countries in the world, with an average concentration of fine particulate matter ($PM_{2.5}$) in the atmosphere of 42.5 micrograms per 1 cubic meter of air (mcg/m^3) during 2023. **$PM_{2.5}$** is 2.5 micrometers or smaller and can be deeply absorbed into the lungs and cause substantial health risks. With this $PM_{2.5}$ concentration, Iraq far exceeded WHO's annual air quality guideline value (IQAir, 2024).

HEALTHCARE SYSTEM

FINANCING, INSURANCE, AND COST

Hospitals and healthcare settings are funded via a combination of public and private sectors. The **public sector** is a government-managed system that provides services at no or minimal cost. **Private sectors** include privately owned hospitals, pharmacies, labs, and clinics that operate for profit, often charging more while purportedly providing better services than public hospitals. Additionally, international investments contribute to the funding. For example, the International Finance Corporation (IFC), a member of the World Bank Group, invested millions in the construction of a new hospital in Erbil in Iraq's Kurdistan region. Construction of the new hospital, which is referred to as the **2021 Seema Hospital project**, cost $92 million. The Seema Hospital is one of few newer facilities with high quality healthcare resources. It has 161 beds and oncology, radiotherapy, and burn centers (IFC, 2020).

Conflicts, economic barriers, and mismanagement have significantly damaged Iraq's once leading Middle Eastern healthcare system. After the Iran–Iraq War, the Gulf War, and the 2003 U.S. invasion, the system's decline led to a rise in personal healthcare spending. Out-of-pocket expenditures make up almost 50% of Iraq's total health expenses, underscoring the financial strain on individuals (WHO, 2024). High personal healthcare costs and lack of expense coverage stem from the country's absence of a unified national health insurance system. As of 2022, roughly 96% of Iraqis had no health insurance, depending only on a neglected general healthcare system with finite services. Although health insurance programs are available for some employees, they offer minimal coverage and are not easily accessible. Iraq is an oil-rich country, which allows it to convey an upper-middle-income status, although its facilities and socioeconomic developments are not at a similar standard. The World Bank has urged reforms to improve living standards, emphasizing the need for a shift from conflict to rehabilitation, state dominance to market orientation, oil dependence to diversification, and isolation to global integration (Arab Reform Initiative, 2024).

Iraq's healthcare system faces significant challenges related to medical care costs, which contribute to widespread inaccessibility and financial strain for its citizens. A staggering 85% of Iraqis report that they find healthcare services unaffordable, leading to delays in seeking necessary medical attention (Arab Reform Initiative, 2024). However, among those seeking medical care, 85% visit private facilities, with 46.3% choosing private clinics and 18.6% opting for private hospitals. This trend highlights a strong inclination toward the private sector, despite its higher expenses, due to superior access to specialists, treatments, medications, and overall care. Regardless, affordability remains a significant barrier to accessing healthcare, particularly among groups like IDPs and refugees. On average, Iraqi households allocate about 8% of their income to healthcare, which is a considerable amount given their often-restricted financial means (Shabila et al., 2024). The Iraqi Health Insurance Law (IHIL) was introduced in 2020 to manage these challenges by enhancing coverage and access. The IHIL requires major reforms, such as forming a **Health Commission** to transfer services from public hospitals to private ones. However, political instability and lack of funds have hindered its implementation. Without prominent alterations and investments, access and affordability gaps will likely grow and worsen health inequalities nationwide (Arab Reform Initiative, 2024). Therefore, the Social Security Law was implemented in 2023 to expand medical insurance to more public employees, including independent workers and employees with unregulated jobs (Social Security Administration, 2024).

EDUCATION AND TRAINING

In Iraq, medical professionals must receive comprehensive training to deliver healthcare services. The Iraqi education system follows the 6-year British curriculum taught in the English language, where there are 3 preclinical years and 3 clinical years. Following the 6 years of education in an accredited medical program, physicians must have an additional year of internship and further specialized postgraduate training in a specified residency program. Residency can last from 4 to 6 years depending on the specialty. Cardiologists, anesthesiologists, and surgeons typically require longer training and residencies. Unlike the United States, where most physicians have an MD, it is required in Iraq that doctors have only a bachelor of medicine, bachelor of surgery, or master of medicine (Al-Shamsi, 2017). Nurses can attend a 3-year nursing program to earn a nursing diploma or complete a 4-year bachelor in nursing degree program. Both nursing programs require additional practical training. Pharmacists must enroll in a 5-year pharmacy school and, with the completion of their coursework, have options in different specialties. Other common healthcare professions include paramedics, radiologists, chemical and laboratory analysts, and physical therapists. All professions require the minimum completion of a specified 4-year bachelor's degree at an accredited university. These educational and training programs ensure healthcare professionals are well-prepared to address Iraq's diverse medical needs in a variety of clinical settings.

SHORTAGE AND GAPS

Although there is a notable lack of medical staff, Iraq's healthcare system primarily relies on public sector workers, including doctors and nurses. The country's shortage of medical professionals is partly due to exceptionally low acceptance rates to the limited number of medical schools, which total 32 accredited medical programs nationwide. As of 2022, Iraq had approximately 10 doctors per 10,00 people, which is well below the global average of 17 per 10,000. The shortage worsens as many skilled professionals relocate for better prospects in other well-developed countries (WHO, 2024). Because most public hospitals and medical centers are located in cities, rural regions are left with insufficient access to healthcare. In many cases, public hospitals struggle to meet the demands of the population due to overcrowding, long waiting times, and a lack of medical equipment. Better funded private facilities are available; however, they are usually restricted to those who can personally pay the expenses of private healthcare.

CONCLUSION

After years of insecurity, Iraq's healthcare system faces political instability, poor budget distribution, lack of preventive care, medical worker shortages, and unequal healthcare access, mainly in rural and conflict-affected regions. To improve public health, Iraq should enshrine a health insurance system, shift to climate-resilient medical facilities, and develop additional and enhanced healthcare and road infrastructures to decrease the number of avoidable deaths in the country. These efforts, along with global partnerships, can lead to a successful and fair healthcare system in Iraq.

LEARNING ACTIVITIES

CourseConnect

To access self-assessment questions and interactive, competency-based learning activities for this chapter, visit www.springerpub.com/courseconnect. See inside front cover and tear-out for CourseConnect details.

REFERENCES

Ahmed, D. (2022). The study of mental illness in Iraq and its common trends: A systematic review. *Global Psychiatry Archives, 5*(1), 26–35. https://doi.org/10.52095/gp.2022.3774.1026

Alatrany, S., Falaiyah, A. M., Zuhairawi, R. H. M., Ogden, R., ALi Sayyid Aldrraji, H., Alatrany, A. S. S., Al-Jumeily, D. (2023). A cross-sectional analysis of the predictors of COVID-19 vaccine uptake and vaccine hesitancy in Iraq. *PLoS One, 18*(3), e0282523–e0282523. https://doi.org/10.1371/journal.pone.0282523

Al-Shamsi, M. (2017). Medical education in Iraq: Issues and challenges. *International Journal of Medical Education, 8*(PMC5357542), 88–90. https://doi.org/10.5116/ijme.58b1.c927

Arab Reform Initiative. (2024) *Publications*. https://www.arab-reform.net/

Atlantic Council. (2024). *Shaping the global future together*. https://www.atlanticcouncil.org/

Chambers, R. L., & Kennedy, H. (2024). *Iraq*. Britannica. https://www.britannica.com/place/Iraq

Central Intelligence Agency. (2024). *Iraq—The world factbook*. https://www.cia.gov/the-world-factbook/countries/iraq/

Dagher, M. (2020). *Iraqi stability and its free-falling middle class.* Center for Strategic & International Studies. https://www.csis.org/analysis/iraqi-stability-and-its-free-falling-middle-class

Institute for Health Metrics and Evaluation. (2021). *Country profiles: Iraq.* University of Washington. https://www.healthdata.org/research-analysis/health-by-location/profiles/iraq

International Finance Corporation. (2020). *IFC investment to increase access to health care services in Kurdistan region in Iraq.* https://www.ifc.org/en/pressroom/2020/ifc-investment-to-increase-access-to-health-care-services-in-kurdistan-region-of-iraq

IQAir. (2024). *Explore your air quality.* https://www.iqair.com/

Iraq Embassy. (2024). *Welcome to embassy of the Republic of Iraq in Washington, D.C.* https://www.iraqiembassy.us/

The New Arab. (2023). *Nearly 70% of Iraq affected by desertification.* https://www.newarab.com/news/over-70-percent-iraq-affected-desertification

Saied, A. A., Ahmed, S. K., Metwally, A. A., & Aiash, H. (2023). Iraq's mental health crisis: A way forward? *The Lancet, 402*(10409), 1235–1236. https://doi.org/10.1016/s0140-6736(23)01283-7

Shabila, N. P., Mahmood, K. A., M-Amin, K. M., Mahmood, K. I., & Saleh, A. M. (2024). Healthcare-seeking behavior and out-of-pocket payments in Erbil, Kurdistan Region of Iraq. *Journal of Health Population and Nutrition, 43*(1), 1235–1236. https://doi.org/10.1186/s41043-024-00616-1

Social Security Adminstration. (2024). *International update.* https://www.ssa.gov/policy/docs/progdesc/intl_update/2024-03/index.html

UN Data Portal. (n.d.). *UN population division data portal.* United Nations. https://population.un.org/dataportal/home/

UN High Commissioner for Refugees. (2023). *Web archive.* https://webarchive.archive.unhcr.org/

UN Development Programme. (2024). *Human development reports.* https://hdr.undp.org/

UNESCO. (2024). *UNESCO.* https://www.unesco.org/en

UNICEF. (n.d.). *Iraq.* https://www.unicef.org/iraq/

UN Population Fund. (2024). *UNFPA - United nations population fund.* https://www.unfpa.org/

U.S. Department of State. (2023). *U.S. Department of State home page.* https://www.state.gov/

World Bank Group. (2024). *The World Bank open data.* https://data.worldbank.org/

World Health Organization. (2024). *The world health data hub.* https://data.who.int/

Younis, M. S., & John, A. (2023). Insight of suicide in Iraq: A coroner's report. *Middle East Current Psychiatry, 30*(1). https://doi.org/10.1186/s43045-023-00320-6

PART XI. Health and Healthcare in South Asia

CHAPTER 43

OVERVIEW OF SOUTH ASIA

Sheena Malla, James Giallella, and Thomas Foley

GEOGRAPHY

South Asia is the most populated Asian subregion, comprising eight autonomous countries: Sri Lanka, Bangladesh, India, Afghanistan, Pakistan, Bhutan, Nepal, and the Maldives (Figure 43.1). The region is peninsula shaped and bordered by the Indian Ocean, Bay of Bengal, and Arabian Sea. Important geographic features include the Himalayan, Hindu Kush, and Karakoram Mountain Ranges, the Thar Desert, and the Indus, Ganges, and Brahmaputra Rivers (Sivaramamurti et al., 2025). Major cities include Delhi (India), Karachi (Pakistan), and Dhaka (Bangladesh). South Asia has the distinction of being the most densely populated area in the world (UN Data Portal, n.d.). In addition, South Asia is one of the world's most vulnerable region to climate change. Heat waves, drought, water and food scarcity, cyclones, and floods threaten the way of life in much of South Asia (World Bank Group, 2025).

BRIEF HISTORY

The history of South Asia can be traced back to the Stone Age when some of the first known cultures, such as the Madrasian and Soanian, emerged. Human culture further progressed in South Asia during the Bronze and Iron Ages. These early historical periods marked important developments in human civilization regarding tools, infrastructure, and materials. Societies that thrived during these periods include the **Indus Valley Civilization**, which is recognized as one of the world's earliest urban civilizations, and the Maurya Empire. The Classical Period saw the rise and spread of the **Gupta Empire**. The Gupta Empire brought urban, religious, artistic, agricultural, scientific, and technological innovations. During this time period, the decimal numeral system was invented and Jainism, Buddhism, and Islam developed as new religions and spread across the region. During the Early Modern Period, the Mughal Empire established itself as an organized regional power with international influence. At its height, the Mughal Empire ruled over most of South Asia and was the world's leading economic force. This was a time of significant innovation, and gave us architectural wonders such as the Taj Mahal (Figure 43.2). The Mughal Empire was weakened and collapsed during the Colonial Period.

During the Colonial Period, the **British East India Company** (BEIC), which acted on behalf of the British Crown, became the dominant power in the Indian peninsula. Official British rule over most of South Asia, which was known as the **British Raj**, began in 1857 after a failed rebellion against the BEIC. Following World War II, the British Raj was dissolved in 1947 and the region was partitioned into separate nations: India and East and West Pakistan. The **1947 Partition of India** displaced millions of people along Hindu and Muslim religious lines, leading to violence, refugee crises, and social inequities that continue to impact the region today. In 1971, East Pakistan gained independence, becoming the People's Republic of Bangladesh. While conflicts and inequities persist, post-colonial South Asia has been a period of remarkable growth (Sivaramamurti et al., 2025).

FIGURE 43.1 Map of South Asia.

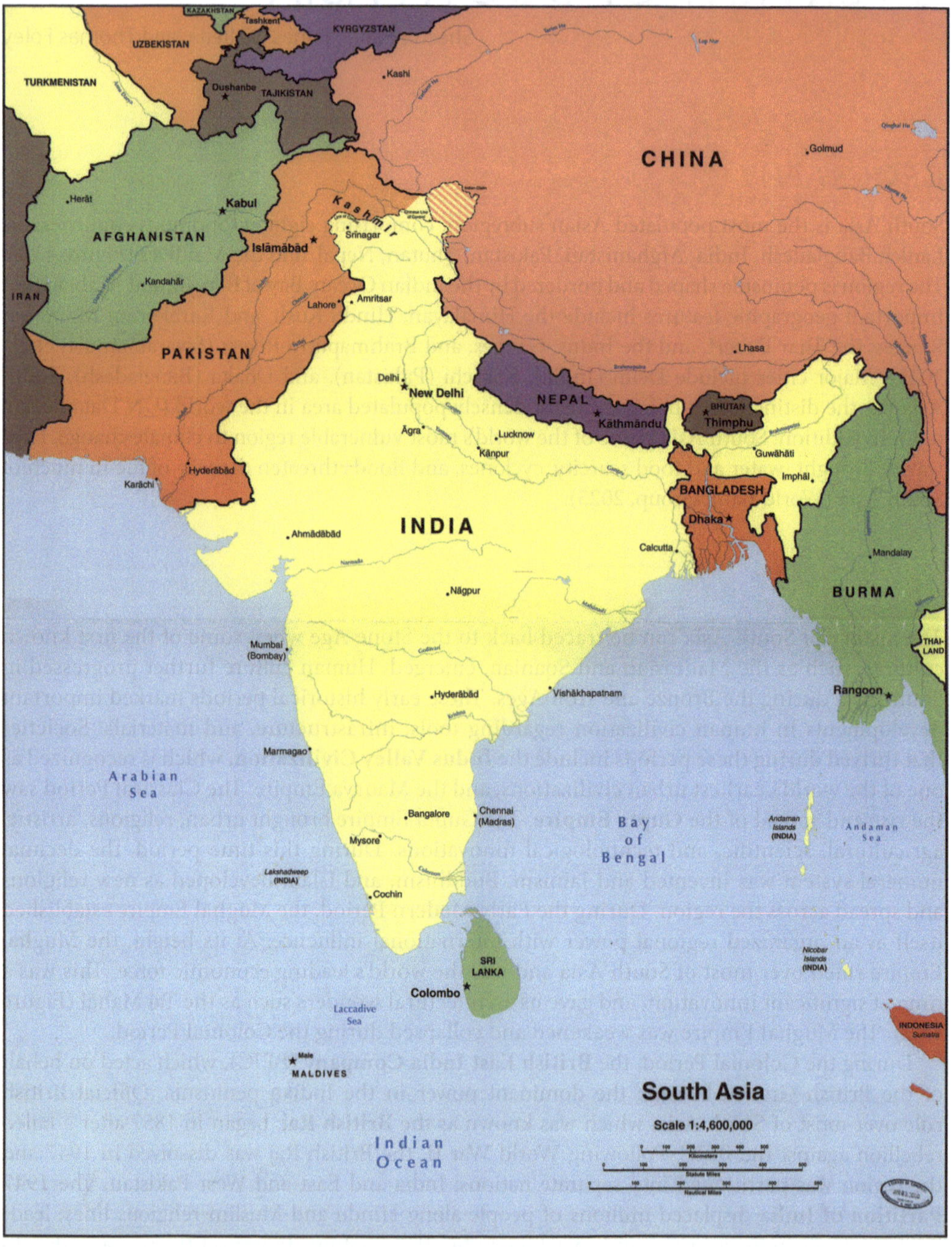

Source: United States Central Intelligence Agency. (1998). *South Asia*. https://www.loc.gov/item/2001622357/

FIGURE 43.2 The Taj Mahal.

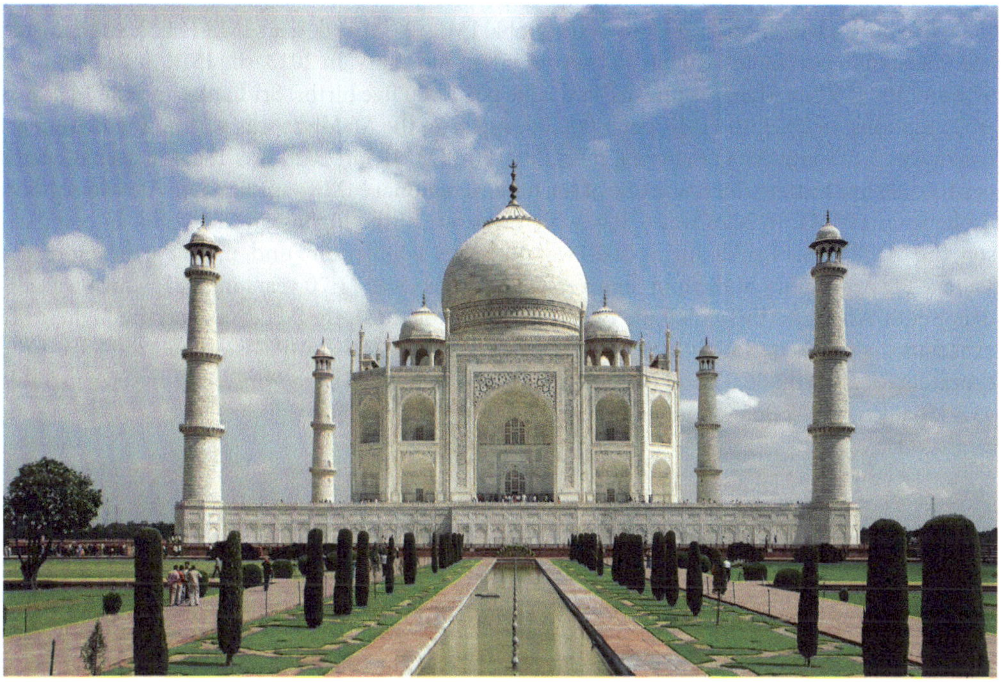

Source: Forget, Y. (2010). *Taj Mahal*. https://en.wikipedia.org/wiki/File:Taj_Mahal_(Edited).jpeg

POPULATION AND HEALTH OUTCOMES

In 2023, South Asia had a population of 2.04 billion people, accounting for approximately one quarter of the world's population and 43% of Asia's population. India's population was nearly 1.44 billion, making it the most populous country in the world, accounting for approximately 70% of South Asia's population, 30% of Asia's population, and 17% of the world's population. Pakistan and Bangladesh are also among the world's most populous countries. In 2023, there were approximately 247.5 million people in Pakistan and 171.4 million people in Bangladesh. South Asia's large population is also relatively young. In 2023, the median age in South Asia was 26.8 years, which was lower than the global median age (30.4 years) and Asia's median age (31.7 years). Sri Lanka and the Maldives are exceptions in South Asia. In 2023, the median age in Sri Lanka was 32.8 years and the median age for the Maldives was 31.1 years. Afghanistan and Pakistan are extremely youthful nations. In 2023, the median age in Afghanistan was 16.9 years and the median age in Pakistan was 20.3 years. Contributing to South Asia's younger population is a high crude birth rate, which was 18.2 births per 1,000 people in 2023. Afghanistan's 2023 birth rate of 35.4 births per 1,000 people was one of the highest in the world (UN Data Portal, n.d.).

With the exception of Afghanistan, the leading causes of mortality in South Asia during 2021 were a mixture of noncommunicable diseases (NCDs) and infectious diseases. The two NCDs that most significantly affected South Asia in 2021 were ischemic heart disease and stroke. Although these chronic diseases are still prevalent in all South Asian countries, COVID-19 was the leading cause of mortality in India, Iran, Nepal, and Pakistan during 2021. Afghanistan's leading cause of mortality in 2021 was conflict and terror. Neonatal disorders, diabetes, cirrhosis of the liver, chronic obstructive pulmonary disease (COPD), tuberculosis, diarrheal diseases, and lower respiratory tract infections also cause significant mortality in South Asia, reflecting a lower-income region that struggles to control infectious diseases, promote infant and maternal health, and combat rising incidences of NCDs (Institute for Health Metrics and Evaluation [IHME], 2024).

Improving infant and maternal health and increasing life expectancy are priorities in much of South Asia. In 2023, the infant mortality rate (IMR) in South Asia was 27.9 infant deaths per 1,000 live births, which was higher than the global IMR (27.3) and Asia's IMR (21.3). Afghanistan and Pakistan in particular struggle to prevent infant mortality. In 2023, the IMR in Pakistan was 49.4 and the IMR in Afghanistan was 44 deaths per 1,000 live births. Sri Lanka and the Maldives are exceptions. In 2023, the IMR per 1,000 live births in the Maldives was 4.3 and the IMR in Sri Lanka was 5.1. South Asia's maternal mortality ratio (MMR) in 2020 was 134.4 maternal deaths per 100,000 live births, which was one of the highest regional MMRs among non-African regions. Afghanistan's MMR in 2020 was 620.4, which was one of the highest in the world. In comparison, the MMR in Sri Lanka during 2020 was 28.8 (UN Population Fund, n.d.). Furthermore, the average life expectancy at birth in South Asian countries was 71.70 years in 2023, which was less than South Asia's and the global life expectancy. During 2023, the Maldives had the highest life expectancy at birth in South Asia at 81.04 years. Afghanistan and Pakistan had the lowest life expectancies at birth: 66.03 and 67.65 years, respectively (UN Data Portal, n.d.). Refer to Table 43.1 for a list of key regional population and health statistics.

SOCIOECONOMIC FACTORS

South Asia is predominantly rural. In 2023, only 33% of South Asians lived in urban areas. As a predominantly rural region, South Asia struggles economically. During 2023, India had one of the largest gross domestic products (GDPs) s in the world; however, its per-capita GDP was only $2,480, emphasizing the inequities that exist in India. The Maldives is an exception in South Asia. During 2023, the Maldives' per-capita GDP was $12,530, making it the only South Asian country

TABLE 43.1 SOUTH ASIA POPULATION AND HEALTH DATA

REGION/ COUNTRY	POPULATION (2023)	LIFE EXPECTANCY AT BIRTH IN YEARS (2023)	INFANT MORTALITY RATE PER 1,000 LIVE BIRTHS (2023)	MATERNAL MORTALITY RATIO PER 100,000 POPULATION (2020)	LEADING CAUSE OF MORTALITY (2021)
South Asia	2.04 billion	71.70	27.9	134.4	—
Afghanistan	41.45 million	66.03	44.0	620.4	Conflict and terror
Bangladesh	171.46 million	74.67	22.8	123	Stroke
Bhutan	786,000	72.98	19.3	59.9	Ischemic heart disease
India	1.44 billion	72.00	22.6	102.7	COVID-19
Maldives	525,000	81.04	4.3	56.7	Ischemic heart disease
Nepal	29.69 million	70.35	21.9	174.4	COVID-19
Pakistan	247.5 million	67.65	49.4	154.2	COVID-19
Sri Lanka	22.97 million	77.48	5.1	28.8	Stroke

Sources: Adapted from Institute for Health Metrics and Evaluation. (2024). *Health research by location: Country profiles*. University of Washington. https://www.healthdata.org/research-analysis/health-by-location/profiles; UN Data Portal. (n.d.). *UN population division data portal*. United Nations. https://population.un.org/dataportal/home/; UN Population Fund. (n.d.). *Data portal*. United Nations. https://www.unfpa.org/data

with a per-capita GDP greater than $4,000. In 2023, the per-capita GDP in Afghanistan, one of the world's poorest countries, was $416 (World Bank Group, n.d.). Continued post-colonial social and economic growth are necessary to increase health equity in South Asia.

LEARNING ACTIVITIES

CourseConnect

To access self-assessment questions and interactive, competency-based learning activities for this chapter, visit www.springerpub.com/courseconnect. See inside front cover and tear-out for CourseConnect details.

REFERENCES

Institute for Health Metrics and Evaluation. (2024). *Health research by location: Country profiles*. University of Washington. https://www.healthdata.org/research-analysis/health-by-location/profiles

Sivaramamurti, C., Yefremov, Y. K., Alexeeva, N. N., & Ryabchikov, A. M. (2025). *South Asia*. Encyclopedia Britannica. https://www.britannica.com/place/South-Asia

World Bank Group. (n.d.). *The World Bank open data*. The World Bank Group. https://data.worldbank.org/

World Bank Group. (2025). *Climate and development in South Asia*. https://www.worldbank.org/en/region/sar/brief/integrating-climate-and-development-in-south-asia/integrating-climate-and-development-in-south-asia-region

UN Data Portal. (n.d.). *UN population division data portal*. United Nations. https://population.un.org/dataportal/home/

UN Population Fund. (n.d.). *Data portal*. United Nations. https://www.unfpa.org/data

CHAPTER 44

BANGLADESH

Sharifa Nasreen and Taufique Joarder

GEOGRAPHIC FEATURES

Bangladesh, officially named the People's Republic of Bangladesh, is a South Asian country with a total surface area of more than 147,000 square kilometers (91,341 square miles; World Bank Group, n.d.). Administratively, Bangladesh has eight divisions (Dhaka, Chittagong, Khulan, Rajshahi, Barisal, Sylhet, and Rangpur), 64 districts, 495 Upazilas (subdistricts), 4,554 unions, 40,987 wards, and approximately 87,320 villages. There are 12 city corporations and 330 municipalities (Directorate General of Health Service [DGHS], 2023). Bangladesh includes

- mostly rich, fertile, flat land with more than 75% of the land less than 3 meters (10 feet) above mean sea level, and thus prone to floods and cyclones;
- the Ganges, Brahmaputra, and Meghna Rivers which form one of the largest deltas in the world;
- hills in the northeast and southeast, and the Bay of Bengal in the south;
- the world's largest mangrove forest, the Sundarbans; and
- a tribal population of over 1.2 million with 45 tribal groups, notably Chakma, Garo, Hajong, Khasia, Magh, Santal, Rakhain, Manipuri, and Murong (Banglapedia, 2024).

DEMOGRAPHIC FEATURES

POPULATION

Bangladesh is one of the most densely populated countries in the world (1,329 people per square kilometer or 0.6 square mile). From 2000 to 2023, the population in Bangladesh increased from 134.5 million to 171.5 million people (UN Data Portal, n.d.). The growth rate declined to 1.1% in 2022 (UN Data Portal, n.d.) due to aggressive family planning measures. The total fertility rate decreased from 3.28 births per woman in 2000 to 2.16 births per woman in 2023 (UN Data Portal, n.d.). The crude birth rate decreased from 29.6 live births per 1,000 people in 2000 to 17.3 live births per 1,000 people in 2023 (UN Data Portal, n.d.).

AGE

The median age in Bangladesh increased from 19.7 years in 2000 to 25.3 in 2023. The proportion of the population aged 15 to 64 years increased from 63% in 2000 to 74% in 2023. The **age dependency ratio** was 38% in 2022 (UN Data Portal, n.d.). Bangladesh has a young population, indicating the need for good education and job opportunities to reap the benefit of this demographic dividend.

MIGRATION

Bangladesh has experienced negative net migration since it gained independence in 1971—the lowest was 52,640 in 1983 and highest was nearly 1.4 million in 2008. While negative net migration decreased significantly during the pandemic in 2020 to just over 61,000, it increased again postpandemic and reached around 310,000 in 2023 (UN Data Portal, n.d.).

ETHNICITY, RACE, SEX, AND GENDER

Ethnically, the population of Bangladesh is an intermixture of Dravidian, Proto-Australoid, Mongoloid, and Aryan (Banglapedia, 2024). In 2022, approximately 50.5% of the population was categorized as female, 49.5% male, and 0.005% third gender; the male-female ratio was 98:100 (DGHS, 2023).

RURAL/URBAN RESIDENCE, LANGUAGE, AND RELIGION

The majority of the population (68.5%) lives in rural areas, while 31.5% live in urban areas. **Bengali** is the national language, spoken by 99.5% of the population, with English as the second most spoken language. Religion-wise, 91% of the population is Muslim, 7.95% Hindu, 0.61% Buddhist, 0.3% Christian, and 0.1% others (Banglapedia, 2024).

BRIEF COUNTRY HISTORY

Bangladesh's history is characterized by cultural richness and a quest for sovereignty. Inhabited for millennia, the region saw early civilizations along the Ganges–Brahmaputra delta. Known as Bengal, it was part of the Maurya and Gupta Empires. King Shashanka, in the seventh century, established the Gauda Kingdom. The Pala and Sena dynasties later promoted Buddhism and Hinduism, respectively (Roy, 1979). Islam's arrival in the eighth century and the Bengal Sultanate in the 14th century shaped Bengali society. The Mughal Empire's annexation brought prosperity, though local chieftains like the Bara-Bhuiyans resisted their rule (Ahmed et al., 2022).

The Battle of Plassey in 1757 marked the beginning of British colonial rule, leading to economic exploitation and famines, with millions perishing in the Great Bengal Famine of 1770 and the Bengal Famine of 1943. Other European powers also influenced local politics. Resistance to British rule included the Sepoy Mutiny of 1857, the Faraizi Movement, and peasant revolts. In 1947, the partition of British India created Pakistan, including East Pakistan (now Bangladesh), where disparities led to the 1971 Bangladesh Liberation War and independence (Ahmed et al., 2022).

Postindependence, Bangladesh has progressed economically and socially, becoming a poverty reduction model. Yet, it faces climate change threats like cyclones and rising sea levels, along with human rights and democratic governance challenges as it moves forward in the 21st century.

HEALTH OUTCOMES

Bangladesh made remarkable improvements in health indicators over the past 52 years while experiencing demographic and epidemiologic transitions. However, Bangladesh is facing the **double burden of disease**—communicable diseases and noncommunicable diseases (NCDs)—because of increasing sedentary lifestyles and unhealthy diets (i.e., calorie-dense and poorly nutritious) in the young and middle-aged population (Islam et al., 2023).

LIFE EXPECTANCY AT BIRTH

Since independence in 1971, Bangladesh made significant gains in life expectancy at birth, raising it to 49.2 years. Since then, life expectancy at birth in Bangladesh has continued to increase—from 62.05 years in 2000 to 74.67 years in 2023. Females have higher life expectancy at birth compared to males (76.4 years versus 73 years; UN Data Portal, n.d.).

LEADING CAUSES OF MORTALITY

The age-standardized mortality rate in Bangladesh decreased substantially since 1990, from 1,509 deaths per 100,000 people in 1990 to 714.4 in 2019 (Islam et al., 2023). A significant reduction in deaths due to communicable diseases such as diarrheal diseases, tuberculosis, lower respiratory infections, and malaria was achieved between 1990 and 2019 (Figure 44.1). Nevertheless, the top

FIGURE 44.1 Age-standardized death rate for the 10 leading causes of death in Bangladesh, 1990 and 2019.

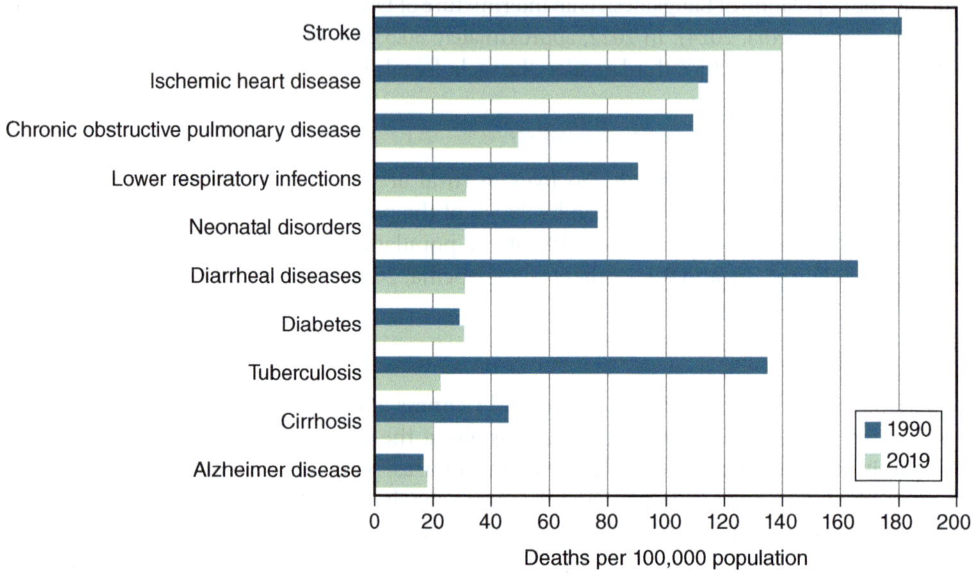

Source: GBD 2019 Bangladesh Burden of Disease Collaborators. (2023). The burden of diseases and risk factors in Bangladesh, 1990–2019: A systematic analysis for the Global Burden of Disease Study 2019. *The Lancet Global Health, 11*(12), e1931–e1942. https://doi.org/10.1016/S2214-109X(23)00432-1

10 causes of death in 2019 included stroke, ischemic heart disease, chronic obstructive pulmonary disease, lower respiratory infections, neonatal disorders, diarrheal diseases, diabetes, tuberculosis, cirrhosis, and Alzheimer disease (Islam et al., 2023).

NONCOMMUNICABLE DISEASES

Bangladesh is facing challenges in addressing the rising burden of noncommunicable diseases (NCDs), with the health system primarily designed to address communicable diseases in children and women within primary healthcare. NCDs account for 70% of deaths, including 19% of probable premature deaths (World Health Organization [WHO], 2022).

Major chronic diseases in Bangladesh include cardiovascular diseases, diabetes, chronic obstructive pulmonary diseases, and cancer (DGHS, 2023). However, there is a lack of national-level comprehensive data on the burden of chronic diseases in the country. During 2017–2018, 28% of women and 26% of men aged 18 years and older had hypertension, and 10% of women and 11% of men had elevated blood glucose level. More than half of hypertensive women and two thirds of hypertensive men were not aware of their elevated blood pressure, whereas 60% of men and women were unaware of their elevated blood sugar level. The prevalence of hypertension, diabetes, and obesity is higher in urban areas than in rural areas (National Institute of Population Research and Training [NIPORT] and ICF, 2020).

Bangladesh has no population-based cancer registry; therefore, lacks accurate cancer prevalence and incidence rate data. There were an estimated 167,256 new cancer cases in 2022 in Bangladesh. The estimated leading cancers were esophageal, lip, oral cavity, and lung (40% of all cancers) in males, and breast, uterine cervix, and esophageal (43% of all cancers) in females (Ferlay et al., 2024).

COMMUNICABLE DISEASES

Deaths due to lower respiratory infections, diarrheal diseases, tuberculosis, enteric fever, acute hepatitis, and malaria have been reduced significantly between 2010 and 2019; nevertheless, they still cause a notable health burden (Institute for Health Metrics and Evaluation [IHME], n.d.).

Bangladesh achieved high vaccine coverage of children through the expanded program on Immunization (EPI) to reduce morbidity and mortality from vaccine-preventable diseases. Emerging infectious diseases such as dengue and Nipah virus infection are of concern. Bangladesh is experiencing a rise in dengue cases and mortality in recent years and experienced a large outbreak in 2019. Longer monsoons with erratic rainfall, rising temperature, and decreasing humidity levels, together with urbanization, are attributed to the rise and risk of dengue spread in the country, and will also impact other mosquito-borne diseases such as chikungunya and malaria (Mahmud et al., 2021).

COVID-19

As of October 2023, Bangladesh had 1.4% case fatality and death rate of 17.88 per 100,000 population due to COVID-19 (Johns Hopkins University of Medicine Coronavirus Research Center, 2023). COVID-19 has infected more than 2 million people in Bangladesh and more than 29,000 have died as of April 2024 (KFF, 2024).

INFANT AND MATERNAL MORTALITY

The infant mortality rate in Bangladesh has been decreasing steadily from 66.2 infant deaths per 1,000 live births in 2000 to 22.6 infant deaths per 1,000 live births in 2023. Males have a higher infant mortality rate (24.7 per 1,000 live births) than females (20.8 per 1,000 live births; UN Data Portal, n.d.). The maternal mortality ratio in Bangladesh has improved from 441 per 100,000 live births in 2000 to 123.0 per 100,000 live births in 2010 (World Bank Group, n.d.).

MENTAL ILLNESSES

In 2019, the prevalence of mental illness among Bangladeshi adults was 18.7%, with the highest prevalence (20.2%) among individuals aged 60 years and older and the lowest prevalence (11%) among adults age 18 to 29 years. Women (21.5%) had a higher prevalence compared to men (15.7%). Depression was the most common mental illness (6.7%) followed by anxiety disorders (4.7%). There is a high prevalence of stigma associated with mental illness and males suffer more stigma than females. The overall treatment gap in adults is 91%. The overall prevalence of mental illness in children age 7 to 17 years is higher in boys (13.7%) than girls (11.5%), and higher in rural children (12.9%) than urban children (11.5%; National Institute of Mental Health [NIMH], 2021).

DETERMINANTS OF HEALTH

HEALTH BEHAVIORS

Health behavior risk factors such as tobacco use, poor dietary intake, and physical inactivity are the drivers of the increasing chronic disease burden in Bangladesh.

Tobacco Use

Age-standardized prevalence of tobacco use among individuals age 15 years and older in Bangladesh is 34.7% (World Bank Group, n.d.). The prevalence of tobacco use (any form) in adults decreased from 51% in 2010 to 39.4% in 2022. Nearly 20% of adults (41.7% of men and 0.5% of women) smoke tobacco products, while 24.8% of adults (24.2% of men and 25.2% of women) consume smokeless tobacco products such as chewing tobacco, snuff, **khoinee**, and **kimam** (DGHS, 2023).

Poor Dietary Intake

The majority of adults in Bangladesh do not meet the recommended dietary intake of fruits and vegetables, as 96.2% of adults eat less than 5 servings of fruits and/or vegetables on average per day. Nearly 37% of adults add salt while eating meals and 13% consume processed food with high salt content (DGHS, 2023).

Physical Inactivity

Nearly 20% of the adult population do not meet the recommended level of physical activity (150 minutes or more of moderate-intensity activity per week or equivalent) and a higher proportion of women (23.9%) than men (14.6%) do not meet the recommended level of physical activity (DGHS, 2023).

Alcohol Abuse

The prevalence of alcohol consumption among adults in Bangladesh is low (1.5%). However, binge drinking is rising and alcohol intoxication cases are reported from time to time. Among the youth, substance abuse such as abuse of narcotic drugs is an emerging social problem (DGHS, 2023).

TOP 10 MORTALITY RISK FACTORS

The leading risk factors associated with age-standardized mortality include high blood pressure, high fasting plasma glucose, smoking, household air pollution, ambient particulate matter, high low-density lipoprotein (LDL) cholesterol, high body mass index, diet low in fiber, low birth weight, and kidney dysfunction (Islam et al., 2023).

SOCIAL AND ECONOMIC FACTORS

Bangladesh is a lower-middle-income country. The gross domestic product (GDP) of Bangladesh is $460.2 billion and the per-capita GDP is $2,688 (World Bank Group, n.d.), with 18.7% of the population living below the national poverty line, and 5.8% of the employed population below $2.15 purchasing power parity per day (2023; Asian Development Bank, 2024). During 2023, unemployment was 4.5% in Bangladesh (World Bank Group, n.d.).

Educational Attainment

The overall literacy rate among individuals age 7 years and older in Bangladesh is 74.8%, with a higher rate in males (76.1%) than in females (72.9%), and in urban areas (81.5%) than in rural areas (71.7%; Bangladesh Bureau of Statistics, 2023).

REFUGEE POPULATION

Bangladesh hosts nearly 1 million **Forcibly Displaced Myanmar Nationals (FDMNs)** from Myanmar's Rakhine State at the world's largest refugee settlement in Cox's Bazar, which borders Myanmar. Although static health centers have been established in and around the camps by the collaborative efforts among the government, private sector, civil society, and international development agencies, challenges remain in providing healthcare to this large FDMN population. There have been outbreaks of diphtheria and measles that were dealt with by vaccination campaigns (DGHS, 2023).

HEALTHCARE SYSTEM

HEALTHCARE DELIVERY

Facility

The healthcare system in Bangladesh is multifaceted and operates under the Ministry of Health and Family Welfare (MoHFW). While MoHFW is the policy- and decision-making body, the implementation of those decisions is the responsibility of the Directorate Generals and other such implementing agencies. The DGHS, the main health service provision agency of the country, and the Directorate General of Family Planning (DGFP), responsible for maternal and child health and nutrition in addition to family planning, are among the 10 such agencies (DGHS, 2023).

The health service structure of Bangladesh features a tiered structure with various healthcare providers serving different levels of the community (Table 44.1). At the grassroots, Satellite Clinics and Community Clinics deliver basic health services, emphasizing preventive care and health education (Hasan et al., 2024). Basic health services are supplemented by domiciliary services provided by a large number of Community Health Workers (CHWs) known as Health Assistants (recruited under the DGHS, each covering 6,000 people) and Family Welfare Assistants (recruited under the DGFP, each covering 500 eligible couples; Joardar et al., 2020). Union Health and Family Welfare Centers and other primary centers offer outpatient care at the union level. Upazila Health Complexes provide comprehensive services at the subdistrict level and are often the first point of contact for health issues. Secondary care is available at District Hospitals, which offer extensive medical services, including emergency care and hospitalization. Tertiary care hospitals, located in major cities and the capital, provide specialized treatments and advanced medical procedures (Hasan et al., 2024).

In addition to the public health network predominantly serving the rural and semiurban populations, Bangladesh has a growing private healthcare sector. This includes private practices, clinics, modern hospitals, and nongovernment organization (NGO)-operated facilities, as well as traditional healers and informal providers like village doctors and drug-shop attendants, who are often the first point of care for the impoverished (Hasan et al., 2024). **Urban healthcare**, particularly primary care, is managed by the Ministry of Local Government, Rural Development and Cooperatives, which outsources services to NGOs under the Urban Primary Healthcare Services Delivery Project, encompassing city corporations and municipalities (Hasan et al., 2024; WHO, 2015).

TABLE 44.1 HEALTHCARE DELIVERY SYSTEM IN BANGLADESH

LEVEL OF HEALTHCARE DELIVERY	ADMINISTRATIVE UNIT/LOCATION	AVERAGE CATCHMENT POPULATION SIZE	DELIVERY SETTING
Primary	Village	3,000–4,000	Satellite clinic[a,b]
	Ward	6,000–8,000	Community clinic[b]
	Union[c]	24,000–30,000	Union Health and Family Welfare Center (UHFWC) Union subcenter Rural health center
	Upazila[c]	250,000	31–50-bed Upazila health complex 30-bed hospital 20-bed trauma hospital
Secondary	District[c]	2,500,000	District hospital 10–20-bed maternal and child welfare center General hospital
Tertiary	Division, district[c]	9,100,104–44,215,759 (lowest–highest in a division)	Medical college hospital 100-bed maternal and child health hospital and fertility services and training center
	National, division[c]	—	Medical university Postgraduate medical institute and hospital Public health institute Super specialized hospital

[a]Outreach activity, no permanent infrastructure.
[b]Provides outpatient service alone.
[c]Outpatient and inpatient service.

FINANCING

Bangladesh's per-capita total health expenditure increased from $10 in 2000 to $54 in 2020, with 68.5% derived from individual out-of-pocket (OOP) payments. Private healthcare facilities rely heavily on OOP payments, accounting for 89% of their funding. Of OOP payments, 64.4% go to the pharmacies or retail drug outlets, followed by 11.7% to medical and diagnostic laboratories, and 10.8% to medical practices. Among the total pharmaceutical expenditure, a whopping 94% is borne by the households, while only 5.6% by the government. Curative care occupies 47% of the government health expenditure, while preventive care only 15% (DGHS, 2023). Secondary care poses a significant financial risk, with 55% of individuals facing potential catastrophic expenses for surgical care and 44% at risk of impoverishment due to such costs.

Bangladesh's health financing mechanisms, aside from government budgets, scarcely employ prepayment methods like health insurance, making up only 0.2% of the total health expenditure. Community-led initiatives have been launched to provide affordable services (WHO, 2015). The government's pilot program, a health protection scheme called Shasthyo Shurokhsha Karmasuchi (SSK), has now expanded to several districts including Dhaka and offers free quality healthcare to the poorest households (DGHS, 2023; WHO, 2015). Additionally, government employees benefit from limited social insurance schemes. Bangladesh has also explored health insurance for microfinance clients since the 1990s, with notable organizations involved in health microinsurance (WHO, 2015).

While the national healthcare system theoretically serves all citizens, many remain untreated due to public service deficiencies. Private sector involvement has grown since the 1980s, but costs often exceed what the poor can afford. The healthcare financing strategy strives to improve the situation by decreasing OOP payments to 32% of total health expenditures and increasing state spending to 30%, among other targets, by 2032 (WHO, 2015).

PROVIDERS, HEALTHCARE EDUCATION, AND TRAINING

Bangladesh has a pluralistic healthcare system comprising allopathic, homeopathic, **unani** (traditional Muslim medicine originating from Greece), and ayurvedic healthcare providers working in the formal public and private sectors, as well as other providers in the informal sector (Nuruzzaman et al., 2022). Providers in the formal sector receive formal education or training from government-recognized institutes and are regulated. Providers in the informal sector do not have any formal education or training, are not recognized, and are not regulated; however, they are the predominant providers in the country, particularly in the rural areas. Health worker education and training are provided through different public and private institutions (Table 44.2). Allopathic healthcare, the modern biomedical system, is the mainstream healthcare delivery method in Bangladesh. It includes physicians, dentists, nurses, midwives, and domiciliary health workers in rural areas. The doctor-population density in Bangladesh is one registered doctor per 1,230 people (DGHS, 2023). There are 0.6 nurses and midwives per 1,000 people in Bangladesh (World Bank Group, n.d.).

Homeopathic, unani, and ayurvedic practitioners provide care in both formal and informal sectors. Traditional healthcare providers in Bangladesh include faith healers, kabiraj, totka, herbalists, bone setters, tooth extractors, and practitioners of folk medicine. Other providers in the informal sector include traditional birth attendants, village doctors, dental technicians without formal education or training, laboratory technicians without formal education or training, and sellers of allopathic medicine from drug stores (Nuruzzaman et al., 2022).

Overall, health worker density is 9.9 per 100,000 population (World Bank Group, n.d.). There is a rural–urban discrepancy in the availability of health workers employed by the government. Approximately 75% of the doctors and nurses work in urban areas (Nuruzzaman et al., 2022).

HEALTHCARE QUALITY AND ACCESS

Public perception of Bangladesh's public healthcare system is notably negative, with criticisms focusing on long waiting times, staff absenteeism, unprofessional behavior, and the exclusion of

TABLE 44.2 HEALTHCARE PROVIDERS, TRAINING, AND EDUCATION IN BANGLADESH

FORMAL SECTOR (FORMAL EDUCATION OR TRAINING FROM GOVERNMENT-RECOGNIZED INSTITUTE, REGULATED)				
CATEGORY	**PROVIDER**	**INSTITUTE**	**DEGREE AND LENGTH OF TRAINING**	**NUMBER OF REGISTERED PROVIDERS**
Allopathic	Physician	Medical college	Bachelor of medicine and bachelor of surgery (MBBS), 5 years	124,849
	Dentist	Dental college	Bachelor of dental surgery (BDS), 5 years	13,546
	Nurse and midwife	Nursing college	BSc in nursing, 4 years	95,415
	Nursing institute (nursing and midwifery)		Diploma, 3 years	
	Sub-assistant community medical officer (SACMO)	SACMO training school	Diploma, 3 years	
	Medical assistant	Medical assistant training schools		
	Medical technologist	Institute of health technology–pharmacy	Diploma, 3 years	
	Pharmacist	Universities	Bachelor, 4–5 years	
	Domiciliary workers: family welfare assistant, family planning inspector, health inspector, assistant health inspector, community paramedic, skilled birth attendant			
Homeopathy, Unani, ayurvedic	Homeopathic, Unani, ayurvedic medicine and surgery practitioner	Medical colleges	Bachelor	Homeopathy: 3,405 Unani: 780 Ayurvedic: 648
		College	Diploma	Homeopathy: 38,054 Unani: 3,262 Ayurvedic: 1,331
	Unani, Ayurvedic certified provider	—	Certificate, 1-month training	Unani: 4,333 Ayurvedic: 3,497

INFORMAL SECTOR (NO FORMAL EDUCATION OR TRAINING, NONRECOGNIZED, NONREGULATED)

- Homeopathy, unani, and ayurvedic providers without any formal education or training
- Traditional providers: faith healers, kabiraj, totka, herbalists, bone setters, tooth extractors, practitioners of folk medicine
- Untrained physiotherapist
- Drug or medicine seller
- Traditional birth attendant
- Village doctor
- Dental technician without formal education or training
- Laboratory technician without formal education or training

Sources: Adapted from Bangladesh Nursing & Midwifery Council. (2024). *Data sheet of registered nurses, midwives and allied professionals in Bangladesh.* https://bnmc.gov.bd/sites/default/files/files/bnmc.portal.gov.bd/miscellaneous_info/6e93ccb9_e0c6_4a12_a5a1_38269198d7cf/2024-05-14-07-08-727073c1ae0653606c03853cbb1d596b.jpg; Directorate General of Health Service. (2023). *Health Bulletin 2022*. Management Information System, Directorate General of Health Service, Government of the People's Republic of Bangladesh, Ministry of Health and Family Welfare; Nuruzzaman, M., Zapata, T., McIsaac, M., Wangmo, S., Islam, M. J., Almamun, M., Alam, S., Talukder, M. H. K., & Dussault, G. (2022). Informing investment in health workforce in Bangladesh: A health labour market analysis. *Human Resources for Health, 20*(1), 73. https://doi.org/10.1186/s12960-022-00769-2

marginalized groups (Omer et al., 2011). The private healthcare sector is swiftly growing, and with no legal barriers to dual practice, 80% of doctors work in both the public and private sectors (Gruen et al., 2002). Private physicians spend an average of 6.02 minutes per outpatient consultation compared to 4.04 minutes in the public sector, and score higher on the Responsiveness of Physicians Scale (ROP-Scale; Joarder et al., 2017). Nevertheless, the quality of care in both sectors is substandard, characterized by insufficient quality control, limited professional knowledge, and poor practice application. Issues of accountability, absenteeism, corruption, and subpar performance plague both public and private providers, leading to widespread reports of malpractice and patient dissatisfaction (WHO, 2015).

Bangladesh lacks a structured referral system, with patients often choosing healthcare providers based on convenience, availability, and cost (WHO, 2015). Serious health issues typically lead to direct visits to public facilities for secondary or tertiary care, bypassing formal referrals. This fragmented referral network results in a high rate of self-referral to tertiary hospitals, with 59% of patients bypassing the system entirely (Hasan et al., 2024).

CONCLUSION

Bangladesh has made significant strides in improving the health sector since its independence. The country has achieved remarkable success in reducing child mortality rates, improving maternal health, and combating infectious diseases through extensive immunization programs. Further improvements are needed toward making healthcare responsive, accountable, affordable, accessible, and equitable, and to better equip it to address emerging health issues such as chronic diseases and emerging infections, mental health, the health of the slowly aging population, and environmental health. To substantially improve the healthcare system in the country and the health and well-being of its population, the government must increase multisectoral coordination between different public and private stakeholders; provide stricter regulation and oversight of private services; explore context-specific innovative health financing solutions, such as introducing sin tax, using corporate social responsibility (CSR) money in health, and channeling **Zakat** (annual charitable contribution obligated by the Islamic faith) for health services for the poor. Additionally, community empowerment along with higher local level planning and decision-making authority for the upazila and district level health facilities with emphasis on preventive, promotive, rehabilitative, and palliative care on top of the existing curative-focused health services, and leveraging the benefits of digital health would also support the population's health and well-being.

LEARNING ACTIVITIES

CourseConnect

To access self-assessment questions and interactive, competency-based learning activities for this chapter, visit www.springerpub.com/courseconnect. See inside front cover and tear-out for CourseConnect details.

REFERENCES

Ahmed, A. F. S., Chowdhury, B. M., Khan, A. M., Chowdhury, A. M., & Shahed, S. M. (Eds.). (2022). *Bangladesh national culture and heritage: An introductory reader* (1st ed.). The University Press Limited (UPL).

Asian Development Bank. (2024). *Poverty data: Bangladesh*. https://www.adb.org/where-we-work/bangladesh/poverty#:~:text=In%20Bangladesh%2C%2018.7%25%20of%20the,died%20before%20their%205th%20birthday

Bangladesh Bureau of Statistics. (2023). *Population and housing census 2022*. National Report (Vol. I). https://bbs.portal.gov.bd/sites/default/files/files/bbs.portal.gov.bd/page/b343a8b4_956b_45ca_872f_4cf9b2f1a6e0/2024-01-31-15-51-b53c55dd692233ae401ba013060b9cbb.pdf

Banglapedia. (2024). *Bangladesh*. https://en.banglapedia.org/index.php/Bangladesh
Directorate General of Health Service. (2023). *Health bulletin 2022*. Dhaka: Management Information System, Directorate General of Health Service, Government of the People's Republic of Bangladesh, Ministry of Health and Family Welfare.
Ferlay, J., Ervik, M., Lam, F., Laversanne, M., Colombet, M., Mery, L., Piñeros, M., Znaor, A., Soerjomataram, I., & Bray, F. (2024). *Global cancer observatory: Cancer today*. https://gco.iarc.who.int/media/globocan/factsheets/populations/900-world-fact-sheet.pdf
Gruen, R., Anwar, R., Begum, T., Killingsworth, J. R., & Normand, C. (2002). Dual job holding practitioners in Bangladesh: An exploration. *Social Science & Medicine, 54*(2), 267–279. https://doi.org/10.1016/s0277-9536(01)00026-0
Hasan, M. J., Rafi, M. A., Nishat, N. H., Islam, I., Afrin, N., Ghosh, B., Kabir, E., Akhter, S. Z., Poushi, M. Z., Shahnoor, S. A. B., Fardous, J., Tabassum, T., Islam, S., Kalam, S. B., Aslam, M. T., Joarder, T. (2024). Patient self-referral patterns in a developing country: Characteristics, prevalence, and predictors. *BMC Health Serv Res, 24*(1), 651. https://doi.org/10.1186/s12913-024-11115-8
Institute for Health Metrics and Evaluation. (n.d.). *Country profile Bangladesh*. https://www.healthdata.org/research-analysis/health-by-location/profiles/bangladesh
Joardar, T., Javadi, D., Gergen, J., & Perry, H. B. (2020). The government family welfare assistants, health assistants, and community health care providers in Bangladesh. In H. B. Perry (Ed.), *Health for the people: National community health worker programs from Afghanistan to Zimbabwe*. The Maternal and Child Survival Program (MCSP), USAID.
Joarder, T., George, A., Sarker, M., Ahmed, S., & Peters, D. H. (2017). Who are more responsive? Mixed-methods comparison of public and private sector physicians in rural Bangladesh. *Health Policy Plan, 32*(suppl_3), iii14–iii24. https://doi.org/10.1093/heapol/czx111
Johns Hopkins University of Medicine Coronavirus Research Center. (2023). *Mortality analyses*. https://coronavirus.jhu.edu/data/mortality
KFF. (2024). *Global COVID-19 tracker*. https://www.kff.org/coronavirus-covid-19/issue-brief/global-covid-19-tracker/
Mahmud, I., Raza, W. A., & Hossain, M. R. (2021). *Climate afflictions*. International Development in Focus. World Bank. http://hdl.handle.net/10986/36333
National Institute of Mental Health. (2021). *National mental health survey 2019*. National Institute of Mental Health. https://nimh.gov.bd/wp-content/uploads/2021/11/Mental-Health-Survey-Report.pdf
National Institute of Population Research and Training and ICF. (2020). *Bangladesh demographic and health survey 2017–18*. https://dhsprogram.com/pubs/pdf/FR344/FR344.pdf
Nuruzzaman, M., Zapata, T., McIsaac, M., Wangmo, S., Islam, M. J., Almamun, M., Alam, S., Talukder, M. H. K., & Dussault, G. (2022). Informing investment in health workforce in Bangladesh: A health labour market analysis. *Human Resources for Health, 20*(1), 73. https://doi.org/10.1186/s12960-022-00769-2
Omer, K., Cockcroft, A., & Andersson, N. (2011). Impact of a hospital improvement initiative in Bangladesh on patient experiences and satisfaction with services: Two cross-sectional studies. *BMC Health Services Research, 11*(2), S10. https://doi.org/10.1186/1472-6963-11-S2-S10
Roy, N. (1979). *Bangaleer Itihas: Aadi Parba* [A Bengali book on the history of the Bengalee: Early period]. Dey's Publishing.
UN Data Portal. (n.d.). *UN population division data portal*. https://population.un.org/dataportal/home/
World Bank Group. (n.d.). *World Bank open data*. https://data.worldbank.org/
World Health Organization. (2015). *Bangladesh health system review, Vol 5(3)*. WHO Regional Office for the Western Pacific.
World Health Organization. (2022). *Noncommunicable diseases progress monitor 2022*. https://iris.who.int/bitstream/handle/10665/353048/9789240047761-eng.pdf

CHAPTER 45

INDIA

Reethee Madona Antony, Sundeep Venkatesan, and Gurpreet Singh

INTRODUCTION

India covers an expanse of 3,287,000 square kilometers (1,269,219 square miles). It is the seventh largest and the second most populous country in the world with 1.4 billion people as of July 2023 (Central Intelligence Agency [CIA], 2025). Its diverse geographic features include the Himalayan Mountain ranges in the north, arid Thar Desert in the northwest, dense rain forests in northeast, the Deccan Plateau, and coastal areas. The Indian peninsula is surrounded by the Arabian Sea, the Bay of Bengal Sea, and the Indian Ocean. The country's topography is influenced by rivers such as the Ganges, Brahmaputra, Yamuna, Godavari, and Kaveri (Figure 45.1).

FIGURE 45.1 India.

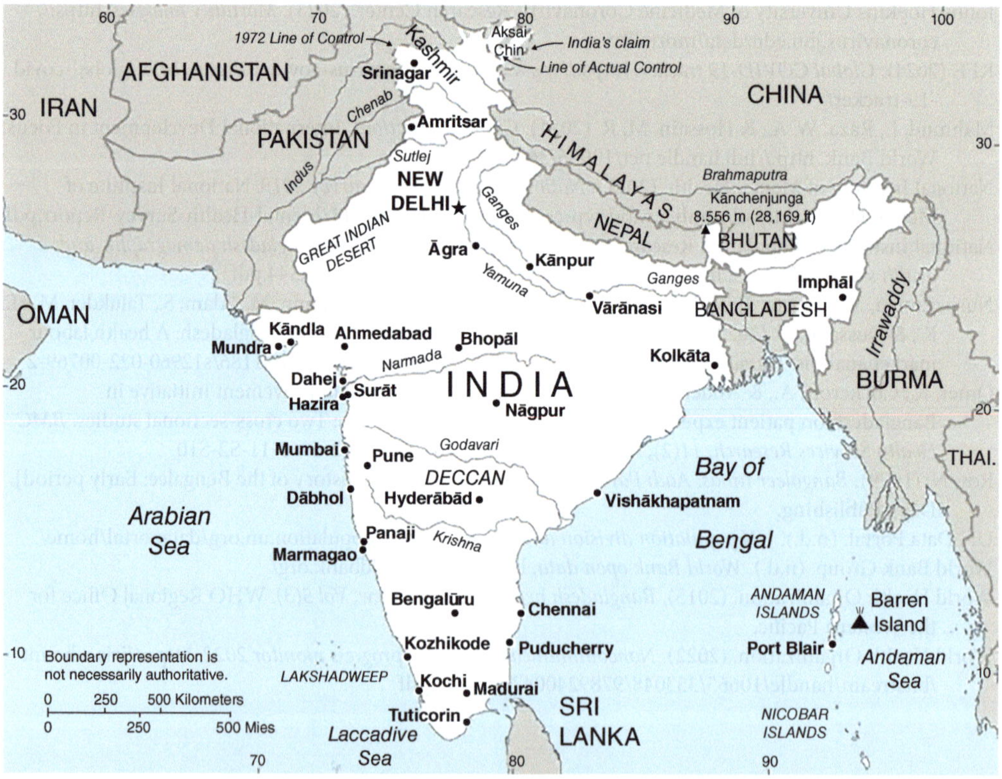

Source: From Central Intelligence Agency. (2021/2023). *The world factbook: India.* https://www.cia.gov/

DEMOGRAPHICS, CULTURAL BELIEFS, AND HISTORICAL SIGNIFICANCE

India has a rich cultural heritage with a history of over 5,000 years. Its people are multiracial, multireligious, and multilingual (Table 45.1). India is a secular country, and it serves as the birthplace for many religions including Hinduism, Buddhism, Jainism, and Sikhism. India is the world's most linguistically diverse country with 22 languages recognized by the Government of India as official languages. Furthermore, 197 languages are endangered (Government of India, 2024).

The historical significance of health and medicinal systems in India dates back prior to the Indus valley civilization (3000 BCE to 1500 BCE), making it one of the most ancient civilizations in the world; for example, **Siddha**, a medicinal system practiced in South India, is 10,000 years old (Patil et al., 2014). The Chakra Samhita, a text which was written in 600 BCE, describes **Shalyapahartrika**—a branch of medicine specializing in surgery.

Throughout India's history, foreign invasions, trade, and the change of empires have repeatedly influenced the culture, religion, education system, music, art, language, politics, cuisine, leisure, and health systems in India. One clear example is the adoption of Unani medicine, a medicinal system in India derived from the word "Ionion" which means "Greek" (Parveen et al., 2020). Unani has its origin in Greece, was practiced by Hippocrates, and reached India through Arab practitioners and scholars when they came to India for refuge following invasions in Persia and Central Asia (Ahmad et al., 2024). At a macro-level, since independence from Britain was achieved on August 15, 1947, there has been immense growth in the areas of healthcare, education, economy, and technology. At a micro level, many individuals still engage in **Suriyanamaskaaram,** performing a set of yoga **asanas** (exercises) early in the morning facing the direction of sunrise.

There are diverse leisure activities that can be related to health in India. Some of these include music and outdoor pursuits. Engaging in music dates back to 1000 BCE. Raja and Bhalla (2021) observed a significant association between Indian musical training and the mathematical skills

TABLE 45.1 DEMOGRAPHIC DISTRIBUTION IN INDIA

Geographical divisions	28 states and 8 union territories
Age distribution	41% of the population is under 20 years of age
Mean age	28 years of age
Birth and death rates	17.7 births per 1,000 people; 9.65 deaths per 1,000 people
In- and out-migration	4.88 million migrants living in India (0.4%); net immigration rate 10.12 immigrants per 1,000 population
Gender distribution	940 females for every 1,000 males Transgender Indians: 488,000 adults; 55,000 children
Racial/ethnic groups	Indo-Aryans (72%), Dravidians (25%), Mongoloids, and Indigenous communities (3%)
Religious composition of the population	Hinduism 79.8%, Islam 14.2%, Christianity 2.3%, Sikhism 1.7%, Buddhism 0.7%, Jainism 0.4%
Language composition of the population	Indo-European 78.07%, Dravidian 19.64%, Austro-Asiatic 1.11%, Tibeto-Burman and Semito-Hamitic <2%; 7.1% trilingual, 26.01% bilingual

Sources: Adapted from World Bank Group. (2025). *India*. https://data.worldbank.org/country/india; Central Intelligence Agency. (2025). *The world factbook: India*. https://www.cia.gov/; Government of India. (2024). *Government of India*. https://www.india.gov.in/, https://nhm.gov.in/ and https://ndma.gov.in/; Singh, M. (2019). Religion in India: Religious composition of population and religious regions. *Research Journal Arts, 18*(1), 63–80. https://shorturl.at/ZGzjl

of children; those exposed to Indian musical training had significantly higher mathematical sills when compared to those who had no exposure to music. In terms of outdoor activities, pilgrimages are an ancient outdoor pursuit and tradition in India with over 100 spiritual sites. Some other outdoor pursuits include hiking, trekking, mountaineering, skiing, rafting in the northern rivers, kayaking on the seas, paragliding, and scuba diving.

HEALTH OUTCOMES

Life expectancy from birth has increased by more than 30 years since the formation of the Republic of India after the dissolution of the British Raj. In 1950, life expectancy from birth was 41.7 years. In 2023, life expectancy from birth was approximately 72 years (UN Data Portal, 2023). The World Health Organization (WHO, 2024) estimates that noncommunicable diseases (NCDs) are responsible for approximately 63% of all deaths in India. According to the Institute for Health Metrics and Evaluation (IHME, 2021), the top 10 causes of mortality in India, in order of decreasing prevalence, are COVID-19, ischemic heart disease, chronic obstructive pulmonary disease, stroke, diarrheal diseases, lower respiratory infections, tuberculosis, neonatal disorders, diabetes mellitus, and chronic liver diseases.

Various long-standing infectious diseases, such as smallpox, guinea worm, polio, leprosy, cholera, and plague, have been controlled and eradicated from the community. However, diseases, such as dengue, malaria, typhoid, and tuberculosis, are still the common causes of febrile illness among people in India (Ram & Thakur, 2022).

According to the World Bank Group, the maternal mortality ratio (MMR) was 154 per 100,000 live births in 2013 and 103 per 100,000 live births in 2020, indicating that the MMR has reduced in the last few years. About 1.30 million maternal deaths occurred between 1997 and 2020, with about 23,800 in 2020, with most occurring in poorer states (63%) and among women age 20 to 29 years (58%). The main cause of maternal death was obstetric hemorrhages (47%; higher in poorer states). The World Bank Group reported an infant mortality rate (IMR) in India of 26 deaths per 1,000 births as of 2022. Child mortality rate is 33.1 deaths per 1,000 live births for children under 5 years of age and 29.2 deaths per 1,000 live births for children under 1 year of age (IHME, 2021).

The overall weighted prevalence of **mental morbidity**, a metric that adjusts for demographic factors (e.g., age distribution, regional differences) in a population, provides a more representative estimate of how many people are affected by mental illness. In India, this prevalence was 10.6% for those over 18 years of age, and the lifetime prevalence was 13.7% (WHO, 2022). Also, the age-standardized suicide rate in India is 21.1 per 100,000 population (WHO, 2024). There are only 0.3 psychiatrists per 100,000 population in India, well below the global median of nine psychiatrists per 100,000 population (WHO, 2017). The Indian government has taken steps to address mental health concerns through initiatives such as the National Mental Health Programme (NMHP) and the Mental Healthcare Act of 2017. There is an urgent need in India for increased investment in mental health services, improved access to care, and efforts to reduce stigma surrounding mental illness (Meghrajani et al., 2023).

DETERMINANTS OF HEALTH

Leading mortality risk factors in India include malnutrition, air pollution, hypertension, dietary risks, tobacco, high fasting plasma glucose, occupational risks, WaSH (**Wa**ter, **S**anitation, **H**ygiene), hypercholesterolemia, and kidney dysfunction (IHME, 2021). In order to improve the health and life expectancy of the entire population, it is crucial to address these risk factors.

Many segments of the population still adhere to traditional practices, such as Ayurveda and yoga. Every region of the country has its own culinary traditions, including aromatic spices in the north and coconut-infused dishes in the south. Lifestyle changes result in an increase in sedentary habits and dietary patterns that have led to the increase in NCDs as a result of rapid urbanization and modernization.

While India's national gross domestic product (GDP) was $3.14 trillion in 2022, the per-capita GDP was only $2,410.90 (World Bank Group, 2025). Although India has a significant GDP, poverty, income inequality, malnutrition, and hunger remain as major challenges. According to the 2023 Global Hunger Index, India ranks 111 out of 125 countries, with 21.9% of the population are below the national poverty line, indicating serious concern (World Bank Group, 2025).

The literacy rate is 76% among adults and 97% among the youth in ages 15 to 24 years (World Bank Group, 2025). The overall unemployment rate is 4.5% and among youth it is 15.5% (International Labor Organization, 2023). Advances have been made to promote inclusivity, equality, and social justice (Government of India, 2024). However, marginalized communities such as Dalits, Adivasis, women, religious minorities, and LGBTQ+ individuals continue to face systemic discrimination and exclusion despite legislative efforts and constitutional provisions. For example, the recent revision to the 2016 Transgender Persons (Protection of Rights) Bill in 2018 requires transgender Indians to have undergone Gender Affirming Surgery (GAS) before changing their gender on legal documents (Pandya & Redcay, 2021).

Environmental and climate conditions influence health. There has been an 8.45% decrease in India's annual rainfall despite complex weather patterns (Amarasinghe et al., 2020). Between 2020 and 2022, 51% of natural hazards were caused by floods and droughts. In 2015, there were more than 2,500 deaths due to heat waves (Government of India, 2024). Heat waves cause dehydration, exhaustion, and heat stroke, and exacerbates existing conditions such as cardiovascular, cerebrovascular, and respiratory conditions.

HEALTHCARE EDUCATION SYSTEM

In India, the educational requirement to earn an allopathic medical degree includes a bachelor of medicine and bachelor of surgery (MBBS) degree which consists of a 5.5 year curriculum, including preclinical studies followed by clinical training plus a 1-year internship. Specialization includes educational degrees such as doctor of medicine (MD) and master of surgery (MS), and super-specialization such as doctorate of medicine (DM) and master of chirurgical (MCh). The completion duration for the specialization degrees is 3 years each. The educational degrees for traditional systems include Ayurveda (bachelor of Ayurvedic medicine and surgery [BAMS]), Unani (bachelor of Unani medicine and surgery [BUMS]), Siddha (bachelor of Siddha medicine and surgery [BSMS]), and Homeopathy (bachelor of homeopathic medicine and surgery [BHMS]).

Admission to medical colleges is based on competitive exams like the National Eligibility cum Entrance Test (NEET); minimum marks in physics, chemistry, and biology; or through donation/management-based seats. However, donation-based admissions face criticism for favoring wealth over merit. All practitioners must be licensed by state medical councils. Oversight is managed by the Central Council of Indian Medicine (CCIM) and Central Council of Homeopathy (CCH).

HEALTHCARE INFRASTRUCTURE, PRACTICES, AND COMPLEMENTARY MEDICINE

A hierarchy of public health infrastructure exists in India: subcenters, primary healthcare centers, community health centers, taluk (i.e., a subdivision of a district) hospitals, district hospitals, and super-specialty hospitals. The system can also be broadly classified into primary, secondary, and tertiary care. As of March 2021, there are over 43,000 subcenters, 9,000 primary health centers, and 1,300 community centers (Government of India, 2024). Along with public facilities, private health care systems consist of hospitals, polyclinics, nursing homes, dispensaries, and general practitioners.

The education system for the health professions in India encounters challenges such as faculty scarcity, and logistical constraints for remote education. India faces a shortage of healthcare professionals, including doctors, nurses, and allied health workers, especially in rural areas. World Bank Group data report 0.7 physicians per 1,000 patients in India as of 2020, well below the WHO recommendation of 2.5 per 1,000 patients, which outlines the severe shortage of accessibility based on numbers (World Bank Group, 2025). The data from community health centers (CHCs) reveal an even bigger mismatch with a shortfall of 79.9% specialists as compared to the requirement. Also, 68% of the sanctioned posts of specialists at CHCs are vacant (Government of India, 2024).

In 2014, the government of India established the Ministry of Ayurveda, Yoga, Unani, Siddha, and Homeopathy (AYUSH). These traditional systems often utilize herbal remedies, dietary modifications, lifestyle practices, and therapeutic techniques (Government of India, 2024). Complementary medicine refers to the medicinal system used along with allopathy. Recent practices involve blending allopathy and ayurveda. The 2022 to 2023 annual report from the Government of India included a study in which AYUSH medicines were provided to front-line workers including the Delhi police officers during the COVID-19 pandemic. They served as the experimental group while the control group was the general population. Results showed that the experimental group had a significantly lower COVID-positive rate relative to the control group ($p = .003$), indicating a lower risk by 55.6% (Government of India, 2024). A number of hospitals have both allopathy doctors and doctors in AYUSH who co-treat the patients. Other medicinal systems prevalent in India include Reiki, chiropractice, Pranic healing, acupressure, and acupuncture.

GAPS AND CHALLENGES IN HEALTHCARE

As of 2020, a mandate requires private sector employees not covered by the Employees State Insurance to obtain a government-regulated health insurance plan through their employer, overseen by the Insurance Regulatory and Development Authority. Similarly, employees within the public sector receive health insurance coverage through the Central Government Health Plan, ensuring broader access to healthcare services across various employment sectors. The National Health Mission (Government of India, 2024) is an initiative designed to address health disparities and improve overall health outcomes. The accessibility to healthcare insurance and out-of-pockets costs for individuals in low socioeconomic status and for older adults without pensions are a concern. Out-of-pocket healthcare costs are predicted to increase to 55.7% in India by 2030 (Sahoo, Rout, et al., 2023).

Access to healthcare in India is a complex issue influenced by various factors such as socioeconomic status, geographic location, infrastructure, and government policies. Public insurance accounts for 32% compared to 68% of private expenditure. The inception of government health insurance schemes Rashtriya Swasthya Bima Yojana in 2008, Ayushman Bharat in 2018, and Pradhan Mantri Jan Arogya Yojana (PM-JAY) are considered some of the milestones in healthcare in India. Regardless of continuous efforts, about 83% of the population lacks any form of protection against healthcare expenses. Furthermore, 86% of rural residents and 81% of urban dwellers remain uncovered by any health expenditure support system (Kumar & Duggirala, 2021).

India's thriving medical tourism market—valued at $2.89 billion in 2020 (Government of India, 2024)—testifies to the country's growing reputation for quality healthcare. In 2019, over 690,000 foreign tourists visited India for medical treatments according to the India Tourism Statistics at a Glance 2020 report, published by the India Brand Equity Foundation (IBEF), an initiative of the Ministry of Commerce and Industry.

India ranks 10th in the Medical Tourism Index (MTI) for 2020/2021 out of 46 destinations identified by the Medical Tourism Association. Despite this robust medical tourism sector, the budgeted health allocation and expenditure in India remain less than 2.5% of the GDP. While over 89 crore rupees have been allocated to the healthcare sector in 2023/2024 (less than 2.5% of GDP), lack of public awareness of the health schemes and reduced access to healthcare, there is underutilization of these government funds and approximately 70% of health-related expenses are still paid out of pocket (Sahoo, Kumar, et al., 2023). The underutilization of funds is provided as the rationale for reallocation of funds to different sectors, other than healthcare. If awareness of health schemes increases among the public and more individuals use the government funding, the out-of-pocket expenditures will reduce which will be beneficial to India's economy. Research has shown that transition of a health system from out-of-pocket expenditures to government-predominated health system leads to improved health system outcomes (Gabani et al., 2023).

One area for growth in healthcare practice is to work on the intersectionality between healthcare and education, specifically in school settings. It is important to have an occupational therapist, physical therapist, speech pathologist, counselor, and nurse in every school for an inclusive environment. In 2012, the Ministry of Social Justice and Empowerment created the Department of Empowerment of Persons with Disabilities (Divyangjan) to address issues related to disability effectively.

The overall prevalence of disability in the entire population is 4.52%. Of these, 44.7% of people living with disabilities have challenges with locomotion, 20.28% with mental status, 14.55% with speech, 12.02% with vision, and 8.45% with hearing (Pattnaik et al., 2023). Individuals living with disabilities have fewer years of schooling (Pattnaik et al., 2023). For example, not all schools in India have an occupational therapist, physical, therapist, speech therapist, special educator, nurse, and counselor. Furthermore, not all schools in India have replaced stairways with ramps. The lack of inclusivity, transportation difficulties, and barriers in environment serve as challenges for individuals for special needs to pursue higher education. A government initiative to improve inclusivity is the National Institute for Open Schooling (NIOS). However, NIOS is still a separate stream of education and its integration into mainstream education is warranted.

There is a need to establish long-term care in India, such as skilled nursing facilities, to increase assisted living services and improve rehabilitation and inclusivity. Figure 45.2 displays the changing trends in Indian population distribution across ages and gender. The right side indicates distribution of males and the left side females. The *y*-axis represents the ages in years, and the *x*-axis represents the population. The three lines: red, blue, and green indicate the data for the 3 years—1990, 2019, and 2100, respectively. The red line is relatively linear, whereas the blue line indicates the 2019 population with more individuals specifically in the age range 5 to 30 years.

FIGURE 45.2 Population age structure for males and females in 1990, 2019, and 2100.

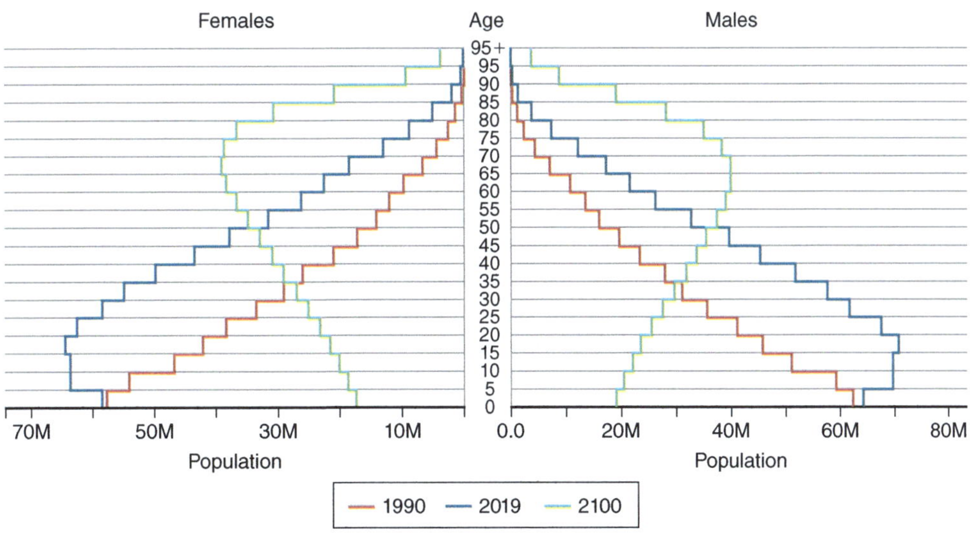

Source: Institute for Health Metrics and Evaluation. (2021). *India*. https://www.healthdata.org/research-analysis/health-by-location/profiles/india

This group of individuals in the upcoming decades will be the aging population, as represented by the green line.

Poor health outcomes are likely to result if the current challenges of increased out-of-pocket expenditure, reduced number of professionals per 1,000 individuals, poor accessibility to healthcare, and uninsured individuals remain unaddressed before the bottleneck phenomenon occurs in the upcoming decades. Hence, it is important to address the current challenges. Addressing these healthcare shortage areas requires targeted interventions, including increased investments in healthcare infrastructure, incentivizing healthcare professionals to work in underserved areas, and leveraging technology to bridge geographic barriers to care delivery.

RECENT DEVELOPMENTS IN HEALTHCARE INNOVATIONS

To improve healthcare access for different segments of the population, the Indian government has introduced several targeted programs. One such initiative, Janani Shishu Suraksha Karyakram is a government initiative to provide free maternity and newborn care to infants in public hospitals. Another initiative is Mukhyamantri Santwana Harish Scheme launched in 2018 by the government that provides free treatment for road accident victims in both private and public hospitals.

Telemedicine and telehealth in India were initiated by Indian Space Research Organization (ISRO) by connecting rural populations with urban hospitals through the Indian National Satellite System (INSAT). ISRO then expanded this project to Village Resource Centres (VRCs); currently there are 461 VRCs providing telehealth and telemedicine (Government of India, 2024). The recent developments include several projects such as OncoNET (launched by the National Cancer Network), Integrated Disease Surveillance Project (IDSP), National Rural Telemedicine Network, and INDIAai (the national Artificial Intelligence portal of India; Bajpai & Wadhwa, 2021; Shah, 2023). The Indian Council of Medical Research and the University of Germany collaborated to start the Arogyasree, an internet-based mobile telemedicine platform. They also developed an echocardiography jacket to monitor the heart health of individuals who live in rural areas (Government of India, 2024). A teleoncology network exists in Kerala for more than 10,000 cancer patients annually who regularly use this communication to keep up with their oncology physician. During Maha Kumbhamelas and other festivals, the state government of Uttar Pradesh uses telemedicine.

Additionally, several startups in India leverage AI for diagnostic imaging solutions, including Predible Health (Bajpai & Wadhwa, 2021). Through AI-powered medical imaging, Predible empowers clinicians to understand cancer comprehensively by developing patient-centric, organ-specific cancer care workflows. States like Tamil Nadu, Maharashtra, Karnataka, and West Bengal have their own AI initiatives to enhance their healthcare.

Digital health includes monitoring/measuring health parameters through digital equipment, accessing online health information, using health and fitness apps and gadgets (such as Arogya-Setu, smartwatches, etc.). India has developed numerous healthcare apps that help individuals take control of their health. As part of the National Health Assurance Scheme (Ayushman Bharat), eligible citizens can receive digital health cards and digital applications that allow patients to schedule doctor appointments and order medications. However, these services require internet access, device accessibility, digital literacy, and robust data protection. Unfortunately, per World Bank Group data from 2021, only 46% of the entire Indian population has access to the internet, a challenge to implementation of effective digital health and telemedicine. Also, government schemes such as Assistance to Persons with Disabilities for Purchase/Fitting of Aids/Appliances (ADIP; Government of India, 2024) are beneficial in some ways but provide only the basic prosthetics for those in need. Consumers, in contrast, often appreciate other government schemes such as the Arogyashree under which several state governments can provide free cochlear implants to individuals.

Precision medicine and genomics are gaining traction in India, with initiatives to personalize healthcare interventions based on genetic data. One recent study is an initiative to create a database called IndiGenomes (Jain et al., 2021). Precision medicine is characterized by individualized interventions that consider contextual factors and individual differences, thereby improving patient outcomes.

CONCLUSION

Increased life expectancy serves as one indicator of the improvements in healthcare in India. One ongoing initiative by the government is to improve health services in rural India. Further, with the launch of government-based insurance schemes, more people in India are enrolling in health insurance plans as public awareness increases. One recommendation would be to make health insurance schemes affordable, accessible, and mandatory for all individuals. Another recommendation, which is an essential need, is to integrate rehabilitative services by health professionals in all schools. Inclusive education is the key to generating a more diverse healthcare workforce and a better healthcare system for future India. Overall, the country has grown as a nation in the healthcare sector. There are increasing needs, but it is evident that the government is expanding their efforts to make healthcare accessible and efficient.

LEARNING ACTIVITIES

CourseConnect

To access self-assessment questions and interactive, competency-based learning activities for this chapter, visit www.springerpub.com/courseconnect. See inside front cover and tear-out for CourseConnect details.

REFERENCES

Ahmad, A., Naqvi, S. B. K., & Sultana, N. (2024). Exploring the roots: The historical journey and evolution of the Unani system of medicine. *Journal of Emerging Technologies and Innovative Research (JETIR), 11*(6), a432–a442. https://www.researchgate.net/profile/Ashfaque-Ahmad-8/publication/381164367_Exploring_the_Roots_The_Historical_Journey_and_Evolution_of_the_Unani_System_of_Medicine/links/666051baa54c5f0b944e9951/Exploring-the-Roots-The-Historical-Journey-and-Evolution-of-the-Unani-System-of-Medicine.pdf

Amarasinghe, U., Amarnath, G., Alahacoon, N., & Ghosh, S. (2020). How do floods and drought impact economic growth and human development at the sub-national level in India? *Climate, 8*(11), 123. https://doi.org/10.3390/cli8110123

Bajpai, N., & Wadhwa, M. (2021). *Artificial intelligence and healthcare in India (No. 43).* ICT India Working Paper. https://www.econstor.eu/bitstream/10419/249832/1/ICT-India-Working-Paper-43.pdf

Central Intelligence Agency. (2025). *The world factbook: India*. https://www.cia.gov/the-world-factbook/countries/india/

Gabani, J., Mazumdar, S., & Suhrcke, M. (2023). The effect of health financing systems on health system outcomes: A cross-country panel analysis. *Health Economics, 32*(3), 574–619. https://doi.org/10.1002/hec.4635

Government of India. (2024). *Government of India*. https://ndma.gov.in/

Institute for Health Metrics and Evaluation. (2021). *India*. https://www.healthdata.org/research-analysis/health-by-location/profiles/india

International Labor Organization. (2023). *India*. https://www.ilo.org/india

Jain, A., Bhoyar, R. C., Pandhare, K., Mishra, A., Sharma, D., Imran, M., Senthivel, V., Divakar, M. K., Rophina, M., Jolly, B., Batra, A., Sharma, S., Siwach, S., Jadhao, A. G., Palande, N. V., Jha, G. N., Ashrafi, N., Mishra, P. K., Vidhya, A. K., . . . & Sivasubbu, S. (2021). IndiGenomes: A comprehensive resource of genetic variants from over 1000 Indian genomes. *Nucleic Acids Research, 49*(D1), D1225–D1232. https://doi.org/10.1093/nar/gkaa923

Kumar, R., & Duggirala, A. (2021). Health insurance as a healthcare financing mechanism in India: Key strategic insights and a business model perspective. *Vikalpa, 46*(2), 112–128. https://doi.org/10.1177/02560909211027089

Meghrajani, V. R., Marathe, M., Sharma, R., Potdukhe, A., Wanjari, M. B., & Taksande, A. B. (2023). A comprehensive analysis of mental health problems in India and the role of mental asylums. *Cureus, 15*(7), e42559. https://doi.org/10.7759/cureus.42559

Pandya, A. K., & Redcay, A. (2021). Access to health services: Barriers faced by the transgender population in India. *Journal of Gay & Lesbian Mental Health, 25*(2), 132–154. https://doi.org/10.1080/19359705.2020.1850592

Parveen, A., Parveen, R., Akhatar, A., Parveen, B., Siddiqui, K. M., & Iqbal, M. (2020). Concepts and quality considerations in the Unani system of medicine. *Journal of AOAC International, 103*(3), 609–633. https://doi.org/10.5740/jaoacint.19-0284

Patil, S. B., Patil, M. S., Chittam, K. P., & Wagh, R. D. (2014). A review on Ayurveda and Siddha: Indian systems of medicine. *Pharma Science Monitor, 5*(2), 40–49. http://www.pharmasm.com/pdf_files/20140430131319_05_minal.pdf

Pattnaik, S., Murmu, J., Agrawal, R., Rehman, T., Kanungo, S., & Pati, S. (2023). Prevalence, pattern and determinants of disabilities in India: Insights from NFHS-5 (2019–21). *Frontiers in Public Health, 11*, 1036499. https://doi.org/10.3389/fpubh.2023.1036499

Raja, V., & Bhalla, D. O. (2021). Impact of Carnatic music training on the mathematical ability of children. *Early Child Development and Care, 191*(12), 1911–1921. https://doi.org/10.1080/03004430.2020.1832484

Ram, B., & Thakur, R. (2022). Epidemiology and economic burden of continuing challenge of infectious diseases in India: Analysis of socio-demographic differentials. *Frontiers in Public Health, 10*, 901276. https://doi.org/10.3389/fpubh.2022.901276

Sahoo, P. M., Kumar, V., Rout, H. S., & Tripathi, T. (2023). Budgeting for health: India's policy priorities and investment trends. *Orissa Journal of Commerce, 44*(2), 150–161. https://shorturl.at/bsNAQ

Sahoo, P. M., Rout, H. S., & Jakovljevic, M. (2023). Consequences of India's population aging to its healthcare financing and provision. *Journal of Medical Economics, 26*(1), 308–315. https://doi.org/10.1080/13696998.2023.2178164

Shah, A. M. (2023). Telemedicine in India: A perspective, collaboration, and knowledge sharing. *National Journal of Physiology, Pharmacy and Pharmacology, 13*(8), 1597–1597. https://www.researchgate.net/profile/Amit-Shah/publication/372554381_Telemedicine_in_India_A_perspective_collaboration_and_knowledge_sharing/links/64e0a131caf5ff5cd0c75e44/Telemedicine-in-India-A-perspective-collaboration-and-knowledge-sharing.pdf

UN Data Portal. (2023). *India*. https://data.un.org/en/iso/in.html

World Bank Group. (2025). *India*. https://data.worldbank.org/country/india

World Health Organization. (2022). *Addressing mental health in India*. https://www.who.int/publications/i/item/9789290210177

World Health Organization. (2024). *India*. https://data.who.int/countries/356

CHAPTER 46

NEPAL

Amit Bhandari

INTRODUCTION

Located in South Asia, Nepal is a country diverse in its geography, demography, climate zones, and fauna and flora. It has been in existence as a unified nation for over 25 years. A low-and middle-income country with a health system that has delivered improved outcomes with regard to communicable diseases and maternal and child health, Nepal now is faced with a double burden due to a rapid increase in noncommunicable diseases (NCDs) and communicable diseases and maternal and child health problems, both still remaining major issues despite the progress. Aggregate progress masks disparities and inequalities in access to services and developmental outcomes.

GEOGRAPHY, DEMOGRAPHICS, AND SOCIOCULTURAL CONTEXT

GEOGRAPHY

Nepal, a federal democratic republic, is a landlocked country with China to the north and India to the south, east, and west. It is roughly trapezoidal shape with an area of 147,516 square kilometers (91,662 square miles) ranking 93rd in the world by land size (World Population Review, 2024). Figure 46.1 shows the official flag of Nepal, and Figure 46.2 shows its administrative map.

FIGURE 46.1 Official flag of Nepal.

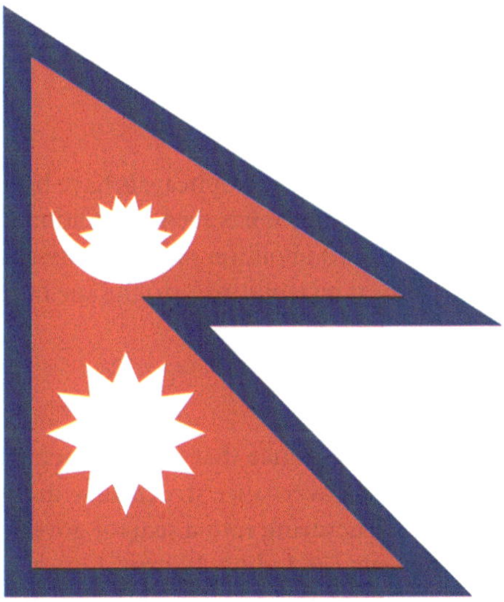

Source: Pumbaa80. (2007). *Flag of Federal Democratic Republic of Nepal*. https://commons.wikimedia.org/w/index.php?curid=343693

FIGURE 46.2 Administrative map of Nepal.

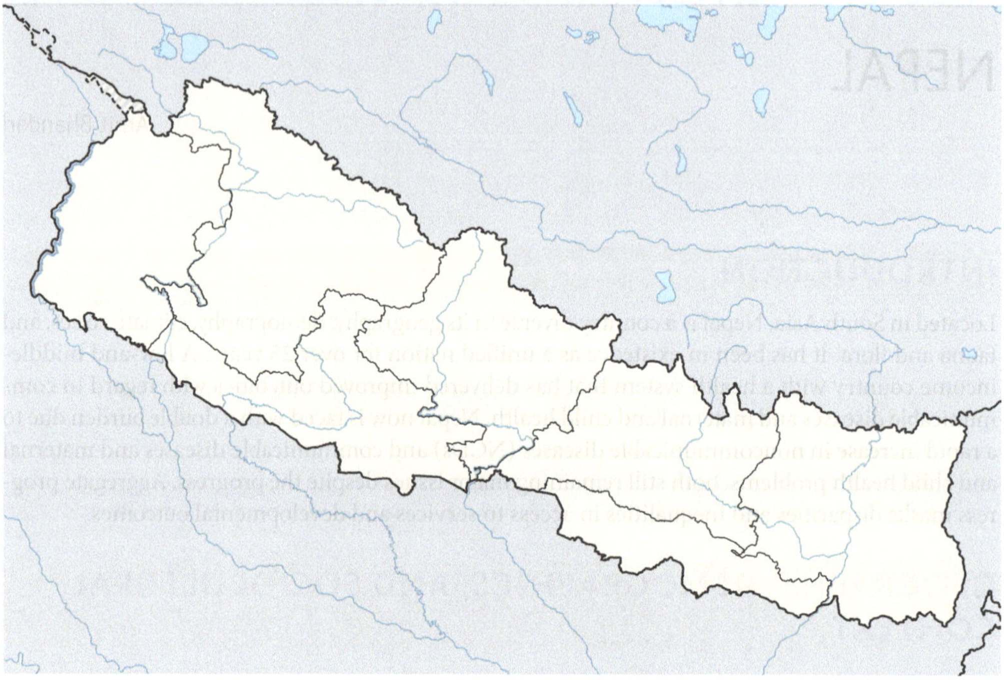

Source: NordNordWest. (2018). *Map of Nepal*. https://commons.wikimedia.org/wiki/File:Nepal_adm_location_map.svg

Nepal is a multiethnic, multilingual, multireligious, and multicultural state, with **Nepali** as the official language. It has a diverse geography and climate that includes tropical, fertile plains; subtropical, temperate, and subalpine forested hills; and alpine and nival mountains hosting eight of the world's 10 tallest mountains in the Himalayas—including Mount Everest (8,849 meters; 29,032 feet), the highest point on Earth—and rich flora and fauna in each of the ecological zones.

POLITICAL CONTEXT

Nepal was unified as a kingdom in the middle of the 18th century. Political upheavals have been a common feature throughout the country's history. Most recently, Nepal has seen restoration of democracy (early 1990s), decade-long civil war (1996 to 2006), and abolition of monarchy and declaration of the republic (2006). Nepal continues to face political instability due to the sociopolitical transition, with changes in government a frequent phenomenon.

GOVERNANCE MODEL

Abolishing the monarchy and a unitary, centralized model of governance that was in place for more than two and one-half decades, Nepal adopted a federalized governance structure with the promulgation of a new Constitution in 2015, subsequently restructuring into a federal government, seven provincial governments, and 753 local governments (including 460 rural municipalities, 276 urban municipalities, 11 submetropolises, and 6 metropolises—collectively known as municipalities). It was underpinned by devolution of power, bringing significant shifts in the health systems as well. Each local unit is composed of wards. There are 6,743 wards in total (The Asia Foundation [TAF], 2017).

DEMOGRAPHY

With a population of 29.2 million (females 51.1% and males 48.9%), Nepal's total population density is 198 people per 1 square kilometer (0.62 square miles), and annual population growth rate of 0.92%. Nepal ranks 49th in the list of countries by population with a share of 0.38% of the world population (Worldometer, 2024). The 2021 census recorded 2,928 people (0.01%) of other genders (sexual and gender minorities) among the total population. People living with disability account for 2.2% of the population. The share of urban and peri-urban population has increased from 63.2% in 2011 to 66.2% in 2021. The net migration rate is –4.21 migrants per 1,000 population (Government of Nepal [GoN] & National Statistics Office [NSO], 2022).

DEMOGRAPHIC SHIFT

Nepal has rapidly transitioned from a high-mortality, high-fertility to a low-mortality, low-fertility society, with rapid "aging" of the population in the last few decades (GoN National Planning Commission [NPC] & UNICEF, 2017). The declining mortality and fertility rates and increasing life expectancy have changed the structure of Nepal's demographic pyramid and dependency ratio. Table 46.1 shows the changes in life expectancy, fertility, birth, and death rates every two decades from 1960 to 2022. Figure 46.3 shows the population pyramid in 2021 (GoN & NSO, 2022). Data from consecutive censuses have shown a decline in annual population growth rate from 2.25% in 2001 to 1.35% in 2011, and to 0.92% in 2021 with the population increasing by 3.3 million between 2001 and 2011 and by only 2.7 million between 2011 to 2021. From 1952 to 1954 to 2011, the median age increased by about 2 years at each census, and then by 4 years from 2011 to 2021. In 2021 the median age was 26 years. Over the years, the number of children (0 to 14 years old) has been declining while the number of working age (15 to 64 years old) and older persons (65 years and older) has increased. In 2021, children made up 27.8% of the population, 15 to 64 year olds 65.2%, and persons over 65 years old 6.9%, resulting in a dependency ratio of 53.3%, which is significantly less than the 67.2% in 2011. Nepal has already entered the **demographic window of opportunity** and is anticipating a demographic dividend. (The demographic window of opportunity opens when the ratio is 60 dependents or less to every 100 working-age people.) It is population is experiencing an age structure with a larger share of working-age population that is highly favorable for accelerated economic growth and development of the country. Nepal's sex ratio at birth has increased from 103 males to 100 females in 1952 to 1954, to 106 males to 100 females in 2011, and 112 males to 100 females in 2021. The 2021 ratio is significantly higher than the "natural" sex ratio at birth of 105 and demonstrates a higher tendency of missing females at birth in Nepal (GoN/NSO, 2024).

CASTE, ETHNICITY, RELIGION, AND LANGUAGE

Nepal has a rich diversity of castes and ethnicities, religions, and languages. There are 142 castes and ethnic groups, but no one group consists of more than 20% of the total population: Chhetris comprise 16.5% of the population, Brahmans-Hill 11.3%, Magars 6.9%, Tharus 6.2%, Tamangs 5.6%, and Bishwakarmas 5.0%. Of the 10 religions followed in the country, Hinduism is predominant,

TABLE 46.1 TRENDS OF DEMOGRAPHIC INDICATORS IN NEPAL

INDICATOR	1960	1980	2000	2022
Life expectancy at birth (years)	39	48	63	70
Total fertility rate (births per woman)	6.0	5.6	3.9	2.0
Crude birth rate (births per 1,000 people)	45	41	31	20
Crude death rate (deaths per 1,000 people)	25	17	8	7

Source: World Bank Group. (n.d.). *Nepal*. https://data.worldbank.org/country/NP

FIGURE 46.3 Nepal's population pyramid (population by 5 year age group and sex).

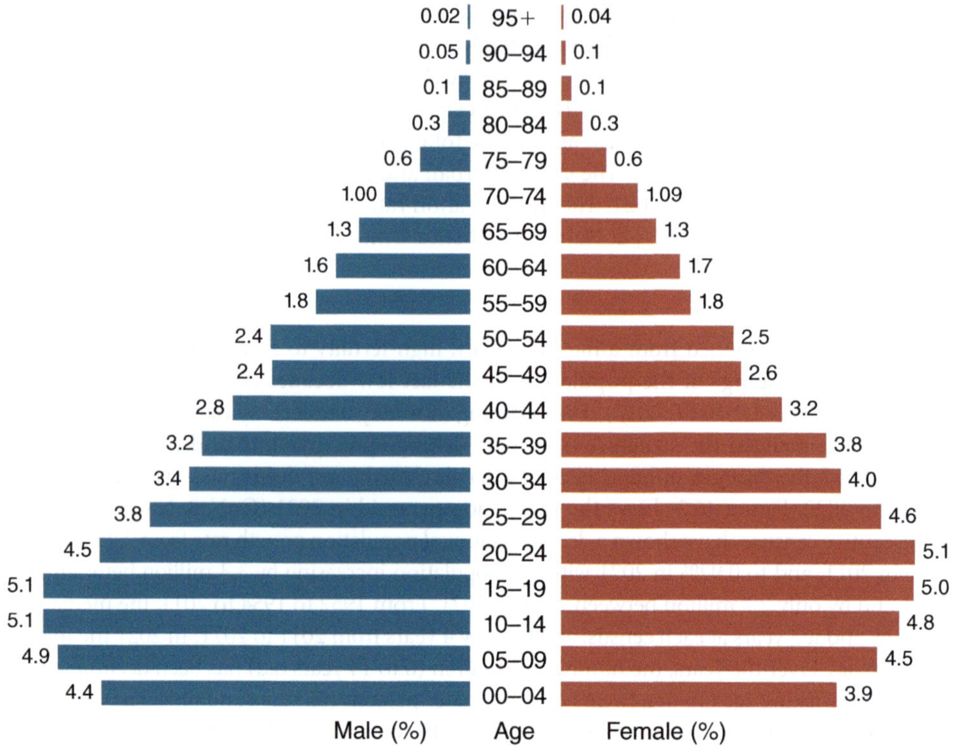

Source: Adapted from Nepal Health Research Council. (2021). *Report of national mental health survey 2020*. Nepal Health Research Council, Government of Nepal. https://censusnepal.cbs.gov.np/results/population

comprising 81.2% of the population; 8.2% of the population practice Buddhism, 5.1% Islam, 3.2% Kirat, 1.8% Christian, and others. Of the 124 languages spoken in Nepal, Nepali is spoken by 44.8% of the population followed by Maithali at 11.1% and Bhojpuri at 6.2% (GoN/NSO, 2022).

HEALTH OUTCOMES

MATERNAL AND CHILD HEALTH

Nepal has made steady and significant progress in health outcomes over the past few decades—such as the reduction in maternal and child mortalities and fertility, and the rise in the life expectancy—despite political turmoil and historically weak economy (see Table 46.2). The trend of service utilization for institutional births reflects the progress Nepal has made in improving access to maternal and child health services. Since 1996, health facility–based deliveries have steadily increased from 8% to 79%, and home deliveries declined from 91% to 19% (Ministry of Health and Population [MoHP], New ERA, & ICF, 2023). Nepal was one of the few countries in South Asia to achieve the Millennium Development Goal (MDG) 4 target to reduce child mortality by two thirds. The political commitment by the GoN in the past few decades to strengthen the health system, particularly community-based health services, has been a major reason for the achievement (Merchant et al., 2016). Although significant progress is evident, challenges remain in access, equity, quality, and affordability of healthcare, making it increasingly difficult to sustain the gains in health outcomes. Access to reproductive, maternal, neonatal, child health, and nutrition services has stagnated in recent decades. For example, the contraceptive prevalence rate

TABLE 46.2 TREND OF REPRODUCTIVE, MATERNAL, AND CHILD HEALTH OUTCOMES AS SHOWN BY POPULATION SURVEYS FROM 1996 TO 2022

INDICATOR	1996 NFHS	2001 NDHS	2006 NDHS	2011 NDHS	2016 NDHS	2022 NDHS	2030 SDG TARGET
Maternal mortality ratio (per 100,000 live births)	539	n/a	281	n/a	259	151	70
5-year-olds or younger mortality rate (per 1,000 live births)	118	91	61	54	39	33	20
Infant mortality rate (per 1,000 live births)	78	64	48	46	32	28	n/a
Neonatal mortality rate (per 1,000 live births)	50	39	33	33	21	21	12
Contraceptive (modern method) prevalence rate (%)	26	35	44	43	43	43	60
Institutional delivery (%)	8	10	20	44	64	79	90

NFHS, Nepal Family Health Survey; NDHS, Napal Demographic and Health Survey; SDG, Sustainable Development Goals.

Source: Adapted from Government of Nepal National Statistics Office. (2022). *Nepal population and housing census 2021.* https://censusnepal.cbs.gov.np/results/population; Ministry of Health and Population, Nepal. (2022). *Nepal demographic and health survey 2022: Key indicators report.* https://dhsprogram.com/pubs/pdf/PR142/PR142.pdf; Ministry of Health and Population, Department of Health Services. (2024). *Annual health report for fiscal year 2022–2023.* https://hdl.handle.net/20.500.14356/2682

(modern methods) has remained around 44% since 2006, and the prevalence of stunting in children under 5 years old remains high—at 25% as of 2021—with the rates varying both by province and socioeconomic groups, reflecting inequitable access to healthcare. Despite considerable expansion of healthcare delivery structures and increased availability of services in the past few decades, the quality of healthcare remains poor due to weaknesses in the health system (MoHP, New ERA, & ICF, 2022).

NONCOMMUNICABLE DISEASES

The causes of the death have seen a transition in the past few decades. The proportion of deaths due to NCDs more than doubled between 1990 (31.3% of total deaths) and 2019 (71.1% of total deaths), while deaths due to communicable, maternal, neonatal, and nutritional (CMNN) diseases have seen a steady decline over the same period (from 62.5% to 21.1% of total deaths between 1990 and 2019). In 2019, the remaining 7.8% of total deaths were due to injuries. The top 10 causes of death are given in Figure 46.4. Among NCDs, cardiovascular diseases are the leading cause of deaths (24% of total deaths). Among CMNN diseases, lower respiratory infections are the leading cause of death (4.5% of total deaths), followed by drug-susceptible tuberculosis (3.5% of total deaths). Among injuries, falls are the leading cause of death (2.0% of total deaths). The younger population bears a greater

FIGURE 46.4 Leading causes of death in Nepal, 2011 and 2021.

Cause	2011 rank	2021 rank	Change in deaths per 100K, 2011–2021
COVID-19	–	1	↑ +143.5
Ischemic heart disease	1	2	↑ +13.7
COPD	2	3	↑ +16.1
Stroke	4	4	↑ +7.7
Neonatal disorders	3	5	↓ −18.9
Lower respiratory infection	5	6	↓ −15.4
Tuberculosis	6	7	↓ −7.2
Diabetes	10	8	↑ +6.6
Cirrhosis liver	8	9	↑ +1.4
Asthma	9	10	↑ +1.1

● Communicable, maternal, neonatal, and nutritional diseases
● Noncommunicable diseases

Source: Institute for Health Metrics and Evaluation. (n.d.). *Health research by location: Country profiles*. https://www.healthdata.org/research-analysis/health-by-location/profiles

burden of mortality due to CMNN diseases while the older population's burden of mortality is due to NCDs. Deaths due to injuries are more common in young adults (Nepal Health Research Council [NHRC], MoHP, Institute for Health Metrics and Evaluation [IHME], Monitoring Evaluation and Operational Research [MEOR], 2021). Increasing life expectancy, demographic and epidemiologic transition, rampant urbanization, and changes in lifestyle all account to this rising burden of NCDs. The increasing disease burden is associated with decreasing quality of life, increase in disability adjusted life years (DALYs), and catastrophic health expenditures (MoHP/DoHS, 2024).

MENTAL HEALTH

In Nepal, one in 10 adults has had some mental disorder in their lifetime, while 4.3% of adults,and 5.2% of adolescents currently have some mental disorder. The prevalence of suicidality (including current suicidal thoughts, lifetime suicidal attempt, and future likelihood of suicidal thoughts) is 7.2%. Vulnerable groups, such as poor, hard-to-reach populations, the homeless, conflict affected, survivors of violence, minority groups, transgender and nonbinary populations, prisoners, and people in humanitarian settings, have higher risks of having mental health problems (NHRC, 2021). The suicide mortality rate in Nepal is nine per 100,000 population (World Health Organization [WHO], 2024). The proportional contribution of mental disorders to the total disease burden has tripled in the three decades between 1990 (1.79% of all DALYs) and 2019 (5.5% of all DALYs; Dhungana et al., 2023). Over the past few years, several initiatives have been taken to improve mental health services in Nepal, such as including mental health services in the basic healthcare package. Effective implementation of mental health services in primary care has been challenging due to limited mental health awareness, low perceived need for services, and high level of stigma which negatively affects help-seeking and hence early detection and management of mental health conditions (Devkota et al., 2021; Luitel et al., 2020).

COVID-19

In January 2020, just a few weeks after the cases in China were first announced, Nepal reported its first case of COVID-19 infection. As of July 2022, Nepal had close to 1 million laboratory confirmed cases and nearly 12,000 COVID-19 related deaths registered in the system (MoHP/DoHS, 2024). The COVID-19 pandemic exposed weaknesses in Nepal's health system, particularly in its readiness to mitigate the impact of the unprecedented health crisis. The weak health system of the country was badly affected due to the disruption in the global supply chain of medical products, including closure of the borders and restrictions on internal movements during the COVID-19 pandemic (Bhandari & Ellis-Petersen, 2021; MoHP, 2021). Hospitals were overstretched and were not able to cater to elevated levels of demand. The pandemic also impacted negatively on routine service delivery (WHO Regional Office for South-East Asia, 2021) and quality of care (Government of Nepal [GoN], MoHP, 2022), leading to worsened health outcomes, for example, excess maternal deaths (Integrated Health Information Management Section, 2021). Despite initial challenges, Nepal succeeded with a swift resumption of the health services and vaccinating a significant proportion of the population to halt the spread of the disease. Many of the indicators bounced back to normalcy after response measures and service continuity were prioritized (MoHP/DoHS, 2022).

DETERMINANTS OF HEALTH

ECONOMY AND HUMAN DEVELOPMENT

Nepal has had a relatively modest economic growth rate in recent decades, averaging 4.9% between 2009 and 2019 however, it has been lower post-COVID-19, with 1.9% in 2023 (World Bank Group, 2024). The per-capita gross domestic product (GDP) is $1,337 and its annual growth is 3.8% (World Bank Group, 2022). Nepal is in the medium human development category with a Human Development Index of 0.587 (GoN/NPC & UNDP, 2020). The literacy rate of the total population aged 5 years and older in the country is 76.2% (83.6% for males and 69.4% for females). Poverty levels have shown a decline over the decades, but still one in five people lived below the national poverty line in 2022 (Asian Development Bank, 2024). Of the total population aged 10 years and older, 65.5% are economically active (GON/NSO, 2022). Modeled estimates for 2023 by International Labor Organization (ILO) show that 11% of the total labor force is unemployed (World Bank Group, 2024). Two thirds of the total employment is dependent on agriculture and there is a slow transformation from an agriculture-based economy to the modern economy (KC et al., 2020). Out migration for labor is common with one third of the households having at least one member in foreign countries (CBS, 2018).

FOOD SECURITY AND NUTRITION

Food security in Nepal has improved considerably in the recent decades. However, 13% of the population still experiences moderate to severe food insecurity, with poor and rural populations more food insecure. Malnutrition in children and women remains a serious concern. One quarter of children under 5 years of age are stunted (25%), 19% are underweight, 8% are wasted, 1% are overweight, and two in five are anemic (43%). Over one quarter of adolescent girls age 15 to 19 years and 10% of women age 20 to 49 years are of short stature, and similar percentages of the population are thin. Similarly, 35% of women and 6% of adolescent girls are overweight or obese. One in three women age 15 to 49 years are anemic (34%). Good dietary practices—such as early, exclusive, and continued breastfeeding of babies under 6 months of age, and consumption of meals with minimum dietary diversity by children under 5 and women of reproductive age—remain suboptimal, whereas consumption of sweet beverages and unhealthy foods are high (between 43% and 69%) among both populations groups (MoHP, New ERA, & ICF, 2023).

WATER AND SANITATION

Access to clean water has improved over the decades; however, sanitation facilities are poor and biofuel still remains a major source for cooking. Only 57.0% of total households use a tap/piped water supply as the main source of drinking water, followed by 29.8% using water this is tube well/hand pump. A small proportion still use unsafe sources such as uncovered wells or rivers/streams (2.5%; GON/NSO, 2022). Just over one half of the population has access to safely managed sanitation services (World Bank Group, n.d.-a). Firewood is still a main source of fuel for cooking for over half of the total households (51.0%), followed by liquefied petroleum gas (44.3%). Only 0.5% of the total households use electricity as the main source of fuel for cooking (GoN/NSO, 2022).

SEX, GENDER, AND OTHER SOCIOCULTURAL DISCRIMINATION

Nepal has seen notable progress in human development; however, large disparities persist across gender, region, and social groups. Remarkable progress has been made on the protection and promotion of women's rights and gender equality (the gender development index is 0.886). Still, fairly moderate gender inequality remains (the gender inequality index is 0.479) and deeply rooted sociocultural norms impede better outcomes. Women experience lower progress than men in education and income (GoN/NPC & UNDP, 2020). Nepal continues to have many cultural norms and beliefs that hinder the advancement of women and marginalized groups, some of which are child marriage, domestic violence, **chhaupadi** (a tradition of menstrual exile that obstructs women and girls' access to education, healthcare, community, and safety), dowry, discrimination based on caste, and accusations of witchcraft. Discriminatory beliefs and practices reinforce objectification of girls and women.

Despite substantial progress in the health sector, healthcare is not distributed equally across the various gender and social groups. Sexual and gender minority populations find access to crucial HIV and healthcare services challenging due to social and structural barriers (U.S. Agency for International Development [USAID], 2020). Though the constitution guarantees the principles of equality and nondiscrimination and laws prohibit untouchability and discrimination on the grounds of caste, the caste system in Nepal perpetuates a form of segregation and oppression against the **Dalits** (the so-called lower castes), who make up approximately 13.8% of the population (Amnesty International, 2024). Child marriage is one of the harmful practices in the society, with 35.1% of women age 20 to 24 years married before 18 years of age. Poorer women are more likely to be married in childhood compared to wealthier women (GoN/NSO, 2022).

CLIMATE CHANGE AND DISASTER

Nepal's diverse geoclimatic system, which combines heavy monsoons, steep terrain, and remoteness, makes it vulnerable to climate-related events and natural disasters (World Bank Group, n.d.-b). Millions are estimated to be at risk from the impacts of climate change including reductions in agricultural production, food insecurity, strained water resources, loss of forest and biodiversity, reduced tourism and damaged infrastructure, and their associated impacts on health (MoHP, n.d.). Heat-related morbidity and mortality, nutrition risks, and vector- and water-borne diseases are the major climate-associated risks for Nepal. These risks are not evenly distributed in the population, with some groups at greater risk than others. The health systems preparedness and capacity to manage the changes in hazards, exposure, and susceptibility that impact health outcomes are low (MoHP, 2021). Nepal experienced a devastating earthquake in 2015 which took nearly 10,000 lives and impacted the livelihoods of hundreds of thousands. Other natural disasters, forest fires, and disease outbreaks are also a common occurrence.

MORTALITY RISK FACTORS

Risk factors are the key drivers of injuries and diseases that cause burden and deaths. Deaths due to behavioral and environmental/occupational factors have declined during 1990 to 2019, while those due to metabolic risk factors have been constantly increasing. In 2019, of the total deaths, 38.1% were due to behavioral risk factors, 31.2% were due to environmental/occupational risk factors, and 22.9% were due to metabolic risk factors. The top five risk factors for deaths are: (a) smoking (17.7%), (b) high blood pressure (12.3%), (c) household air pollution from solid fuels (11.2%), (d) ambient air pollution (9.3%), and (e) high fasting plasma glucose (8.0%; NHRC, MoHP, IHME, & MEOR, 2021).

HEALTHCARE BACKGROUND

HEALTH GOVERNANCE

Health is enshrined as a fundamental right in the 2015 Constitution of Nepal and ensuring access to basic healthcare, free of cost to users, is the State's responsibility. Nepal's legal and policy framework for the health sector is geared toward fulfilling the constitutional provisions to ensure easy availability of and equal access to quality healthcare for all without financial hardship, and achieve Universal Health Coverage (UHC), in line with the country's commitment to achieve SDGs by 2030. Under the new federal structure, health is a concurrent function among the three levels of government—federal, provincial, and local. The primary function of the federal government is to set national level goals, policies, legal frameworks, and standards for the health sector; finance basic healthcare; and provide tertiary level services. Provinces also perform similar functions to the federal level but within their own territory and under the policy and legal provisions defined by the federal level. Delivering basic healthcare services free of charge to users is an exclusive function of the local governments. However, in practice, higher levels of public health facilities are also engaged in providing basic healthcare services. The Basic Healthcare Services (BHS) package includes a prioritized set of promotive, preventive, basic curative and rehabilitative services and covers immunization, reproductive and maternal, newborn and child health and nutrition, family planning, safe abortion, infectious diseases, non-communicable diseases and physical distortions, mental health, geriatrics, general emergency care, promotional health, and aspects of Ayurveda and other traditional healthcare. Local governments have major responsibility when it comes to delivering basic services; however, weak institutional and human resource capacities have meant that there is little practice of contextualized and results-oriented programming for comprehensive, effective, and equitable healthcare delivery (Bhandari et al., 2020).

ORGANIZATION OF HEALTHCARE DELIVERY

Figure 46.5 gives a schematic outline of the organization of government healthcare delivery system in Nepal. At the federal level, there are several divisions under the MoHP, which is responsible for managing the policy framework, planning, setting standards, coordination, monitoring, and supervision. Immediate implementation and further planning are conducted through three departments: Department of Health Services (DoHS), Department of Ayurveda and Alternative Medicine, and Department of Drug Administration. These departments, through their respective deconcentrated entities, provide guidance to their provincial counterparts under the provincial ministries, which in turn support health offices at the district and health coordination units at the local level. Public institutions—including basic healthcare service centers (BHSCs) and basic hospitals at the local level; primary and secondary (general) hospitals at the provincial level; and tertiary, super-specialized, and academia/teaching hospitals at the federal levelare mandated to deliver health services to the populace. The service provision extends further into communities through female community health volunteers (FCHVs), and school and community health nurses. The government healthcare delivery encompasses both allopathic, and Ayurvedic and alternative medicine, extending beyond curative services to include promotive, preventive, rehabilitative, and palliative dimensions as well. Private health facilities operate at all levels, complementing public institutions (MoHP/DoHS, 2024).

HEALTHCARE NETWORK

With the federal restructuring, health facilities are expanded to widen the network of the public health facilities up to the ward level, but human resources are scant and the functionality of health facilities remains poor. The policy provisions to expand the healthcare network have contributed to widening access to healthcare, but concerns are growing on the quality as well as efficiency of the systems. Nepal's public sector healthcare delivery system has over 8,000 healthcare facilities

FIGURE 46.5 Organization of the government healthcare delivery system in Nepal.

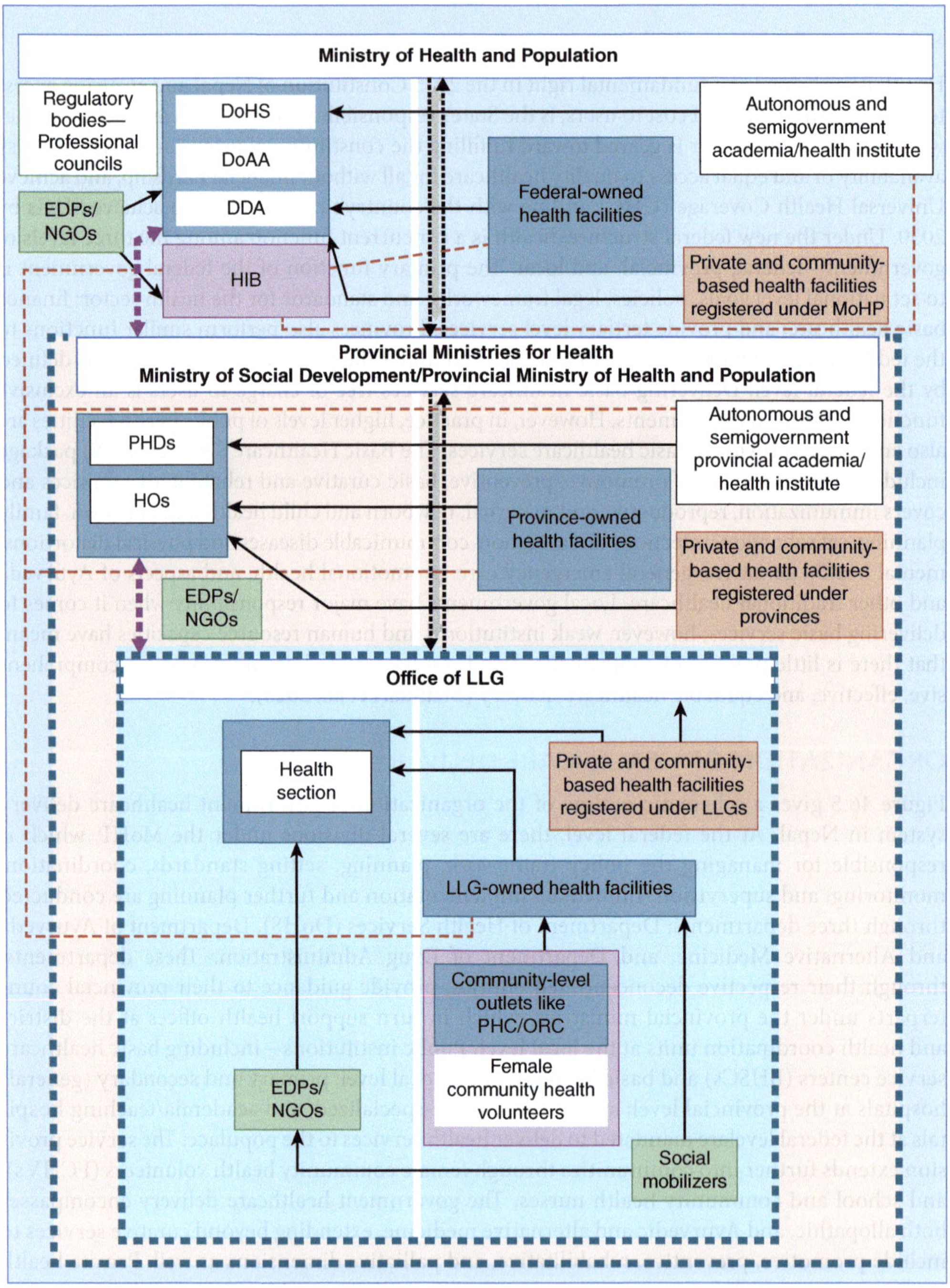

DDA, Department of Drug Administration; DoAA, Department of Ayurveda and Alternative Medicine; DoHS, Department of Health Services; EDP, external development partners; HIB, health insurance board; HO, health office; LLG, local-level government; NGO, nongovernmental organization; ORC, outreach center; PHC, primary healthcare; PHD, provincial health directorate.

Source: Ministry of Health and Population–Department of Health Services. (2024). *Annual health report for fiscal year 2022–2023*. https://dohs.gov.np/content/21/annual-health-report-2079-80-ahr/

offering different levels of care, and there are 2,551 facilities in the nonpublic sector (which comprises hospitals and healthcare facilities run by private entities, communities, and cooperatives; MoHP/DoHS, 2024). Public sector health facilities are under different levels of government; their distribution is given in Table 46.3. Basic healthcare services (primary care) are mostly provided by public sector facilities, while the majority of the curative healthcare is provided by the private sector (estimated at around 70% of all curative service utilization).

HEALTH REFORMS AND GLOBAL COMMITMENTS

Nepal has adopted the Sector Wide Approach (SWAp) in the health sector for the past two decades to enhance country leadership and effectively use development cooperation to drive reforms. This has entailed coordinating, harmonizing, and aligning development partners' investments (financial and technical assistance) and policy engagement around country-led, periodic national health sector strategies and plans, underpinned by overarching monitoring and evaluation (M&E) frameworks. Since the shift to SWAp, health sector programs and priorities have been defined and guided by medium term periodic sector strategies: (a) Nepal Health Sector Strategy (NHSS): An Agenda for Reform (NHSS, 2004 to 2009); (b) Nepal Health Sector Strategy II (NHSS II, 2010 to 2015); (c) Nepal Health Sector Strategy III (NHSS III), 2016 to 2022; and (d) Nepal Health Sector Strategic Plan (NHS-SP), 2023 to 2023. The first two sector programs were aligned with the global commitment to the Millennium Development Goals (MDGs), while the third was developed when the country was recovering from the devasting earthquake of April 2015 and was transitioning toward federalism. The third and the fourth programs are aligned with Nepal's commitment to the UN's Sustainable Development Goals (SDGs). The SWAp modality has been considered successful in Nepal given the implementation of reforms and remarkable progress in achieving health outcomes, such as the MDG targets for maternal and child health (Ministry of Finance [MoF], 2018).

UNIVERSAL HEALTH COVERAGE

The Constitution and the periodic strategies and sectoral plans provide the legal and policy foundation and espouse the strategic priorities, directions, and objectives for achieving the UHC in Nepal. The policies envisage increasing population, services, and financial coverage through a mix of approaches: providing (tax-funded) basic health services free of cost to users (a constitutional right of citizens); universal enrollment in social health insurance for services beyond basic health; and strengthening health systems to improve service quality and equity. In 2016, the Government of Nepal (GoN) introduced the National Health Insurance Program, governed and implemented by the Health Insurance Board, as a major vehicle to improve financial protection and service delivery. However, progress has been slow. More than 7 years into implementation, the insurance program's geographic expansion to cover all 753 municipalities has just been achieved, but the

TABLE 46.3 HEALTH FACILITIES TYPE AND NUMBER BY LEVEL OF GOVERNMENT

LOCAL LEVEL	PROVINCIAL LEVEL	FEDERAL LEVEL
Basic health service centers[a]: 7,582 Basic hospitals (5, 10, 15 beds): 246	General hospitals (25–50 beds): 333 General hospitals (100–300 beds): 79	Specialized hospitals (100+ beds): 28 Super-specialty hospitals (50+ beds): 22 Teaching hospitals, academy and others (300+ beds): 29
Other types of health facilities (including Ayurveda, homeopathic, etc.): 2,164		

[a] Basic health service centers include: primary health care centers, health posts, community heath units, and urban health centers.

Source: Ministry of Health and Population-Department of Health Services. (2024). *Annual health report for fiscal year 2022–2023*. https://dohs.gov.np/content/21/annual-health-report-2079-80-ahr/

population coverage remains low at 16%, and the renewal rate is only 76% (Ministry of Health and Population [MoHP]/Department of Health Services [DoHS], 2024). The program provides an annual coverage of up to (approximately) $750 for a family of five at a premium of $26. There are also other health protection schemes, such as maternity incentives schemes which provide cash transfers to women delivering in health facilities as a transport allowance (between $7 and $21, depending on the geographic remoteness), in addition to reimbursing the health facility for those not covered by health insurance ($19 for normal delivery and $75 for cesarean section). An impoverished citizens' treatment scheme provides a one-time cash grant of $750 to people suffering from eight selected diseases (kidney disease, heart disease, cancer, head injury, spinal injury, Parkinson disease, Alzheimer disease, and sickle cell anemia). There are also other social security schemes which provide health insurance coverage to formal sector employees, in addition to other security benefits. Penetration of private health insurance is negligible. Only a negligible fraction of the population purchase private health insurance.

HEALTHCARE FINANCING

Despite a reasonably conducive policy environment, progress toward free provision of basic healthcare services and multiple and fragmented social health security schemes is slow. There are disparities in access to care, and out-of-pocket expenditure (OOPE) on healthcare remains high, indicating regressive financing structure for health services. General Government Health Expenditure stands at 0.5% of GDP or $16.9 per capita, one of the lowest in the South Asia region. Nepal's per-capita health spending remains below the global estimates of $86 considered necessary for universal coverage of essential health services. With inadequate levels of public financing for health, OOPE in Nepal is high, causing financial catastrophe and impoverishment. OOPE accounted for 58% and 54% of the current health expenditure in fiscal years 2018/2019 and 2019/2020, respectively (MoHP, 2023). The share of OOPE on health is highest among the poor quintile households, with an estimated 0.5 million Nepalese pushed into poverty ($1.90 level; WHO, 2021). Similarly, 10.7% of people spend more than 10% of their household's total expenditure on healthcare indicating financial catastrophe.

HEALTHCARE PRACTICES

Health services in Nepal encompass allopathic as well as traditional medicine, and include Ayurvedic, Homeopathic, Unani, Naturopathy, Amchi, acupuncture/acupressure, yoga, and other Indigenous practices. Allopathic medicine is increasingly used and has become the mainstay for healthcare. An estimated two thirds of the population in Nepal, however, will rely on traditional medicine at some point in their life, mainly due to its accessibility, affordability, and links to the cultural practices. The traditional medical system in Nepal has deep cultural and religious roots. Ayurveda is the oldest and most popular, which the government recognizes and provides along with homeopathic services. Delivery of traditional medicine at the national, provincial, and local levels— through a network of two Ayurveda hospitals, 14 zonal Ayurveda dispensaries, 61 district Ayurveda health centers, and 305 Ayurveda dispensaries that provide services at no or nominal charge—is managed by the Department of Ayurveda and Alternative Medicine (Giri & Malla, 2023). There have not been any programs to offer integrative medicine through the public health facilities.

CONCLUSIONS

Nepal's health system has delivered some remarkable health outcomes relative to the context of poor economy, climatic and other disasters, and sociocultural and political challenges. With a demographic shift toward an aging population, an epidemiologic transition underpinning a double burden of diseases, widespread inequities and health disparities, and poor levels of social health protection, Nepal is faced with steeper challenges ahead to improve the health outcomes of its populace. In addition to strengthening systems, enhancing resilience, and augmenting financial protection for health, a holistic approach to address the social determinants of health are equally crucial.

LEARNING ACTIVITIES

CourseConnect

To access self-assessment questions and interactive, competency-based learning activities for this chapter, visit www.springerpub.com/courseconnect. See inside front cover and tear-out for CourseConnect details.

REFERENCES

Amnesty International. (2024). *Nepal: Systemic descent-based discrimination against Dalits needs urgent action: New report.* https://www.amnesty.org/en/latest/news/2024/05/descent-based-discrimination-against-dalits-in-nepal/#:~:text=The%20constitution%20of%20Nepal%20guarantees,on%20the%20grounds%20of%20caste

Asian Development Bank. (2024). *Poverty data: Nepal* (2022). https://www.adb.org/where-we-work/nepal/poverty

Australian Government-The Asia Foundation Partnership on Subnational Governance in Nepal. (2017). *Diagnostic study of local governance in federal Nepal 2017.* https://asiafoundation.org/wp-content/uploads/2018/07/Diagnostic-Study-of-Local-Governance-in-Federal-Nepal-07112018.pdf

Bhandari, A., Pokhrel, S., Paudel, P., Rijal, K., Sigdel, S., & Bista, R. (2020). *Local health governance: Situational and political economy analysis report, Kathmandu, Nepal: Public policy Pathshala and the Asia Foundation.* https://asiafoundation.org/wp-content/uploads/2021/03/Nepal_Local-Health-Governance-Situational-and-Political-Economy-Analysis-Report_en.pdf

Bhandari, R., & Ellis-Petersen, H. (2021, May 10). *'A hopeless situation': Oxygen shortage fuels Nepal's Covid crisis.* The Guardian. https://www.theguardian.com/world/2021/may/10/hopeless-situation-oxygen-shortage-fuels-nepal-covid-crisis

Central Bureau of Statistics. (2018). *Nepal labour force survey 2017/2018.* Central Bureau of Statistics.

Devkota, G., Basnet, P., Thapa, B., & Subedi, M. (2021). Factors affecting utilization of mental health services from primary health care (PHC) facilities of western hilly district of Nepal. *PLoS One, 16*(4), e0250694. https://doi.org/10.1371/journal.pone.0250694

Dhungana, R. R., Pandey, A. R., Joshi, S., Luitel, N. P., Marahatta, K., Aryal, K. K., & Dhimal, M. (2023). The burden of mental disorders in Nepal between 1990 and 2019: Findings from the global Burden of Disease Study 2019. *Cambridge Prisms: Global Mental Health, 10*, e61. https://doi.org/10.1017/gmh.2023.55

Giri, B., & Malla, A. (2023). An overview of healthcare system of traditional medicine in Nepal. *World Journal of Advanced Healthcare Research, 7*, 44–47. https://www.researchgate.net/publication/379957844_AN_OVERVIEW_OF_HEALTHCARE_SYSTEM_OF_TRADITIONAL_MEDICINE_IN_NEPAL

Government of Nepal, Ministry of Health and Population. (2022, May). *Health sector response to COVID-19 pandemic in Nepal* [Report]. Nepal Health Sector Support Programme. https://www.nhssp.org.np/Resources/EA/Health%20Sector%20Response%20to%20COVID-19-Report-%20May%202022.pdf

Government of Nepal/National Planning Commission & UNICEF. (2017). *Demographic changes of Nepal: Trends and policy implications.* https://www.undp.org/nepal/publications/sustainable-development-goals-status-and-roadmap-2016-2030

Government of Nepal & National Statistics Office. (2022). *Nepal population and housing census 2021.* https://censusnepal.cbs.gov.np/results/population

Government of Nepal & National Statistics Office. (2024). *Nepal population and housing census 2021—Population composition of Nepal.* https://censusnepal.cbs.gov.np/results/files/result-folder/Final_Population_compostion_12_2.pdf

Integrated Health Information Management Section. (2021). *Assess impact of COVID-19 pandemic in selected health services with estimation of "excess maternal deaths."* Integrated Health Information Management Section, Department of Health Services.

KC, P., Dhakal, S. C., & Chhetri, R. K. (2020). Changing pattern of employment in Nepal. *Journal Institute of Agriculture and Animal Science, 36*, 75–84. https://doi.org/10.3126/jiaas.v36i1.48385

Luitel, N. P., Breuer, E., Adhikari, A., Kohrt, B. A., Lund, C., Komproe, I. H., & Jordans, M. J. D. (2020). Process evaluation of a district mental healthcare plan in Nepal: A mixed-methods case study. *BJPsych Open, 6*(4), e77. https://doi.org/10.1192/bjo.2020.60

Merchant, H. F., Devlin, K., & Egan, K. F. (2016). *Nepal's community-based health system model: Structure, strategies, and learning.* Advancing Partners & Communities.

Ministry of Finance. (2018). *An assessment of sector wide approach in the health and education sectors of Nepal.* Ministry of Finance, Kathmandu Nepal. https://mof.gov.np/content/1403/an-assessment-of-sector-wide-approach--swap-/

Ministry of Health and Population. (n.d.). *Climate change and health.* https://climate.mohp.gov.np/34-scroll/index.php?option=com_content&view=article&id=160&catid=2

Ministry of Health and Population. (2021). *Progress of the health and population sector: National joint annual review report 2021.* https://www.nhssp.org.np/Resources/HPP/NJAR%20Report-%202021-Final.pdf

Ministry of Health and Population. (2022). *Health sector response to COVID-19 pandemic in Nepal.* https://www.nhssp.org.np/Resources/EA/Health%20Sector%20Response%20to%20COVID-19-Report-%20May%202022.pdf

Ministry of Health and Population. (2023). *Nepal national health accounts 2018/19 – 2019/20.* Ministry of Health and Population, Government of Nepal. https://drive.google.com/file/d/1whatUaO1aHkYE8c8pXTVp8CZoydEwV6U/view

Ministry of Health and Population/Department of Health Services. (2022). *Annual health report for fiscal year 2020–2021.* https://dohs.gov.np/content/40/annual-health-report-2077-78/

Ministry of Health and Population/Department of Health Services. (2024). *Annual health report for fiscal year 2022–2023.* https://dohs.gov.np/content/21/annual-health-report-2079-80-ahr/

Ministry of Health and Population, New ERA, & ICF. (2022). *Nepal health facility survey 2021 final report.* https://dhsprogram.com/pubs/pdf/SPA35/SPA35.pdf

Ministry of Health and Population, New ERA, & ICF. (2023). *Nepal demographic and health survey 2022.* Ministry of Health and Population. https://www.dhsprogram.com/pubs/pdf/FR379/FR379.pdf

Ministry of Health and Population & National Statistics Office. (2022). *National population and housing census 2021: Nepal maternal mortality study 2021.* Ministry of Health and Population; National Statistics Office.

Nepal Health Research Council. (2021). *Report of national mental health survey 2020.* Health Research Council, Government of Nepal. https://nhrc.gov.np/wp-content/uploads/2022/10/National-Mental-Health-Survey-Report2020.pdf

Nepal Health Research Council, Ministry of Health and Population, Institute for Health Metrics and Evaluation, Monitoring Evaluation and Operational Research. (2021). *Nepal burden of disease 2019: A country report based on the 2019 global burden of disease study.* https://nhrc.gov.np/wp-content/uploads/2022/02/BoD-Report-Book-includ-Cover-mail-6_compressed.pdf

U.S. Agency for International Development. (2020). *Nepal and Camris international, Nepal gender equality and social inclusion analysis 2020.* USAID.

World Bank Group. (2022). *UHC service coverage index.* World Health Organization, Global Health Observatory Data Repository. https://data.worldbank.org/indicator/SH.UHC.SRVS.CV.XD?locations=NP

World Bank Group. (2024). *The world bank in Nepal.* https://www.worldbank.org/en/country/nepal/overview

World Bank Group. (n.d.-a). *Nepal, country profile.* https://data.worldbank.org/country/NP

World Bank Group. (n.d.-b). *Nepal – vulnerability.* Climate Change Knowledge Portal. https://climateknowledgeportal.worldbank.org/country/nepal/vulnerability

World Health Organization. (2021). *Monitoring progress on universal health coverage and the health-related Sustainable Development Goals in the South- East Asia Region: 2021 Update.* WHO South-East Asia Region. https://iris.who.int/handle/10665/344764

World Health Organization. (2024). *Suicide mortality rate – Nepal.* https://data.who.int/indicators/i/16BBF41

World Health Organization Regional Office for South-East Asia. (2021). *Monitoring progress on universal health coverage and the health-related sustainable development goals in the South- East Asia Region.* https://iris.who.int/handle/10665/344764

World Population Review. (2024). *Where is Nepal in the world?* https://worldpopulationreview.com/countries/nepal/location

Worldometer. (2024). *Nepal demographics*. https://www.worldometers.info/demographics/nepal-demographics/

CHAPTER 47

PAKISTAN

Imran Bari, Uzma Rahim Khan, Mishalle Kayani, Fouzia Farooq, and Adnan A. Hyder

INTRODUCTION

Pakistan has a multifaceted healthcare system with government and private facilities functioning concurrently, and strong complementary and alternative medicine like homeopathy, **Hikmat** (traditional medicine), and spiritual healers (Ahmad et al., 2021). Traditionally, the healthcare delivery system has been jointly managed by federal and provincial governments, and districts have been tasked with implementation at the local level. The Pakistani health sector grapples with numerous challenges, including the escalating burden of a growing population with a total fertility rate of 3.5 births per woman (World Bank Group, 2021), a shortage of healthcare professionals, and insufficient funding, all of which hinder the delivery of quality healthcare services.

GEOGRAPHY AND POPULATION

GEOGRAPHIC FEATURES

Pakistan is located between the regions of South Asia, Central Asia, and the greater Middle East (Haleem, 2013). It borders Afghanistan and Iran in the west, India in the east, and China in the far northeast. The main river is the Indus, which flows through the entire country and is fed by the combined waters of three of the five rivers of Punjab—Chenab, Jhelum, and Ravi. Pakistan is a diverse country occupying over 880,000 square kilometers (546,806 square miles) and characterized by a vast range of topography, ecosystems, socioeconomic conditions, and climactic zones (World Bank Group, 2020). The country lies in a temperate zone, and like its topography, the climate varies as well. It is generally dry and hot near the coast and along the lowland plains of the Indus River and progressively cooler in the country's northern part (World Bank Group, 2020).

The country is divided into four provinces: Punjab, Sindh, Balochistan, and Khyber Pakhtunkhwa (Figure 47.1). Additionally, it has three territories: the Islamabad Capital Territory, Azad Jammu and Kashmir, and Gilgit-Baltistan (Permanent Committee on Geographical Names, 2024).

DEMOGRAPHIC FEATURES

As of 2022, Pakistan's population is approximately 235 million, making it the fifth largest country in the world in terms of population size (World Bank Group, 2022). The population pyramid illustrates a demographic structure with a substantial youth bulge, indicating that most of the population, approximately 66%, is under the age of 30 (Pakistan Bureau of Statistics [PBS], 2021). Sixty-four percent of the population resides in rural areas, while 36% resides in urban areas of Pakistan (PBS, 2021). Females comprise about 49.98% of the population, while males account for 50.02% (PBS, 2021). While the PBS has not reported the recent numbers for the transgender population, based on the last census (PBS, 2021a), approximately 10,418 transgender persons were recorded, although the actual number might be far greater.

FIGURE 47.1 Map of Pakistan.

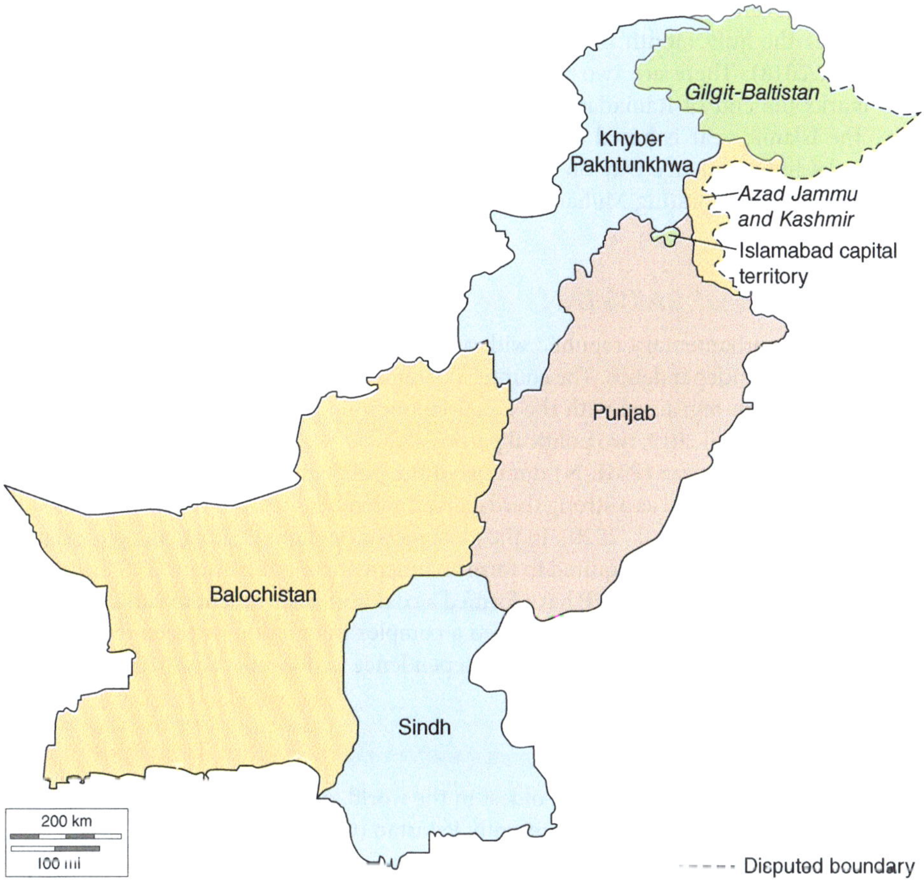

Source: UK Government. (2023). *Pakistan toponymic factfile.* UK Government. https://assets.publishing.service.gov.uk/media/650bf4cb27d43b0014375a60/Pakistan_Toponymic_Factfile.pdf

ETHNIC GROUPS, RELIGION, AND LANGUAGE

Pakistan has a multicultural society and hosts one of the largest refugee populations in the world, mainly from Afghanistan (Haleem, 2013). There are six major ethnic groups in the country. Among these, Punjabis make up roughly 44.7% of the population, followed by Pashtuns (Pathan) at 15.4%, Sindhis at 14.1%, Saraikis at 8.4%, "Muhajirs" at 7.6%, Baloch at 3.6%, and other groups accounting for 6.3% of the population (Central Intelligence Agency [CIA], 2024). Islam is the predominant religion in the country, with approximately 96.5% of the population identifying as Muslim; the rest is a mix of Christian, Hindu, Sikhs, Parsis (Zoroastrians), Bahá'ís, Buddhists, and Jains (Cultural Atlas, 2024).

Urdu and English are the two major languages, with Urdu being spoken or understood by 75% of Pakistanis. After reaching independence in 1947, Pakistan recognized only English as the official language (Permanent Committee on Geographical Names, 2024). However, in 2015, the Supreme Court of Pakistan directed federal and provincial governments to adopt Urdu as the official language (Permanent Committee on Geographical Names, 2024). Punjabi is also one of the most widely spoken first languages in Pakistan; other recognized languages include Baluchi, Pashto, Punjabi, Seraili, and Sindhi (Permanent Committee on Geographical Names, 2024).

CULTURE AND TRADITIONS

Pakistan observes several celebrations. Like other countries with large Muslim populations, Pakistan observes the holy month of Ramadan where observant Muslims fast from sunrise to sunset (Bada, 2018). There are two major Islamic holidays observed in Pakistan: Eid-al-Fitr, which marks the end of Ramadan, and Eid-al-Adha, which marks the end of the Hajj/Pilgrimage. The Islamic year is based on a lunar calendar. Aside from religious celebrations, the nation marks Independence Day on August 14, and December 25 is also celebrated as a national holiday, commemorating Muhammad Ali Jinnah's birthday (the founder of Pakistan; Bada, 2018).

POLITICAL SYSTEM OF PAKISTAN

Pakistan is a federal parliamentary republic with an electoral system that has undergone many manifestations since its independence. The country operates on a multiparty system, and in 2018, 120 political parties were registered with the Election Commission of Pakistan (ECP; Siddiqui et al., 2020). From 1988 until 2013, two political parties, namely People's Party Pakistan (PPP) and Pakistan Muslim League-Nawaz (PML-N) dominated the political landscape. In 2018, Pakistan Tehreek-e-Insaaf (PTI) emerged as a strong third-party contender, securing the majority of votes in the 2018 elections (Siddiqui et al., 2020). In the most recent elections of 2024, no political party won an absolute majority, which is required to form an independent government (U.S. Institute of Peace, n.d.). At present PML-N and PPP have formed a coalition government to run the country. Pakistan's political landscape has largely witnessed a complex interaction between the military–bureaucratic elite and the political elite since its independence (Siddiqui et al., 2020).

BRIEF COUNTRY HISTORY

The **Indus Valley civilization** is one of the oldest in the world, dating back approximately 5,000 years and spreading over much of what is presently Pakistan (CIA, 2024). The area has witnessed multiple invasions over the centuries from Persians, Greeks, Scythians, Arabs, Afghans, and Turks. In the 16th and 17th centuries, the Mughal Empire largely ruled, while the British dominated in the 18th century. In 1947, British India was divided into the Muslim state of Pakistan (with West and East sections) and a largely Hindu state of India. Several wars were fought between India and Pakistan, and to date, tensions exist. In 1971, East Pakistan became a separate nation presently known as Bangladesh.

HEALTH OUTCOMES

Health outcomes in Pakistan are influenced by various socioeconomic disparities, infrastructure challenges, and public health policies. While progress has been made over the years, in certain areas, especially those with limited healthcare access, significant hurdles persist.

LIFE EXPECTANCY

Pakistan has seen improvements in life expectancy over the last two decades. Life expectancy increased from 61.1 years in 1990 to 65.9 years in 2019, an increase of 7.9% (GBD 2019 Pakistan Collaborators, 2023). The gap in health life expectancy (HALE) between men and women has also decreased, as women's life expectancy increased by 8.22% during this period, compared to 7.44% for men (GBD 2019 Pakistan Collaborators, 2023). Despite improvements, Pakistan's life expectancy still falls below that of its neighboring countries—India (69.4 years), Bangladesh (72.3 years), Sri Lanka (76.8 years), and China (76.7 years; Ministry of Finance, Government of Pakistan, 2021).

LEADING CAUSES OF MORTALITY

Pakistan has a double burden of disease (having both communicable and noncommunicable diseases [NCDs]). Nearly 40% of the total burden of disease accounts for communicable/infectious diseases that mostly affect children, including respiratory diseases, diarrheal diseases, tuberculosis, malaria, and childhood clusters (measles, pertussis, and polio; GBD 2019 Pakistan Collaborators, 2023). Another 12% is due to reproductive health problems and specific nutritional deficiencies (Figure 47.2). The remaining burden of diseases is comprised mainly of noncommunicable/degenerative diseases, including cardiovascular diseases, diabetes, cancers, and other NCDs. Predominant causes of mortality in Pakistan include neonatal disorders, ischemic heart disease, stroke, diarrheal diseases, and lower respiratory infections (World Health Organization [WHO], 2024). The top two contributors of mortality among babies are low birth weight and preterm birth (GBD 2019 Pakistan Collaborators, 2023). Additionally, with a rise in pollution and climate change, particulate matter pollution has also been a leading risk factor contributing to the growing disease burden in the country from 1990 to 2019.

NONCOMMUNICABLE DISEASES

The country is, at present, witnessing an epidemiologic transition as the burden of disease shifts from communicable diseases to NCDs. Cardiovascular disease, cancers, and diabetes were identified as the leading NCDs contributing to the mortality burden in 2019 as shown in Figure 47.2 (GBD 2019 Pakistan Collaborators, 2023). The forecasted burden for 2040 in Pakistan shows a rapid increase in all three diseases with the estimation that they will become the overall leading causes of death in Pakistan by 2040 (GBD 2019 Pakistan Collaborators, 2023). Given this projection and with the current demographic structure of Pakistan, which has a significantly large population below the age of 40 years, preventive interventions targeting the NCD burden need to focus on informing the youth and young adults about changes in lifestyle choices and behaviors.

COMMUNICABLE DISEASES

In addition to NCDs, communicable diseases contribute significantly to the loss of lives in the country. The burden of tuberculosis and hepatitis is higher than expected and reducing the prevalence of these diseases is complicated by the fact that in most parts of the country, prescription medication and injections are not regulated (GBD 2019 Pakistan Collaborators, 2023). Pakistan also remains one of the last countries, in addition to Afghanistan, where polio is still an endemic virus. Since 1994, Pakistan has undertaken several initiatives aimed at polio eradication and while the burden of polio is quite low currently, a persistent and concerted effort is required for complete eradication.

MENTAL ILLNESS, ILLEGAL DRUG USE, AND SELF-HARM

Mental health remains a challenging situation in Pakistan as 10% to 20% of children and adolescents in the country have behavioral and mental disorders (Shah et al., 2022). About 9.99 per 1,000 people in Pakistan have epilepsy. Approximately 6.45 million people in Pakistan use illegal drugs, of which 70% are men age 15 to 40 years, with the most common illegal drugs as marijuana, benzodiazepines, heroin, and methamphetamine (Shah et al., 2022). Suicide and self-harm have also become a growing concern in Pakistan. Evidence indicates that females under 35 years of age—usually married housewives with low socioeconomic statuswere more likely to engage in self-harm. For suicides, the risk factors pointed to married males under the age of 35 years with low socioeconomic status (Shahid & Hyder, 2008).

MATERNAL INFANT MORTALITY

Although maternal and infant mortality rates have been declining over the years, there are still substantial concerns regarding these indicators, which reflect gaps in reproductive health services

FIGURE 47.2 Heat map of leading causes of all-age deaths in Pakistan and subnational locations, 2019.

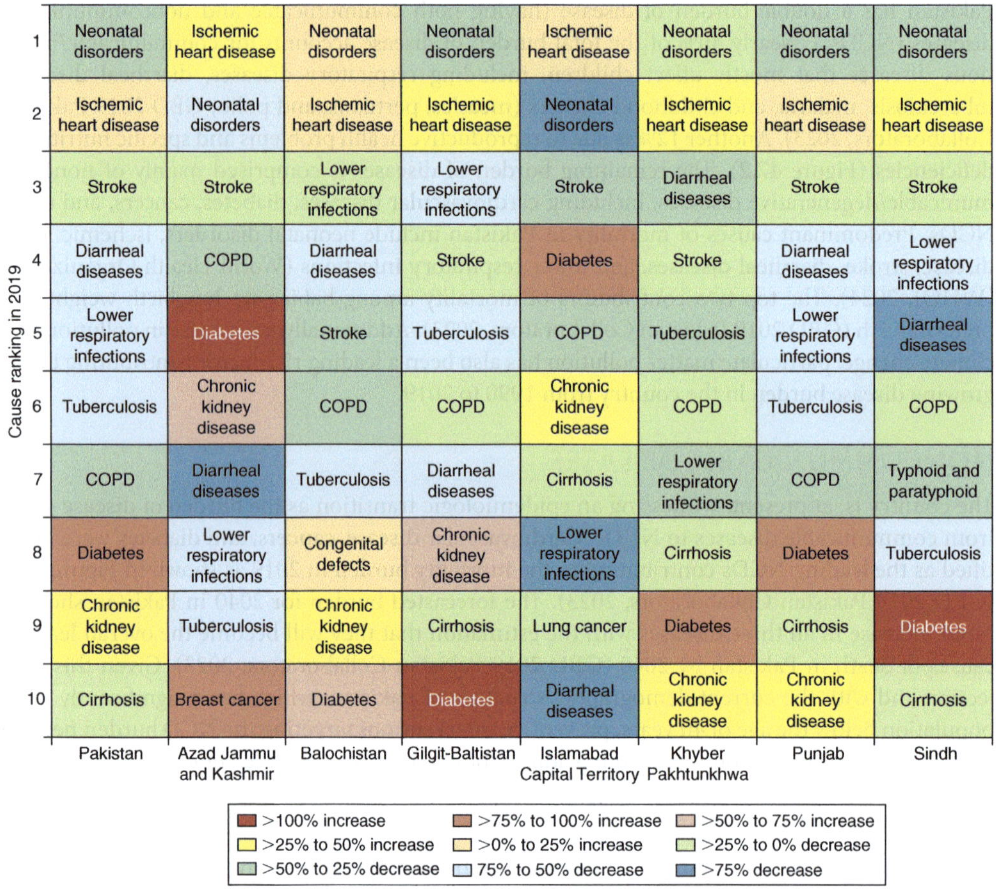

COPD, chronic obstructive pulmonary disease.

Source: GBD 2019 Pakistan Collaborators. (2023). The state of health in Pakistan and its provinces and territories, 1990–2019: A systematic analysis for the Global Burden of Disease Study 2019. *The Lancet Global Health, 11*(2), e229–e243. https://doi.org/10.1016/S2214-109X(22)00497-1

and prenatal care. The 2019 Pakistan Maternal Mortality Survey (PMMS) found that the maternal mortality ratio is 186 deaths per 100,000 live births (National Institute of Population Studies & Demographic and Health Surveys Program, 2020). According to the Pakistan Demographic and Health Survey (PDHS) of 2017 to 2018, the neonatal mortality rate in the country is 42 deaths per 1,000 live births, the infant mortality rate is 62 deaths per 1,000 live births, and the under-5 years mortality rate is 74 deaths per 1,000 live births (National Institute of Population Studies & ICF, 2019). The under-5 years mortality rate also varies by region, with 85 deaths per 1,000 live births in Punjab, 77 in Sindh, 64 in Khyber Pakhtunkhwa, and 78 in Balochistan (UNICEF, 2020).

DETERMINANTS OF HEALTH

ECONOMIC PROFILE

Pakistan is a low-middle income country with a gross domestic product (GDP) of $374.4 billion and an annual GDP growth rate of 4.7% (World Bank Group, 2022). The per-capita GDP per is $1,588.88 (World Bank Group, 2022). In 2022, the unemployment rate was 5.6% and inflation was recorded at 19.9% (World Bank Group, 2022).

In recent years, Pakistan's economy has drastically shrunk due to catastrophic floods and disrupted external support, which has caused public investment to plunge and private investment and industry to dwindle (Asian Development Bank, 2024). This economic downturn has been exacerbated by inflation, which has reached a five-decade high of 29.2% in Fiscal Year 2023 (Asian Development Bank, 2024). Supply disruptions and currency depreciation have driven up food and energy prices, adding to the strain on the economy, which in turn have led to low investments in the country (Asian Development Bank, 2024).

POVERTY

In Pakistan, poverty is a deeply entrenched issue, affecting millions of citizens and depriving them of the ability to meet basic needs such as food, shelter, and healthcare. As of 2023, poverty reached 37.2% ($3.65/day) in Pakistan (World Bank Group, 2023). The rate is slightly lower than the figures for 2018 but accounting for the population growth in the country, there are approximately 3 million more poor people than in 2018 (World Bank Group, 2023).

EDUCATION AND LITERACY

In 2022, Pakistan's literacy rate was 62.8%, higher among males (73.4%) than among females (51.9%; Ministry of Finance, Government of Pakistan, 2021). However, disparities in literacy rates not only persist between genders but also show variation across different regions and between urban and rural areas. In rural settings, the literacy rate was 54%, contrasting with the urban rate of 77.3% in 2022. Moreover, significant variations exist among provinces: Punjab had a literacy rate of 66.3%, followed by Sindh at 61.8%, Khyber Pakhtunkhwa at 55.1%, and Baluchistan at 54.5% (Ministry of Finance, Government of Pakistan, 2023). Furthermore, the rate of primary school (grades 1–5) or higher secondary school (grades 6–10) completion stands at 51%, with a notable disparity favoring males over females.

Pakistan has a high population growth rate, which poses a major challenge to the education sector. According to sources, approximately 43% of the population aged 15 and above is illiterate (Asian Development Bank, 2019). Despite these low literacy rates and education attainment scenarios, the government of Pakistan spends only 1.7% of its GDP on education (Ministry of Finance, Government of Pakistan, 2021).

MALNUTRITION

In Pakistan, 45% of the burden of mortality in children can be attributed to childhood malnutrition (Bhutta et al., 2013). According to Pakistan's National Nutrition Survey of 2018, the stunting and wasting rates of children under 5 years old were 40.2% and 17.7%, respectively, and about 29% of children are underweight (Ministry of National Health Services, Regulations and Coordination, 2019). Only 36% of children are exclusively breastfed for the first 6 months of life and, as a result, more than half the children under 5 years of age are deficient in vitamin A, 40% are deficient in both zinc and vitamin D, and nearly 62% are anemic (UNICEF, 2018). Addressing the issue of malnutrition requires a comprehensive approach that includes improving healthcare services, promoting proper nutrition practices, and addressing socioeconomic disparities.

HEALTH BEHAVIORS

In 2022, an estimated 25.4 million Pakistanis age 15 years and over used tobacco products (Tobacconomics, 2022). Among adolescents age 11 to 17 years, 85% of males and 89% of females are physically inactive (WHO, 2022). Among adults over the age of 18, 24% of males and 43% of females are physically inactive, while 30% of males and 50% of females in the 70 and over age group are physically inactive (WHO, 2022). In terms of achieving the diet-related NCD targets,

Pakistan has shown limited progress. Approximately 13.4% of adult women (age 18 years and over) and 7.5% of adult men are living with obesity (Global Nutrition Report, 2019).

CLIMATE CHANGE AND HEALTH

Pakistan is highly vulnerable to climate effects, posing serious challenges not only to the economy but also to the population's health. The impacts of climate change are increasingly visible through more frequent occurrences of droughts, floods, changes in precipitation patterns, decreased availability of freshwater, and loss of biodiversity (World Bank Group, n.d.; Ministry of Finance, Government of Pakistan, 2021). The country is also projected to see a 6.1°C (42.9°F) rise in average annual temperature from 1990 to 2100. As a result of this, a substantial increase in heat-related deaths, with the number of deaths in the elderly (65 years and older) is projected to increase from under 10 per 100,000 annually in 1961 to 1990 to approximately 63 per 100,000 by 2080 (World Bank Group, n.d.). Climate change is also contributing to the increased risk of vector-borne diseases like malaria and dengue, which could affect up to 46 million people annually by 2070 (Riaz et al., 2022). Currently, Pakistan is grappling with alarmingly high levels of air pollution, with certain urban areas consistently experiencing hazardous pollution levels throughout the year (Ministry of Finance, Government of Pakistan, 2021).

HEALTHCARE SYSTEM IN PAKISTAN

HEALTHCARE DELIVERY

Pakistan has kept the British healthcare system, which consists of the Beveridge model, since its partition from Britain in 1947 (Muhammad et al., 2023). This is characterized by a multifaceted healthcare delivery system divided into the public and private sectors. The public healthcare sector comprises a three-tier system: primary, secondary, and tertiary. At the first level, Basic Health Units (BHUs) and Rural Health Centers (RHCs) provide primary and secondary healthcare services, while Tehsil Headquarters Hospitals (THQs), district Headquarters Hospitals (DHQs), and teaching hospitals provide inpatient and specialized care (Figure 47.3; WHO, Regional Office for the Eastern Mediterranean, n.d.).

According to the Pakistani constitution, except for federally administered areas, provincial governments are mandated to manage healthcare. Traditionally, healthcare delivery has been jointly administered by the federal and provincial governments, with districts responsible for implementation. Services are organized through preventive, promotional, curative, and rehabilitative services (WHO, Regional Office for the Eastern Mediterranean, n.d.). The healthcare delivery system of Pakistan is represented in Figure 47.3. At the community level, healthcare is provided through a referral system where Lady Health Workers (LHWs) refer cases to first-level care facilities (BHUs and RHCs), and depending on the severity of the cases, referrals are made to secondary- and tertiary-level facilities. The referral system has not worked successfully as patients have reported dissatisfaction with the services offered at the nearest first-level care facilities (Siddiqi et al., 2001).

The private sector helps bridge the gap between the rising demand and limited public health facilities. The number of private hospitals, clinics, and diagnostic laboratories has increased considerably over the years. Despite the presence of both public and private healthcare systems, the quality of care is sometimes questionable, particularly in the public sector. Moreover, the private sector is often associated with high costs, rendering healthcare services inaccessible to a significant portion of the population (Muhammad et al., 2023).

A critical component of the healthcare system in Pakistan includes the Emergency Medical Services (EMS), established in 2006, which provides prehospital emergency care across the nation to over 220 million people (Baig et al., 2024) The EMS system is governed by the provincial

FIGURE 47.3 Healthcare delivery system of Pakistan.

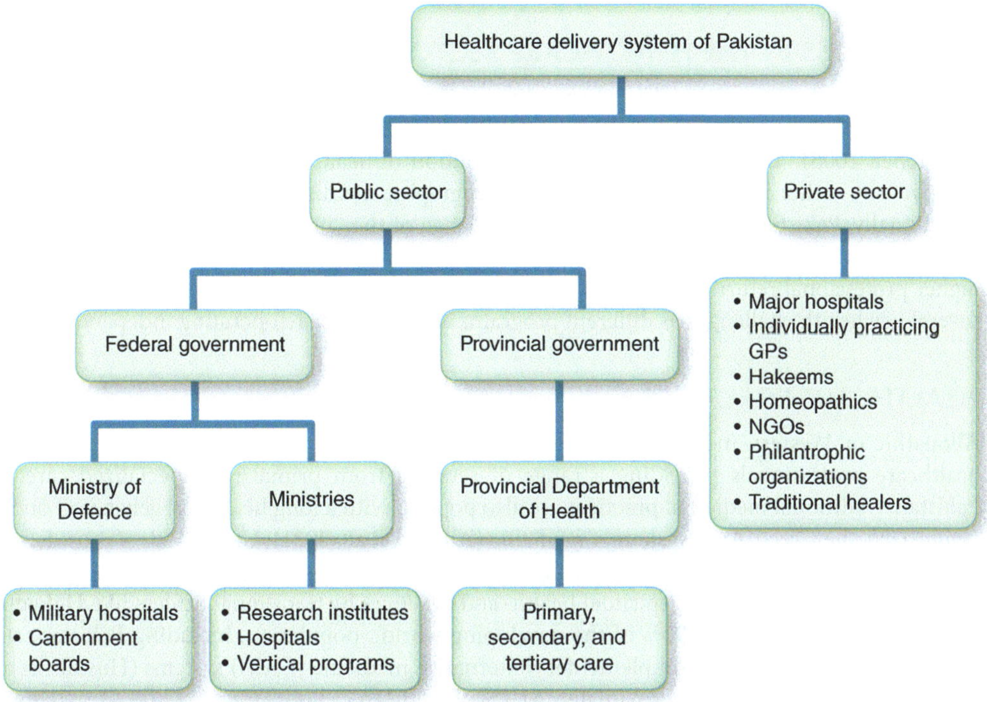

GP, general practitioner; NGO, nongovernmental organization.

Source: Nazakat, S., & Sajid, M. (2022). Comparison and analysis of health care delivery system: Pakistan versus Russia. *Global Social Sciences Review, 7*, 184–195. https://doi.org/10.31703/gssr.2022(VII-II).18

governments, whereas ambulance services are operated through a mix of private, not-for-profit, and philanthropic organizations.

HEALTHCARE INFRASTRUCTURE

The national health infrastructure comprises 1,201 hospitals, 5,518 BHUs, 683 RHCs, 5,802 dispensaries, 731 maternity and child health centers, and 347 tuberculosis centers; the total availability of beds in these health facilities is estimated to be 123,394 (WHO, Regional Office for the Eastern Mediterranean, n.d.). In addition, more than 95,000 LHWs provide healthcare services to communities in rural areas.

Data from 2017 show that the total health workforce includes 195,896 registered doctors, 18,333 registered dentists, and 99,228 registered nurses (WHO, Regional Office for the Eastern Mediterranean, n.d.). The population per doctor is 997, per dentist is 10,658, and per bed is 1,584.

HEALTHCARE FUNDING

The public healthcare system suffers from insufficient funding. The country spends approximately 1.2% of its GDP on health, which is much lower than the 6% that is recommended by WHO (Muhammad et al., 2023). This has inevitably led to a shortage of hospitals, doctors, nurses, and medical equipment in the public sector (Muhammad et al., 2023). Although the government introduced a national health insurance scheme in 2018 through the Sehat Sahulat Program (SSP) to reduce out-of-pocket payments and increase access to healthcare services, particularly for marginalized communities, the country is still struggling in terms of implementation and reach (Hasan et al., 2022).

CHALLENGES IN THE HEALTHCARE SECTOR

In addition to the low national-level spending, private-sector healthcare is quite costly for the general population, with 78% of the population paying for healthcare out-of-pocket (Shaikh & Hatcher, 2005). There is an inequitable distribution of healthcare resources with a focus on curative care rather than preventive care, and geographic maldistribution favoring urban areas. Additionally, Pakistan is grappling with the challenge of the "brain drain" phenomenon, where healthcare professionals are leaving the country in search of better career opportunities and higher professional returns (Khan et al., 2023). The country lacks coordinated efforts to address several key health challenges as different programs and facilities are operating independently.

HEALTHCARE PRACTICES

Allopathic or Western medicine is widely practiced, with a network of hospitals, clinics, and healthcare professionals providing a range of services from primary to specialized care. In Pakistan, traditional medicinal practices are also popular with a long history largely based on the *Unani Tibb*, the Greco-Arab system of medicine (Ahmad et al., 2021). Unani Tibb is considered a first-line treatment among many tribal communities (Ahmad et al., 2021). Other traditional practices include herbal remedies, spiritual health, and practices by traditional healers like **Hakeems** (Ahmad et al., 2021). Over 80% of the developing world's population, including Pakistan, still depends on traditional and complementary/alternative medicine (CAM) systems (Hussain et al., 2012). Surveys reports that approximately 51.7% of Pakistanis choose CAM, while 48.3% choose allopathic biomedicine (Shaikh & Thatcher, 2005).

HEALTHCARE INNOVATIONS

In recent years, telemedicine initiatives have gained traction in Pakistan, enabling remote consultations and healthcare access, especially in underserved areas. In a study conducted at a tertiary healthcare facility in Karachi providing telemental health services, participants highlighted several benefits of virtual consultations such as the cost-effectiveness of the service and the destigmatization of mental health (Asad et al., 2024). Concerns related to privacy and issues with access to technology were some challenges identified by the participants (Asad et al., 2024). Digital health records and information systems are being developed to streamline healthcare delivery, ensuring better coordination and continuity of care. In tandem, several public health initiatives, such as vaccination drives and disease eradication programs, showcase innovation in preventive healthcare. Moreover, research and development in biotechnology and pharmaceuticals contribute to advancements in medical treatments.

CONCLUSION

This brief overview reveals a multifaceted healthcare landscape in Pakistan shaped by demographics, culture, economics, and health practices. Progress has been made in health systems, but persistent challenges require ongoing attention. To improve the healthcare system and overall health status of the country, to strengthen the primary healthcare infrastructure, particularly in rural and underserved areas, and to encourage community engagement and participatory approaches to healthcare planning and delivery, education and investment in mental health services and awareness campaigns are critical. There is evidence that the social determinants of health are increasingly important in healthcare. Improving education, reducing poverty, and addressing gender disparities in Pakistan are crucial aspects that should be prioritized by the government.

LEARNING ACTIVITIES

CourseConnect

To access self-assessment questions and interactive, competency-based learning activities for this chapter, visit www.springerpub.com/courseconnect. See inside front cover and tear-out for CourseConnect details.

REFERENCES

Ahmad, K., Ahmad, M., Huber, F. K., & Weckerle, C. S. (2021). Traditional medicinal knowledge and practices among the tribal communities of Thakht-e-Sulaiman Hills, Pakistan. *BMC Complementary Medicine and Therapies, 21*(1), 230. https://doi.org/10.1186/s12906-021-03403-1

Asad, N., Pirani, S., Osama, K., & Nadeem, T. (2024). Patients' experiences with tele-mental health services during COVID-19 in Pakistan. *Eastern Mediterrianean Health Journal, 30*(4), 283–291. https://doi.org/10.26719/2024.30.4.283

Asian Development Bank. (2019). *School education in Pakistan: A sector assessment*. https://www.adb.org/documents/pakistan-school-education-sector-assessment

Asian Development Bank. (2024). *Asian Development Outlook April 2024: Pakistan*. https://www.adb.org/sites/default/files/publication/957856/pak-ado-april-2024.pdf?

Bada, F. (2018). *Pakistani culture, customs, and traditions*. WorldAtlas. https://www.worldatlas.com/articles/pakistani-culture-customs-and-traditions.html

Baig, M. N. A., Khan, N., Naseer, R., Akhter, S., Shaikh, A. J., & Razzak, J. A. (2024). Pakistan's emergency medical services (EMS) system & out-of-hospital-cardiac-arrest (OHCA): A narrative review of an EMS system of a low middle income country in context of OHCA. *Resuscitation Plus, 8*, 100627. https://doi.org/10.1016/j.resplu.2024.100627

Bhutta, Z. A., Das, J. K., Rizvi, A., Gaffey, M. F., Walker, N., Horton, S., Webb, P., Lartey, A., Black, R. E., The Lancet Nutrition Interventions Review Group, & the Maternal and Child Nutrition Study Group. (2013). Evidence-based interventions for improvement of maternal and child nutrition: What can be done and at what cost? *The Lancet, 382*(9890), 452–477. https://doi.org/10.1016/s0140-6736(13)60996-4

Central Intelligence Agency. (2024). *Pakistan—People and society*. The World Factbook. https://www.cia.gov/the-world-factbook/countries/pakistan/

Cultural Atlas. (2024). *Pakistani—Religion*. https://culturalatlas.sbs.com.au/pakistani-culture/pakistani-culture-religion

GBD 2019 Pakistan Collaborators. (2023). The state of health in Pakistan and its provinces and territories, 1990–2019: A systematic analysis for the Global Burden of Disease Study 2019. *The Lancet Global Health, 11*(2), e229–e243. https://doi.org/10.1016/S2214-109X(22)00497-1

Global Nutrition Report. (2019). *Country nutrition profile: Pakistan*. https://globalnutritionreport.org/resources/nutrition-profiles/asia/southern-asia/pakistan/

Haleem, S. (2013). *Pakistan—Culture smart! The essential guide to customs and culture*. Kuperard.

Hasan, S. S., Mustafa, Z. U., Kow, C. S., & Merchant, H. A. (2022). "Sehat sahulat program": A leap into the universal health coverage in Pakistan. *International Journal of Environmental Research Public Health, 9*(12), 6998. https://doi.org/10.3390/ijerph19126998

Hussain, S. S., Malik, F., Khalid, N., Qayyum, A. M., & Riaz, H. (2012). Alternative and traditional medicines systems in pakistan: History, regulation, trends, usefulness, challenges, prospects and limitations. *IntechOpen*. https://doi.org/10.5772/28224

Khan, S. J., Asif, M., Aslam, S., Khan, W. J., & Hamza, S. A. (2023). Pakistan's healthcare system: A review of major challenges and the first comprehensive universal health coverage initiative. *Cureus, 15*(9), 44641. https://doi.org/10.7759/cureus.44641

Ministry of Finance, Government of Pakistan. (2021). *Pakistan Economic Survey 2020–21*. Economic Adviser's Wing, Ministry of Finance. https://www.finance.gov.pk/survey/chapters_21/PES_2020_21.pdf

Ministry of Finance, Government of Pakistan. (2023). *Economic survey of Pakistan 2022–23*. Government of Pakistan. https://www.finance.gov.pk/survey/chapter_25/10_Education.pdf

Ministry of National Health Services, Regulations and Coordination. (2019). *National nutrition survey 2018: Key findings report (Volume 1)*. United Nations Children's Fund and Aga Khan University. https://www.unicef.org/pakistan/media/2861/file/NNS%20KFR.pdf

Muhammad, Q., Eiman, H., Fazal, F., Ibrahim, M., & Gondal, M. F. (2023). Healthcare in Pakistan: Navigating challenges and building a brighter future. *Cureus, 15*(6), e40218. https://doi.org/10.7759/cureus.40218

National Institute of Population Studies & Demographic and Health Surveys Program. (2020). *Pakistan maternal mortality survey 2019: Summary report*. https://dhsprogram.com/pubs/pdf/SR267/SR267.pdf

National Institute of Population Studies & ICF. (2019). *Pakistan demographic and health survey 2017–18: Key demographic and health indicators*. https://www.dhsprogram.com/pubs/pdf/FR354/FR354.pdf

Pakistan Bureau of Statistics. (2021a). *Final results of census-2017*. https://www.pbs.gov.pk/content/final-results-census-2017-0

Pakistan Bureau of Statistics. (2021b). *Percentage distribution of population by age, sex and area: Pakistan*. https://www.pbs.gov.pk/sites/default/files/labour_force/publications/lfs2020_21/tables/Table_1.pdf

Permanent Committee on Geographical Names. (2024). *Pakistan: Toponymic factfile*. https://assets.publishing.service.gov.uk/media/6717aaa7d29a0f082ac9c174/Pakistan_Toponymic_Factfile.pdf

Riaz, K., Ahmad, M., Gul, S., Malik, M. H. B. A., & Ur Rehman, M. E. (2022). Climate change and its implications on health and the healthcare system: A perspective from Pakistan. *Annals of Medicine and Surgery, 81*, 104507. https://doi.org/10.1016/j.amsu.2022.104507

Shah, S. M., Sun, T., Xu, W., Jiang, W., & Yuan, Y. (2022). The mental health of China and Pakistan, mental health laws and COVID-19 mental health policies: A comparative review. In Y. Xu & J. Chen (Eds.), *General psychiatry* (Vol. 35, Issue 5). BMJ Publishing Group.

Shahid, M., & Hyder, A. A. (2008). Deliberate self-harm and suicide: A review from Pakistan. *International Journal of Injury Control Safety Promotion, 15*(4), 233–241. https://doi.org/10.1080/17457300802149811

Shaikh, B. T., & Hatcher, J. (2005). Complementary and alternative medicine in Pakistan: Prospects and limitations. *Evidence Based Complement Alternative Medicine, 2*(2), 139–142. https://doi.org/10.1093/ecam/neh088

Siddiqi, S., Kielmann, A., Khan, M., Ali, N., Ghaffar, A., Sheikh, U., & Mumtaz, Z. (2001). The effectiveness of patient referral in Pakistan. *Health Policy Plan, 16*(2), 193–18. https://doi.org/10.1093/heapol/16.2.193

Siddiqui, N., Mufti, M., & Shafqat, S. (2020). Introduction: Pakistan's political parties in an era of transition. In N. Siddiqui, M. Mufti, & S. Shafqat (Eds.), *Pakistan's political parties: Surviving between dictatorship and democracy* (pp. 1–20). Georgetown University Press.

Tobacconomics. (2022). *Research: Tobacco taxes in Pakistan (fact sheet)*. https://tobacconomics.org/research/tobacco-taxes-in-pakistan/

UNICEF. (2018). *Pakistan: Nutrition*. https://www.unicef.org/pakistan/nutrition-0

UNICEF. (2020). *Situation analysis update 2020—Children in Pakistan*. https://www.unicef.org/pakistan/media/5301/file/Situation%20Analysis%20Update%202020:%20Children%20in%20Pakistan.pdf

U.S. Institute of Peace. (n.d.). *Understanding Pakistan's election results*. https://www.usip.org/publications/2024/02/understanding-pakistans-election-results

World Bank Group. (n.d.). *Pakistan country profile — Climate change knowledge portal*. https://climateknowledgeportal.worldbank.org/sites/default/files/2021-05/15078-WB_Pakistan%20Country%20Profile-WEB.pdf

World Bank Group. (2020). *Pakistan–Climate data, historical*. Climate Change Knowledge Portal. https://climateknowledgeportal.worldbank.org/country/pakistan/climate-data-historical

World Bank Group. (2021). *Fertility rate, total (births per woman)*. Gender Data Portal. https://genderdata.worldbank.org/en/indicator/sp-dyn-tfrt-in

World Bank Group. (2022). *Population, total – Pakistan*. World Development Indicators. https://databankfiles.worldbank.org/public/ddpext_download/POP.pdf?utm_source=chatgpt.com

World Bank Group. (2023). *Global poverty estimates for Pakistan — 2023 (people living under $3.65/day, 2017 PPP)*. https://databankfiles.worldbank.org/public/ddpext_download/poverty/987B9C90-CB9F-4D93-AE8C-750588BF00QA/current/Global_POVEQ_PAK.pdf

World Health Organization, Regional Office for the Eastern Mediterranean. (n.d.). *Health service delivery—Pakistan*. WHO EMRO. https://www.emro.who.int/pak/programmes/service-delivery.html

World Health Organization. (2022). *Physical inactivity profile 2022 – Pakistan*. https://cdn.who.int/media/docs/default-source/country-profiles/physical-activity/physical-activity-pak-2022.pdf?sfvrsn=9c04

World Health Organization. (2024). *Global health estimates 2021: Deaths by cause, age, sex, by country and by region, 2000–2021* [Data portal]. https://www.who.int/data/gho/data/themes/mortality-and-global-health-estimates/ghe-leading-causes-of-death

PART XII: Health and Healthcare in East Asia

CHAPTER 48

OVERVIEW OF EAST ASIA

Sophie Whittington and Thomas Foley

GEOGRAPHY

East Asia is the second most populous subregion of Asia. It includes China, Japan, North Korea, South Korea, Mongolia, and Taiwan. The diverse territory of East Asia consists of important geographic features such as the Himalaya Mountains, Yangtze River, Gobi Desert, Mongolian–Manchurian Steppe, and Japan Sea. East Asia includes both sparsely populated rural areas such as across much of Mongolia and Western China, and highly dense urban areas such as in Taiwan, Macau, and Hong Kong. East Asia is also home to some of the world's most populous and influential cities, including Tokyo and Osaka in Japan, Seoul in South Korea, and Beijing and Shanghai in China (Britannica, 2024). Figure 48.1 is a map of East Asia.

BRIEF HISTORY

East Asia has a rich and complex history. The traditions, beliefs, and practices predominant in East Asia, especially from early Chinese culture, have had a significant global influence. China is recognized as a **cradle of civilization**, a place where civilization emerged independently, and one of the world's earliest civilizations. China existed for more than a thousand years prior to the emergence of other East Asian nations. The **Han Dynasty** ruled China for more than four centuries, marking

FIGURE 48.1 Map of East Asia.

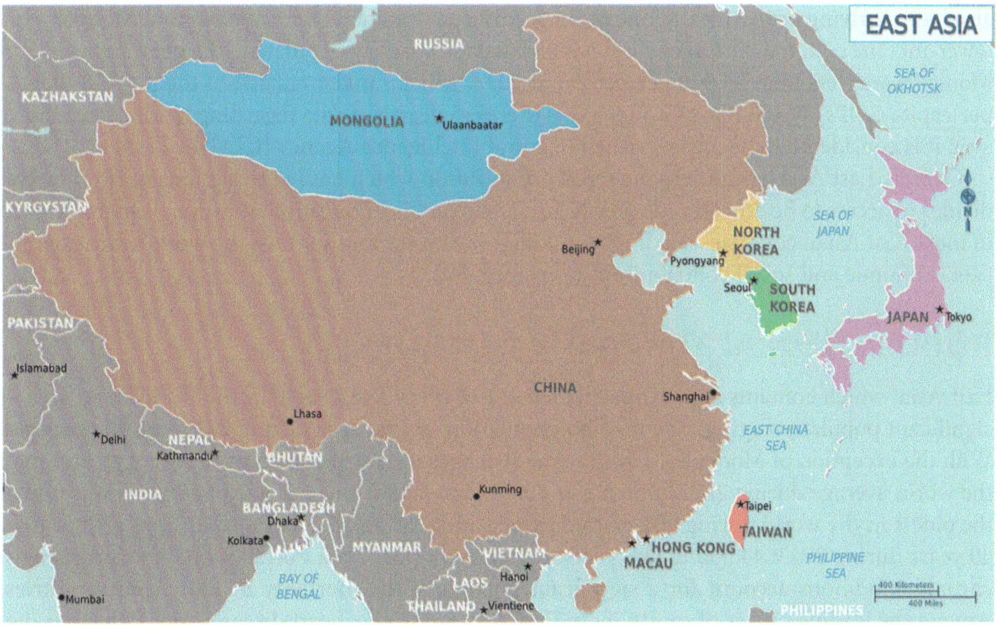

Source: Cacahuate. (2008). *Map of East Asia*. https://commons.wikimedia.org/wiki/File:Map_of_East_Asia.png.

the height of Imperial China's expansion and strength. The **Chinese Revolution of 1911** led to the establishment of the **Republic of China**, signifying the end of dynastic rule in China (Fairbank & Goldman, 2006). Japan replaced Imperial China as the leading power in the region and seized control of Taiwan from China during the latter part of the 19th century and then Korea during the early part of the 20th century. After Japan was defeated by the Allied Forces during World War II, it ceded control of Taiwan and Korea (Gordon, 2014). The Allied Powers divided unified Korea into two separate regions: North Korea, which was initially occupied and later supported by the Soviet Union, and South Korea, which was initially occupied and later supported by the United States. The Republic of Korea in South Korea and the **Democratic People's Republic of Korea** in North Korea were established in 1948. The two Koreas remain separated by the Korean Demilitarized Zone and ideological differences based on Soviet and U.S. influences (Cumings, 2005). Control of Taiwan was returned to China; however, the defeat of the Republic of China by the **Chinese Communist Party** in 1949 complicated claims to rule on the island nation of Taiwan. The Republic of China fled from mainland China to Taiwan and established their control over Taiwan while the Chinese Communist Party took control of mainland China and established the present-day **People's Republic of China** (Fairbank & Goldman, 2006). Following a history of influence and occupation by China and the former Soviet Union, Mongolia established an independent democracy and market economy in the early 1990s, which it has since maintained (Rossabi, 2014).

SOCIOECONOMIC FACTORS

East Asia's socioeconomic landscape is characterized by diverse economic and social development. While China has the world's second largest gross domestic product (GDP) behind only the United States, its per-capita GDP represents more of a middle-income nation. The inequity between its national GDP (approximately \$18.9 trillion in 2023) and per-capita distribution (\$12,600 in 2023) is a product of its large population and social inequities. Japan and South Korea, along with China, rank among the world leaders in GDP. The equity in Japan and South Korea are much more favorable, however, when compared to China. The per-capita GDPs in Japan and South Korea during 2023 were both slightly more than \$33,000 per person. Taiwan also has a thriving economy and one of the leading per-capita GDPs in the region. Mongolia is a lower-income country, typical of rural nations that are sparsely populated. The per-capita GDP in Mongolia was less than \$6,000 per person in 2023, which ranked outside of the top 100 highest per-capita GDPs (World Bank Group, n.d.). There is a dearth of data regarding North Korea; however, it is considered to be impoverished (Central Intelligence Agency [CIA], 2024).

Overall, East Asia has undergone rapid urbanization which has led to significant rural–urban divides in access to healthcare, education, and quality of life. Education, however, is highly valued in most East Asian countries, leading to a skilled workforce and some of the world's most significant economic and social contributions (Lansford, 2023).

POPULATION AND HEALTH OUTCOMES

East Asia, which contains approximately one out of every five people in the world, is an area of significant population aging. The median population in East Asia during 2023 was 40 years old. With the exception of Mongolia, all of the median ages in East Asian countries were greater than the world average during 2023, which was 30.4 years. Japan's median age of 49 years was one of the oldest in the world during 2023. South Korea and Taiwan also had median ages greater than 40 years during 2023: 44.5 and 43.5 years, respectively (UN Data Portal, n.d.). Not surprisingly, chronic conditions account for a significant portion of the mortality in East Asian countries. Among the leading causes of mortality in East Asia are stroke, heart disease, and Alzheimer disease (Institute for Health Metrics and Evaluation [IHME], 2024).

While a significant increase in preventable chronic disease morbidity and mortality is an issue in East Asian countries, the region has favorable health outcomes when compared to other regions. Life expectancy from birth in East Asia was nearly 79 years in 2023. The infant mortality rate was 5.1 infant deaths per 1,000 live births in 2023 (UN Data Portal, n.d.). The maternal mortality ratio was 24 maternal deaths per 100,000 live births in 2020 (UN Population Fund, n.d.). Japan and South Korea are among world leaders in life expectancy and preventing maternal and infant mortality. While it is extremely important for East Asian countries to address the increasing incidences of preventable chronic diseases and to ensure the quality of life among their aging populations, there is much for the global community to learn about healthy living from the cultures within East Asia. Refer to Table 48.1 for information about East Asia's population and health.

TABLE 48.1 EAST ASIA POPULATION AND HEALTH DATA

REGION/ COUNTRY	POPULATION (2023)	LIFE EXPECTANCY AT BIRTH IN YEARS (2023)	INFANT MORTALITY RATE PER 1,000 BIRTHS (2023)	MATERNAL MORTALITY RATIO PER 100,000 BIRTHS (2020)	LEADING CAUSE OF MORTALITY (2021)
East Asia	1.66 billion	78.89	5.1	24	—
China	1.42 billion	77.95	5.1	23	Stroke
Japan	124 million	84.71	1.6	4.3	Alzheimer disease
Mongolia	3.43 million	71.33	10.6	39.5	Heart disease
North Korea	26.43 million	73.64	14.5	106.7	Stroke
South Korea	51.75 million	84.33	2.1	8.1	Stroke
Taiwan	23.32 million	80.56	3	13	Heart disease

Sources: Institute for Health Metrics and Evaluation. (n.d.). *Health research by location: Country profiles.* https://www.healthdata.org/research-analysis/health-by-location/profiles; UN Data Portal. (n.d.). *UN Population Division Data Portal*. United Nations. https://population.un.org/dataportal/home/; United Nations Population Fund. (2024). *Data portal*. United Nations. https://www.unfpa.org/data.

LEARNING ACTIVITIES

CourseConnect >

To access self-assessment questions and interactive, competency-based learning activities for this chapter, visit www.springerpub.com/courseconnect. See inside front cover and tear-out for CourseConnect details.

REFERENCES

Britannica. (2024). *East Asia*. www.britannica.com/place/East-Asia

Central Intelligence Agency. (2024). *Korea, North: The world factbook*. https://www.cia.gov/the-world-factbook/countries/

Cumings, B. (2005). *Korea's place in the sun: A modern history*. W. W. Norton & Company.
Fairbank, J. K., & Goldman, M. (2006). *China: A new history* (2nd enlarged ed.). Belknap Press of Harvard University Press.
Gordon, A. (2014). *A modern history of Japan: From Tokugawa times to the present* (3rd ed.). Oxford University Press.
Institute for Health Metrics and Evaluation. (n.d.). *Health research by location: Country profiles*. University of Washington. https://www.healthdata.org/research-analysis/health-by-location/profiles
Lansford, T. (2023). *Political handbook of the world 2022–2023*. CQ Press.
Rossabi, M. (2014). *Modern Mongolia: From khans to commissars to capitalists*. University of California Press.
UN Data Portal. (n.d.). *UN Population Division data portal*. United Nations. https://population.un.org/dataportal/home/
UN Population Fund. (2024). *Data portal*. United Nations. https://www.unfpa.org/data.
World Bank Group. (n.d.). *The World Bank open data*. https://data.worldbank.org/.

CHAPTER 49

JAPAN

Akiko S. Hosler

GEOGRAPHY AND POPULATION

Japan is an island nation consisting of five major islands—Hokkaido, Honshu, Shikoku, Kyushu, and Okinawa—and over 14,000 small islands along the Pacific Ring of Fire. Northernmost Hokkaido has a humid continental climate with cold winters, while southernmost Okinawa has a subtropical climate. Northern Honshu is known as one of the snowiest regions in the world, and the entire country is prone to earthquakes. Japan's territory is 377,975 square kilometers (234,862 square miles). While the land area of Japan is 67% forests and 12% agricultural, most of Japan's 124.4 million inhabitants concentrate in coastal urban areas (National Statistics Center, 2024).

In 2023, the median age of the Japanese was 49 years, an increase of more than 10 years since 1994, and 29.5.2% of its population was 65 years or older (United Nations, 2024). Coupled with low total fertility rates, which have fluctuated between 1.30 and 1.45 in the last 10 years, a shrinking population and increasing proportions of the elderly are major concerns (Ministry of Health, Labour, and Welfare [MHLW], 2024). Approximately 3,224,000 foreign nationals resided in Japan in 2023. The three largest foreign national groups were Chinese, Vietnamese, and South Korean (National Statistics Center, 2024).

POLITICS, LANGUAGE, CULTURE, AND RELIGION

Japan is an industrialized democratic nation with a **parliamentary constitutional monarchy** type of government like the United Kingdom. Under Japan's constitution, the Emperor assumes a ceremonial role while the Prime Minister, who is nominated by the Parliament, holds executive power. Japanese is the de facto national language of Japan. While Japanese culture, from traditional arts, crafts, and cuisine to contemporary popular culture, is widely recognized and appreciated, Japanese religious life is not well understood, in part due to the unique history and status of religions in Japan. In 2022, 84,206 Shinto shrines and 76,701 Buddhist temples existed in Japan (Agency for Cultural Affairs, 2023). **Shinto** is the Indigenous religion of Japan while Buddhism was introduced in the sixth century. The Japanese, historically, practiced the two religions concurrently. Still today most Japanese people participate in both Shinto and Buddhist rituals for commemorating major life events and celebrating calendar events while not officially affiliated with any specific religion. Some health-related behaviors and beliefs in Japan have roots in religion, such as handwashing and environmental hygiene practices (Shinto) and a vegan diet (Buddhism).

HEALTH OUTCOMES

LIFE EXPECTANCY AT BIRTH

Japan's life expectancy has been increasing steadily over several decades, and, since the mid-1980s, Japan has been the nation with the longest life expectancy in the world. In 2023, life expectancy at birth was 84.7 years. Female life expectancy at birth was 87.74 while men's life expectancy at birth was 81.69 (United Nations, 2024). Reasons for exceptional life expectancy are multifactorial, drawing upon several of the main determinants of health.

LEADING CAUSES OF DEATH

In 2022, the top five leading causes of death among Japanese men were cancer, heart disease, **cerebrovascular disease** (stroke), pneumonia, and dementia. Among Japanese women, they were cancer, heart disease, dementia, cerebrovascular disease, and pneumonia. Cancers of the lung, colon, and stomach were the three leading cancer deaths in men, while cancers of the colon, lung, and pancreas were the three leading cancer deaths in women (MHLW, 2024). Although cerebrovascular disease was the leading cause of death in Japan in the 1960s and 1970s, it declined dramatically since then, largely due to successful nationwide sodium reduction campaigns (Kokubo, 2017). During 2022, suicide was the number one cause of death in men 10 to 44 years of age and in women 10 to 34 years of age. Suicide death rates for the Japanese overall have been in decline, from 40.0 per 100,000 in 2003 to 22.9 per 100,000 in 2019 (MHLW, 2024), but are still approximately 1.6 times higher than the U.S. rate of 14.5 per 100,000 (Centers for Disease Control and Prevention [CDC], 2024). Homicides are rare in Japan, with a homicide death rate of 0.23 per 100,000 in 2022 (MHLW, 2024). The U.S. homicide death rate, 7.8 per 100,000, was approximately 34 times greater than the Japanese rate in the same year (CDC, 2024).

MATERNAL AND INFANT MORTALITY

In Japan during 2023, the infant mortality rate was 1.6 infant deaths per 1,000 live births and the under-5 years mortality rate was 2.3 newborn deaths prior to per 1,00 live births (United Nations, 2024). The maternal mortality ratio in 2020 was 4.0 maternal deaths per 100,000 live births. Japanese infant and under-5 years mortality rates and maternal mortality ratio are among the lowest (under 5%) in the world and the lowest among the **G7 nations**, which include Canada, France, Germany, Italy, Japan, the United Kingdom, and the United States (World Bank Group, 2024).

Japan started a comprehensive maternal child health improvement program in 1948, featuring a "mother and child handbook" to educate pregnant women about pregnancy-related health practices and schedules and to keep track of all prenatal and postnatal care (Nakamura, 2007). The handbook is still in use today, and its concept has been exported to many nations.

COMMUNICABLE DISEASES

Like other industrialized nations, communicable diseases are no longer the leading causes of death in Japan. In terms of morbidity, the five leading reportable communicable diseases in Japan in 2021 were pulmonary tuberculosis (TB), syphilis (all stages), enterohemorrhagic *Escherichia coli* (*E. coli*) infection, Legionnaires' disease, and carbapenem-resistant *Enterobacterales* (CRE) infection. TB cases declined from 31,483 cases in 2011 to 16,299 cases in 2021. Syphilis has increased disproportionately in recent years; the total cases of syphilis in 2021 (n = 7,978) were more than 10 times greater than those in 2010 (n = 621). Japan was affected by COVID-19 early on as the first confirmed case was reported on January 16, 2020 (National Institute of Infectious Diseases [NIID], 2024). A total of 33,320,438 COVID-19 cases and 72,997 COVID-related deaths were reported as of March 10, 2023. Japan's COVID-19 mortality rate (57.72 per 100,000) was the lowest among the 20 countries most affected by the COVID-19 and about 1/6 of the United States' COVID-19 mortality rate (Johns Hopkins Coronavirus Resource Center, 2024).

NONCOMMUNICABLE DISEASES AND MENTAL HEALTH

In Japan, noncommunicable diseases (NCDs) are the major causes of death, decreased quality of life, and disability. The Japanese medical community considers most NCDs and some mental and emotional disorders as **lifestyle-related diseases**. A nationwide patient survey revealed that common lifestyle-related diseases (excluding dental and eye conditions) are hypertension, hyperlipidemia, type 2 diabetes, cancer, heart disease, asthma, cerebrovascular disease, mood and emotional disorders (including bipolar disorder), osteoporosis, atopic dermatitis (eczema), neurosis (phobia, panic disorder, obsessive-compulsive disorder [OCD], stress-related disorders), and sleeping disorder (Japan Preventive Association of Lifestyle-related Disease [JPALD], 2024). The most common cancer sites are prostate, colon, stomach, and lung in men and breast, colon, lung, and stomach in women (MHLW, 2024). Since 2008, Japan has had a nationwide program to prevent cardiometabolic diseases in adults 40 to 74 years of age through annual checkups and lifestyle counseling. The program has shown measurable reductions in major risk factors (Tsushita et al., 2018).

DETERMINANTS OF HEALTH

Japan is a wealthy nation with the third highest annual gross domestic product (GDP; $4.231 trillion) in the world (World Bank Group, 2024). The ratio of the average income of the richest 10% to the poorest 10% is 4.5 times, which is the lowest ratio in the world (United Nations, 2024). Furthermore, Japan's richest 1% has 18.2% of the nation's wealth, which is also the lowest among industrialized nations (Credit Suisse Research Institute, 2023). The percentage of adults 25 to 64 years of age who had attained any postsecondary degree was 56% in 2021, the second highest among major nations in the world. In addition, 99% of Japanese adults are literate (Organisation for Economic Co-operation and Development [OECD], 2024). The 2023 unemployment rate in Japan was 2.6%, the lowest among the G7 nations (World Bank Group, 2024). The high educational attainment, stable economy, and relative lack of inequality are believed to be the foundation for Japan's favorable health outcomes. However, health disparities do exist in Japan, and experts often focus on differences in individuals' health behaviors for explanation. The following are major lifestyle risk factors and the improvement goals of Healthy Japan 21 (Third Phase), a national health promotion campaign similar to the United States's *Healthy People*.

SMOKING

In 2020, smoking prevalence was 16.7% among all adults, 27.1.% in men and 7.6% in women (MHLW, 2024). Smoking prevalence in women stabilized below 10% for several decades, while men's smoking prevalence peaked in 1966 at 83.7% and declined incrementally to the current level, but is still higher compared to other G7 nations (JPALD, 2024). The current targets are to reduce smoking prevalence to 12% in all adults, and eliminate smoking by pregnant women (MHLW, 2024).

PHYSICAL ACTIVITY

According to the 2019 National Health and Nutrition Survey, 34.1% of adult men and 25.1% of adult women engaged in regular physical activity. Men in their 40s and women in their 30s had the lowest prevalence of regular physical activity, with 8.5% and 9.5%, respectively. Walking is a recommended form of physical activity, and the average daily steps were 6,793 in men and 5,832 steps in women in 2019 (JPALD, 2024). Health behavior targets are to increase the physical activity prevalence to 40% and daily steps to 7,100 (MHLW, 2024).

DIET AND NUTRITION

The traditional Japanese diet features a wide variety of fish/seafood, seasonal vegetables, and soy products with minimal amounts of animal protein and fat. The Japanese diet is considered to be healthier than typical Western diets, evidenced by a relatively low prevalence of obesity and obesity-related diseases. In 2021, 23% of Japanese adults were overweight and 5% were obese. In comparison, 30% of U.S. adults were overweight and 43% were obese (OECD, 2024). Maintaining a nutritionally balanced diet in modern Japan, however, can be a challenge. During 2019, approximately 45% of Japanese men and 49% of Japanese women reported having a meal containing a staple starch (rice, noodles, or bread), a side dish of plant-based foods, and another side dish of protein at least twice daily (JPALD, 2024). The goal of Healthy Japan 21 is to increase this proportion to 50% or higher (MHLW, 2024).

HEALTHCARE SYSTEM

Japan's favorable health outcomes are also a result of successful government policy that guarantees equal access to affordable, diverse, and high-quality healthcare while achieving cost containment. Japan has had universal healthcare coverage since 1961 (Ikegami et al., 2011). Japan's per-capita healthcare spending was $4,388 in 2020, the second lowest among the G7 nations. The United State's per-capita healthcare spending is approximately 2.7 times greater than Japan's spending (World Bank Group, 2024).

HEALTH INSURANCE AND HEALTH FINANCING

There are three types of health insurance plans in Japan; **Citizens Health Insurance** for self-employed individuals and people who do not work, various employer-based insurance plans, and Insurance for the Elderly. The eligibility for enrollment is determined by public assistance status, age (75 and above), and employment status (Figure 49.1). All residents in Japan, including non-citizens staying in Japan for 3 months or longer, are required by law to enroll in a health plan. Individuals who are on public assistance (1.7% of the population) are the exception. Their medical costs are paid directly by the government. In 2020, a majority of Japanese residents (approximately 59%) were covered by employer-based plans (Matsuda, 2020). The government provides subsidies for Citizens Health Insurance, Insurance for the Elderly, and employer-based insurance plans administered by medium and small companies. Regardless of health insurance type, all essential medical care, mental health care, home care, hospice care, prescription drugs, dental care, and many other auxiliary services and products are covered. The major source of healthcare

FIGURE 49.1 Health insurance eligibility in Japan.

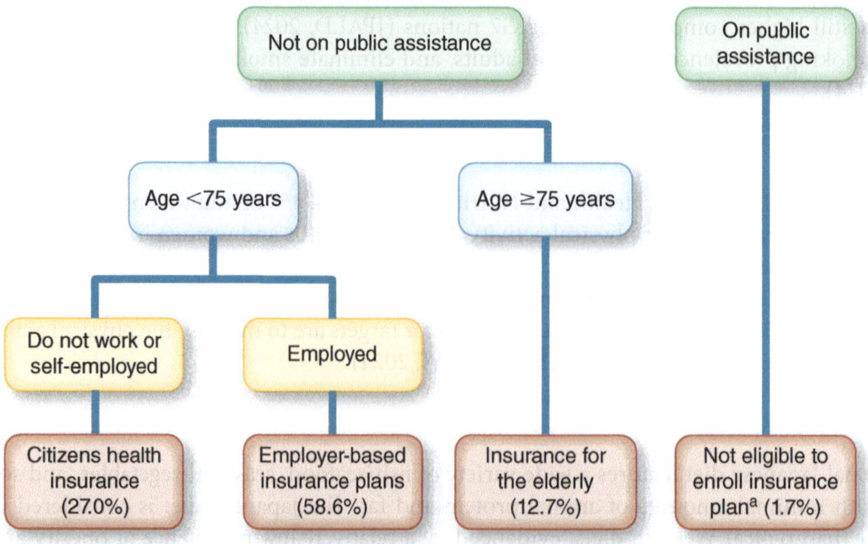

[a] Medical cost directly paid by the government.

Source: Data from Matsuda, R. (2020). *Japan*. In R. Tikkanen, R. Osborn, E. Mossialos, A. Djordjevic, G. A. Wharton (Eds.), *International health care system profiles*. Commonwealth Fund. https://www.commonwealthfund.org/international-health-policy-center/countries/japan

cost containment in Japan is the uniform fee schedule. Fees for almost all clinical services, products, and prescription drugs delivered by healthcare providers are fixed at affordable prices by the **national fee schedule**, which are revised every 2 years through negotiations between the government and various stakeholders (Ikegami et al., 2011). The current rate of out-of-pocket expense to providers (copayment) is 10% to 30% of the total cost, and this rate depends on the age of enrollees and other factors. There are safety net systems to reimburse out-of-pocket expenses exceeding the monthly and annual thresholds. The insurance premium is equity-based and has a sliding scale based on income and age.

HEALTHCARE FACILITIES AND DELIVERY

In 2022, there were 113,415 healthcare facilities in Japan, including 7,100 general hospitals, 1,056 mental hospitals, and 105,259 medical clinics (MHLW, 2024). The available hospital beds per 100,000 population was 12.6, the second highest among major industrialized nations. The average length of hospital stay was 16.0 days in 2019, a 14% reduction since 2009, but still the second highest among industrialized nations. In comparison, the average length of stay in the United States was 5.5 days (OECD, 2024). Patients in Japan have free access to specialty care, as the health insurance plans do not have strict gatekeeping provisions. This contributes to an accurate diagnosis and initiation of advanced treatment at an early stage of disease progression but causes overcrowding in some specialty care facilities. Starting in 2022, patients without referrals are required to pay a fixed fee to access specialty care at designated large community and research hospitals (Government of Japan, 2024). In addition, reflecting a rapidly aging society, Japan has a growing elder care sector. In 2022, there were 13,797 senior long-term care facilities, 75,818 various home care organizations, 19,394 senior daycare facilities, and 14,139 group homes for dementia patients (MHLW, 2024). To continue the current level of healthcare cost containment, improving efficiencies in all sectors of healthcare is a high priority.

HEALTHCARE WORKFORCE

Healthcare and elder care workers accounted for 13.3% of the Japanese workforce in 2021 (MHLW, 2024). The five largest healthcare professions licensed by the national government (excluding elder care and dental professions) are registered nurses, physicians, pharmacists, licensed practical nurses, and acupuncturists (Figure 49.2). The most popular physician specialty is internal medicine, followed by orthopedic surgery and pediatrics (MHLW, 2024). Japan's physician–patient ratio is still relatively low, with 2.6 physicians per 1,000 residents in 2020 (World Bank Group, 2024). Government policy aims to increase all types of healthcare professionals in response to the growing elderly population. More than 80 medical colleges (6-year programs) accept approximately 9,500 students annually. There is an effort to increase female medical students (MHLW, 2024). For nursing education, there is a mixture of 4-year college programs ($n = 300$), 2- or 3-year vocational school programs ($n = 547$), and 5-year combined high school and vocational programs ($n = 79$; Ministry of Education, Culture, Sports, Science and Technology [MEXT], 2024). Four-year college graduates are on the rise, and they accounted for 42.2% of all new nursing graduates in 2022. Pharmacists are the fastest-growing licensed healthcare professionals as the number of pharmacists in Japan doubled during the last 20 years. Since 2006, all pharmacy programs switched from 4-year to 6-year programs. Currently, 79 colleges accept over 12,700 pharmacy students annually, and about two thirds of them are women (MHLW, 2024).

COMPLEMENTARY MEDICINE

As shown in Figure 49.2, four types of complementary medicine practitioners that utilize traditional healthcare practices—acupuncturists, **moxibustionists** (a practitioner who uses heat therapy by burning plants at or near the skin), **Anma and Shiatsu** (massage) therapists, and **Judo therapists** (bonesetters)—are among the top 10 largest licensed healthcare professionals

FIGURE 49.2 Healthcare professions in Japan.

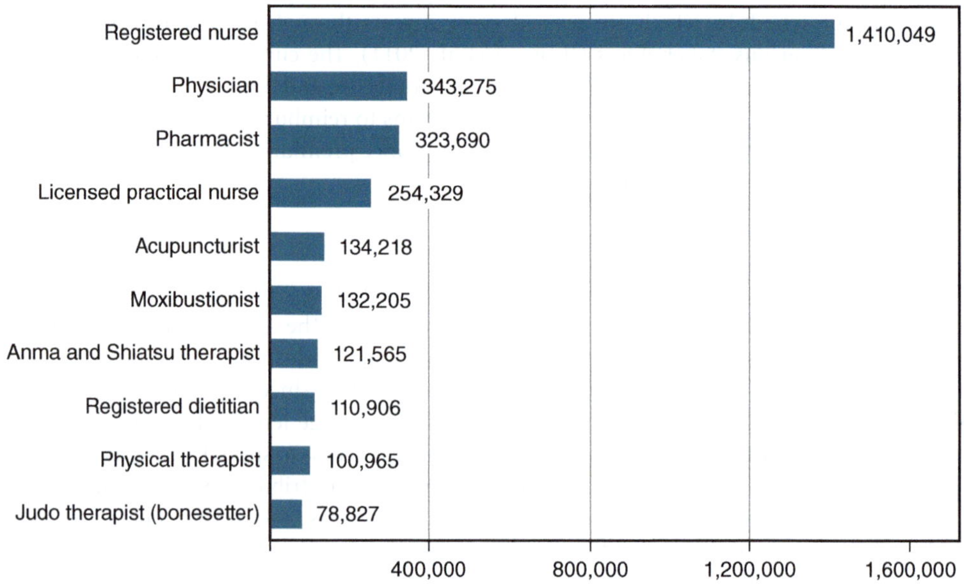

Source: Ministry of Health, Labour, and Welfare. (2024). *Statistics and white paper*. MHLW. https://www.mhlw.go.jp/toukei_hakusho/

in Japan. Licensing of these professionals by the government started in 1947 (Shiatsu was added in 1970), and services provided by them are covered by health insurance plans if ordered by a physician. In addition, the Japanese ***Pharmacopeia*** (book describing how substances are used as medicines) includes 294 traditional herbal prescriptions for a variety of health conditions, and 148 of the herbal prescriptions are covered by health insurance plans (MHLW, 2024). A study of hospital clinic patients in Tokyo found that 50% of their respondents used complementary medicine in the previous year, indicating wide acceptance of complementary medicine in Japan (Hori et al., 2008).

CONCLUSION

Japan is a healthy nation indicated by various objective health outcome measures that are ranked on a global scale. The relative lack of social inequality, high educational attainment, and stable economy, combined with a healthy dietary tradition and government policy that ensures affordable, accessible, and diverse high-quality healthcare are the key reasons Japan's health outcomes are favorable on a global scale. The major health challenges in Japan include low total fertility rates, a rapidly aging population, and anticipated increases in healthcare demands and expenditures. The Japanese government is responding to these challenges by increasing the number of healthcare workers, improving the efficiency of healthcare, and promoting healthy behaviors.

LEARNING ACTIVITIES

CourseConnect >

To access self-assessment questions and interactive, competency-based learning activities for this chapter, visit www.springerpub.com/courseconnect. See inside front cover and tear-out for CourseConnect details.

REFERENCES

Agency for Cultural Affairs. (2023). *Yearbook of religion 2023*. Agency for Cultural Affairs. https://www.bunka.go.jp/tokei_hakusho_shuppan/hakusho_nenjihokokusho/shukyo_nenkan/index.html

Centers for Disease Control and Prevention. (2024). *National center for health statistics—FastStats*. CDC. https://www.cdc.gov/nchs/fastats/default.htm

Credit Suisse Research Institute. (2023). *Global wealth report 2023*. UBS.

Government of Japan. (2024). *Public relations office online: Healthcare*. Government of Japan. https://www.gov-online.go.jp/health_medical_welfare/medical/

Hori, S., Mihaylov, I., Vasconcelos, J. C., McCoubrie, M. (2008). Patterns of complementary and alternative medicine use amongst outpatients in Tokyo, Japan. *BMC Complementary and Alternative Medicine, 8*(14), 1–9. https://doi.org/10.1186/1472-6882-8-14

Ikegami, N., Yoo, B. K., Hashimoto, H., Matsumoto, M., Ogata, H., Babazono, A., Watanabe, R., Shibuya, K., Yang, B. M., Reich, M. R., Kobayashi, Y. (2011). Japanese universal health coverage: Evolution, achievements, and challenges. *The Lancet, 378*(9796), 1106–1115. https://doi.org/10.1016/S0140-6736(11)60828-3

Japan Preventive Association of Lifestyle-related Disease. (2024). *Lifestyle-related disease surveys and statistics*. JPALD. https://seikatsusyukanbyo.com/statistics/2023/010698.php

Johns Hopkins Coronavirus Resource Center. (2024). *Latest data by region*. Johns Hopkins University. https://coronavirus.jhu.edu/region

Kokubo, Y. (2017). The changes of stroke morbidity and mortality in Japan and abroad. *Journal of the Japanese Society of Cardiovascular Disease Prevention, 52*, 223–232. https://www.jacd.info/library/jjcdp/review/52-3_01_%20kokubo.pdf

Matsuda, R. (2020). *Japan*. In R. Tikkanen, R. Osborn, E. Mossialos, A. Djordjevic, G. A. Wharton (Eds). *International health care system profiles*. Commonwealth Fund. https://www.commonwealthfund.org/international-health-policy-center/countries/japan

Ministry of Education, Culture, Sports, Science and Technology. (2024). *Directory of MEXT-accredited schools for training healthcare professionals*. MEXT. https://www.mext.go.jp/a_menu/koutou/kango/1353401.htm

Ministry of Health, Labour, and Welfare. (2024). *Statistics and white paper*. MHLW. https://www.mhlw.go.jp/toukei_hakusho/

Nakamura, Y. (2007). Maternal and child health handbook in global perspective. *Seisan to Gijutu, 59*(2), 87–90. http://seisan.server-shared.com/592/592-87.pdf

National Institute of Infectious Diseases. (2024). *Annual surveillance of infectious diseases*. NIID. https://www.niid.go.jp/niid/ja/ydata

National Statistics Center. (2024). *e-Stat portal site of official statistics of Japan*. https://www.e-stat.go.jp/

Organisation for Economic Co-operation and Development. (2024). *Publications: Insights and context to inform policies and global dialogue*. https://www.oecd.org/en/publications.html

Tsushita, K., Hosler, A. S., Miura, K., Ito, Y., Fukuda, Y., Kitamura, A., & Tatara, K. (2018). Rationale and descriptive analysis of specific health guidance: The nationwide lifestyle intervention program targeting metabolic syndrome in Japan. *Journal of Atherosclerosis and Thrombosis, 25*(4), 308–322. https://www.jstage.jst.go.jp/article/jat/25/4/25_42010/_pdf

United Nations. (2024). *UN data: A world of information*. United Nations. https://data.un.org/Default.aspx

World Bank Group. (2024). *World Bank open data*. World Bank. https://data.worldbank.org/

CHAPTER 50

CHINA

Jia Sun, Carl Condé, and Jiahao Wang

GEOGRAPHY AND POPULATION

The **People's Republic of China** is one of the largest countries in the world, spanning 9,596,960 square kilometers (5,963,274 square miles; Central Intelligence Agency [CIA], 2024). China consists of two **semiautonomous special administrative districts** (Hong Kong and Macau), four **directly controlled municipalities** (Beijing, Chongqing, Shanghai, and Tianjin), five **autonomous regions** (Guangxi Zhuang, Inter Mongolia, Ningxia Hui, Tibet, and Xinjiang Uyghur), and 23 provinces (The State Council, The People's Republic of China, 2024). China also includes some of the world's most remarkable geographic features, including the Gobi Desert, the Yellow and Yangtze Rivers, and the Himalaya, Karakoram, Pamir, and Tian Shan mountain ranges. Figure 50.1 is an administrative map of China.

FIGURE 50.1 Administrative division of the People's Republic of China.

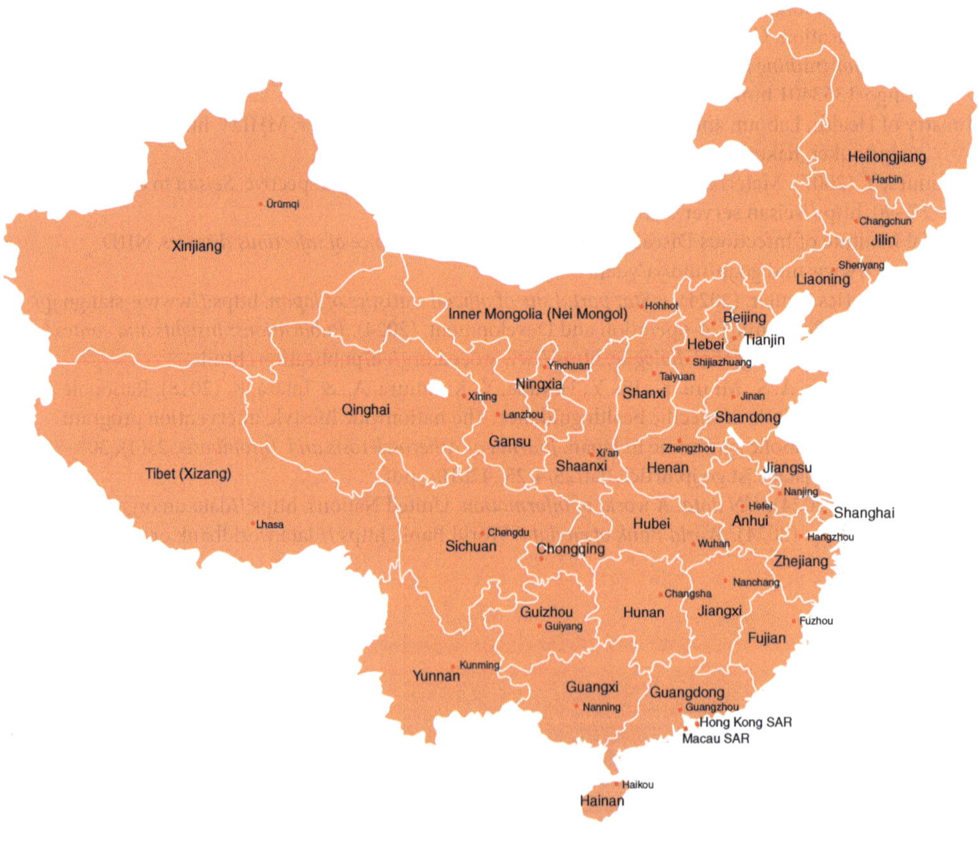

Source: Sameboat. (2024, February 28). *China provinces numbered.* from https://commons.wikimedia.org/w/index.php?title=File:China_administrative_de_facto.svg&oldid=856644410

China's population of approximately 1.42 billion in 2023 ranked second in the world behind India (UN Data Portal, n.d.) However, most of the population is densely centered in coastal urban areas in Eastern China (CIA, 2024). The uneven distribution of China's population is influenced by geography, particularly the **Hu Huanyong Line**, which divides the drier, sparsely populated west from the wetter, densely populated east (Li et al., 2018). The **Qinghai-Tibetan Plateau**, known as the "roof of the world," also contributes to this imbalance due to its high elevation and harsh living conditions (People's Republic of China, Central Government, 2005). The Han ethnic group makes up 91.11% of the population, while minority ethnic groups, mainly living along China's borders, have a faster growth rate (National Bureau of Statistics [NBS], 2021). China is a multilingual, multidialect, and multiscript nation with diverse religions such as Buddhism, Taoism, Islam, Catholicism, and Christianity—each with centuries to millennia of history within the country. While the ruling party of China is officially atheist, there are about 100 million believers and numerous formal and informal places of worship (The State Council, The People's Republic of China, 2024). Approximately 64% of China's population lived in urban areas during 2021 (NBS, 2021). Despite being a developing country, China is facing rapid population aging, with a declining working-age population (ages 15 to 59) and an increasing older adult population (NBS, 2024). Combined with a low immigration rate, this trend is expected to lead to labor shortages (NBS, 2021). China is believed to have the largest LGBTQ population globally, though no official statistics exist (Wang et al., 2019).

HEALTH OUTCOMES

There have been substantial **demographic** and **epidemiologic** transitions in China (Wang, 2022). Following World War II, fertility rates surged and mortality rates declined (Zheng, 2021). The **One-Child Policy**, which limited families to one child between 1979 to 2015, then led to a sharp drop in fertility. Mortality rates continued to decline due to economic growth, healthcare improvements, and better living standards (Cook & Dummer, 2004). Concurrently, the causes of death transitioned from communicable diseases to noncommunicable diseases (NCDs), with infectious diseases decreasing from 12% to less than 3% of deaths by the 1990s, while chronic diseases rose by 17% (Wang, 2022). These transitions reflect China's broader socioeconomic development and public health advancements (Cook & Dummer, 2004). In 2021, China's leading causes of death were stroke, heart diseases, lung cancer, chronic obstructive pulmonary disease (COPD) Alzheimer disease, stomach cancer, esophageal cancer, colorectal cancer, and road injuries. Leading risk factors of mortality in China during 2021 included tobacco use, metabolic conditions (high blood pressure, plasma glucose, body mass index, and low-density lipoprotein cholesterol), poor diet, air pollution, occupational hazards, kidney dysfunction, and alcohol abuse (Institute for Health Metrics and Evaluation [IHME], n.d.). Life expectancy at birth in China during 2023 was 77.95 years, which was almost 5 more years of life expectancy when compared to global life expectancy, but approximately 1 year less than regional (East Asia) life expectancy during 2023 (UN Data Portal, n.d.).

MENTAL HEALTH

Mental health care in China dates back to 2,600 BCE, with traditional therapies and family caregiving playing key roles. Modern mental health care began in the late 19th century with Western influence, and the formal system was established in 1958. By 2015, 16.6% of Chinese adults had mental health disorders, primarily anxiety, mood, and substance use disorders. Despite expanded government efforts, four out of five people do not seek professional mental health help, often relying on informal care. In 2021, mental health disorders ranked as the 11th leading cause of death in China, with higher rates among women. The government has improved access and insurance coverage, but disparities and financial burdens persist, particularly in less developed areas of China (Xu et al., 2022).

COMMUNICABLE AND NONCOMMUNICABLE DISEASES

The Chinese government has focused on preventing and controlling infectious diseases by integrating traditional Chinese medicine with modern Western approaches, including vaccines and antibiotics. Investments in public health infrastructure have led to a decline in diseases like cholera and typhoid. However, respiratory diseases and sexually transmitted infections have resurged, especially due to urbanization and environmental issues, with rising mortality rates among the poor and vulnerable populations (Cook & Dummer, 2004). Disparities persist based on age, gender, and economic status (Du et al., 2023). The mortality rate from NCDs in China has risen significantly, from 533 deaths per 100,000 in 2012 to 685 per 100,000 in 2018, with heart disease being the leading cause. Men and people living in rural areas are disproportionately affected. Despite a slight decrease in 2021, NCDs remain China's leading cause of death. The prevalence of NCDs is also increasing, linked to low health literacy, urbanization, and unhealthy lifestyles. While efforts to manage and treat NCDs have improved, disparities persist, particularly among men, younger individuals, and rural populations (Peng et al., 2024). Furthermore, China exhibits significantly higher levels of NCDs than countries with a similar **Sociodemographic Index**, which is a composite index of development based on a country's fertility rate, mean education, and per-capita income (Zhou et al., 2019).

MATERNAL AND INFANT MORTALITY

In 1949, China began prioritizing maternal and infant health. As a result, the maternal mortality ratio decreased from 1,500 maternal deaths per 100,000 live births in 1950 (Di et al., 2017) to 23 maternal deaths in 2020 (UN Population Fund, n.d.). The infant mortality rate decreased from 127.1 infant deaths per 1,000 live births in 1950 to 5.1 infant deaths in 2023 (UN Data Portal, n.d.). Comprehensive healthcare programs narrowed regional disparities and raised hospital delivery rates to 99.9% in 2018. The focus now shifts to providing high-quality healthcare services (Qiao et al., 2021).

DETERMINANTS OF HEALTH

SOCIOECONOMIC STATUS

China's gross domestic product (GDP) is the second largest in the world, nearly reaching $18 billion in 2023. However, China's per-capita GDP was only $12,614 in 2023, which ranked 70th globally (World Bank Group, n.d.). China ranked 97th globally in equitable wealth distribution, indicating a notable gap between economic strength and individual prosperity (World Bank Group, 2024). Education and literacy rates in China have improved significantly in recent years. In 2021, 15.5% of the population had a college degree (NBS, 2021). However, these advancements are unevenly distributed, with notable regional disparities, as rural areas in the west lag far behind eastern urban areas. The unemployment rate in China during 2023 was approximately 5% (NBS, 2024). Local residents had a slightly higher unemployment rate than migrants (State Council Information Office, 2024).

LIFESTYLE

In recent years, Chinese diets have shifted from predominantly grain based to being more diverse, including more plant-based and animal-derived foods due to economic growth. Food security and environmental sustainability challenges persist, particularly in rural areas. While food security in urban areas is rapidly improving, caloric intake is exceeding recommended levels, creating new dietary issues (Han et al., 2023). The Chinese government advances healthy lifestyles through a three-tier network managed by the China Centers for Disease Control and Prevention (China CDC). Supported by central funding, this initiative coordinates with provincial offices and employs both traditional media and platforms such as WeChat and Weibo.

Efforts emphasize balanced living, including reduced salt and sugar intake, exercise, oral health, and mental well-being (China CDC, 2024). Drug use has significantly decreased due to government efforts, but smoking, physical inactivity, and alcohol consumption remain high despite progress (National Health Commission [NHC], 2015).

SOCIAL AND NATURAL ENVIRONMENT

Human history in China spans over 1.7 million years. China's openness to diverse cultures is evident in its political systems, ethnic groups, and cultural practices. Confucianism, originating in the early feudal period, emphasized family responsibility over community or government reliance (Park & Chesla, 2007). Buddhism has also influenced China. Communism reached China in recent years and led to its current socialist system with Chinese characteristics (Wang & Pan, 2021). As a result, China is currently governed by the Communist Party, which operates within a framework involving eight other minor parties (People's Republic of China, Central Government, 2005).

Environmental factors, including natural toxins and pollution, significantly threaten food security and exacerbate disease burdens in China, with climate change worsening these issues (Yang et al., 2010). Recently, the country has made notable progress through technological advancements, policy measures, and improvements in sewage treatment, emissions control, and renewable energy. By 2022, reductions in carbon emissions and increased forest coverage highlighted China's commitment to climate action (Zhou, 2013).

HEALTHCARE SYSTEM

HISTORICAL BACKGROUND OF HEALTHCARE

In 1949, China was among the world's poorest countries and life expectancy at birth was only 35 years. The main healthcare challenges for the government were establishing a robust healthcare system to cover the large, dispersed rural population and funding hospital investments. Over the next 29 years, the government implemented a tiered healthcare network and funded hospitals, ensuring health services were available from counties to villages. This effort raised life expectancy by 30 years, despite the country remaining among the world's poorest nations. By 1978, China experienced significant economic growth and life expectancy matched the global average. In recent years, rising healthcare costs driven by profit motives and excessive testing and prescriptions have prompted government interventions to reduce expenses (Lin, 2021).

HEALTHCARE DELIVERY, FINANCE, INSURANCE, AND PAYMENT

Modern China's healthcare system is centrally managed by the government, prioritizing basic services for all citizens. The National People's Congress oversees its regulations, while the State Council and the Central Committee of the Communist Party implement significant reforms. In 2018, the State Council established the NHC to oversee policy, medical reform, and public health. Healthcare costs are managed by the State Medical Insurance Administration, with funding from the Ministry of Finance. The State Market Regulatory Administration approves drugs, the China CDC supports local centers, and local governments manage health services to ensure quality, safety, and equity. As of 2018, China had approximately 10,000 public hospitals and 20,000 private hospitals. Approximately 25,000 hospitals were not-for-profit, while 12,600 were for-profit. Primary healthcare in China is provided by village doctors, general practitioners (GPs), and hospital professionals. Village doctors work independently and offer after-hours care voluntarily, while GPs collaborate with hospital nurses. Patients are encouraged to use local services with lower cost-sharing but can still see GPs or specialists without referrals. As of 2018, there were about half a million public primary care clinics, half a million private village clinics, and 1 million village doctors. There were more than 300,000 licensed and assistant GPs. Emergency departments in hospitals provide after-hours care with minimal extra costs. A significant gap exists in integrating mental health care with primary care, and China faces a scarcity of long-term care resources, with hospice care being rare and often uninsured (Fang et al., 2020).

In 2018, healthcare accounted for 7% of China's GDP, comprising 28% from government funding, 28% from out-of-pocket payments, and 44% from various sources such as public and private insurance and donations. Public healthcare insurance is the major source of funding and includes the **Urban Employee Basic Medical Insurance,** which is mandatory for urban workers, and the **Urban–Rural Resident Basic Medical Insurance**, which covers rural residents and the urban self-employed or unemployed. These insurance schemes cover medical services, prescription drugs, and traditional Chinese medicine, but not home care or durable medical equipment. Dental and vision care are partially covered, and preventive services are partially government funded. Coverage for care and prescriptions varies by plan, with modest outpatient copayments ($1 to $3). No cap is placed on out-of-pocket spending, which was $332 per capita in 2018. Public insurance has reimbursement limits and requires deductibles. Long-term care is supported by local subsidies and new pilot programs. A safety net assists those unable to afford public insurance, prioritizing catastrophic care. Private insurance, preferred by the wealthy, covers additional costs. The government promotes private insurance and encourages foreign participation (Fang et al., 2020).

HEALTHCARE TRAINING AND EDUCATION

China faces a shortage of physicians, especially in rural areas, so the government promotes medical training and service in these regions by waiving tuition fees and relaxing entry requirements for students who commit to working in rural areas for at least 6 years. Nationwide, government-subsidized medical school tuition is less than $2,800 per year. Currently, China does not have private medical schools (Fang et al., 2020).

HEALTHCARE COST, QUALITY, AND ACCESS

The Chinese government regulates primary care fees in public health institutions to prevent overbilling. Private clinics and hospitals, however, can charge above these rates. Patients pay deductibles and copayments upfront, and hospitals bill insurers for the rest. China's healthcare costs have surged, with per-capita expenditures increasing 3.5 times from 2004 to 2018. The government attributes this increase to healthcare reforms, a growing older adult population, economic growth, and technological advancements. To control costs, the government has limited new hospital construction and high-tech equipment acquisition. It has also reformed the payment system, moving from the fee-for-service model to value-based models. Additionally, the government promotes community hospitals over more expensive tertiary care facilities, encouraging competition based on quality, technology, and copayment rates. The price of prescription drugs was regulated by the "zero markups" campaign. The Department of Health Care Quality, under the National Health Commission, oversees the healthcare system in China. Every 5 years, the National Health Service Survey reports on key quality indicators from patients and providers. Hospitals must be accredited by local health authorities, and physicians are licensed through affiliated hospitals. Although national hospital rankings exist, there are no financial incentives for quality improvement and individual provider information lacks transparency in China (Fang et al., 2020).

China has improved healthcare accessibility but still faces significant disparities. Despite progress from health insurance reforms, gaps remain due to inconsistent oversight and targeted programs. Urban areas have better-equipped hospitals, while rural areas face shortages and undertrained doctors. The absence of a national electronic health records (EHR) standard results in varied, noninteroperable systems. Although some regions are planning regional EHRs, many patients rarely use them (Fang et al., 2020).

HEALTHCARE PRACTICE

OVERVIEW

Ancient Chinese public health practices influenced medicine and social norms into the 20th century. Christian medical missionaries, however, introduced allopathic medicine and Western health management, shifting health ideology to link individuals with the national status. This transition emphasized a robust, centralized state for national development, disease prevention, and well-being. Recently, this ideology evolved to include monitoring citizen behavior and managing public health infrastructure, goals consistent since the 20th century (Fu, 2022).

ALLOPATHIC MEDICINE

In contemporary China, allopathic medicine, which relies on biomedical research and scientific technologies, is the mainstream healthcare practice and forms the foundation of the country's modern public health infrastructure. Known as "Western Medicine" in China, it was first introduced by Christian missionaries in the 19th century. It did not clinically outperform traditional Chinese medicine until the advent of antibiotics, vaccines, anesthetics, surgical, and ophthalmic technologies. Its widespread acceptance led to the establishment of allopathic medicine-based hospitals and medical schools in colonized territories. Eventually, China's governments adopted allopathic principles to establish a public health system that persists despite political changes (Dubey & Kumar, 2025).

TRADITIONAL CHINESE, COMPLEMENTARY, AND ALTERNATIVE MEDICINE

Traditional Chinese medicine (TCM) aims for overall wellness rather than just symptom relief. It includes herbal medicine, pulse diagnosis, acupuncture, orthopedics, and health preservation, based on thousands of years of clinical experience and insights. TCM's approach observes body changes; considers behavior, diet, and environmental factors; and promotes a holistic view to harmonize body functions. European interest in TCM grew through Christian missionaries, resulting in the translation of over 60 texts (1700–1840). Classified as complementary and alternative medicine (CAM) in China due to its divergence from modern scientific norms, TCM faced discrimination and decline in some regions. In response, the government promoted TCM by establishing hospitals, certifying practitioners, advancing research, and integrating TCM into health insurance. Today, China's healthcare system offers both TCM and allopathic medicine with a combined approach often preferred for greater effectiveness (Dubey & Kumar, 2025). Scientific methods are increasingly applied to TCM research, highlighted by Tu Youyou's Nobel Prize work on the use of artemisinin to treat malaria (Su & Miller, 2015).

HEALTHCARE INNOVATIONS

Due to high demand, securing appointments at tertiary hospitals can be difficult. To address this, the government formed medical alliances led by a tertiary hospital and supported by secondary and primary care facilities. These alliances aim to reduce unnecessary tertiary hospital visits, improve efficiency, and lower costs. They enable seamless referrals and transitions among care levels and use a unified electronic health records system for streamlined access to patient data. China has three main alliance models: the Zhenjiang model (local health bureau ownership), the Wuhan model (tertiary hospital manages all), and the Shanghai model (autonomous hospitals with separate ownership). The Shanghai model is the most common (Fang et al., 2020).

CONCLUSION

In recent decades, the dramatic improvements in the accessibility of healthcare services and the comprehensive overhaul of China's healthcare system are notable. As a developing nation with the second largest population globally, China has made significant strides in enhancing life expectancy, reducing infant and maternal mortality, establishing healthcare facilities, optimizing insurance systems, and integrating TCM with allopathic practices. Despite these advancements, China's current health outcomes, while improved compared to the past, still fall short of those in more developed countries, particularly in areas such as insurance coverage, affordability, rural healthcare access, and disease prevention. Given the escalating issues related to aging and low fertility rates in China, the future of its healthcare system faces considerable challenges. It would be prudent for the healthcare system to adopt more effective measures to address the rising demand for healthcare services.

LEARNING ACTIVITIES

CourseConnect

To access self-assessment questions and interactive, competency-based learning activities for this chapter, visit www.springerpub.com/courseconnect. See inside front cover and tear-out for CourseConnect details.

REFERENCES

Central Intelligence Agency. (2024). *China*. https://www.cia.gov/the-world-factbook/countries/china/#geography

China Centers for Disease Control and Prevention. (2024). *Introduction to China healthy lifestyle for all.* https://www.chinacdc.cn/jiankang121/mryw/

Cook, I. G., & Dummer, T. J. (2004). Changing health in China: Re-evaluating the epidemiological transition model. *Health Policy, 67*(3), 329–343. https://doi.org/10.1016/j.healthpol.2003.07.005

Di, J, Yang Q., & Jin, X. (2017). Combating maternal mortality in China: Experience, challenges, and opportunities. *Global Health Journal, 1*(3), 20–33. https://doi.org/10.1016/S2414-6447(19)30096-X

Du, M., Wang, R., Yuan, J., Lv, X., Yan, W., Liu, Q., Qin, C., Xiang, N., Zhu, L., Liang, W., Liu, M., & Liu, J. (2023). Trends and disparities in 44 national notifiable infectious diseases in China: An analysis of national surveillance data from 2010 to 2019. *Journal of Medical Virology, 95*(1), e28353. https://doi.org/10.1002/jmv.28353

Dubey, R.K., & Kumar, B. (2025). A comprehensive overview of traditional Chinese medicine (TCM). *Chinese Journal of Applied Physiology, 41*, e20250015. https://doi.org/10.62958/j.cjap.2025.015

Fang, H., Tikkanen, R., Osborn, R., Mossialos, E., Djordjevic, A., & Wharton, G. A. (2020). *China*. The Commonwealth Fund. https://www.commonwealthfund.org/international-health-policy-center/countries/china

Fu, J.-C. (2022). *Health and medicine in modern China.* Oxford Research. https://oxfordre.com/asianhistory/display/10.1093/acrefore/9780190277727.001.0001/acrefore-9780190277727-e-137

Han, Z., Zheng, X., Hou, L., Xiao, N., & Deng, X. (2023). Changes in China's food security driven by nutrition security and resource constraints. *Environment Development & Sustainability, 26*, 7927–7945. https://doi.org/10.1007/s10668-023-03042-1

Institute for Health Metrics and Evaluation. (n.d.). *Country profiles: China*. https://www.healthdata.org/research-analysis/health-by-location/profiles/china

Li, M., He, B., Guo, R., Li, Y., Chen, Y., & Fan, Y. (2018). Study on population distribution pattern at the county level of China. *Sustainability, 10*(3598), 1–16. https://doi.org/10.3390/su10103598

Lin, Y. (2021). *The development and reform exploration of China's healthcare system*. Institute of New Structural Economics. https://www.nse.pku.edu.cn/sylm/xwsd/511323.htm

National Bureau of Statistics. (2021). *The 7th national census bulletin*. The State Council. https://www.gov.cn/guoqing/2021-05/13/content_5606149.htm

National Bureau of Statistics. (2024). *National data*. National Bureau of Statistics. https://data.stats.gov.cn/easyquery.htm?cn=C01

National Health Commission. (2015). *Report on the nutrition and chronic disease status of Chinese residents*. http://www.nhc.gov.cn/jkj/s5879/201506/4505528e65f3460fb88685081ff158a2.shtml

Park, M., & Chesla, C. (2007). Revisiting confucianism as a conceptual framework for Asian family study. *Journal of Family Nursing, 13*(3), 293–311. https://doi.org/10.1177/1074840707304400

Peng, W., Chen, S., Chen, X., Ma, Y., Wang, T., Sun, X., Wang, Y., Ding, G., & Wang, Y. (2024). Trends in major non-communicable diseases and related risk factors in China 2002–2019: An analysis of nationally representative survey data. *The Lancet Regional Health West Pacific, 43*, 100809. https://doi.org/10.1016/j.lanwpc.2023.100809

People's Republic of China, Central Government. (2005). *The multi-party cooperation and political consultation system under the leadership of the Communist Party of China*. https://www.gov.cn/test/2005-05/25/content_639.htm

Qiao, J., Wang, Y., Li, X., Jiang, F., Zhang, Y., Ma, J., Song, Y., Ma, J., Fu, W., Pang, R., Zhu, Z., Zhang, J., Qian, X., Wang, L., Wu, J., Chang, H. M., Leung, P. C. K., Mao, M., Ma, D., . . . Hesketh, T. (2021). A *Lancet* Commission on 70 years of women's reproductive, maternal, newborn, child, and adolescent health in China. *The Lancet, 397*(10293), 2497–2536. https://doi.org/10.1016/S0140-6736(20)32708-2

State Council Information Office. (2024). *Press conference on the national economic performance in 2023 held by the state council information office*. The Central People's Government of the People's Republic of China. https://www.gov.cn/zhengce/202401/content_6926623.htm

State Council, The People's Republic of China. (2024). *Overview of China*. https://www.gov.cn/guoqing/

Su, X.Z., & Miller, L.H. (2015). The discovery of artemisinin and the Nobel prize in physiology or medicine. *Science China Life Sciences, 58*, 1175–1179. https://link.springer.com/article/10.1007/s11427-015-4948-7

UN Data Portal. (n.d.). *UN Population Division data portal*. United Nations. https://population.un.org/dataportal/home/

UN Population Fund. (n.d.). *UNFPA—United Nations Population Fund*. https://www.unfpa.org/

Wang, H. (2022). Disease burden: Progresses made, current state, future challenges, and ppportunities. *China CDC Weekly, 4*(13), 280–283. https://doi.org/10.46234/ccdcw2022.070

Wang, Y., Hu, Z., Peng, K., Xin, Y., Yang, Y., Drescher, J., & Chen, R. (2019). Discrimination against LGBT populations in China. *Lancet Public Health, 4*(9), e440–e441. https://doi.org/10.1016/S2468-2667(19)30153-7

Wang, Z., & Pan, J. (2021). *A hundred years in retrospect and lessons learned: The comintern and its relationship with the Chinese revolution*. Institute of Political Science CASS. http://chinaps.cass.cn/gjshj/202107/t20210719_5348282.shtml

World Bank Group. (2024). *Gini index*. The World Bank. https://data.worldbank.org/indicator/SI.POV.GINI?end=2023&most_recent_value_desc=false&start=1963&view=chart

World Bank Group. (n.d.). *The World Bank open data*. https://data.worldbank.org/

Xu, Z., Gahr, M., Xiang, Y., Kingdon, D., Rusch, N., & Wang, G. (2022). The state of mental health care in China. *Asian Journal of Psychiatry, 69*, 102975. https://doi.org/10.1016/j.ajp.2021.102975

Yang, L., Wang, W., Tan, J., Liang, T., & Dong, Y.-s. (2010). Overview on the research works in the field of environmental geography and human health. *Geographical Research, 29*(9), 1571–1583. https://doi.org/10.11821/yj2010090004

Zheng, Z. (2021). From the past to the future: What we learn from China's 2020 Census. *China Population and Development Studies, 5*, 101–106. https://doi.org/https://doi.org/10.1007/s42379-021-00084-8

Zhou, M., Wang, H., Zeng, X., Yin, P., Zhu, J., Chen, W., Li, X., Wang, L., Wang, L., Liu, Y., Liu, J., Zhang, M., Qi, J., Yu, S., Afshin, A., Gakidou, E., Glenn, S., Krish, V. S., Miller-Petrie, M. K., . . . Liang, X. (2019). Mortality, morbidity, and risk factors in China and its provinces, 1990–2017: A systematic analysis for the Global Burden of Disease Study 2017. *Lancet, 394*(10204), 1145–1158. https://doi.org/10.1016/S0140-6736(19)30427-1

Zhou, S. (2013). *The development process and achievements of environmental protection in China*. Ministry of Ecology and Environment of the People's Republic of China. https://www.mee.gov.cn/gkml/sthjbgw/qt/201310/t20131009_261311.htm

CHAPTER 51

SOUTH KOREA

Suk-Young Kang

INTRODUCTION

South Korea, officially the Republic of Korea, has a single-payer healthcare system organized through the **National Health Insurance Service (NHIS)**. Figure 51.1 shows the structure of the NHIS. South Korea's healthcare policy was developed to fulfil the World Health Organization's (WHO) definition of **universal health coverage (UHC)**: "All people have access to the full range of quality health services they need, when and where they need them, without financial hardship.

FIGURE 51.1 The structure of the National Health Insurance Service.

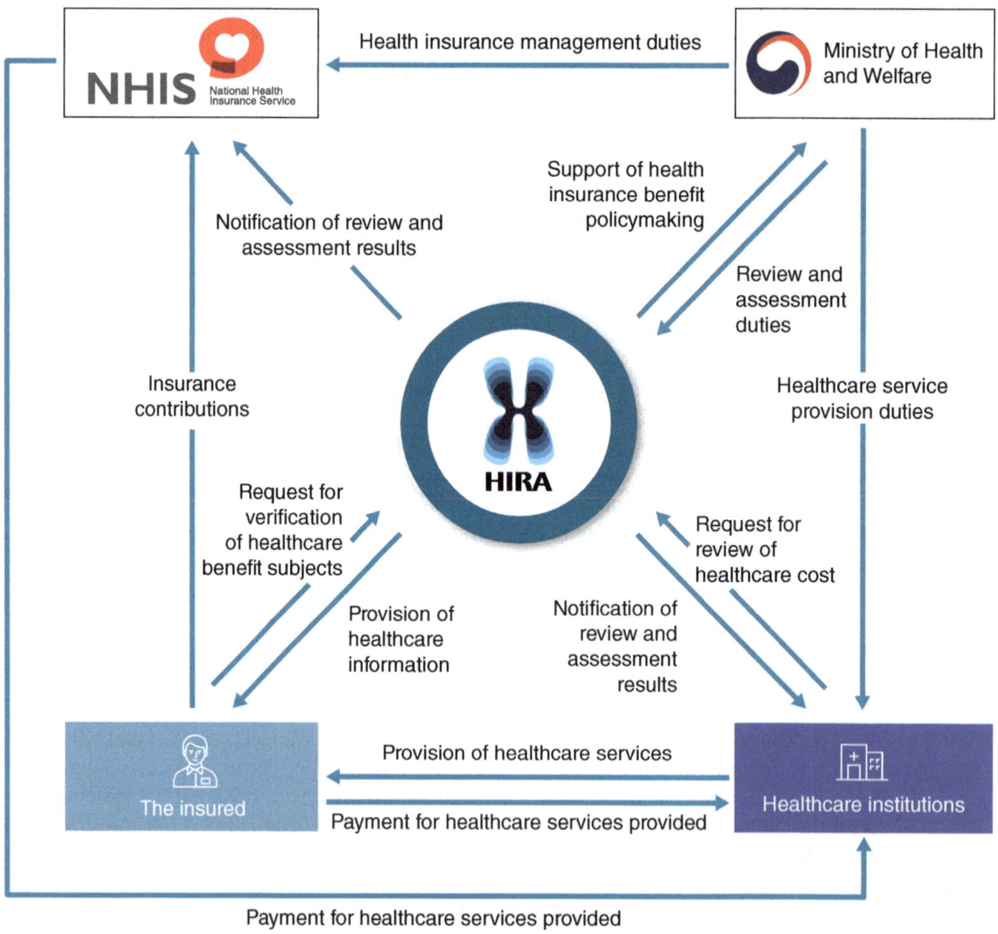

HIRA, Health Insurance Review and Assessment Service; NHIS, National Health Insurance Service.

Source: Health Insurance Review and Assessment Service. (2021). *What we do: Healthcare system in Korea*. https://www.hira.or.kr/dummy.do?pgmid=HIRAJ010000006000

It covers the full continuum of essential health services, from health promotion to prevention, treatment, rehabilitation, and palliative care" (WHO, 2025).

UHC in South Korea was accomplished in a very short time period between 1977 and 1989 (Jeong, 2011). However, the NHIS covered only 64.5% of healthcare costs in 2021 (Statistics Korea, n.d.). Patients were responsible for 35.5% of costs, either personally or through private insurance. In addition, long-term care costs can be very high for South Koreans.

GEOGRAPHY AND POPULATION

South Korea is relatively small, with a total surface area of 100,432 square kilometers (62,405 square miles), which is almost one-hundredth of the size of the United States. The population is predominately urban, comprising 81% of the entire population (World Bank Group, 2023). There were approximately 57.75 million people in South Korea in 2023. Since 2020, the population has decreased due to low and declining birthrates, which decreased from 5.2 live births per 1,000 people in 2020 to 4.6 in 2023 (UN Data Portal, n.d.). In 2022, the total fertility rate (TFR) decreased to 0.78 live births per 1,000 women, the lowest rate since 1970, when birth statistics began to be collected (Academy of Korean Studies [AKS], 2023). South Korea's TFR was the lowest among all of the Organisation for Economic Co-operation and Development (OECD) members. Population replacement requires a TRF above 2.1 children per woman (OECD, 2024)

South Korea's population is also rapidly aging. The median age of the South Korean population increased from 17.7 years in 1954 to 44.5 years in 2023 (UN Data Portal, n.d.). In 2000, adults age 65 and older accounted for approximately 7% of the population; in 2023, adults age 65 and older accounted for more than 18% of the total population (UN Data Portal, n.d.). Like other parts of the world, an aging population challenges the Korean healthcare system. In particular, Korean society has started to see changes in caring for older parents, shifting from a family duty to a shared governmental role. The family has traditionally served as the primary care support system for older Koreans; however, rapid modernization has diminished the influence of traditional values, which historically kept generations closely connected. Younger generations are now less bound by longstanding beliefs, including the sense of duty to care for their elders (Kang & Kim, 2015).

South Korea was a demographically homogeneous country until a few years after the 1988 Seoul Olympics. It now has a more diverse population with migrants from other countries, including people who fled from North Korea—in 2019, there was an estimated 30,000 people who fled North Korea living in South Korea (Jung et al., 2019). Koreans comprise 96% of the population, with other groups making up the remaining 4%.

The official spoken language is Korean, which is a distinctive native language and writing system. The Korean alphabet was created in 1443, during King Sejong's reign (Lee, 2013). The majority of the Korean population can use this language. However, with population diversity comes a growing need to provide more culturally and linguistically appropriate healthcare.

BRIEF COUNTRY HISTORY

The Korean Peninsula, a landmass about as large as Britain, has its own unique history. Its languages and the ancestry of about 85 million modern-day Koreans are estimated to have unfolded for more than 2,000 years (Park, 2022). The Korean peninsula neighbors China and Russia, and across the East Sea, it faces Japan. Korea's geopolitics necessitate delicate relations with major powers. Despite this, Koreans maintain a distinct history and culture (Park & Kang, 2007).

From 2333 BCE to the early 10th century, there were several important civilizations, including the Gojoseon (or "Old Chosŏn"), the Three Kingdoms, and the Era of Northern and Southern States. In 912 CE, a united monarchy (Goryeo) was established, later replaced by another monarchy (Joseon) in 1392, which, for the most part, kept an independent political system and distinctive culture for hundreds of years (Park, 2022).

Korea endured extended periods of foreign control and political fragmentation starting in the late modern period. From 1910 to 1945, Korea was under Japanese occupation, followed by division and control by the United States and the Soviet Union. Since 1948, two states have coexisted: South Korea (Republic of Korea) and North Korea (Democratic People's Republic of Korea). Following the Korean War (1950–1953), North Korea transformed into a secluded dictatorship, while South Korea developed into a lively democracy, playing a significant role in the global political and economic landscape (Park, 2022).

After the Korean War, the South Korean government faced the arduous task of reviving the nation's shattered industrial capacity and stabilizing livelihoods. They turned to foreign aid, notably receiving $3.1 billion from the United States between 1945 and 1961. This aid kickstarted Korea's economic growth, laying the groundwork for its capitalist development with a focus on consumer goods (Song et al., 2019).

Substantial economic progress began with Park Chunghee's regime following a military coup in 1961. The first economic development plan (1962–1966) was aimed at industrialization and self-sufficiency, surpassing its gross domestic product (GDP) growth target by 7.8%. The economic success led to a demand for medical insurance. The second economic plan (1967) focused on modernizing industries, leading to a staggering 17.9% GDP growth, driven by advancements in basic and export industries. The third plan (1972–1976) prioritized heavy chemical industry development, targeting $10 billion in exports and $1,000 per-capita GDP by 1981. Korea exceeded these goals by 1977. With heavy industrial exports surpassing light industry by 1984, Korea experienced growth despite challenges like overinvestment, oil crises, and political unrest (Song et al., 2019).

In the 1990s, the Kim Young-sam administration created the New Five-Year Economic Plan and Korea became a member of the OECD. However, the 1997 financial crisis, triggered by trade deficits and mismanagement, necessitated International Money Fund (IMF) intervention. Kim Dae-jung's administration tackled the crisis through neoliberal policies, structural reforms, and public cooperation. Since then, Korea's economy has thrived, notably in the semiconductor sector. By 2016, Korea ranked as the world's 11th largest economy, with a GDP of $1.41 trillion. Despite economic growth, challenges such as high living costs and inflation have persisted, leading to a relatively low standard of living and a declining fertility rate (Song et al., 2019). Still, Korea's journey from postwar recovery to economic prominence showcases resilience and strategic policymaking, albeit with ongoing socioeconomic challenges. Most healthcare policies have been aligned with this economic growth.

HEALTH OUTCOMES

LIFE EXPECTANCY AT BIRTH

South Korea's life expectancy at birth of 21 years in 1950 was affected by the Korean War (1950–1953). Since that time, life expectancy at birth in South Korea has increased dramatically. Life expectancy increased nearly 40 years, from 46.9 years in 1954 to 84.3 years in 2023 (UN Data Portal, 2024), which is greater than the OECD average (OECD, 2023). Women in South Korea have greater life expectancy than men. In 2023, female life expectancy at birth was 87.16 years while male life expectancy was 81.19 years (UN Data Portal, n.d.).

LEADING CAUSES OF MORTALITY

In 2019, noncommunicable diseases (NCDs) accounted for nearly four of every five deaths. Communicable, maternal, perinatal, and nutritional conditions accounted for 12.8% of all deaths and injuries accounted for 9.3% (WHO, 2024). In 2021, the leading causes of death included cancer, heart disease, pneumonia, cerebrovascular disease (stroke), suicide, diabetes, Alzheimer disease, liver disease, sepsis, and hypertensive disease. These leading causes accounted for 66%

of all deaths, with the top four (cancer, heart disease, pneumonia, and cerebrovascular disease) making up 50.3% of all deaths (AKS, 2023).

INFANT AND MATERNAL MORTALITY

In Korea, the quality of maternal health has increased substantially from 1950 to 2023. The maternal mortality ratio has improved over several decades from 39.3 maternal deaths per 100,000 live births in 1985 to eight maternal deaths per 100,000 live births in 2020 (WHO, 2023).

The infant mortality rate has been steadily decreasing in Korea, in alignment with economic growth. In 1950, infant mortality was 178.7 infant deaths per 1,000 live births. By 1994, infant mortality was 9.8 in 1994. In 2023, the infant mortality rate in Korea was 2.1 infant deaths per 1,000 live births, which is one of the lowest infant mortality rates in the world (UN Data Portal, n.d.).

MENTAL ILLNESSES

The 2021 mental health survey by South Korea's Ministry of Health and Welfare found that one in three men (32.7%) and nearly one in four women (22.9%) experienced mental illness in their lifetime. This means that over one quarter of adults in South Korea have dealt with mental health issues at some point (National Center for Mental Health [NCMH], 2021). Only 12.1% of individuals diagnosed with mental disorders (such as alcohol abuse, nicotine abuse, depression, and/or anxiety) sought professional assistance, indicating a potential lack of awareness about mental health issues and barriers to seeking support (NCMH, 2021, p. 27).

In 2021, South Korea's age-standardized suicide rate was 24.1 per 100,000, which was the highest among OECD member countries. It was more than twice the OECD average (10.7 people), and the only OECD nation with a rate greater than 20. Lithuania (18.5 suicides per 100,000 people) had the second highest suicide rate among OECD nations (OECD, 2024).

COVID-19

Koreans have a strong inclination toward trusting their government. This attitude enabled the South Korean government to effectively carry out intense contact tracking and monitoring measures, utilizing advanced technology such as mobile applications and surveillance systems, throughout the COVID-19 pandemic. The effort resulted in one of the lowest COVID-19 death rates in the world. As of March 2023, more than 30 million people in South Korea had been infected with COVID-19 and approximately 34,000 had died of the disease (Johns Hopkins Coronavirus Resource Center, 2024).

SOCIAL DETERMINANTS OF HEALTH

HEALTH BEHAVIORS

A lifestyle risk score was developed with five individual unhealthy behaviors associated with increased morbidity and mortality: smoking, alcohol abuse, unhealthy weight, physical inactivity, and insufficient/prolonged sleep (Lee et al., 2020). The most prevalent risk factors in South Korea were insufficient/prolonged sleep, followed by physical inactivity, weight, smoking, and drinking.

The National Sleep Foundation's recommended sleep duration for both the young and for older adults is 7 to 9 hours (Hirshkowitz et al., 2015). Many Koreans experience insufficient sleep. The national average is 7.2 hours (429.4 minutes) on weekdays (Jang et al., 2023). One in four adults are regarded as getting inadequate physical activity. Obesity prevalence is 7.0%, which is much lower than the OECD average of 25.7%. Smoking prevalence is 15.4%, close to the OECD average of 16% (OECD, 2023). Alcohol consumption is lower than the OECD average. In 2023, some local authorities began to enforce a ban on drinking in public places. Legally, however, the punishment is relatively lenient, and accidents by drunken drivers is a significant social issue in South Korea.

SOCIAL AND ECONOMIC FACTORS

In 2022, South Korea's nominal GDP was $1.67 trillion and the per-capita GDP was $32,422.60. South Korea's 2022 per-capita GDP ranked well above the world's average of $12,687; however, lower than the OECD member average (World Bank Group, 2024). Even though the size of the South Korean economy has improved over time, income and financial resource gaps are getting larger. The average income of the richest 20% is 6.5 times more than the lowest 20% (Austin & Sokolowsky, 2021). The costs of housing and raising children are very high, a key reason for low fertility rates. In addition, South Korea has the worst gender pay gap in the OECD. Korean women are paid only two thirds (63%) of a man's income (OECD, 2017).

Based on a relative poverty measure of children living in a household earning less than 60% of the median income, 11.5% of children are in poverty (Austin & Sokolowsky, 2021). Almost 40% of people over age 65 live below the OECD's poverty line, which is set at half the national median income. While a country's old-adult poverty rate is typically higher than its full population, it is exceptionally high in South Korea (Lee, 2023), making health-service use harder for older adults.

HEALTHCARE SYSTEM

OVERVIEW

The healthcare system in South Korea has three main components; the National Health Insurance Service (NHIS) Program, **Medical Aid Program**, and Long-Term Care Insurance Program (LTCI). The NHIS program ensures healthcare access and coverage to all citizens. Primary funding sources for the NHIS come from government subsidies and contributions by the insured (Song et al., 2019). The Medical Aid Program utilizes government subsidies to provide healthcare services to those with low incomes. The LTCI Program offers services to older adults (Health Insurance Review and Assessment Service [HIRA], 2021).

ACCESS, QUALITY, AND COST

The entire population receives essential services. Satisfaction with healthcare availability is 78%, higher than the OECD average of 67%. However, financial coverage is near the bottom of all OECD countries, except for Greece and Brazil. Mandatory prepayment covers 62% of spending versus the OECD average of 76%. Out-of-pocket spending constitutes 29% of health expenditures, higher than the OECD average of 18% (OECD, 2023). South Korea's per-person healthcare expenditure is $4,570, closely matching the OECD average of $4,986. This accounts for 9.7% of the country's GDP, slightly higher than the OECD average of 9.2%.

In 2006, approximately 96% of the total population was insured in one of two ways: employee insured or self-employed insured. The employee insured group includes the immediate family members of the insured individual. These employees contribute 5.08% of their average salary, with the contribution rate adjusted annually. The self-employed insured group consists of those not classified as employee insured, and their contribution is determined based on income, property, living standards, and level of economic activity. A small percent of the population receives support from the Medical Aid Program (Song et al., 2019). Koreans living overseas and foreigners working in South Korea must reside in the country for 6 months before applying for NHIS, which offers the same coverage as it does for Korean citizens (NHIS, 2020).

DELIVERY

According to an OECD report (2023), there are 2.6 practicing doctors and 8.8 practicing nurses per 1,000 population in South Korea. The OECD average is 3.7 and 9.2, respectively. Korea has 12.8 hospital beds per 1,000 population, while the OECD average is 4.3 hospitals. In 2021, there were

772,104 health professionals. Per AKS (2023, p. 16): "The number of licensed nurses accounted for the largest share at 235,041 (30.4%), followed by nurses' aides at 210,810 (27.3%), medical doctors (including dentists and Korean traditional medicine doctors) at 156,892 (20.3%), and medical technologists at 156,217 (20.2%)." In South Korea, patients can choose their providers. However, the uneven distribution of medical services among regions is a significant issue. Most private medical facilities are profit driven and concentrated in urban areas, resulting in 92.1% of physicians and 90.8% of hospital beds being located where 79.7% of the population resides (Song et al., 2019).

A BRIEF HISTORY OF THE NATIONAL HEALTH INSURANCE SERVICE

NHIS was enacted in 1963 but not enforced until 1977. Prior to 1977, patients had to pay for all healthcare except for industrial accidents. The high cost of medical visits led patients to opt for medications that did not require a doctor's prescription to treat minor symptoms, which was legal until pharmaceutical reforms were implemented in 2000 (Jeong, 2005). When Korea's NHIS was introduced in 1977, it was only available to large corporations with 500 or more workers. The Medical Aid Program also started in 1977. Combined, they initially provided health insurance to 10% of the population (Jeong, 2011).

Universal coverage was enacted by July 1989. With universal coverage, enhancing the range of benefits became the focus of healthcare improvement. In October 1989, the benefits package was expanded to include prescription drugs. The number of treatment days allowed were increased to 180 days per year by 1994. All restrictions were eliminated in 2000 (Jeong, 2011). In January 2000, the South Korean parliament passed a law separating prescribing and dispensing drugs to address high costs and misuse/overuse, marking a drastic transformation of the health system (Jeong, 2005; Kwon & Reich, 2005). In July 2000, more than 350 insurance entities were merged into a single organization and designated as a branch of the National Health Insurance Corporation (NHIC; Jeong, 2011; Kwon, 2017).

In April 2007, the Korean National assembly passed the **National Long-Term Care Insurance (NLTCI) for the Elderly Act**, which went into effect on July 1, 2008. NLTCI covers services to older adults such as physical and household-activity support for daily life challenges, thereby improving quality of life. Long-term care and commonly associated issues, such as dementia and stroke, have traditionally been managed by the family. This system seeks to distribute care responsibility between the state and society according to the principle of social solidarity. In addition, it provides benefits not only for older adults, but for all generations, including the people directly responsible for providing long-term care and their children (Kwon, 2017). Although the NLTCI policy has other advantages, it primarily acts as a support mechanism, complementing family-based care for elderly individuals rather than substituting it, and making limited contributions to gender equality (Carson, 2023).

CONCLUSION

The South Korean government developed the country's healthcare system after the society gained economic improvements following the Korean War. This healthcare system has gone through several reforms to address emerging issues. The quality of South Korea's modern healthcare system is very high. Still, questions remain about the health disparities found between the Seoul region and areas far outside of Seoul. Regional inequality in access to medical care services, the low birthrate, high prices of some drugs, suicide rates, low utilization of mental health services, and persistent challenges for long-term older adult care are healthcare issues South Korea needs to address. To address these healthcare concerns and continue enhancing the healthcare system, key stakeholders, sometimes with opposing interests, need to work together.

LEARNING ACTIVITIES

CourseConnect

To access self-assessment questions and interactive, competency-based learning activities for this chapter, visit www.springerpub.com/courseconnect. See inside front cover and tear-out for CourseConnect details.

REFERENCES

Academy of Korean Studies. (2023). *InfoKorea 2023: An essential guide for educators.* https://www.mofa.go.kr/eng/wpge/m_5723/contents.do

Austin, A. & Sokolowsky, T. (2021, October 27). *Don't be fooled, Squid Game fans; the United States is more unequal than South Korea on several measures.* Center for Economic and Policy Research. https://cepr.net/dont-be-fooled-squid-game-fans-the-united-states-is-more-unequal-than-south-korea-on-several-measures/

Carson, A. (2023). A pressure release valve: South Korean long-term care policy as supplemental to family elder care. *Journal of Aging and Social Policy, 35*(6), 756–779. https://doi.org/10.1080/08959420.2022.2133318

Health Insurance Review and Assessment Service. (2021). *What we do: Healthcare system in Korea.* https://www.hira.or.kr/dummy.do?pgmid=HIRAJ010000006000

Hirshkowitz, M., Whiton, K., Albert, S. M., Alessi, C., Bruni, O., DonCarlos, L., Hazen, N., Herman, J., Katz, E. S., Kheirandish-Gozal, L., Neubauer, D. N., O'Donnell, A. E., Ohayon, M., Peever, J., Rawding, R., Sachdeva, R. C., Setters, B., Vitiello, M. V., Ware, J. C., & Hillard, P. J. A. (2015). National Sleep Foundation's sleep time duration recommendations: Methodology and results summary. *Sleep Health, 1*(1), 40–43. https://doi.org/10.1016/j.sleh.2014.12.010

Jang, Y., Jun, J. S., & Jung, K-Y. (2023). Trends in sleep duration in Korea: The Korean time use survey. *Sleep Medicine, 106*, 24–28. https://doi.org/10.1016/j.sleep.2023.01.025

Jeong, H. S. (2005). Health care reform and change in public–private mix of financing: A Korean case. *Health Policy, 74*(2), 133–145. https://doi.org/10.1016/j.healthpol.2004.12.017

Jeong, H. S. (2011). Korea's national health insurance—Lesson from the past three decades. *Health Affairs, 30*(1), 136–144. https://doi.org/10.1377/hlthaff.2008.0816

Johns Hopkins Coronavirus Resource Center. (2024). *Mortality analyses.* https://coronavirus.jhu.edu/data/mortality

Jung, K., Haggard, S., & Choi, C. (2019). Value systems and adaptation: A typology of North Korean defectors. *International Journal of Korean Unification Studies, 28*(2), 67–96.

Kang, S. Y., & Kim, J. K. (2015). Successful aging and economic security among older Koreans. In S. T. Cheng, I. Chi, H. H. Fung, L. W. Li, & J. Woo (Eds.), *Successful aging: Asian perspectives.* Springer. https://doi.org/10.1007/978-94-017-9331-5

Kwon, J. H. (2017). 10 years since the introduction of long-term care insurance for the older population: Implications seen through major issues from the birth of the law to the development of the system. *Medical Policy Forum, 15*(2), 8–14.

Kwon, S. & Reich, M. R. (2005). The changing process and politics of health policy in Korea. *Journal of Health Politics, Policy, and Law, 30*(6), 1003–1026. https://doi.org/10.1215/03616878-30-6-1003

Lee, D. H., Nam, J. Y., Kwon, S., Keum, N. N., Lee, J-T., Shin, M-J., & Oh, H. (2020). Lifestyle risk score and mortality in Korean adults: A population-based cohort study. *Scientific Report, 10*, 10260. https://doi.org/10.1038/s41598-020-66742-y

Lee, J-Y. (2013). *Understanding Korea Series No.1: Hangeul.* The Academy of Korean Studies.

Lee, S-H. (2023, September 25). *Assessing old-age poverty with income and assets: Generational insights and policy directions.* Korea Development Institute. https://www.kdi.re.kr/eng/research/focusView?pub_no=18121

National Center for Mental Health. (2021). *National mental health survey 2021: Adult mental health survey 2021.* National Center for Mental Health. https://mhs.ncmh.go.kr/

National Health Insurance Service. (2020). *National Health Insurance: Guidance for foreigners.* https://www.nhis.or.kr/english/wbheaa02900m01.do

Organisation for Economic Co-operation and Development. (2017). *The pursuit of gender equality: An uphill battle. How does Korea compare.* https://www.oecd.org/korea/Gender2017-KOR-en.pdf

Organisation for Economic Co-operation and Development. (2023). *Health at a glance 2023: OECD indicators.* OECD Publishing, Paris. https://doi.org/10.1787/7a7afb35-en
Organisation for Economic Co-operation and Development. (2024). *Data indicators.* https://data.oecd.org
Park, E. Y. (2022). *Korea: A history.* Stanford University Press.
Park, S. J., & Kang, S. Y. (2007). Social work practice with Korean nursing home residents and their families. In P. Kolb (Ed.), *Social work practice with racially and ethnically diverse nursing home residents and their families* (pp. 162–190). Columbia University Press.
Song, H. J., Jeon, D. J., Lim, K. H., Kim, I. H., Lee, K. H., Choi, E. D., Chun, Y. S., Suh, Y. H., Chun, W. Y., Hahn, M., & Chung, C. H. (2019). *Understanding Korea series No.10: A history of Korea* (D. Kane, J.C. An, & K. Seidel, Trans.). The Academy of Korean Studies.
Statistics Korea. (n.d.). *Statistics Korea.* https://kostat.go.kr/anse/
UN Data Portal (n.d.). *Republic of Korea.* https://population.un.org/dataportal/home?df=f4655af1-c356-49db-9ced-be9871fc65c2
World Health Organization. (2023). *Maternal mortality ratio (per 100,000 live births).* https://data.who.int/indicators/i/AC597B1
World Health Organization. (2024). *Republic of Korea: Health data overview.* https://data.who.int/countries/410
World Health Organization. (2025). *Universal health coverage.* https://www.who.int/health-topics/universal-health-coverage#tab=tab_1
World Bank Group. (2023). *World Bank open data.* https://data.worldbank.org/
World Bank Group. (2024). *Fertility rate, total (births per woman).* https://data.worldbank.org/indicator/SP.DYN.TFRT.IN?end=2021&locations=KR&start=1960&view=chart

CHAPTER 52

TAIWAN

Mei-Hsiu Chen

GEOGRAPHY AND POPULATION

Taiwan, officially called the **Republic of China** (used interchangeably herein) is a democratic country located in the western Pacific region between Japan (to the north) and the Philippines (to the south). It is a small island nation, which consists of the main island of Taiwan, five smaller residential islands (Penghu, Kinmen, Matsu, Green Island, and Orchid Island), and many other islets. The total area of Taiwan is 36,197 square kilometers (Republic of China, 2024). Because the major island of Taiwan is in the tropical-to-temporal spectrum of climate zones, agricultural development is very advanced with rice as the primary grain. Due to the high mountains spanning from north to south in the middle of Taiwan Island, the west side of the island is much more populated and better developed than the east side. Taiwan Island sits on the edges of tectonic plates (part of the Ring of Fire) in the Pacific Ocean and experiences frequent earthquakes such as the 7.4-magnitude earthquake in April 2024. It also regularly experiences typhoons during the summer months.

Taiwan's population increased 3.6% from 22.6 million in 2003 to 23.4 million in 2023. Its population density of 647 persons per square kilometer (0.6 square miles) is among the top 20 highest in the world (Republic of China, 2024c). However, its crude birth rate decreased from 10.06 births per 1,000 in 2003 to 5.81 births per 1,000 in 2023, while adults age 65 and older doubled from 9.2% in 2003 to 18.3% in 2023 (Department of Household Registration, Ministry of the Interior, 2024). As shown in Figure 52.1, the median age increased from 32 years in 2003 to 42 years in 2023.

CULTURE

The Han people account for 96.4% of Taiwan's population and use Mandarin, Holo, and Hakka as primary languages. There are 16 Indigenous Malayo–Polynesian tribes that together account for 2.5% of the total population. There are 42 recognized languages among the Indigenous Malay–Polynesian people. New immigrants account for 1.1% of the population and are primarily from China and Southeast Asian countries (Republic of China, 2024). For written language, Taiwan is the only country to use traditional Chinese characters where each character retains its history. In addition, Taiwan has developed its own sign language, called Taiwanese Sign Language.

The freedom of religion and the right to belief are protected by the Constitution of the Republic of China, thus there is a wide spectrum of religions and religious beliefs. A total of 22 different religions are recognized in Taiwan. Chinese folk religions, Buddhism, and Taoism are the three most popular religions. Because of the fusion of traditional tenets such as Buddhism and Confucianism with modern culture, important cultural events and celebrations are mostly tied with the Lunar Calendar and the 24 Solar Terms. Specifically, the **Lunar New Year** is considered a family holiday where families get together on Lunar New Year's Eve and enjoy feasts together along with family-friendly games. Other important celebrations include the **Mid-Autumn Festival**, which is celebrated with traditional moon cakes and barbeque, and the **Dragon Boat Festival**, which is celebrated with dumplings wrapped in bamboo leaves and dragon boat racing.

The political system in Taiwan is a multiparty democracy that directly elects a president and a vice president every 4 years by each voter casting one ballot. The two largest political parties are the Kuo Ming Tang (KMT) and the Democratic Progressive Party (DPP). Members of the

FIGURE 52.1 Age distributions in Taiwan, 2003 and 2022.

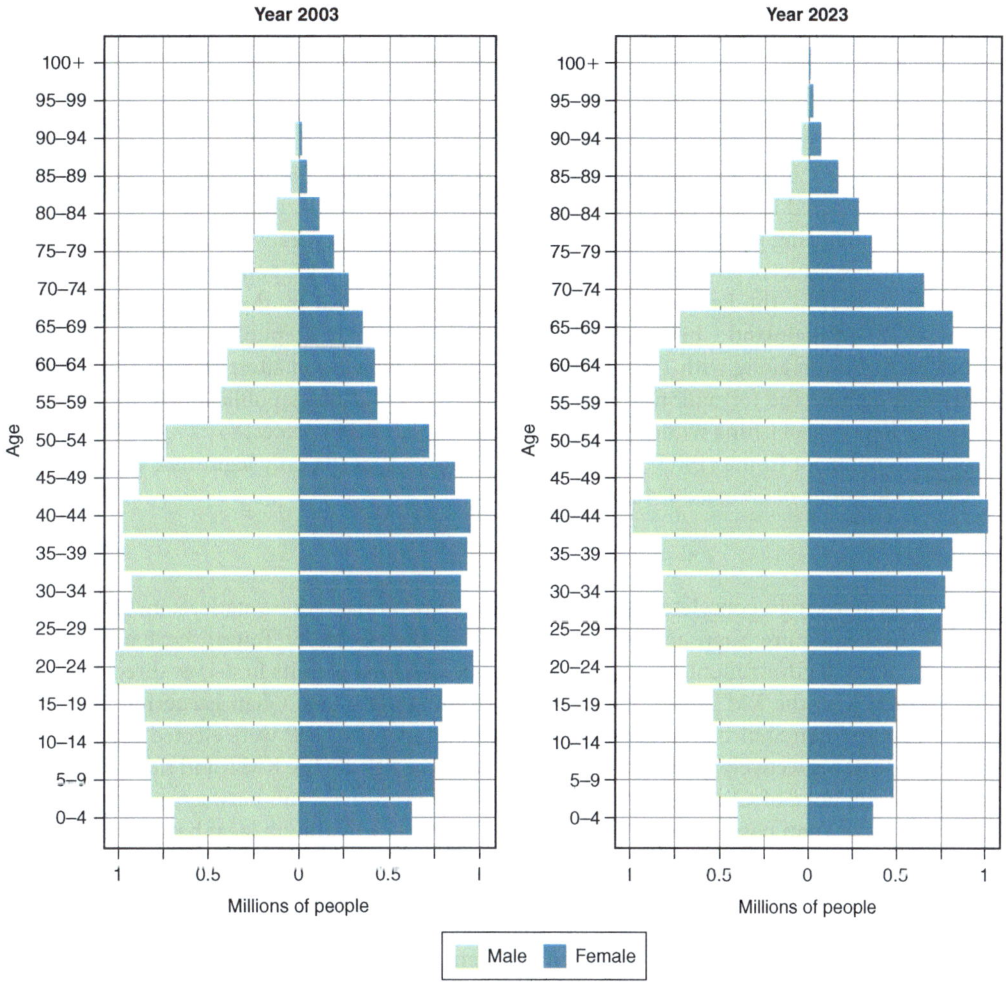

Source: Department of Household Registration, Ministry of Interior. (2024). *Demographics*. https://www.ris.gov.tw/app/portal/346

Legislative Yuan branch of the government are elected by each voter casting two ballots, one for the local district and one for the at-large seats every 4 years. Citizens can also exercise the power of ratifying Constitutional Amendments through referenda. The governing tasks and the checks-and-balances are carried out in the central government that consists of the president and five major branches (called **Yuans**): the Executive Yuan, Legislative Yuan, Judicial Yuan, Examination Yuan, and Control Yuan (Republic of China, 2024a).

BRIEF HISTORY

TAIWAN HISTORY

Taiwan has been home to Indigenous Malayo–Polynesian peoples for many millennia. Small groups of Chinese merchants, fishermen, and pirates visiting Taiwan were documented in the 16th century. Also during the 16th century, European sailors referred to the island as Ilha

Formosa, or beautiful island. In the 17th century, Taiwan was intermittingly occupied by Dutch and Spanish explorers and Chinese loyalists of the Ming Dynasty. From 1895 to 1945, Taiwan was under Japanese rule as part of the Treaty of Shimonoseki (National Museum of Taiwan History, n.d.).

REPUBLIC OF CHINA IN TAIWAN

The Republic of China was founded in mainland China by revolutionaries against the Qing Dynasty and elected its first president in 1912. After World War II, the Republic of China took over Taiwan following Japan's surrender in 1945. After the takeover, Taiwan natives were excluded from the higher ranks of governing officials which led to a large-scale political uprising of Taiwan residents in 1947—"The February 28 Incident." Following defeat by the Chinese Communist's Party (CCP) on mainland China in 1949, the government of the Republic of China completely relocated to Taiwan along with 1.2 million people from China. Soon after, **martial law** went into effect and banned the formation of new political parties and news publications until 1987. In 1971, the Republic of China withdrew from the United Nations in protest to its recognition of the People's Republic of China (PRC), formerly called the CCP, as the only legitimate representative of China (Republic of China, 2024d).

ROAD TO DEMOCRACY

Since 1991, following a complete re-election of all congressional representatives, including members of the Legislature Yuan and National Assembly, the people of Taiwan have achieved full representation in government. In 1996, the Republic of China held its first-ever direct presidential election, with the KMT's Lee Teng-hui and running mate Lien Chan garnering 54% of the vote. In 2000, Chen Shui-bian and Annette Hsiu-lien Lu of the DPP were elected president and vice president, respectively, ending more than 50 years of rule by the KMT and marking the first transfer of Republic of China government executive power in Taiwan between political parties. The Legislative Yuan passed the Referendum Act in 2003, providing a legal basis for citizens to vote directly on issues of local or national importance, a huge milestone for a country going from martial law to full democracy. In 2 years, a constitutional amendment was passed halving the number of Legislative Yuan seats and introducing the single-district, two-votes system for legislative elections that provides voter involvement, both locally and nationally. In 2016, the DPP Chairperson Tsai Ing-wen and academic Chen Chien-jen were elected president and vice president, respectively, of the Republic of China, marking the first time a female was elected president. The DPP went on to win the next two presidential elections (2020 and 2024), the first time that a party has held the office for three consecutive terms since Taiwan began direct presidential elections in 1996 (Republic of China, 2024b).

WELFARE

Taiwan's 9-year compulsory education system was launched in 1968 at a time when few countries had done so. This set the stage for a well-educated population and is also a major contributing factor in the peaceful transition from martial law to full democracy. The **National Health Insurance (NHI) program** started in 1995 and provides health insurance for the entire population. In 2002, Taiwan became a member of the World Trade Organization. In 2009, Taiwan attended the World Health Assembly as an observer, its first UN activity since its withdrawal in 1971. In 2017, the **Indigenous Languages Development Act** was enacted to preserve and promote the native tongues of Taiwan's 16 officially recognized Indigenous tribes. In 2019, the Taiwan became the first Asian country to legalize same-sex marriages (Republic of China, 2024a). The Republic of China is also well known for its high-tech manufacturing brawn in such achievements as the Taiwan Semiconductor Manufacturing Company (TSMC), agriculture advancements, and culinary traditions and innovations such as pineapple cakes and bubble tea.

HEALTH OUTCOMES

Life expectancy at birth in Taiwan during 2023 was 80.56 years, an increase of 4.42 years from 76.14 years during 2000. Women are consistently projected to outlive men by about 5 years—83.61 versus 77.63 years in 2023 (UN Data Portal, n.d.). As of 2022, the top five causes of death were cancer, cardiovascular disease, COVID-19, pneumonia, and stroke. The leading cancer deaths for men were lung, liver, and colorectal; the leading cancer deaths for females were lung, colorectal, and breast (Ministry of Health and Welfare [MoHW], 2023). Figure 52.2 shows the 10 leading causes of death and the 11 leading cancers in 2022 in comparison with 2012 (MoHW, 2023).

Taiwan has low infant and maternal mortality. In 2023, Taiwan's infant mortality rate was three infant deaths per 1,000 live births. The maternity maternal mortality ratio slightly increased from 8.5 maternal deaths per 100,000 live births in 2012 to 13.1 in 2022, perhaps due in part to increasing maternity age (Republic of China, 2023b). In 2019, a total of 2.8 million people (11.8% of the

FIGURE 52.2 Leading causes of death and leading cancer deaths in Taiwan, 2022 and 2012.

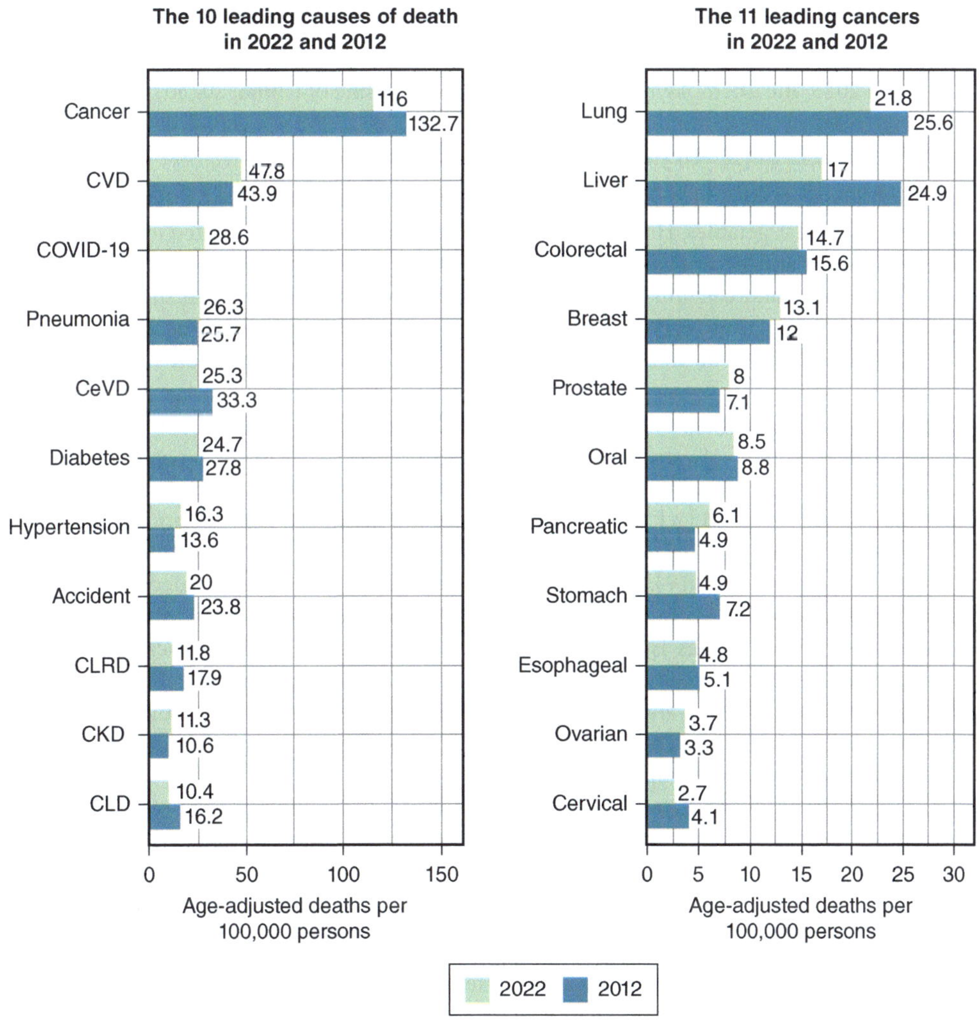

CeVD, cerebrovascular disease; CKD, chronic kidney disease; CLD, chronic liver disease; CLRD, chronic lower respiratory disease; CVD, cardiovascular disease.

Source: Ministry of Health and Welfare. (2023). *111 Chinese death statistics*. https://www.mohw.gov.tw/cp-16-74869-1.html

total population) sought medical help for mental health, among them 56% were females (Mental Health's Day Report, 2021).

DETERMINANTS OF HEALTH

SOCIOECONOMIC DETERMINANTS

The nominal gross domestic product (GDP) for the Republic of China in 2022 was $653 billion, which ranked comparably to Poland and Switzerland. Its per-capita GDP in 2022 was $32,756, which is slightly less than half that of the United States, but represents similar purchasing power parity as the Bahamas and South Korea (Republic of China, 2024a). The poverty rate steadily decreased from 1.53% in 2012 to 1.24% in 2022 (Republic of China, 2023c). Because the 9-year compulsory education system has been in effect since 1968, Taiwan has an extremely high literacy rate (98.96% in 2019) that continues to climb. The majority of people who are illiterate are age 65 and older. For those age 15 and up, 30.0% have a high school diploma and 46.5% have at least an associate degree (11.1% associate degree, 27.9% bachelor's degree, 7.5% advanced degree) as their highest level of education. Approximately 48% of males and 45% of females have at least an associate degree (Republic of China, 2020). The unemployment rates generally hover between 3.0% and 4.0%; in 2023, the unemployment rate was 3.48% (Republic of China, 2023d).

BEHAVIORAL DETERMINANTS

A balanced diet and physical activities are keys to a healthy life. Traditional Taiwanese diets are rich in seafood and vegetables. However, Western cultural influence has resulted in an increase in sedentary lifestyles and dietary intake of excessive total calories and saturated fat. At the same time, intake of potassium and calcium is insufficient. Because of unhealthy cultural shifts, the Health Promotion Administration (HPA) in the Republic of China began publishing healthy dietary intake guidelines to prevent and manage various diseases (Health Promotion Administration, n.d.). The HPA also enacts measures to promote physical activity. The percentages of women and men exercising regularly (defined as 30 minutes or more 3 times a week, with moderate strength) increased slightly from 35.6% and 27.0% in 2013 to 38.7% and 31.5% in 2023, respectively.

Cigarette smoking (including secondhand smoke), excessive alcohol intake, consumption of betel nuts, poor diet, and lack of physical activities are the major contributing mortality risk factors in Taiwan. Lung cancer deaths have been the number one cancer deaths for both men and women. However, the smoking rate among men age 18 and older has decreased steadily from 48.2% in 2002 to 24.4% in 2022, and among women from 5.3% in 2002 to 3.7% in 2022. The decline in smoking rates is attributed to increased taxation, public education, smoking cessation measures, and a smoking ban at public places (Report on Smoking Behavior, 2023). Historically, because smoking and alcohol consumption are parts of tribal celebration activities for the Indigenous Malayo–Polynesian people, specifically tailored educational outreach has been designed for those vulnerable populations.

The Taiwanese culture of chewing betel nuts contributes to the high rate of oral cancer deaths for men. In 2018, 6.2% of men age 18 and older chewed betel nuts, with the highest usage rates among men age 30 to 50 and those with low educational attainment (MoHW, 2023).

ENVIRONMENTAL DETERMINANTS

Due to climate change, the average air and sea temperatures have steadily increased over the last 100 years in Taiwan Island. As a result, the summer seasons are lengthened while the winter seasons are shortened. The overall rainfall in Taiwan Island has been steadily increasing and has induced higher chances of flooding and periods of drought. The rising sea level and the drought-induced depletion of underground water can cause salt water to seep through aquifers and pollute the water essential for agriculture in the coastal areas. Increased temperature also diminishes wind speed, and the air quality is projected to worsen because pollutants, such as fine particulate matter ($PM_{2.5}$) and ozone, are less likely to be dispersed (National Environmental Research Academy, 2024).

HEALTHCARE SYSTEM

OVERVIEW

The NHI program was started in 1995 by integrating the existing labor, farmers, and government employees' medical insurance systems into a comprehensive social insurance regime that covers the entire population. After several rounds of reorganizations and consolidations, the current 29-year old NHI system is a government-run, single-payer regime.

The NHI program is mandatory for all nationals of the Republic of China who have had a registered domicile in the country for at least 6 months and for all newborns born in Republic of China. The insured individuals are classified into six categories that are largely based on occupations, and the insurance premiums are calculated based on tiers within each category. To accommodate social changes and promote human rights and fairness, the NHI has undergone several statutory amendments expanding coverages to new immigrants, long-term foreign residents, overseas Chinese and foreign students, and military personnel. To further promote equal rights to medical care, inmates in correctional facilities are also eligible as beneficiaries after the second-generation NHI was launched in 2013. Additional requirements for eligibility were also added based on public expectations of social fairness and justice. As of 2022, there were more than 23 million NHI beneficiaries (Republic of China, 2023a).

FINANCES

Since its inception, the NHI has operated under the principles of financial self-sufficiency and pay-as-you-go. At present, the NHI derives its income primarily from premiums paid by the insured, employers, and the government, with a small fraction supplemented by premium overdue charges, contributions from public welfare lottery net revenues, and the tobacco health and welfare surcharge. Social and demographic changes, however, have led to the NHI's expenses growing far faster than premium income does. Broadening sources of income, conserving funds, and premium adjustments have been adopted to stabilize NHI finances and ensure that the NHI can stay soundly operational. The launch of second-generation NHI introduces a key feature of revenue-expenditure linkage to preserve long-term financial stability. The **NHI Committee**, comprised of representatives from key stakeholders such as the insured population, employers, and medical service providers, was established to review the premium rate and make recommendations for government approval every year. The general premium rate that applies directly to the ratable wage is kept at 5.17%. The supplementary premium rate, which applies to supplemental incomes, has been 2.11% since 2021 (Republic of China, 2023a).

DELIVERY

Healthcare services covered by the NHI include outpatient care, inpatient care, traditional Chinese medicine, dental care, child delivery, rehabilitation, home healthcare, and chronic mental illness rehabilitation. Services are delivered by hospitals, clinics, pharmacies, and laboratory test institutions. The scope of medical payments under the NHI includes screening, diagnosis, examination, lab test, surgery, anesthesia, medication, materials, treatment, and nursing, and covers nearly all necessary healthcare services. Pharmacy services include distribution of medications with prescriptions and providing medication education and consultations to ensure safe medication use.

As of 2022, there was a total of 21,860 NHI-contracted hospitals and clinics, which accounted for 92.04% of all hospitals and clinics nationwide. There were 7,184 contracted pharmacies, 744 home care institutions, 250 psychiatric rehabilitation institutions, 16 midwifery institutions, 217 medical testing institutions, 32 physical therapy clinics, eight medical radiological institutions, two occupational therapy clinics, and 12 home respiratory care institutions. In 2022, the average annual number of per-capita outpatient visits was 14.27, the average annual number of hospitalizations per 100 persons was 13.2, and the average annual number of days of hospitalization per capita was 1.24 days (Republic of China, 2023a).

NHI copayments are designed to guide the utilization of medical resources and ensure that hospitals and clinics at different levels carry out their respective duties. Several rounds of adjustments in copayments and revisions to hierarchical referral systems were done to encourage compliance with the referral system, reduce drug waste, and improve medical care efficiency. In addition, to ensure that people can receive continuous, comprehensive medical care locally, the **NHI Family Physician Integrated Care Project** formed community healthcare groups that each contain five or more primary care clinics and a corresponding regional hospital. The community healthcare groups provide 24-hour healthcare counseling hotlines, health education and management, smooth referral and information relays, and continuous care. By 2022, a total of 609 community healthcare groups were in operation, participating primary care clinics numbered 5,678 with a 53.1% participation rate, participating physicians numbered 7,833 with a 46% physician participation rate, and the beneficiaries of community healthcare groups exceeded 6 million persons (Republic of China, 2023a).

GLOBAL BUDGET PAYMENT SYSTEM

Since its inception, the NHI program has utilized a fee-for-service, third-party payment approach and paid medical expenses to hospitals and clinics based on a NHI fee schedule. While several revisions based on scope of reimbursements and recommendations of medical groups were made, the system was still stressed by uncontrolled increases in medical expenses that affected the quality of care. Accordingly, the National Health Insurance Administration (NHIA) followed other leading countries' example by designing payment methods based on the characteristics of different medical care types to change treatment behaviors, such as case payment and pay-for-performance (P4P). The NHIA pays hospitals and clinics based on care quality and outcomes under P4P plans. In addition, the Integrated Delivery System (IDS) implemented by the NHIA in mountain areas and on offshore islands has enhanced integration of the medical service system. To enhance patient health and medical efficiency, the NHIA launched the **Taiwan Diagnosis Related Groups (TW-DRGs)** program in 2010, which divides inpatients into groups based on their conditions and/or demographic characteristics and sets the payment rates accordingly. TW-DRGs has helped mitigate unnecessary waste in medical procedures and improved patient care (Republic of China, 2024b).

By 2002, full-scale global budget payment systems were implemented, providing effective, high-quality medical care using limited health insurance resources. Overall, the system had successfully limited the medical expense growth rate to below 6%—in 2023, the medical expense growth rate was only 3.323%. Quality assurance programs, such as quality satisfaction surveys and complaints and reported case response mechanisms, have also been enacted to ensure that the quality and scope of care available at medical institutions do not change due to the implementation of a global budget payment system.

STRENGTHS AND INNOVATIONS

New diagnostic and treatment items reflecting advances in medical technologies and clinical needs have been added regularly to the NHI, allowing the public to receive up-to-date medical services. As of 2022, the fee schedule contained a total of 4,785 diagnostic and treatment items. Since 2010, the screening of breast, cervical, oral, and colorectal cancers have been fully covered (Health Promotion Administration, n.d.).

To encourage hospitals to place a greater emphasis on the clinical nursing workforce, a program to improve the quality of inpatient nursing care was implemented in 2009. The program includes hiring more nursing staff, increasing pay for night shifts, and subsidizing extra overtime to incentivize nurses to stay on the job. Additional investment was made to adjust the reimbursement rates for inpatient nursing services. This measure has not only increased the payment point values for the nurses' services but also reduced nurses' burdens through the linkage of payments to the nurse–patient ratio.

NHI's P4P plans were designed to provide greater incentives for providers to offer comprehensive care and to improve the quality and effectiveness of care by adjusting medical expenses payments to hospitals and clinics accordingly. Since 2001, the management of several diseases, such as cervical cancer and diabetes, were included in the P4P plans, resulting in more people receiving comprehensive care and decreasing mortality.

In 2013, the **NHI MediCloud System** was established to give providers access to prescriptions and all medical information. With the promotion of individualized cloud service (**My Health Bank**), individuals can also monitor and manage their own health more easily. Cloud technologies have played an important role in containing the spread of COVID-19 via information sharing and overall healthcare management during the pandemic (MoHW, 2023).

CONCLUSION

The healthcare system in the Republic of China is young but has made tremendous progress. Since the inception of the NHI program in 1995, addressing inequalities and maintaining affordability has been its central mission. Regular medical service review of the NHI is carried out to avoid overutilization and ensure medical quality. Shifting the care for chronic diseases to comprehensive care and utilizing technological innovations has made the management and delivery of healthcare in the Taiwan more effective at promoting overall health while containing costs. Continuing education and promoting healthy behaviors will be keys to combat issues arising from population aging and climate change.

LEARNING ACTIVITIES

CourseConnect

To access self-assessment questions and interactive, competency-based learning activities for this chapter, visit www.springerpub.com/courseconnect. See inside front cover and tear-out for CourseConnect details.

REFERENCES

Department of Household Registration, Ministry of the Interior, Republic of China. (2024). *Household registration statistics*. https://www.ris.gov.tw/app/portal/346

Ministry of Health and Welfare. (2023). *111 Chinese death statistics*. https://www.mohw.gov.tw/cp-16-74869-1.html

National Environmental Research Academy. (2024). *Climate change report*. https://www.moenv.gov.tw/nera/7CFA1D364EA6AFE4

National Museum of Taiwan History. (n.d.). *Homepage*. https://www.nmth.gov.tw

Republic of China. (2020). *Educational attainment report*. https://ws.moi.gov.tw/001/Upload/OldFile/news_file/109%E5%B9%B4%E7%AC%AC12%E9%80%B1%E5%85%A7%E6%94%BF%E7%B5%B1%E8%A8%88%E9%80%9A%E5%A0%B1_%E6%95%99%E8%82%B2%E7%A8%8B%E5%BA%A6.pdf

Republic of China. (2021). *Mental health's day report*. https://www.mohw.gov.tw/dl-72387-864eb8f0-64ef-42db-8a12-63169b8b97fc.html

Republic of China. (2023). *Report on smoking behavior*. https://www.hpa.gov.tw/Pages/Detail.aspx?nodeid=1718&pid=9913

Republic of China. (2023a). *Annual report of NHI.* https://www.nhi.gov.tw/en/dl-66546-2d7d3464d48e48a49f3df9c2145d5818-2.pdf

Republic of China. (2023b). *Infant and maternity deaths.* https://www.gender.ey.gov.tw/GecDB/Common/FileDownload.ashx?sn=ZjuYAILSzOJbDTdzlIsO5g%40%40&ext=.pdf

Republic of China. (2023c). *Low-income statistics.* https://dep.mohw.gov.tw/DOS/cp-5342-59468-113.html

Republic of China. (2023d). *Unemployment rates.* https://www.stat.gov.tw/News_Content.aspx?n=2703&s=230291

Republic of China. (2024a). *About Taiwan.* https://www.taiwan.gov.tw/about.php

Republic of China. (2024b). *TW-DRGs overview.* https://www.mohw.gov.tw/cp-115-2552-2.html.

Republic of China. (2024c). *Executive Yuan.* https://www.ey.gov.tw/state/

Republic of China. (2024d). *History.* https://www.taiwan.gov.tw/content_3.php

UN Data Portal. (n.d.). *UN Population Division data portal.* https://population.un.org/dataportal/home/

PART XIII: Health and Healthcare in Southeast Asia

CHAPTER 53

OVERVIEW OF SOUTHEAST ASIA

Ammcise Apply and Thomas Foley

GEOGRAPHY

Covering approximately 13 million square kilometers (8 million square miles), Southeast Asia represents about 10% of Asia's total landmass (Leinbach & Frederick, 2024). It is divided into Mainland Southeast Asia, which spans around 2.3 million square kilometers (1.4 million square miles), and Maritime Southeast Asia, covering over 10.5 million square kilometers (6.5 million square miles; Bradford & Strating, 2023). Mainland Southeast Asia includes Myanmar, Thailand, Lao People's Democratic Republic (Laos), Cambodia, Vietnam, and Peninsular Malaysia. This area is characterized by rugged mountain ranges, such as the Annamite Range and the Shan Hills, that are interspersed with fertile river valleys like the Mekong, Irrawaddy, and Chao Phraya rivers, crucial for agriculture and transportation. Maritime Southeast Asia consists of numerous islands and archipelagos, including Indonesia, the Philippines, East Malaysia, Brunei, Singapore, and Timor-Leste. This subregion features some of the world's largest islands, such as Borneo and Sumatra, and is part of the Pacific Ring of Fire, resulting in significant volcanic and seismic activity (Berglee, 2016).

Climate change profoundly impacts Southeast Asia, leading to high sea levels and more frequent and severe extreme weather events such as floods and landslides. Southeast Asia is also notable for its strategic geographical position between the economic giants of East Asia and South Asia. It is bordered by the Indian Ocean to the west, the Pacific Ocean to the east, and the South China Sea to the south. Its sea routes are among the busiest and play a crucial role in international trade (Leinbach & Frederick, 2024). Figure 53.1 is a map of Southeast Asia.

POPULATION

The population of Southeast Asia was slightly greater than 690 million people in 2023, representing approximately 8.5% of the global population. While Southeast Asia is predominately rural, there are areas with significant population density such as Singapore and the cities of Jakarta on the Indonesian island of Java, Ho Chi Minh City in Vietnam, and Bangkok in Thailand. Indonesia is the Southeast Asian country with the largest population (approximately 281 million people in 2023), while Brunei has the smallest (458,949 people in 2023). Southeast Asia's median age in 2023 was 30.2 years, which was slightly lower than the global median age of 30.4 years. Median ages in Southeast Asia during 2023 ranged from 21 years in Timor-Leste to 39.8 years in Thailand. The birth rate in Southeast Asia during 2023 was 14.9 per 1,000 peope, which was also slightly lower than the global average of 16.3. Birth rates in Southeast Asia varied drastically based on urban–rural and low–high income divides. For example, the birth rates in Thailand and Singapore during 2023 were both 8.2 births per 1,000 people, while the birth rate in Timor-Leste was 22.1 births per 1,000 people (UN Data Portal, n.d.).

BRIEF HISTORY

Southeast Asia's role as a crossroads of trade and culture has attracted various global powers, significantly shaping its political and economic landscape for thousands of years. Early civilizations

FIGURE 53.1 Map of Southeast Asia.

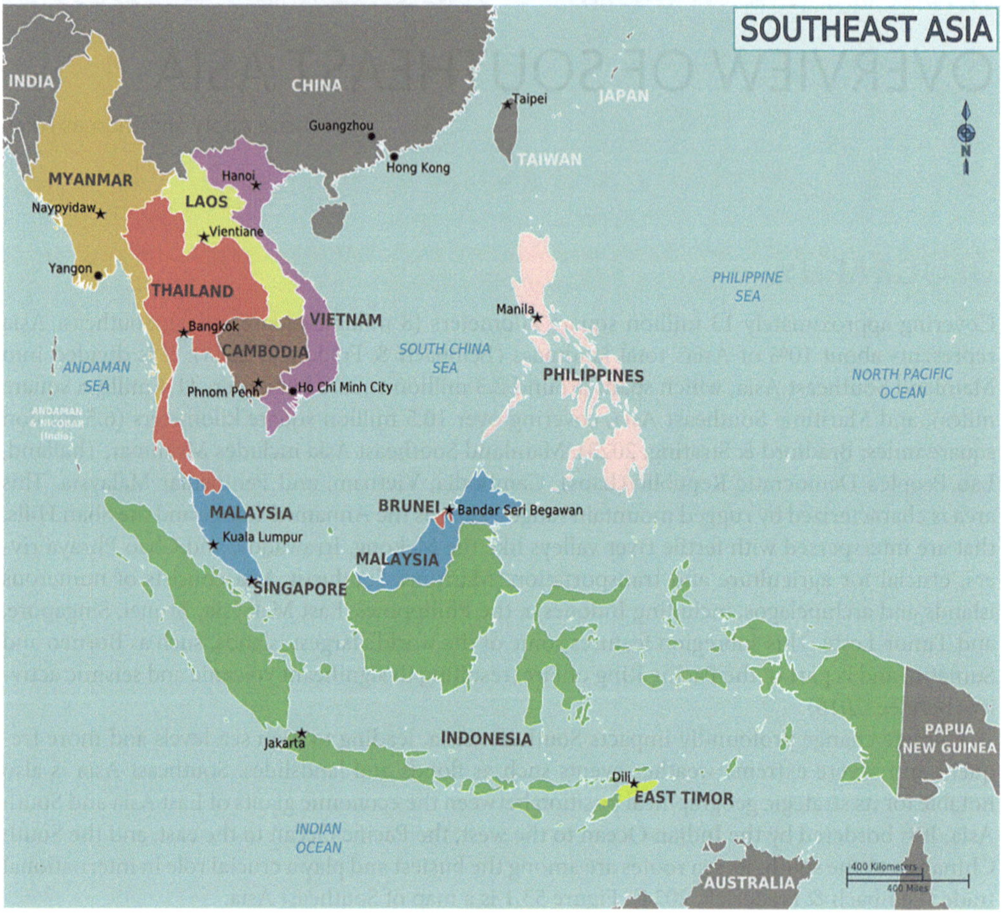

Source: Cacahuate. (2008). *Map of Southeast Asia*. https://commons.wikimedia.org/wiki/File:Map_of_Southeast_Asia.png

such as the Dong Son culture in Vietnam and Ban Chiang in Thailand were advanced in agricultural and metallurgical practices. Indian cultural influences introduced Hinduism and Buddhism, shaping powerful kingdoms like the Funan and the Khmer Empire. From the seventh century, maritime trade routes connected the region with India, China, and the Middle East, spreading Islam in the 13th century and leading to the rise of influential sultanates such as Malacca. European colonization in the 16th century—by the Portuguese, Spanish, Dutch, British, and French, all vying for control over the region's spice trade and strategic locations—led to significant social, economic, and political changes that have shaped modern Southeast Asia. Following World War II, the region saw a wave of decolonization and independence movements such as in Indonesia, the Philippines, Myanmar, and Vietnam (Frederick, 2018). Today, Southeast Asia is a dynamic and diverse region marked by economic growth and cultural richness. The creation of the **Association of Southeast Asian Nations (ASEAN)** in 1967 has played a crucial role in fostering regional cooperation for economic and cultural development and combating political instability and social inequities. The 2021 military coup in Myanmar, however, has challenged the effectiveness of ASEAN (Teekah, 2024).

COMPARATIVE DETERMINANTS OF HEALTH IN SOUTHEAST ASIA

Economic indicators and social determinants of health vary widely across Southeast Asia. Singapore has one of the highest per-capita gross domestic products (GDP) in the world, exceeding $84,700 in 2023, due to its wise economic strategies, which has led to subsequent investments in healthcare. Conversely, Myanmar's low per-capita GDP, which was $1,187.60 per person in 2023, limits resources for healthcare. Singapore, with less than a 1% poverty rate due to comprehensive social welfare programs, contrasts sharply with Myanmar, where approximately 25% of the population lives below the national poverty line. Literacy further illustrates regional disparities, ranging from 70% to 98% between 2019 and 2022. Singapore has achieved a high level of literacy, with a literacy rate of approximately 98%. In contrast, Timor-Leste has a literacy rate of approximately 70%, which can challenge efforts to address poverty and improve health outcomes (World Bank Group, n.d.).

HEALTH OUTCOMES

Southeast Asia presents diverse health outcomes influenced by economic development, healthcare infrastructure, and regional disparities. Life expectancy and infant and maternal mortality vary significantly across the region. Singapore, which is a high-income, urban nation, has extremely low infant and maternal mortality, while low-income Southeast Asian countries such as Timor-Leste and Myanmar have high infant and maternal mortality. Life expectancy at birth in Southeast Asia at 72.13 years was slightly below the world average of 73.17 years in 2023. While Singapore has one of the greatest life expectancies at birth in the world, Myanmar, Laos, Timor-Leste, the Philippines, Cambodia, and Indonesia have life expectancies below the world average (UN Data Portal, n.d.). While chronic diseases account for a large percentage of mortality in Southeast Asia, deaths due to infectious diseases and poor maternal and child healthcare are still prominent issues. Tuberculosis and neonatal disorders were among the top 10 leading causes of mortality in Cambodia, Laos, Myanmar, the Philippines, and Timor-Leste during 2021 (Institute for Health Metrics and Evaluation [IHME], n.d.). Dengue is also a major concern, with a 46% increase in cases from 2015 to 2019. Indonesia, Myanmar, and Thailand are among the top 30 most dengue endemic countries in the world (World Health Organization [WHO], n.d.).

Studying the countries of Southeast Asia provides significant insight into the etiology of health and disease. From the effectiveness of health promotion programs in Singapore to the impact of political instability on Myanmar's healthcare system, there is much for the global community to garner from this region. Table 53.1 includes regional health outcome data.

TABLE 53.1 HEALTH OUTCOMES IN SOUTHEAST ASIA

REGION/ COUNTRY	LIFE EXPECTANCY AT BIRTH (YEARS), 2023	INFANT MORTALITY (PER 1,000 LIVE BIRTHS), 2023	MATERNAL MORTALITY (PER 100,000 LIVE BIRTHS), 2020	LEADING CAUSE OF MORTALITY, 2021
Southeast Asia	72.31	18	134.2	—
Brunei	75.33	8.1	44.2	Heart disease
Cambodia	70.67	19.2	218	Stroke
Indonesia	71.15	17.1	172.9	Stroke
Laos	68.96	31.7	126.1	Stroke
Malaysia	76.66	6.4	21.1	Heart disease

(continued)

TABLE 53.1 HEALTH OUTCOMES IN SOUTHEAST ASIA (*CONTINUED*)

REGION/ COUNTRY	LIFE EXPECTANCY AT BIRTH (YEARS), 2023	INFANT MORTALITY (PER 1,000 LIVE BIRTHS), 2023	MATERNAL MORTALITY (PER 100,000 LIVE BIRTHS), 2020	LEADING CAUSE OF MORTALITY, 2021
Myanmar	75	31.8	178.7	Stroke
Philippines	69.83	20.7	78.2	COVID-19
Singapore	83.74	1.7	7.5	Heart disease
Thailand	76.41	6.2	28.6	Stroke
Timor-Leste	67.69	37.6	203.9	Stroke
Vietnam	74.59	15.1	124.3	Stroke

Sources: Institute for Health Metrics and Evaluation. (n.d.). *Health research by location: Country profiles*. University of Washington. https://www.healthdata.org/research-analysis/health-by-location/profiles; UN Data Portal. (n.d.). *UN Population Division data portal*. https://population.un.org/dataportal/home?df=94a1141a-930a-4648-b73b-a78f739690bc; UN Population Fund. (n.d.). *Data portal*. https://www.unfpa.org/data

LEARNING ACTIVITIES

CourseConnect >

To access self-assessment questions and interactive, competency-based learning activities for this chapter, visit www.springerpub.com/courseconnect. See inside front cover and tear-out for CourseConnect details.

REFERENCES

Berglee, R. (2016). *Southeast Asia in world regional geography*. University of Minnesota, World Regional Geography. https://open.lib.umn.edu/worldgeography/

Bradford, J., & Strating, B. (2023). *Maritime governance policy and priorities in Southeast Asia*. Asia Maritime Transparency Initiative. https://amti.csis.org/maritime-governance-policy-and-priorities-in-southeast-asia/

Frederick, W. H. (2018). History of Southeast Asia. *Encyclopedia Britannica*. https://www.britannica.com/place/history-of-Southeast-Asia-556509

Institute for Health Metrics and Evaluation. (n.d.). *Health research by location: Country profiles*. University of Washington. https://www.healthdata.org/research-analysis/health-by-location/profiles

Leinbach, T. R., & Frederick, W. H. (2024). Southeast Asia. *Encyclopedia Britannica*. https://www.britannica.com/place/Southeast-Asia

Teekah, E. (2024). ASEAN. *Encyclopedia Britannica*. https://www.britannica.com/topic/ASEAN

UN Data Portal. (n.d.). *UN Population Division data portal*. United Nations. https://population.un.org/dataportal/home/

World Bank. (n.d.). *The World Bank open data*. https://data.worldbank.org/

World Health Organization. (n.d.). *Child health in the Southeast Asia region*. https://www.who.int/southeastasia/health-topics/child-health

CHAPTER 54

MYANMAR

Thet Su Htwe and Thomas C. Muller

INTRODUCTION

Blessed with bountiful natural resources, a highly literate populace, and a relatively advanced healthcare system in urban areas, Myanmar (formerly Burma) has for decades been considered a promising candidate for strong economic and social advancement. However, it has not matched the progress of a number of other Southeast Asian countries. As of 2022, Myanmar ranked 144th out of 193 nations in the UN Human Development Index (2024) and 109th of 163 countries in quality of their health and healthcare systems (Statista, 2024). By far the greatest impediment regarding Myanmar's development has been the decades-long violent conflict between the military-controlled national government and a myriad of ethnic groups fighting for greater autonomy, primarily in border areas. As you read this chapter, think about the following question: What are the healthcare challenges facing a developing nation, especially one enmeshed in a civil war?

GEOGRAPHY

At approximately 676,000 square kilometers (420,000 square miles), the Republic of the Union of Myanmar is the largest country on the mainland of Southeast Asia. Its borders do not always reflect what might be considered natural and/or organic geographic fusions, however. Consequently, many of the diverse ethnic groups along those borders share stronger cultural and linguistic ties with the populations of neighboring countries than with other segments of Myanmar. A "horseshoe" of mountains envelopes the western, northern, and eastern sides of the country. The middle section gradually rises in elevation northward from the highly populated coastal and delta plains in the south through the fertile central lowlands surrounding the Irrawaddy River. The mountainous border region in the east that Myanmar shares with Laos and Thailand is known as "**The Golden Triangle**," which is one of the world's largest sources of opium and illicit synthetic drugs (Banks et al., 2008). Although authority has always been strongly vested in the national government, Myanmar is divided for administrative purposes into seven states (Chin, Kachin, Kayin [Karen], Kayah, Mon, Rakhine [Arakan], and Shan) and seven regions (Irrawaddy [Ayeyarwady], Magway, Mandalay, Bago [Pegu], Sagaing, Tanintharyi, and Yangon). The states are largely based on ethnicity, a situation that has contributed to fighting among their populations and the government, as well as conflict among the various ethnic militias themselves (Myanmar National Portal, n.d.).

POPULATION AND DEMOGRAPHICS

POPULATION

The World Bank estimated that the total population of Myanmar in 2022 was approximately 54.2 million people (50.2% female, 49.8% male), with the growth rate holding steady at 0.7% annually. Approximately one quarter of the population was under 15 years of age, while nearly 7% was over 65 (World Bank Group, 2024). The largest cities are Yangon (the former capital, with more than 5.5 million people), Mandalay (more than 1.5 million people), and Nay Pyi Taw (the current capital city with more than 900,000 people). It is estimated that approximately three quarters of the population live in the Irrawaddy River Basin (Banks et. al., 2008), which stretches from the southern delta (where Yangon is located) through the central part of the country. Reflecting the nation's longstanding respect for education, the literacy rate in 2019 for those over 15 years old was 89% (World Bank Group, 2024).

ETHNICITY/RACE, LANGUAGE, AND RELIGION

According to government sources, there are eight "major national ethnic races" (Kachin, Kayah, Kayin [Karen], Chin, Mon, Bamar [approximately 70% of the population], Rakhine [Arakan], and Shan) and a subset of 135 official "ethno-racial" groups (Myanmar National Portal, n.d.). An estimated 75% of the population speaks **Burmese**, which is the country's official language, followed by Shan (11%), Arakanese (6%), Karen (5%), Mon (3%), and Kachin (2.5%). In addition, more than 100 different dialects are spoken, reflecting Myanmar's extremely diverse ethnic and ethnoracial background. English, which was a second language for most adults following independence from British rule, is still often used as a second language for people who do not share a first language. Nearly 90% of the population adheres to Buddhism. Smaller percentages adhere to Christianity, Islam, and Hinduism (Central Intelligence Agency [CIA], 2024). Theravada Buddhism and the Buddhist monkhood have strongly influenced most elements of Burmese life since the 11th century.

HISTORY

OVERVIEW

Dating back to the second century CE, much of the territory that would become the current Myanmar was dominated by small states and kingdoms. Beginning in the 11th century, control was gradually consolidated in various iterations by a cyclical series of monarchical dynasties. Britain took dominion of an ever-increasing portion of the country in three Anglo–Burmese wars from 1824 to 1885, finally eliminating the current monarchy and absorbing all of Burma into the British colony of India in 1886. Britain separated Burma from India in 1937 and gave it its own colonial constitution. Following several years of occupation by Japanese forces during World War II, the country gained independence in 1948 as the Union of Burma (Steinberg et al., 2024). The following is a subsequent historical timeline:

- *1948–1962*: Parliamentary democracy; marked by widespread political fractionalization
- *March 1962*: Military coup
- *1974*: New constitution in pursuit of a "socialist republic" (one-party, military-dominated rule)
- *1988*: Military coup; country's name changed to Myanmar
- *1988–1989*: "People's Power" uprising led by National League for Democracy (NLD)
- *2010–2014*: Gradual political and economic liberalization under military-controlled but officially civilian government
- *2015*: Landslide victory in general election by the NLD, which assumed civilian control of the national government
- *February 2021*: Military coup in the wake of the success of the NLD in the 2020 general elections; parallel "national unity government" announced by members of parliament (from the NLD and other political parties) and various ethnic civilian and military groups

CIVIL CONFLICT

Border areas that are home to minority ethnic groups have experienced major conflicts for decades as local militias have fought against the military in efforts to wrest control from the national government. Conditions generally improved following the gradual transition to civilian government in the second decade of the 21st century. However, in the wake of the coup of February 2021, massive prodemocracy demonstrations broke out throughout the country, prompting a brutal crackdown by the **junta** (group that rules a country after taking it over by force). As a result, many of the prodemocracy proponents formed the People's Defence Force (PDF), which subsequently joined with longstanding ethnic militias to battle the national military. As of mid-2024, the opposition forces controlled more than half of the country (Beech & Cai, 2024).

HEALTH OUTCOMES

Life expectancy in Myanmar has increased steadily since 1960 (Box 54.1), in large part as a result of broad national vaccination campaigns against infectious diseases and greater availability of antibiotics and other drugs (UN Data Portal, n.d.). Not surprisingly, as people have lived longer, the percentage of deaths has risen from noncommunicable conditions (NCDs; Institute for Health Metrics and Evaluation [IHME], n.d.). The leading cause of death is stroke, in part due to a dearth of health screening services, which means that much of the population, especially in rural areas, is unaware of the value of early assessment and treatment of problems such as high blood pressure that often contribute to strokes and other end stage conditions. Finances also contribute to patient reluctance to address mild symptoms early on.

Box 54.1 Key Health Outcomes in Myanmar

- *Life expectancy*: 1960 (43.9 years [42.39 for males, 45.48 for females]); 2022 (67.3 years [64.18 for males, 70.48 for females]; World Bank Group, 2024)
- *Top 10 causes of death (ranked in descending order as of 2019)*: Stroke, ischemic heart disease, chronic obstructive pulmonary disease (COPD), diabetes, tuberculosis, neonatal infections, cirrhosis of the liver, lower respiratory infections, road accidents, chronic kidney disease (World Health Organization [WHO], 2024); note, data are pre-COVID-19 pandemic.
- *Percent of total deaths caused by communicable diseases and maternal, neonatal, and nutrition conditions*: 2000 (43.8%); 2019 (21.6; World Bank Group, 2024)
- *Percent of total deaths caused by NCDs*: 2000 (49%), 2019 (71%; World Bank Group, 2024)
- *Current common infectious diseases*: Malaria (incidence rate of 6.2 per 1,000 population at risk in 2021), tuberculosis (prevalence rate of 475 per 100,000 population in 2022), dengue hemorrhagic fever (31,288 cases in 2017), hepatitis A, typhoid fever, leptospirosis, helminthiasis, elephantiasis, HIV (270,000 people living with HIV in 2022; World Bank Group, 2024)
- *Infectious diseases that have been greatly reduced, by vaccinations*: Measles (444 cases in 2020), mumps (zero cases in 2020), rubella (three cases in 2020), polio (zero cases in 2020), Japanese encephalitis (75 cases in in 2020), tetanus (17 cases of neonatal tetanus in 2020), whooping cough (13 cases in 2019), *Hemophilus influenzae* infections, diphtheria (169 cases in 2020), hepatitis B, meningococcal infections, rotavirus (WHO, 2024)
- *Common NCDs and conditions*: Cardiovascular diseases (ischemic heart disease, hypertensive heart disease, valvular heart disease), hypertension, stroke, chronic obstructive pulmonary disease (COPD), diabetes, cirrhosis of the liver, cancers
- *Infant mortality rate*: 32.5 per 1,000 live births (World Bank Group, 2024)
- *Under-5 mortality rate (from 28 days of life to 5 years of age)*: 40.1 deaths per 1,000 live births (World Bank Group, 2024)
- *Maternal mortality ratio*: 179 per 100,000 live births (World Bank Group, 2024)

The total number of deaths from the COVID-19 pandemic of 2020–2023 was reported at 19,494 out of a total of 641,393 cases (WHO, 2024), although those figures are widely presumed to be low because many cases, especially in rural areas, went unreported and the gathering of reliable data in this and many other health-related areas has been compromised by the civil war.

Infant and maternal deaths are higher in rural areas where access to emergency obstetrics and gynecologic care is limited. The main causes of maternal deaths are postpartum hemorrhage (severe bleeding after childbirth), eclampsia (hypertensive disorder of pregnancy), unsafe deliveries, and unsafe abortions. Reflecting traditional Buddhist and British colonial doctrine on the matter, abortion is illegal in Myanmar except to save the life of the mother. Nevertheless, it was estimated that abortion-related deaths accounted for half of maternal deaths from 2009 to 2011 (WHO, 2024). Illegal abortions are often performed by nonmedical personnel via invasive procedures such as the insertion of metal sticks or toxic substances into the uterus. Abortion pills (misoprostol) are widely available on the lucrative black market.

Meanwhile, older adults, whose population has been increasing steadily over the past two decades, are primarily cared for in extended-family units, although there are some government-funded homes for the aged as well as facilities run by religious and other charity-based organizations. Comprehensive specialized care for the aging is generally considered poor.

Myanmar is also deficient in the treatment of mental illness, in part because there has been a longstanding social stigma surrounding it. A limited number of psychiatrists, primarily in cities, treat conditions such as schizophrenia, psychosis, bipolar disorder, posttraumatic stress disorder (PTSD), and major depression. However, less acute conditions such as anxiety and minor depression often go untreated, reflecting the sentiment among much of the population that such problems represent weaknesses that should be shielded from scrutiny. Despite the imperfections in the approach to mental illness, the 2019 suicide mortality rate of 2.96 per 100,000 population (World Bank Group, 2024) was relatively low by global standards, in part due to Buddhist doctrine on the sanctity of life. Anecdotally, a degree of progress in accepting mental health as an integral part of everyone's overall health has been noted in recent years, as information has become more available through the internet and the efforts of nonprofit mental health advocacy organizations. Other prominent health concerns are teenage pregnancies, road deaths (which are significantly higher among males than females), and neonatal health complications such as prematurity, birth asphyxia and other birth trauma, and congenital abnormalities.

DETERMINANTS OF HEALTH

LEADING MORBIDITY AND MORTALITY RISK FACTORS

During 2021, the top 10 morbidity and mortality risk factors were air pollution, high blood pressure, malnutrition, high fasting plasma glucose, tobacco use, dietary risks, kidney dysfunction, high alcohol use, high body mass index, and elevated low-density lipoprotein levels (IHME, n.d.). It is important to note that the morbidity and mortality risks from metabolic disorders such as hypertension and hyperglycemia are exacerbated by unhealthy behaviors such as tobacco and alcohol use as well as socioenvironmental risk factors like air pollution and malnutrition in Myanmar.

ECONOMIC FACTORS

Following independence, the fledgling parliamentary democracy had little success in combating the nation's economic malaise and ethnic unrest. Subsequent military governments formally pursued socialist economic policies, leaving most nonagricultural production in the hands of state-run enterprises that were heavily dominated by the military and were widely perceived as corrupt.

Among other things, economic strictures hindered effective exploitation of the country's important natural resources, including gas and oil, numerous valuable minerals, gemstones, and lumber. Reforms introduced under the civilian governments in the 2010s showed promise, but the economy suffered seismic shocks from the outbreak of the COVID-19 pandemic in 2020 and the rapid intensification of civil conflict following the February 2021 coup. Refer to Table 54.1 for information on the negative socioeconomic impacts of these twin crises. By mid-2024, the UN Development Program estimated that the poverty rate had nearly doubled to almost 50%, with access to many basic services, including healthcare, having collapsed under severe stress (UN Development Program, 2024). Consequently, declining incomes and inflation constrained the ability of average citizens to cover their often-substantial out-of-pocket expenses for healthcare. Meanwhile, wealthy citizens, who are primarily concentrated in urban areas, enjoyed easier access to both domestic healthcare and treatment by specialists in nearby countries such as Thailand, Singapore, and India.

ENVIRONMENT

In Myanmar, the widespread use of wood as a major fuel for households in rural areas contributes significantly to air pollution, which is a leading morbidity and mortality risk factor. The affiliated deforestation exacerbates the inevitable floods and landslides from the June–September monsoons, which are often marked by cyclones. Such disruptions lead to higher incidences of dysentery, malaria, enteric infections, other vector-borne diseases, heat stroke, injuries, and snake bites. In general, Myanmar is perceived to be poorly prepared to deal with the potential consequences of global climate change, including rising sea levels that could permanently inundate coastal and lowland areas.

RECREATIONAL DRUG AND TOBACCO USE

The use, production, or sale of recreational drugs is strictly prohibited by law. Nevertheless, there were 300,000 to 400,000 drug users in Myanmar in 2012 (UN Office on Drugs and Crime, 2024). In 2020, approximately 44% of adults used tobacco (World Bank Group, 2024) in the form of cigarettes, cigars, and chew, contributing significantly to chronic obstructive pulmonary diseases (COPD), lung cancer, heart disease, cerebrovascular incidents, and other blood-vessel–related conditions. Tangentially, many tobacco users also chew betel leaves for their perceived mood-altering effect. That behavior is tied to oral cancer and other disorders of the mouth and teeth.

TABLE 54.1 ECONOMY OF MYANMAR

ECONOMIC INDICATOR	FISCAL YEAR(S)
GDP	2020 ($79 billion); 2022 ($62.3 billion)
GDP per capita	2020 ($1,480); 2022 ($1,150)
Real GDP growth	2019/2020 (6.6%); 2021/2022 (–12%); 2023/2024 (1%)
CPI inflation	2020/2021 (2.3%); 2023/2024 (18%)
Unemployment	2023 (8.1%)
Poverty rate	2020 (7.6%); 2023 (26.5%)
National defense spending	2020/2021 (10.0% of budget); 2023/2024 (17.0%)
National health spending	2020/2021 (4.7% of budget); 2023/2024 (2.5%)
Foreign direct investment	2017 (7.3% of GDP); 2022 (2.0% of GDP)

Note: Dates containing 2 reference fiscal years from April through March.

CPI, Consumer Price Index; GDP, gross domestic product.

Source: Myanmar Economic Monitor. (2024). *Myanmar economic monitor June 2024*. The World Bank Group. https://documents1.worldbank.org/curated/en/099061124195517221/pdf/P5006631cca59607d182041fae76ab566cc.pdf

EFFECTS OF THE CONFLICT FOLLOWING THE 2021 COUP

Many medical doctors and other healthcare workers joined the initial civil-disobedience movement after the coup and stopped going to work. Eventually, some medical doctors and other healthcare workers left the country. As a result, hospitals and outpatient clinics operated at a reduced level and timely access to services was restricted throughout the country (Box 54.2). Capacity improved somewhat by mid-2023 in urban areas free of conflict, but extreme difficulties continued in the rural conflict zones. Broad international sanctions were imposed following the coup in the hope of pressuring the junta into establishing a timetable for a return to civilian government. However, as has often been the case with such initiatives, the sanctions created unwanted difficulties for average citizens. For example, trade embargoes and supply chain strictures sharply curtailed the availability of important imported medicines and equipment, making it difficult for patients to adequately treat chronic health conditions.

Internal and external displacements have been high since independence as a result of ongoing conflict between ethnic militias and the national military forces. In the wake of the 2021 coup, the number of internal refugees skyrocketed to more than 3 million by mid-2024 (UN High Commissioner for Refugees, 2024). Nearly 1 million more Rohingya refugees lived in camps in Bangladesh and other neighboring countries, having fled intense military repression and attacks since 2017. Healthcare conditions were extremely dire in the internally displaced people camps. Although services in those areas were sometimes provided by doctors, nurses, and midwives who had joined the civil-disobedience movement, refugees were often forced to rely on volunteers from the general public who had gained some basic knowledge by attending online courses or participating in sessions presented by nonprofit organizations. Major humanitarian assistance is needed to meet the survival needs of refugees.

HEALTHCARE SYSTEM

FACILITIES AND PROVIDERS

The nation's Ministry of Health (MoH) oversees a system of separate yet sometimes overlapping public and private sectors (Myanmar National Portal, n.d.). There are more than 1,100 public hospitals, ranging from as few as 16 beds in rural areas to as many as 2,000 beds in urban facilities. Most public hospitals also operate their own outpatient clinics. In addition, there is a wide

BOX 54.2 Effects on Healthcare of Recent Conflict

- More than 50,000 people dead, 26,000 arrested (Beech & Cai, 2024)
- Massive dislocations
- Damage to healthcare facilities in conflict zones from bomb attacks and intense shelling
- Food insecurity and undernourishment in conflict zones, leading to vitamin and mineral deficiencies, insufficient protein levels, diminished immune systems, and maternal and neonatal complications
- Nighttime curfews that limited access to emergency services
- Difficulty in traveling to health facilities in conflict zones because of landmines and road checkpoints
- Strict censorship by the government of the internet and other telecommunications, making it difficult for doctors to communicate with each other or with patients
- Power outages
- Compromised sanitation systems, leading to disease outbreaks
- Closures of schools and universities
- Increased production of opium, a major source of financing for both sides in the conflict (As of 2023, Myanmar was the world's largest producer of opium [UN News, 2024].)

network of nonbedded public healthcare centers that provide outpatient primary and secondary care, including maternal and child services and health education. The public facilities are significantly subsidized by the government, although their patients often spend some of their own money, particularly on supplies and prescription drugs. Still, patient expenses are much higher for private primary care and specialist hospitals and clinics, which tend to serve affluent populations in urban areas and generally offer a wider range of services than the public facilities. Meanwhile, low-cost and no-cost care is available through charity-based hospitals and clinics run by religious and other nonprofit organizations under licenses from the government. Their services, such as free mobile clinics, are especially important in rural areas where the government facilities are often dilapidated and underfunded.

Primary care physicians (general practitioners) are the main healthcare providers in Myanmar. Many of them are at least partly affiliated with public, government-run hospitals and clinics. Patients who can afford the associated fees often seek initial care from private doctors, who treat health conditions in their offices as appropriate and refer patients needing more extensive care to hospitals or specialists. However, such referrals are not required, and patients can go directly to hospitals, clinics, and specialists on their own. In addition to standard primary care, general practitioners are taught surgical and obstetric procedures and other advanced skills as part of their regular university and internship training. They sometimes conduct minor and major surgeries such as appendicectomies, hernia repair, orthopedic plastering, cesarean sections, and vacuum- and forceps-assisted deliveries that are generally performed by specialists in more developed countries. That expanded role of general practitioners is particularly important in underserviced rural areas to which doctors are routinely sent for their first assignment.

HEALTHCARE TRAINING AND EDUCATION

The MoH is the main authoritative body for the training of the healthcare workforce (Myanmar National Portal, n.d.). Most of the medical education systems, including all universities, are public entities. However, there are private programs from which people can earn the required certification for some medical-related jobs such as pharmacy assistants and nurses' aides. The public system, overseen by the MoH through the division of the Department of Human Resources for Health, includes both the allopathic and traditional medicine universities as well as nursing and midwifery training schools. The Ministry of Defense is completely responsible for training the military's doctors and the rest of its healthcare workforce. Under the Department of Traditional Medicine, the University of Traditional Medicine was established in 2001, providing bachelor's and master's degrees. Physicians initially earn bachelor of medicine (MB) and bachelor of surgery (BS) degrees. The standard length of study is 6 years, although only 5 years are required for the degrees in traditional medicine. Graduates of the MB and BS programs must serve a 1-year internship before providing regular service as general practitioners. Doctors who subsequently pursue master's and doctorate degrees must first join the civil service. Postgraduate offerings were expanded recently to provide more intensive training in the fields of family medicine, pediatrics, obstetrics and gynecology, and emergency medicine. In addition, selected graduate candidates from various disciplines are sent overseas to pursue master's or doctorate degrees or to receive short-term specialized training before returning to work in Myanmar.

FINANCE AND INSURANCE

Public hospitals and clinics are subsidized by the government, although patients may be asked to pay part of the expense according to their financial status. Patients also usually pay out of pocket for supplies and prescription drugs. Expenses are much higher in private facilities and are usually completely paid for by the patients. Underscoring the special status of the military in Myanmar, the government provides free healthcare for members of the military and their families at military-only hospitals and clinics. Some government ministries also provide care for their employees. Unlike conditions in other economically similar countries, the health insurance sector in Myanmar has only begun to develop. Some businesses provide their own internal insurance policies to defray a portion of healthcare expenses for their employees. In addition, a few private companies offer health insurance policies for sale to the general public and the government has introduced its own somewhat subsidized polices. The public is not well educated in regard to such options, however, and utilization remains low. Policymakers in the pre-coup civilian government began to consider a comprehensive universal healthcare system, but such consideration stopped in the wake of the 2021 coup.

TRADITIONAL MEDICINE

While British rule left Myanmar with a somewhat Westernized health system, particularly in urban areas, and the Westernized allopathic approach remains the dominant approach to healthcare, traditional medicine plays a significant role in Myanmar. It is highly institutionalized within the healthcare system, starting with the Department of Traditional Medicine, which is one of six main departments in the MoH. Like their counterparts in the allopathic institutions, traditional medicine doctors study basic sciences such as biology, physics, anatomy, physiology, and pathology. However, they also study areas such as botany, zoology, and traditional pharmacology that are unique to their approach to healthcare. Traditional medicine promotes the use of drugs made from indigenous herbs and administered via liquids, powders, tablets, and capsules. Underscoring the formal status of traditional medicine in Myanmar, those medicines are regulated by the national Food and Drug Administration. Proponents of astrology, alchemy, and **scratching** (a process in which the skin is deliberately broken by an object such as a coin to release blood believed to be infiltrated with toxins) are also grouped under the umbrella of traditional medicine (WHO, 2024). For the most part, the traditional medicine doctors perform primary care functions such as treating some viral infectious diseases, chronic conditions, minor wounds, skin conditions, and maternal and child issues. They refer their patients who need more advanced care to hospitals and specialty care, which can be either allopathic or traditional in nature. Many patients choose traditional medicine because of their belief in the efficacy of that practice, as passed on through family lore. In addition, low-income patients sometimes gravitate toward traditional medicine because it is usually much less expensive than private allopathic care.

Allopathic doctors strongly prefer that their patients do not add traditional remedies to their allopathic care for fear of potential harmful interactions. Traditional medicine doctors generally do not have such qualms. If needed, both branches regularly recommend complementary treatments such as massage therapy, acupuncture, and physical therapy, which enjoy longstanding popularity throughout the country. Physicians also encourage their patients to quit smoking, reduce alcohol consumption, engage in mindful meditation and yoga, and increase physical activity.

OTHER PRACTICES

In many suburban areas, privately owned but government-licensed local pharmacies provide minor health services such as testing blood glucose levels and blood pressures. They dispense a wide variety of drugs, but only opioid-derived drugs and drugs used to treat psychiatric conditions are controlled by the government. Antibiotics and other drugs to combat acute and chronic illnesses such as colds and the flu, diabetes, stomach and digestive problems, and skin conditions are not controlled and can be easily purchased from pharmacies and markets without prescriptions. Nonregulated practitioners include spiritual healers, who retain a large and devoted following in Myanmar, in part because their services are relatively inexpensive. Patients travel days to reach their offices for treatment, particularly for chronic NCDs and conditions.

CONCLUSION AND RECOMMENDATIONS

In April of 2024, *The New York Times* described Myanmar as "the most fractured country on earth" (Beech & Cai, 2024). National disunity contributed greatly to major problems in the healthcare system, as did longstanding rural–urban disparities, economic underperformance, and political instability. Progress of any kind depends on resolution of the civil war and installation of a civilian government supported by the country's disparate ethnic communities and regions. Peace would permit the restoration of health services that have been severely compromised since the 2021 military coup. In addition, it would give planners and policymakers the opportunity to address the following long-term needs:

- Build more hospitals and clinics in rural areas and expand the transportation infrastructure to reduce the rural–urban disparity in access to treatment.
- Improve public health education programs that promote healthy living choices, help people better recognize health hazards and properly assess emergency conditions, and encourage wider understanding of reproductive and sexual health.
- Promote healthcare research and innovation through the significant expansion of government funding and public–private initiatives that would, among other things, prepare healthcare professionals to utilize high-tech diagnostic and curative equipment.
- Establish a system of universal healthcare coverage.

LEARNING ACTIVITIES

CourseConnect

To access self-assessment questions and interactive, competency-based learning activities for this chapter, visit www.springerpub.com/courseconnect. See inside front cover and tear-out for CourseConnect details.

REFERENCES

Banks, A. S., Muller, T. C., & Overstreet, W. R. (2008). *Political handbook of the world 2008*. CSA Publications.

Beech, H., & Cai, W. (2024). What's happening in Myanmar's civil war? *The New York Times*. https://www.nytimes.com/interactive/2024/04/20/world/asia/myanmar-civil-war.html?unlocked_article_code=1.qE0.-Uai.HkikpvsxY62I&smid=url-share

Central Intelligence Agency. (2024). *The world factbook: Burma*. https://www.cia.gov/the-world-factbook/

Institute for Health Metrics and Evaluation. (n.d.). *Country profiles: Myanmar*. University of Washington. Seattle, WA. https://www.healthdata.org/research-analysis/health-by-location/profiles/myanmar

Myanmar National Portal. (n.d.). *People and society*. https://myanmar.gov.mm/people-society

Statista. (2024). *Health and health systems ranking of countries worldwide in 2023*. https://www.statista.com/statistics/1376359/health-and-health-system-ranking-of-countries-worldwide/

Steinberg, D. I., Aung, M. H., & Aung-Thwin, M. A. (2024). *Myanmar*. Britannica. https://www.britannica.com/place/Myanmar

UN Data Portal. (n.d.). *UN Population Division data portal*. https://population.un.org/dataportal/home/

UN Development Program. (2024). *Human development report. (2023/2024) Snapshot*. https://hdr.undp.org/system/files/documents/global-report-document/hdr2023-24snapshoten.pdf

UN High Commissioner for Refugees. (2024). *Operational data portal*. https://data.unhcr.org/en/country/mmr

UN News. (2024). *Myanmar overtakes Afghanistan as world's top opium producer*. United Nations. https://news.un.org/en/story/2023/12/1144702#:~:text=Myanmar%20is%20now%20the%20world's,towards%20illicit%20opium%20poppy%20production

UN Office on Drugs and Crime. (2024). *Central committee for drug abuse control.* https://www.unodc.org/roseap/uploads/archive/documents/2013/11/ats-2013/embargoed/2013_Regional_ATS_Report_Myanmar.pdf

World Bank Group. (2024). *World Bank open data.* https://data.worldbank.org/

World Health Organization. (2024). *South-East Asia: Myanmar.* https://www.who.int/myanmar/

CHAPTER 55

VIETNAM

Trang Nguyen, Linh Le, and Thuy Tran

INTRODUCTION

The Socialist Republic of Viet Nam (Vietnam) is considered a developing country with a fast-growing economy that has moved from being one of the world's poorest nations to a middle-income economy in less than 40 years (World Bank Group, n.d.). In the 1980s, under economic reform called **Doi Moi** (or Renovation), Vietnam switched from a centralized, planned economy to a mixed economy called a socialist-oriented market that includes a free market promoting private businesses along with the provision of government services and coordination (Collins & Zhu, 2005). Economic reform has had a large impact on health, healthcare, and the determinants of health in Vietnam.

GEOGRAPHY AND POPULATION

Vietnam is located at the eastern side of Southeast Asia. It is approximately 331,000 square kilometers, including 40% mountains, 42% heavy forest, and less than 20% leveled. Vietnam has a long coast that stretches from Mong Cai in the north to Ha Tien in the South. Vietnam has 58 provinces and five municipalities. Hanoi is the capital of the country. The largest city is Ho Chi Minh City. Vietnam's climate is tropical monsoon with two main seasons, wet and dry (Buttinger & Osborne, 2025).

Vietnam is the world's fifteenth-most populous country even though it is about 30 times smaller than the United States. In 2022, the population of Vietnam was more than 98 million people, representing a 25% increase from 2000 (Ngan, 2023). Vietnam has one of the world's fastest aging populations. Figure 55.1 shows estimated changes in the age distribution of Vietnam's population between 2023 and 2050. Adults aged 55 and older will account for a much larger percentage of the total population (Ngan, 2023).

SOCIAL AND ECONOMIC FACTORS

ECONOMY

Vietnam's GDP in 2023 was nearly $430 billion, which ranked within the top 35 globally. On a per capita basis, the GDP in Vietnam during 2023 was only about $4,350. However, in the last 40 years, Vietnam's per capita GDP grew more than six times (World Bank Group, n.d.). The poverty rate has significantly decreased from 14% in 2010 to 4.2% in 2022. Despite impacts from the COVID-19 pandemic, Vietnam's economy grew 8% in 2022 (Ngan, 2023). The economic improvements accredited to market reforms initiated in 1986 has enhanced the healthcare infrastructure and delivery of healthcare services in Vietnam.

EDUCATION

The literacy rate for people 15 years of age and older was 95.7% in 2021, a 2% increase from the literacy rate in 2010. The average duration of schooling is 10.2 years, second among the Association

FIGURE 55.1 Vietnam estimated population changes by age and sex, 2023–2050.

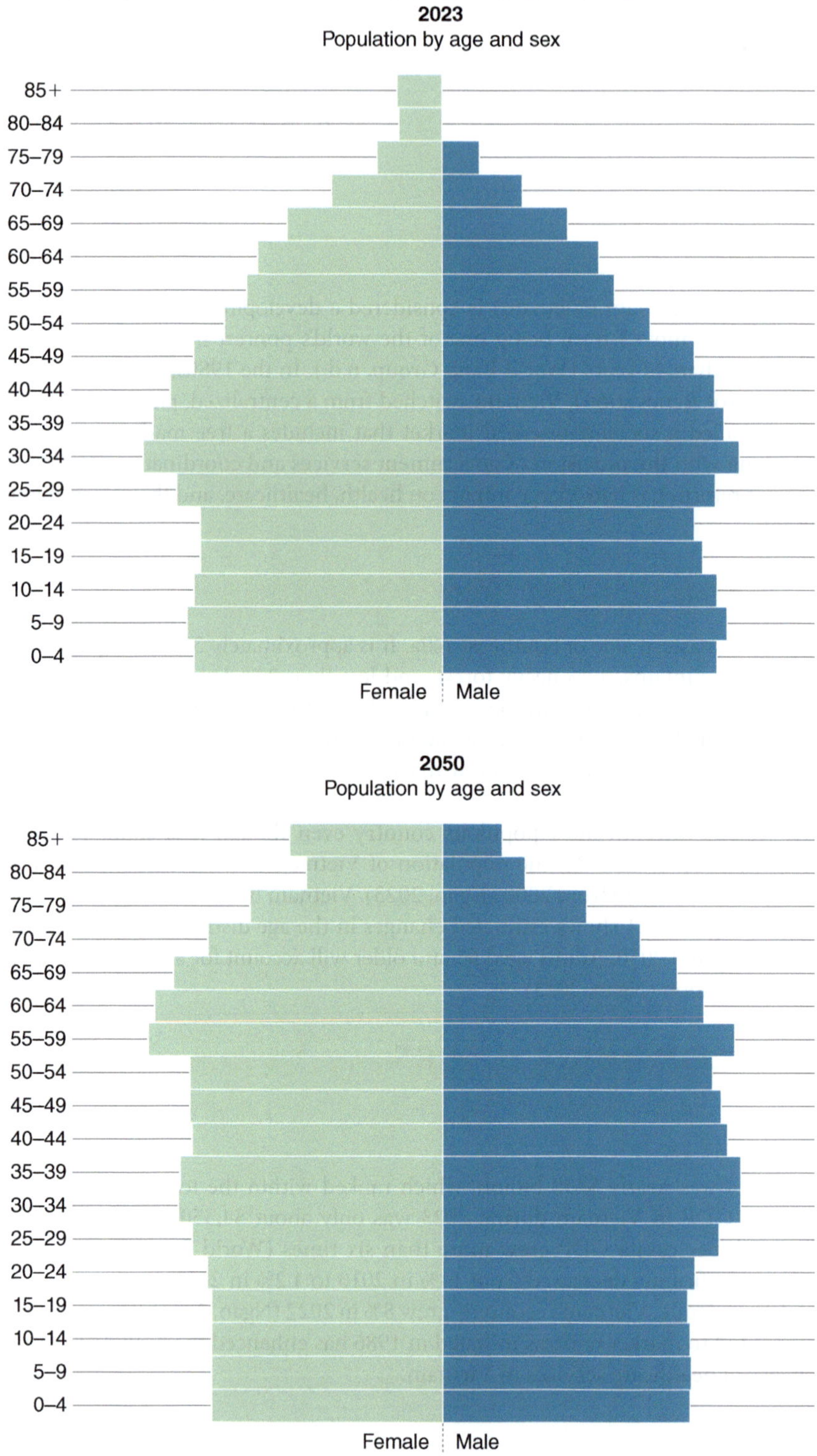

Source: World Health Organization. (2024). *The world health data hub*. https://data.who.int/

of Southeast Asian Nations (ASEAN) countries (World Bank Group, n.d.). ASEAN, established in 1967, promotes regional peace and stability and economic and social progress through cooperation among Southeast Asian member nations and international partners (ASEAN Secretariat, 2024).

INFRASTRUCTURE

There has been significant improvement in public works and utility infrastructure in Vietnam. Approximately 99.4% of the population had electricity in 2019, as compared to only 14% in 1993 (World Bank Group, n.d.). Approximately 97% of the population has access to improved water supplies, which is a drastic improvement from 2000 when only 65% of the population had access to clean water (UNICEF, n.d.). While only 51% of people living in rural areas had access to clean water in 2020, rural access has vastly improved from 1993 when only 17% had access to clean water (World Bank Group, n.d.).

HEALTH OUTCOMES

OVERVIEW

Health outcomes in Vietnam have ameliorated due to improvements in infrastructure and economic conditions. Improved socioeconomic conditions in Vietnam have resulted in large reductions in poverty and hunger, enhanced living conditions such as clean water, better roads, and expanded availability of electricity and modern technologies, as well as increased investments and expansion in the healthcare system, providers, facilities, equipment, and services (Ngan, 2023). Conversely, rapid urbanization, with greater population migration from rural to urban areas, has led to negative environmental changes such as increased exposure to air pollution and limited green space availability and negative lifestyle changes such as increased physical inactivity and dietary intake of sugar, fat, and salt. These environmental and lifestyle changes are determinantal to population health in Vietnam (Nguyen & Trevisan, 2020).

LIFE EXPECTANCY

Life expectancy at birth increased from approximately 69 years in 1990 to 74.6 years in 2023. Females had nearly 10 more years of life expectancy at birth when compared to males; 79.3 compared to 69.9, respectively (UN Data Portal, n.d.). Significant changes in morbidity and mortality have been observed in Vietnam since the 1990s (Figure 55.2). There have been great reductions in morbidity and mortality from unintentional injuries and communicable disease such as lower respiratory infections, childhood vaccine preventable diseases, tuberculosis, and diarrheal diseases. However, morbidity and mortality from preventable noncommunicable diseases such as cardiovascular disease, cancers, chronic obstructive pulmonary disease (COPD), and diabetes mellitus have drastically increased (Nguyen & Trevisan, 2020).

LEADING CAUSES OF MORTALITY

Figure 55.3 shows the leading causes of death in Vietnam during 2011 and 2021 (Institute for Health Metrics and Evaluation [IHME], n.d.). The lists are dominated by preventable noncommunicable diseases; stroke, heart disease, COPD, diabetes, cirrhosis of the liver, chronic kidney disease, and lung cancer. In addition, mortality from these noncommunicbale diseases increased from 2011 to 2021. Stroke and heart disease were the top two leading causes during both years. Injuries and communicable diseases account for a much smaller percentage of mortality in Vietnam as a result of the improving infrastructure and economy. Road injuries and tuberculosis were top 10 leading causes of mortality in Vietnam during both 2011 and 2021; however, the mortality rates from these two causes decreased during this timeframe. In 2021, COVID-19 was the third leading cause of mortality in Vietnam.

FIGURE 55.2 Change in morbidity and mortality pattern in Vietnam.

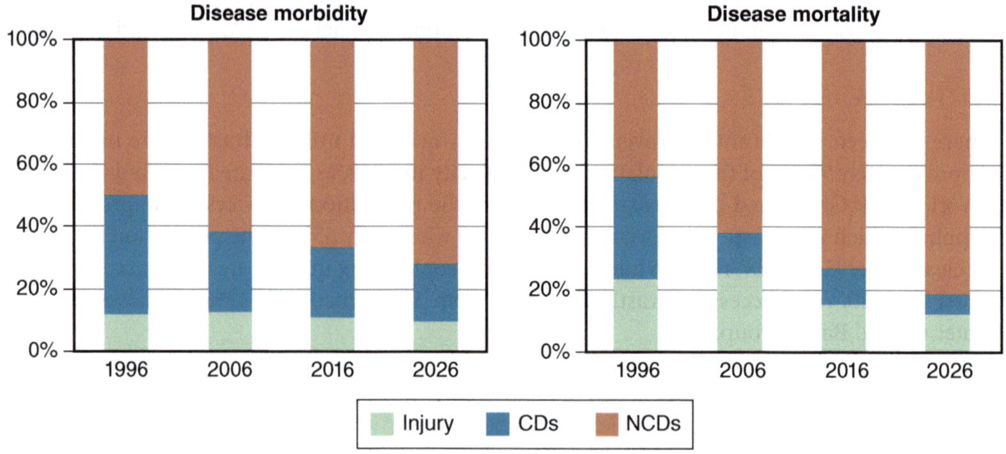

CD, communicable disease; NCD, noncommunicable disease.

Source: Nguyen, T. T., & Trevisan, M. (2020). Vietnam a country in transition: Health challenges. *BMJ Nutrition Prevention and Health, 3*(1), 60–66. https://doi.org/10.1136/bmjnph-2020-000069

FIGURE 55.3 Leading causes of mortality in Vietnam, 2011 and 2021.

Cause	2011 rank	2021 rank	Change in deaths per 100K, 2011–2021
Stroke	1	1	↑ +8.6
Ischemic heart disease	2	2	↑ +8.3
COVID-19	–	3	↑ +36.3
COPD	3	4	↑ +1.4
Diabetes	6	5	↑ +6.8
Cirrhosis liver	8	6	↑ +1.3
Chronic kidney disease	9	7	↑ +5.1
Road injuries	4	8	↓ −3.9
Lung cancer	10	9	↑ +5.3
Tuberculosis	5	10	↓ −6.3

Communicable, maternal, neonatal, and nutritional diseases
Noncommunicable diseases
Injuries

COPD, chronic obstructive pulmonary disease.

Source: Institute for Health Metrics and Evaluation. (n.d.). *Viet Nam*. https://www.healthdata.org/research-analysis/health-by-location/profiles/vietnam

INFANT AND MATERNAL MORTALITY

The infant mortality rate in Vietnam fell more than 50% from 31.4 infant deaths per 1,000 live births in 1993 to 15.1 in 2023 (UN Data Portal, n.d.). Vietnam's maternal mortality ratio (MMR), which has been rapidly decreasing, was lower than the regional and global averages during 2020. The MMR in Vietnam during 2020 was 124.3 infant deaths per 100,000 live births (UN Population Fund, n.d.).

MAJOR COMMUNICABLE DISEASES

In addition to the COVID-19 pandemic, tuberculosis and HIV have resulted in significant communicable disease morbidity and mortality in Vietnam. As of May 2023, Vietnam recorded 11,612,608 confirmed COVID-19 cases and a total of 43,206 deaths. This percent fatality among COVID-19 cases was nearly 3 times lower than the rate in the United States. Vietnam has high COVID-19 vaccination rates, with 92% of the population receiving at least 1 dose (World Health Organization [WHO], 2024). In 2021, there were more than 13,000 new HIV cases in Vietnam, making the cumulative incidence of people living with HIV nearly 214,000 (217.1 per 100,000 population). In 2021, there were 1,856 HIV/AIDS-related deaths (1.9 per 100,000 population) in Vietnam. While there has been a significant decrease in tuberculosis morbidity and mortality in Vietnam, it is still one of the leading causes of mortality in Vietnam. Tuberculosis cases in Vietnam decreased by approximately 40% from 296 tuberculosis cases per 100,000 people in 2000 to 176 cases per 100,000 people in 2022 UNICEF. (n.d.). The percentage of children under 1 year old fully immunized with vaccinations was 96.8% in 2020. However, due to the impact of COVID-19, this percentage decreased to 87.1% in 2021 (WHO, 2024). Monitoring child vaccination rates is necessary to prevent the spread of and deaths from vaccine preventable communicable diseases.

DETERMINANTS OF HEALTH

ENVIRONMENTAL

Air pollution is one of country's leading morbidity and mortality risk factors (IHME, n.d.). The annual mean concentrations of fine particulate matter ($PM_{2.5}$) in Vietnam during 2019 was 20.89 micrograms per cubic meter of air (mcg/m^3), which was more than three times higher than that in the U.S. Vietnam is also one of the most climate change vulnerable nations in the world. It is especially prone to flooding due to intense precipitation, rising sea levels, and low elevation in coastal areas (Central Intelligence Agency [CIA], 2024). Improving drainage in flood-prone, densely-populated urban coastal areas is a priority.

SOCIO-BEHAVIORAL

Tobacco use, dietary risks, and malnutrition are among the leading morbidity and mortality risk factors in Vietnam (IHME, n.d.). More than 1 out of every 5 people 15 years of age and older used tobacco products in 2021. Tobacco use among males was more than 20 times higher than among females (WHO, 2024). With improvements in economic conditions, Vietnamese nutrition has been rapidly changing. A positive effect of economic growth on nutrition has been a decrease in nutritional deficiencies. A negative effect has been a transition away from the traditional Vietnamese diet, which is based on whole foods such as vegetables and whole grains, towards a Westernized diet and fast-food products that are often high in saturated fat, sugar, and sodium and lacking in healthful whole grains, fruits, and vegetables (Nguyen & Trevisan, 2020).

BIOLOGICAL

The prevalence of obesity among Vietnamese adults aged 18+ years increased from 0.2% in 1990 to 2.0% in 2019. In 2019, the percentage of Vietnamese adults aged 30-79 years with hypertension was 29.7%, which is a 17% increase when compared to 1990. Metabolic disorders such as hypertension and hyperglycemia are leading risk factors for morbidity and mortality in Vietnam (IHME, 2021).

HEALTHCARE SYSTEM

HEALTHCARE SYSTEM STRUCTURE

Vietnam's public healthcare structure includes four hierarchical administrative levels; central, provincial, district, and commune (Le et al, 2010). The overall goals of the system are to make the healthcare system universal and affordable for the entire population. Vietnam's healthcare strategies specifically focus on

- preventing and controlling emerging diseases;
- responding to climate change and public health emergencies;
- improving the quality and efficiency of the public health network from the central to the grassroots level in response to changing disease patterns;
- strengthening the healthcare workforce, human resources, and the public health system;
- enhancing maternal and child health;
- improving healthcare quality and equity and patient satisfaction; and
- reducing health disparities (Socialist Republic of Viet Nam, 2024).

The Vietnamese Ministry of Health plays a central role in healthcare and is primarily responsible for managing healthcare activities and services for the country such as developing and issuing health-related laws, policies, protocols, and guidelines. Within the local government at provincial, district, and commune levels, committees are responsible for allocating financial and human resources to support provincial or district health departments in developing and implementing healthcare services. On average, a provincial health department manages from 10 to 20 districts, each overseeing dozens of commune health centers. District health centers and commune health stations operate as primary health service delivery, providing basic services including maternal and child healthcare, family planning, treatment for acute respiratory infections, immunization and treatment of common ailments. District health centers and commune health stations also function as "gatekeepers," providing screening to identify healthcare needs and referring people who require higher levels of care. The district and commune health centers and stations are often referred to as "grassroots healthcare systems" (General Statistics Office, 2022).

HEALTHCARE FINANCE, INSURANCE, AND EXPENDITURES

In the late 1980s, following Doi Moi, the Vietnam healthcare system transitioned from a fully public service system to a mixed public-private provider system. Because of economic reform, more health services, products, and options are offered by the private health sector via the availability of user fee-for-services. This created a competition, enabling people to get better healthcare services (Quan & Taylor-Robinson, 2023).

Vietnam's universal health coverage index is higher than regional and global averages. Approximately 91% of the population was covered by the national health insurance scheme in 2020 (Viet Nam Ministry of Health, n.d.). Although the primary care system is well established with 98.7% of communes having health stations (CHSs), only 72.7% of villages have village health workers and 80% of CHSs provide health services under the social health insurance scheme. The Vietnamese Ministry of Health has implemented a new reform under the Direction of Healthcare Activities to address deficiencies in care by requiring healthcare facilities at higher government administration levels (central and provincial) to support those at lower levels by providing medical services for local communities in primary care settings. Supporting communes and villages will also decrease the number of patients that seek care at crowded central and provincial facilities (Takashima et al, 2017).

HEALTHCARE FACILITIES AND WORKFORCE

Overall, the Vietnamese healthcare system capacity has rapidly expanded during economic reform. There are more than 34,200 operating medical facilities and 460,000 hospital beds. There is also a notable shift from public to private facilities. The percentage of healthcare facilities that are private increased from 68.1% in 2016 to 94.7% in 2020. In 2020, there were 1,029 hospitals in Vietnam, of which 721 were public and 308 were private. There were 29,644 polyclinics, special clinics, family doctor clinics, and health centers in 2020. Of the 29,644 clinics and health centers, only 803 were public facilities. The remaining 28,841 clinics and centers were private (General Statistics Office, 2022).

There has also been a significant increase in healthcare workers because of economic reform. In 2020, there were 603,150 healthcare employees, an increase of 13.3% from 2016. The rate of physicians per 10,000 people increased 57% from 5.3 in 2001 to 8.3 in 2016. The rate of nurses and midwifes per 10,000 people increased from 7.42 in 2001 to 14.5 in 2016. The density of pharmaceutical personnel per 10,000 people increased from 0.75 in 2001 to 3.4 in 2016 (General Statistics Office, 2022).

CHALLENGES AND OPPORTUNITIES

Vietnam has built a healthcare system that is relatively effective in providing services and protecting its people. Vietnam serves as a best-practice model for healthcare systems in low- to middle-income countries. Although significant progress has been made in improving the healthcare system and health outcomes for the entire population over the last several decades, major challenges remain. Rapid population aging and environmental and lifestyle changes have led to increases in chronic diseases such as cardiovascular diseases, diabetes mellitus, and kidney and liver failure. These chronic conditions place significant burdens and demands on individuals and the healthcare system (Nguyen & Trevisan, 2020). Chronic conditions require appropriate primary prevention and secondary and tertiary management policies and strategies, as well as a sufficient healthcare workforce that is well equipped to provide preventive and treatment services. Large disparities exist between urban and rural areas regarding the availability of healthcare professionals and services. Advanced services and treatments are more likely available in urban areas; however, are less affordable for middle- and low-income populations. Therefore, healthcare needs of populations with low income or living in remote locations can go unmet. The lack of a universal computerized information system for managing individual health records could hinder the effectiveness of preventive healthcare strategies such as disease screening, immunization, medication management, and referrals. Furthermore, a universal computerized information system could help mitigate healthcare waste caused by duplications in services and medical errors. Finance of the healthcare system is underbudgeted to adequately meet the population's health needs. Out-of-pocket payment fee-for-services are not affordable for a large portion of the population. Vietnam's universal health insurance has made significant improvement in healthcare coverage and accessibility, mitigating inequitable effects of costly fee-for-services. Improving public healthcare service availability and quality could enable the system to better meet population health needs (Quan & Taylor-Robinson, 2023).

Stigmatization of health issues could hinder progress in the detection, treatment, and prevention of diseases. Developing a healthcare workforce that is well equipped with local knowledge and person-centered skills is necessary to implement a culturally appropriate approach to preventing disease-related stigma. Strengthening the collaboration between the healthcare sector and non-healthcare sectors will help address economic, social, and environmental determinants of health by developing tailored programs that include community education, awareness, and engagement (Socialist Republic of Viet Nam, 2024).

CONCLUSION

Vietnam's healthcare system has vastly improved with political, economic, and educational reforms. Healthcare is more affordable and services are more accessible. Vietnam is taking steps to address challenges in its healthcare system by increasing funds for public healthcare, introducing more private healthcare options, improving efficiency with digital technologies, enhancing healthcare training, and bolstering the healthcare workforce. Requiring support from healthcare facilities at higher levels for those at lower levels will help to reduce the disparities in accessibility and quality of care between urban and rural areas. Emphasis and investment in preventive healthcare is necessary to be prepared for emerging infectious diseases and to address the increase in chronic diseases in a rapidly aging population.

ACKNOWLEDGMENT

The authors would like to thank Dr. Kathleen Kelly, PhD, MPH, MS, FNP, retired dean, School of Health Sciences and associate professor in nursing at The Russell Sage College, for her review and feedback.

LEARNING ACTIVITIES

CourseConnect

To access self-assessment questions and interactive, competency-based learning activities for this chapter, visit www.springerpub.com/courseconnect. See inside front cover and tear-out for CourseConnect details.

REFERENCES

Association of Southeast Asian Nations Secretariat. (2024). *Association of Southeast Asian nations: A community of opportunity for all.* https://asean.org/

Buttinger, J., & Osborne, M. E. (2025). Vietnam. *Britannica.* https://www.britannica.com/place/Vietnam

Central Intelligence Agency. (2024). *Vietnam: The world factbook.* www.cia.gov

Collins, N., & Zhu, Y. (2005). The transformation of HRM in transitional economics: The case of Vietnam. *The Journal of Comparative Asian Development, 4*(1), 161–178. http://doi.org/10.1080/15339114.2005.9678414

General Statistics Office. (2022). *Vietnam health: Figures and assessments from the economic census 2021.* Viet Nam Department of Social and Environmental Statistics. https://www.gso.gov.vn/wp-content/uploads/2024/04/04-Sach-KQ-danh-gia-TDTKT-Y-te-VN-_19x27_.doc-_OK-in_.pdf

Institute for Health Metrics and Evaluation. (2021). *Country profiles: Vietnam.* Institute of Health Metrics and Evaluation. www.healthdata.org

Institute for Health Metrics and Evaluation. (n.d.). *Viet Nam.* https://www.healthdata.org/research-analysis/health-by-location/profiles/vietnam

Le, D. C., Kubo, T., Fujino, Y., Pham, T. M., & Matsuda, S. (2010). Health care system in Vietnam: Current situation and challenges. *Asian Pacific Journal of Disease Management, 4*(2), 23–30. http://doi.org/10.7223/apjdm.4.23

Ngan, NH. (2023). *Vietnam's economic growth slows due to global headwinds and internal constraints.* World Bank Group. https://www.worldbank.org/en/news/press-release/2023/08/10/vietnam-s-economic-growth-slows-due-to-global-headwinds-and-internal-constraints

Nguyen, T. T., & Trevisan, M. (2020). Vietnam a country in transition: Health challenges. *BMJ Nutrition Prevention and Health, 3*(1), 60–66. https://doi.org/10.1136/bmjnph-2020-000069

Quan, N. K., & Taylor-Robinson, A. W. (June 14, 2023). Vietnam's evolving healthcare system: Notable successes and significant challenges. *Cureus, 15*(6), e40414. https://doi.org/10.7759/cureus.40414

Socialist Republic of Viet Nam. (2024). *Government news: National strategy on people's health released.* https://en.baochinhphu.vn/national-strategy-on-peoples-health-released-111240124180120253.htm

Takashima, K., Wada, K., Tra, T. T., & Smith, D. R. (2017). A review of Vietnam's healthcare reform through the Direction of Healthcare Activities (DOHA). *Environmental Health and Preventive Medicine, 22*(1), 74. https://doi.org/10.1186/s12199-017-0682-z

UNICEF. (n.d.). *Viet Nam.* https://data.unicef.org/country/vnm/

UN Data Portal. (n.d.). *UN population division data portal.* https://population.un.org/dataportal/home/

UN Population Fund. (n.d.). *UNFPA - United Nations Population Fund.* https://www.unfpa.org/

Viet Nam Ministry of Health. (n.d.). *Health statistics.* https://moh.gov.vn/thong-ke-y-te

World Bank Group. (n.d.). *The World Bank open data.* https://data.worldbank.org/

World Health Organization. (2024). *The world health data hub.* https://data.who.int/

PART XIV: Health and Healthcare in Oceania

CHAPTER 56

Overview of Oceania

Anna Foucek Tresidder

INTRODUCTION

Oceania encompasses a diverse range of nations with distinct health systems shaped by their geography, history, and socioeconomic conditions. Oceanic health systems are diversely designed as the countries' organizations, people, and actions aim to promote, restore, or maintain health in various ways. Understanding these systems offers valuable insights into the broader dynamics of healthcare in Oceania (World Health Organization [WHO], 2023).

GEOGRAPHY

Oceania is a region defined by its vast expanse of the Pacific Ocean, encompassing thousands of islands and varying geographic conditions (Figure 56.1). Australia and New Zealand are large, developed nations with substantial landmasses, while Papua New Guinea, Tonga, Samoa, and Fiji

FIGURE 56.1 Map of Oceania.

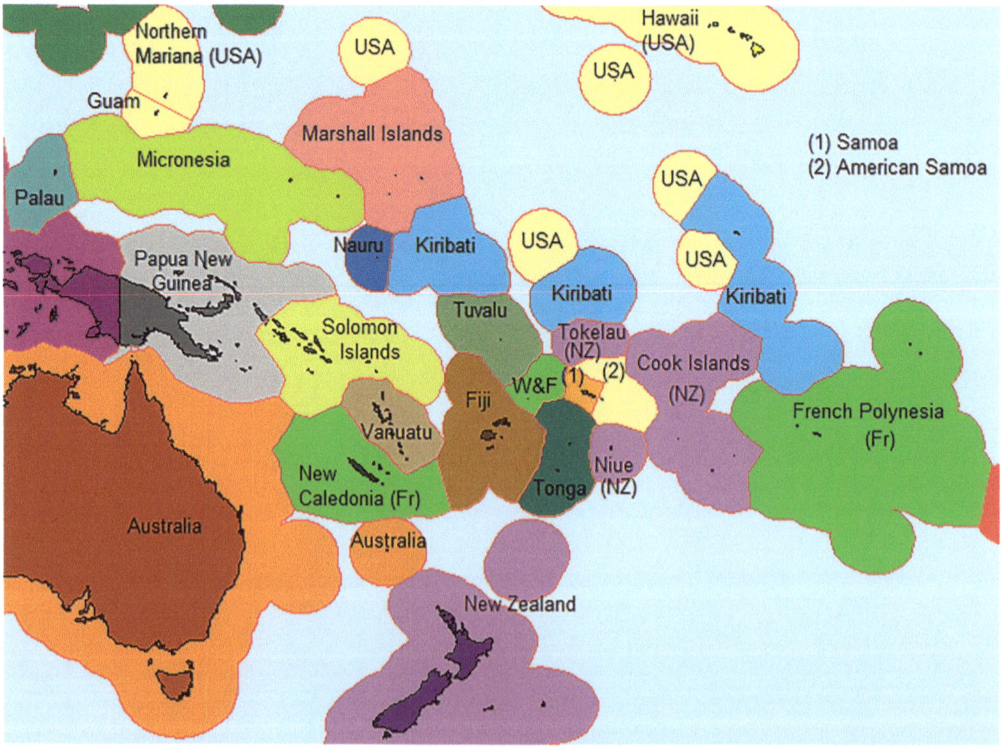

Source: EEZ Borders. (2022). *Oceania political map*. https://commons.wikimedia.org/w/index.php?title=File:Oceania_political_map.png&oldid=726087471

are smaller island nations with more limited resources. Geography significantly influences health-care delivery. Remote areas and dispersed populations present logistical challenges, such as limited transportation networks, shortages of skilled health personnel in remote regions, and difficulties in ensuring consistent supply chains for medical resources, especially in Papua New Guinea, Tonga, Samoa, and Fiji (Papua New Guinea National Department of Health, 2023; WHO, 2021b).

HISTORY

Colonial legacies, Indigenous practices, and modern development have shaped the design of health systems in Oceania. For instance, British colonial influences introduced centralized health administration in Australia and New Zealand, while missionary efforts brought Western medical practices to nations like Tonga and Samoa (Ministry of Health [MoH] New Zealand, 2023; Tonga MoH, 2023). Australia and New Zealand's systems evolved from British colonial influences, adopting universal healthcare frameworks. Papua New Guinea's healthcare system reflects its postcolonial challenges, with underfunded infrastructure and reliance on international aid (Papua New Guinea National Department of Health, 2023). Tonga's health system, influenced by traditional Polynesian practices and missionary health efforts, combines modern and Indigenous approaches (Tonga MoH, 2023). Samoa and Fiji have similarly integrated traditional and Western health practices, with Fiji benefiting from its history as a British colony and Samoa influenced by missionary efforts and traditional Polynesian medicine (MoH Samoa, 2023).

POPULATION

The populations of these countries vary significantly in size and demographics. Australia has approximately 26 million residents, and New Zealand has about 5 million, with aging populations and urbanized societies (Australian Institute of Health and Welfare [AIHW], 2023). Papua New Guinea has over 9 million people, most living in rural areas with limited infrastructure (Papua New Guinea National Department of Health, 2023). Tonga, with a population of around 100,000, is a small, closely knit society where communal living impacts healthcare accessibility and delivery (Tonga MoH, 2023). Fiji and Samoa, with populations of approximately 900,000 and 200,000, respectively, are primarily rural but have more centralized healthcare facilities in urban centers like Suva in Fiji and Apia in Samoa (MoH Fiji, 2023; MoH Samoa, 2023).

SOCIOECONOMIC FACTORS

Socioeconomic conditions play a critical role in health systems across Oceania. Australia and New Zealand, as high-income nations, have robust economies enabling substantial healthcare investment (AIHW, 2023; Organisation for Economic Co-operation and Development [OECD], 2021). Their citizens benefit from advanced medical technologies, well-funded hospitals, and comprehensive health insurance schemes. Conversely, Papua New Guinea faces significant challenges, with over 80% of its population living in rural areas and a per-capita gross domestic product (GDP) among the lowest globally (World Bank Group, 2021a). These economic constraints result in underfunded health infrastructure, limited access to essential medications, and inadequate health workforce capacity (Vallely et al., 2022). As lower-middle-income nations, Tonga, Samoa, and Fiji rely heavily on remittances and external aid, limiting their ability to fund their healthcare systems independently (World Bank Group, 2021b). Samoa and Fiji also face challenges in addressing urban–rural healthcare access and quality disparities (MoH Fiji, 2023).

HEALTH OUTCOMES

Health outcomes reflect the disparities among these nations (Table 56.1). Australia and New Zealand consistently rank high in global health metrics, with 82 and 81 years of life expectancies,

TABLE 56.1 HEALTH OUTCOMES FOR OCEANIA, 2023

COUNTRY	LIFE EXPECTANCY AT BIRTH (YEARS)	INFANT MORTALITY RATE (PER 1,000 LIVE BIRTHS)	MATERNAL MORTALITY RATIO (PER 100,000 LIVE BIRTHS)	LEADING CAUSE OF MORTALITY
Australia	83.2	3.1	4.8	Ischemic heart disease
New Zealand	82.4	3.6	11	Ischemic heart disease
Papua New Guinea	65.5	35.5	145	Lower respiratory infections
Tonga	70.2	14.9	124	Cardiovascular diseases
Samoa	73.4	17.4	127	Cardiovascular diseases
Fiji	67.3	22.5	59	Diabetes mellitus

Sources: Australian Institute of Health and Welfare. (2022). *Australia's mothers and babies: Maternal deaths.* https://www.aihw.gov.au/reports/mothers-babies/maternal-deaths-australia; Central Intelligence Agency. (2021). *Infant mortality rate comparison—The world factbook.* https://www.cia.gov/the-world-factbook/field/infant-mortality-rate/country-comparison; Organisation for Economic Co-operation and Development. (2021). *Infant mortality rates.* https://www.oecd.org/en/data/indicators/infant-mortality-rates.html

respectively (World Bank Group, 2021b). Both countries excel in managing chronic diseases and providing preventive care (AIHW, 2023). Papua New Guinea's health outcomes are among the poorest in Oceania, with high maternal and child mortality rates and a life expectancy of 64 years (UNICEF, 2023a, 2023b; WHO, 2021a). Malaria, tuberculosis, and malnutrition are significant public health challenges. Tonga faces a dual burden of infectious diseases and noncommunicable diseases (NCDs), particularly diabetes and obesity, due to lifestyle changes and imported diets (Tonga MoH, 2023). Public health strategies, such as community health promotion programs and dietary education, are being implemented to combat these challenges (WHO, 2021b). Samoa and Fiji also grapple with high rates of NCDs, especially diabetes and hypertension. Still, Fiji has made strides in addressing health challenges through regional partnerships and public health initiatives (MoH Fiji, 2023).

CONCLUSION

The health systems of Oceania reflect the region's diversity, shaped by geographic, historical, and socioeconomic factors. While Australia and New Zealand lead with advanced systems providing equitable care, Papua New Guinea, Tonga, Samoa, and Fiji face significant challenges in meeting basic health needs. Addressing these disparities requires regional cooperation, sustainable funding, and innovative solutions tailored to each nation's unique contexts. By understanding these dynamics, policymakers can foster more equitable health outcomes across Oceania. The chapters that follow will delve into the design of the health systems of Australia and Papua New Guinea.

LEARNING ACTIVITIES

CourseConnect

To access self-assessment questions and interactive, competency-based learning activities for this chapter, visit www.springerpub.com/courseconnect. See inside front cover and tear-out for CourseConnect details.

REFERENCES

Australian Institute of Health and Welfare. (2022). *Australia's mothers and babies: Maternal deaths*. https://www.aihw.gov.au/reports/mothers-babies/maternal-deaths-australia

Australian Institute of Health and Welfare. (2023). *Australia's health 2023*. https://www.aihw.gov.au

Central Intelligence Agency. (2021). *Infant mortality rate comparison*. The World Factbook. https://www.cia.gov/the-world-factbook/field/infant-mortality-rate/country-comparison

Ministry of Health Fiji. (2023). *Fiji health system overview*. https://www.health.gov.fj

Ministry of Health New Zealand. (2023). *Health system overview*. https://www.health.govt.nz

Ministry of Health Samoa. (2023). *Samoa health profile*. https://www.health.gov.ws

Organisation for Economic Co-operation and Development. (2021). *Infant mortality rates*. https://www.oecd.org/en/data/indicators/infant-mortality-rates.html

Papua New Guinea National Department of Health. (2023). *National health plan 2021–2030*. https://www.health.gov.pg

Tonga Ministry of Health. (2023). *Tonga health system overview*. https://www.health.gov.to

UNICEF. (2023a). *Child mortality*. https://data.unicef.org/wp-content/uploads/2024/03/UNICEF-2023-Child-Mortality-Report-1.pdf

UNICEF. (2023b). *Maternal mortality rates and statistics*. https://data.unicef.org/topic/maternal-health/maternal-mortality/

Vallely, L. M., Calvert, B., De Silva, M., Panisi, L., Babona, D., Bolnga, J., Duro-Aina, T., Noovao-Hill, A., Naidu, S., Leisher, S., Flenady, V., Smith, R. M., Vogel, J. P., & Homer, C. S. E. (2022). Improving maternal and newborn health and reducing stillbirths in the Western Pacific region: Current situation and the way forward. *The Lancet Regional Health, Western Pacific*, 32, 100653. https://doi.org/10.1016/j.lanwpc.2022.100653

World Bank Group. (2021a). *Life expectancy at birth, total (years)*. https://data.worldbank.org/indicator/SP.DYN.LE00.IN

World Bank Group. (2021b). *Mortality rate, infant (per 1,000 live births)*. https://data.worldbank.org/indicator/SP.DYN.IMRT.IN

World Health Organization. (2021a). *Maternal mortality ratio (MMR): Western Pacific Health Data Platform*. https://data.wpro.who.int/maternal-mortality-ratio-mmr

World Health Organization. (2021b). *Papua New Guinea*. https://data.who.int/countries/598

World Health Organization. (2023). *Western Pacific region: Health statistics*. https://www.who.int/westernpacific

CHAPTER 57

AUSTRALIA

Brigitte Tenni, Katherine Gilbert, and Alison Macintyre

GEOGRAPHY, SIZE, DEMOGRAPHICS

Australia is both a country and the world's smallest continent. It is the sixth largest country in the world by land mass with a total surface area of 7.7 million square kilometers (4,784,558 square miles; Australian Bureau of Statistics, 2024a). Since 1901, Australia has been a federation of six states: New South Wales, Victoria, Queensland, South Australia, Western Australia, and Tasmania; and two territories, Northern Territory and the Australian Capital Territory.

Australia is a country of great geographic diversity. Although it is rich in natural resources and has much fertile land, more than one third of Australia is desert. Most Australian cities and farmland are situated in the southwest and southeast coastal areas, where the climate is more temperate. Australia has a population of just over 26 million people and a population density of just 3.5 people per square kilometer (0.6 miles) making it one of the most sparsely populated countries on Earth (Australian Bureau of Statistics, 2024b). This can create significant challenges in terms of equitable healthcare provision to the more remote areas. Australia is also one of the world's most urbanized countries with 89% of its population living in a small number of urban areas (Australian Government, Department of Climate Change, Energy, the Environment and Water, 2013).

Australia has an aging population. The median age of all Australians was 38 years at the last census in 2021 and is projected to increase in the future (Australian Bureau of Statistics, 2023b) presenting potential challenges for healthcare provision. The total fertility rate (TFR) was last at replacement levels in 1975 and has continued to fall since. The TFR reached a low of 1.7 babies per woman in 2001, and increased again to 2.0, before declining to 1.8 in 2016 and to 1.6 in 2022 (Australian Bureau of Statistics, 2023b). Net overseas migration is therefore the key driver of Australia's population growth (Table 57.1).

Australia is a culturally and linguistically diverse country and has a rich mix of cultural backgrounds and heritage, with the number of people living in Australia who were born overseas continuing to increase. Just over 50% of Australians were born overseas or have at least one parent born overseas. The top five places of birth (after Australia) of residents of Australia are England, India, China, New Zealand, and the Philippines (Australian Bureau of Statistics, 2023a). The top five languages, other than English, spoken at home were Mandarin (2.7%), Arabic (1.4%), Vietnamese (1.3%), Cantonese (1.2%), and Punjabi (0.9%; Australian Bureau of Statistics, 2021b). In the year proceeding June 2023, overseas migration contributed a net gain of 518,000 people to Australia's population. This was the largest net overseas migration estimate since records began. This followed 2 years of the largest declines in migrant arrivals due to COVID-19-related border closures (Australian Bureau of Statistics, 2023c). More recently there has been considerable growth in the number of migrants from Nepal, India, Pakistan, Iraq, and the Philippines (Australian Bureau of Statistics, 2023a). Over 40% of Australians identify as Christians, 2.7% as Hindus, and 3.2% as Muslim. While the percentage of those who identify as Christian has decreased over time, the percent of Hindu and Muslims has increased, as has those who report having no religion (40%; Australian Bureau of Statistics, 2022).

TABLE 57.1 KEY DEMOGRAPHIC INFORMATION, AUSTRALIA

Median age, 2021	38.1 years
Percent of population by age, 2023	0–9 years: 12% 10–24 years: 18.2% 25–39 years: 21.5% 40–54 years: 19.3% 55–74 years:21.5% 75 years and over: 7.5%
Total fertility rate, 2023	1.63 children per woman
Top five ancestries (as a proportion of the population), 2021	English: 33.00% Australian: 29.90% Irish: 9.50% Scottish: 8.60% Chinese: 5.50%
Top five most common languages (other than English), 2021	Collectively, Australians speak over 400 languages. Of these, 167 are actively spoken Aboriginal and Torres Strait Islander languages. Mandarin: 2.7% Arabic: 1.4% Vietnamese: 1.3% Cantonese: 1.2% Punjabi: 0.9% 16,242 people used sign language (Auslan) in 2021.
Female to male ratio, 2023	1.00 females per 0.99 males
Intersex, 2023	1.7% of the population
Nonbinary, 2021	0.17% of the population (Responses show the concept of nonbinary sex was not consistently understood and was perceived in different ways by different people. Results cannot be used as a measure of gender diversity, nonbinary genders, or trans populations.)
Gender and sexual orientation, 2019	11% of the Australian population identify as lesbian, gay, bisexual, transgender, or intersex (LGBTI)
Urban population, 2021	89%

Source: Adapted from Australian Bureau of Statistics. (n.d.). *Population*. https://www.abs.gov.au/statistics/people/population

Aboriginal and Torres Strait Islander (hereafter **First Nations**) people are the first peoples of Australia. They comprise hundreds of groups that have their own distinct set of languages, histories, cultural traditions, healthcare systems, and concepts of health. Current research estimates that First Nations peoples have lived in Australia for more than 60,000 years (The Australian Institute of Aboriginal and Torres Strait Islander Studies, 2022). It is estimated that over 750,000 First Nations people inhabited Australia in 1788, at the time of colonization by the British Empire (The Aboriginal Heritage Office, 2024). Colonization has had a devastating impact on First Nations' communities and cultures. First Nations people have been subjected to myriad injustices, including mass killings and displacement from traditional lands to missions and reserves. Many First Nations people lost their lives in the years following colonization as a result of massacres, wars, and resistance (The Victorian Public Sector Commission, 2024). Many more First Nations people died from diseases brought by the colonists such as the flu, measles, tuberculosis, and smallpox (Deadly Story, 2024). Oppressive practices and policies that followed have resulted in complex experiences of trauma and loss and a legacy of intergenerational trauma for First Nations Australians. These practices included the dispossession of First Nations land and the forcible removal of children from their families—the "stolen generations"—between 1800s to 1969 (Darwin et al., 2023).

First Nations people live in urban, regional, and remote areas and are present in all communities, not only on their traditional lands. At the 2021 census, 3.8% of the Australian population identified as First Nations. In 2021, 76,978 First Nations people reported speaking 167 Aboriginal and Torres Strait Islander languages throughout Australia (Australian Bureau of Statistics, 2021a). For First Nations people, self-determination and empowerment, cultural identity, family and kinship, relationships with their traditional lands, knowledge and beliefs, language and participation in cultural activities, and access to traditional lands are key determinants of their health and well-being (Australian Bureau of Statistics, 2021a).

GOVERNANCE

Australia is a representative democracy and a constitutional monarchy with King Charles III as Head of State. He is represented in Australia by the Governor General (Parliament of Australia, 2024). Australia's federal government and the state and territory governments share responsibility for the management of the healthcare system via a complex arrangement of funding, administration and management, and service delivery (Australian Government, Department of Health and Aged Care, 2019). In general, the federal government provides the majority of funding for medical services and subsidizes medicines and health research. The state and territory governments provide the majority of the funds for community health services. The federal government and state and territory governments share responsibility for funding public hospital services (Australian Government, Department of Health and Aged Care, 2019).

HEALTH OUTCOMES

LIFE EXPECTANCY

Life expectancy reflects both the relatively high level of human development in Australia compared to other countries, and continuing inequities. Overall life expectancy at birth for females was 85.3 years and 81.2 years for males between 2020 and 2022 (Australian Bureau of Statistics, 2024d). Although this reflects a small decline (of 0.1 years) in life expectancy due to COVID-19, life expectancy increased by 1.0 years for women and 1.3 years for men across the decade, meaning that Australia has the third highest life expectancy in the world (Australian Bureau of Statistics, 2024d). Yet there are significant inequities in life expectancy, with the Australian Government estimating that the gap between the most advantaged and disadvantaged socioeconomic groups was 6 years for women and 8.7 years for men in 2016 (Australian Government Actuary, 2021). Similarly, First Nations people have a lower life expectancy compared to non-Indigenous Australians with differences of 8.1 years for women and 8.8 years for men in 2020 to 2022 (Australian Bureau of Statistics, 2023d). These differences increase with both remoteness and socioeconomic disadvantage; the gap widens to 12.4 years for both men and women when comparing First Nations and non-Indigenous people living in remote and very remote areas (Australian Bureau of Statistics, 2023d). These inequities are caused and perpetuated by inequities in the determinants of health and gaps in the utilization of healthcare services, as discussed in the following (Australian Institute of Health and Welfare [AIHW], 2024d).

TOP FIVE CAUSES OF DEATH

Australia's top five causes of death for men and women are coronary heart disease, dementia, COVID-19, cerebrovascular disease, and lung cancer, as shown in Table 57.2. There has been minimal change in the top five causes of death over the past 10 years, except for the introduction of COVID-19 (AIHW, 2024c). While the top five causes of death are the same for men and women, women have a higher proportion of deaths attributable to dementia and cerebrovascular disease compared to men (AIHW, 2024b).

NONCOMMUNICABLE DISEASES

Like other countries that have progressed along the epidemiologic and demographic transition, and have an aging population, noncommunicable diseases (NCDs) accounted for seven of the 10 top causes of mortality and 91% of the nonfatal disease burden in Australia in 2022 (AIHW, 2024b). This leads to significant service utilization needs. In 2022/2023 at the primary care level, one in six Australians (16%) had a Chronic Disease Management Service plan to manage a long-term or terminal illness (Australian Institute of Health and Welfare, 2024b). At the hospital level, NCDs accounted for an estimated 55% of hospitalizations and 74% of all bed days (AIHW, 2024).

MENTAL HEALTH

Mental health is a significant public health concern in Australia; suicide is the number one cause of death among persons age 25 to 44 years (AIHW, 2024b) and depressive and anxiety disorders are, respectively, the second and fourth most significant causes of death and disability (Institute for Health Metrics and Evaluation, 2024). In 2018, the burden of disease among First Nations people was 2.3 times that of non-Indigenous Australians, with mental and substance use disorders being the leading contributor to this disease burden (24%; AIHW, 2024a). Utilization of government-subsidized mental health services increased from 7% to 11% of the population between 2012 and 2022 (AIHW, 2024f). Females and young people age 15 to 24 years have the highest

TABLE 57.2 TOP 10 CAUSES OF MORTALITY IN AUSTRALIA, ALL AGES, 2022

	TOTAL	MALES	FEMALES
1	Coronary heart disease	Coronary heart disease	Dementia
2	Dementia	Dementia	Coronary heart disease
3	COVID-19	COVID-19	Cerebrovascular disease
4	Cerebrovascular disease	Lung cancer	COVID-19
5	Lung cancer	Cerebrovascular disease	Lung cancer
6	Chronic obstructive pulmonary disease	Chronic obstructive pulmonary disease	Chronic obstructive pulmonary disease
7	Diabetes	Prostate cancer	Breast cancer
8	Colorectal cancer	Diabetes	Diabetes
9	Other ill-defined causes	Colorectal cancer	Colorectal cancer
10	Accidental falls	Suicide	Heart failure and complications and ill-defined heart disease

Source: Australian Institute of Health and Welfare. (2024). *Australia's health 2024: in brief, catalogue number AUS 249.* https://www.aihw.gov.au/reports/australias-health/australias-health-2024-in-brief/summary

service utilization rates, and young people had the greatest growth in service utilization between 2012 and 2022 (AIHW, 2024).

COVID-19 AS A NEW INFECTIOUS DISEASE

When COVID-19 became the third leading cause of death in 2022, it was the first time an infectious disease was in the top five causes of death in Australia since 1970 (AIHW, 2024b). Efforts to address COVID-19 in Australia have revealed the challenges of collecting comparable information and implementing coherent disease-specific strategies across state-based jurisdictions.

DETERMINANTS OF HEALTH

SOCIAL AND ECONOMIC JUSTICE

Australia's wealth is higher than other advanced economies. In 2023, Australia's economy was the 13th largest in the world, with a per-capita gross domestic product (GDP) of $64,711 compared to the global average of $13,138 (World Bank Group, 2023). With strong universal education, health, and social protection systems, Australia ranked 10th on the UN Human Development Index in 2022 (UN Development Programme [UNDP], 2024). However, while measures of inequality remain small relative to other advanced economies, in 2019 and 2020, there was a significant wealth gap of –20% with the population with the highest incomes holding 41% of the wealth, more than the bottom 60% (UNSW and Australian Council of Social Service, 2024). This impacts health outcomes as noted, as well as the utilization of healthcare as will be discussed further.

Differences in educational attainment, employment, and household income between First Nations people and non-Indigenous Australians are estimated to account for over one third of the health gap experienced by First Nations people already described (AIHW, 2024c). For example, in 2021, 68.1% of First Nations people age 20 to 24 years attained a secondary school qualification or equivalent, compared to 90.7% for non-Indigenous people (AiHW, 2022; Australian Government Productivity Commission, 2024a). The same follows for employment. In 2021, 55.7% of First Nations people age 25 to 64 years were employed compared to 77.7% for non-Indigenous people (Australian Government Productivity Commission, 2024b). Nationally, 35% of First Nations people were in the poorest 20% of households, although this increases to 65% in very remote areas, reflecting the intersecting nature of disadvantage (Australian Government, AIHW, & National Indigenous Australians Agency, 2021).

ENVIRONMENTAL JUSTICE AND CLIMATE CHANGE

Both the built and natural environment impact our health. The Australian population enjoys relatively high access to the built environment including safe housing, clean water and sanitation, safe air, and green spaces, yet the country faces considerable challenges with respect to housing and climate change. In regard to housing, in 2018, 33% of First Nations people lived in a house with a major structural problem, which increased to 50% in very remote areas (AIHW, 2024a). Climate change has increased the frequency of extreme weather events (heatwaves, bushfires, and floods) in Australia, with recent analysis showing extreme weather leads to approximately 912 hospitalizations per year, with one third of hospitalizations among those age over 65 years (AIHW, 2024b). The highest number of hospitalizations due to extreme weather was recorded in 2019 and 2020, when Australia recorded an El Niño (reduced rainfall and warmer temperatures; AIHW, 2024c). Evidence suggests that climate change will impact First Nations people more than non-Indigenous Australians (AIHW, 2024e).

COMMERCIAL DETERMINANTS AND HEALTH BEHAVIORS

An estimated 38% of Australia's burden of disease was attributed to 40 risk factors in 2018, including daily tobacco use, excessive alcohol consumption, obesity status, blood pressure, and insufficient exercise (AIHW, 2024b). Declines have been observed with respect to insufficient exercise (from 68.5% to 46% between 2007 and 2022), excessive alcohol consumption (from 18.6% to 13.1% between 2001 and 2022), and daily smoking (from 22.4% to 10.6% between 2001 and 2022), with declines in daily smoking in part attributable to structural interventions including the introduction of plain packaging and an increase in tobacco taxes (Wilkinson et al., 2019). While increased taxation has been proposed as a method to reduce the consumption of sugar (Breadon & Geraghty, 2024) and alcohol (The Foundation for Alcohol Research and Education [FARE], 2024) at a federal or state level, this has not been adopted, in part due to the strength of the commercial lobby groups in these sectors. Improvements in blood pressure and nutritional intake have stagnated and obesity has increased from 61.2% to 65.8% between 2007/2008 and 2022 (AIHW, 2024b, 2024d). Like the other determinants, First Nations people and remote populations have higher rates of smoking, alcohol intake, and obesity and disadvantaged populations have higher rates of smoking and obesity (AIHW, 2024c).

HISTORICAL/THEORETICAL BACKGROUND OF HEALTHCARE

HEALTHCARE DELIVERY, FINANCE, INSURANCE, AND PAYMENT

Australia has a mixed public–private healthcare system, including a universal, tax-based national health insurance system, called **Medicare**, which finances care for all offered by public and private providers, and a private health insurance system. Between 2017 and 2021, Australia spent 10% to 11% of its GDP on health and increased its health expenditure per capita from $5,814 to $7,055 with economic growth (World Health Organization [WHO], 2022). Globally, this amounted to the fifth-highest expenditure per capita on health in 2021 in the world (WHO, 2022). More than three quarters (76%) of Australia's health spending is government funding. Out-of-pocket costs (OOP), paid at the point of care, constituted 13.8% of total health spending (AIHW, 2023c) and voluntary (but tax-incentivized) private health insurance constituted another 7.2%. Other sources of funding (3.0%) include workers' compensation schemes, motor vehicle insurance, and donations. In 2021 and 2022, hospitals constituted 39.8% of total health spending from all sources (AIHW, 2023c); primary care 34.9% and referred medical care 10.4%.

Primary care is provided by general practitioners (GPs), who mostly operate in private firms and receive payment on a fee-for-service basis from the government via Medicare (with the type and level of reimbursement for each service set out in the **Medical Benefits Scheme [MBS]**), and the patient via an OOP payment that may be charged at the discretion of the private GP. Similarly, prescriptions given by GPs can be filled at pharmacies, which are mostly private, with payment made again via Medicare (as set out in the **Pharmaceutical Benefits Scheme [PBS]**) and an OOP payment made by the patient. Patients with an income-contingent Health Care Card or Seniors Card are exempt from paying OOP at private GPs and at pharmacies for medicines on the PBS. Patients can also seek care from private GP practices that do not charge any patients OOP (referred to as bulk-billing), or community health organizations, such as **Aboriginal Community Controlled Health Organisations (ACCHOs)**, that offer primary care services under a different provider payment model with salaried GPs and no to minimal fees. The term **"bulk billing"** refers to the payment mechanism. If the patient is not charged an OOP, the GP or medical provider will "bulk bill" Medicare for provision of the services. If the patient is charged an OOP, the patient will pay for the full cost of the service, and the patient will receive reimbursement from Medicare. For private GPs, there is no cap on the level of OOP charged to patients (outside of the exemptions noted previously). As all citizens and some visa holders are entitled to Medicare, private health insurance does not offer reimbursement for GP services. However, private insurance does fund dental, allied and mental health (as well as hospital and specialist care as described in the following). Dental care is not covered by Medicare.

Out-of-hospital specialist care is also funded through Medicare (i.e., the federal government) through the MBS and PBS, with the difference between the Medicare payment and the provider fee met by the patient as an OOP and/or, for those covered, by private insurance companies. Public hospitals also receive funding from federal and state governments through Medicare, based on national standards weighted by the activities of each hospital, with patients paying limited OOP. Public hospitals can also seek reimbursement from private health insurance where patients are covered. In 2021 and 2022, private hospitals, which primarily facilitate elective rather than emergency procedures, received a mix of private health insurance payments (47.3%), government funding (33.4%), and other nongovernment funding including OOP (19.3%; AIHW, 2023c).

HEALTHCARE TRAINING AND EDUCATION

Degree-based education for health workers is provided through universities, which are funded through a mix of government funding and student fees, which may be paid upfront or with the support of income-contingent government loans. Some state governments have started paying for health worker degrees, such as nursing, to incentivize enrollment. Both universities and specialty colleges provide post-graduate or continuing education. One of the major challenges in medical education is encouraging more graduates to pursue GP training (primary care), where there are significant workforce shortages (AIHW, 2023c).

HEALTHCARE EQUITY, EFFICIENCY, AND QUALITY

Australia's healthcare system faces several challenges to maintaining and extending equity, alongside addressing the ongoing challenges posed by the epidemiologic and demographic transition, particularly the aging population, and increasing pressure to contain costs on new medical technologies (Duckett, 2022). First, utilization varies by wealth, with people living in the least economically disadvantaged areas more likely to see a dentist, specialist, or GP compared to those living in the most disadvantaged areas; people living in the most disadvantaged areas are more likely to use hospital emergency departments (Australian Bureau of Statistics, 2024c). The most disadvantaged are more likely to delay or not use health services than those more advantaged, as shown in Table 57.3. These data must also be considered in the context of the relationship between the determinants of health and economic disadvantage already noted, meaning that the most disadvantaged are likely to carry a greater share of the burden of disease.

Second, inequities in utilization are in part due to differences in the willingness and capacity to pay OOP and private health insurance (Callander, 2023). Approximately 55% of the population has private health insurance, which may include hospital costs (including specialists) and/or extras (including dental; Australian Competition and Consumer Commission, 2023), including 78.6% of those in the most advantaged quintile, compared to 35.3% in the most disadvantaged (Australian Bureau of Statistics, 2024c). In addition to greater utilization of care among the most economically advantaged as already noted, those with private health insurance have much shorter waiting times for elective surgery in both public and private hospitals; in public hospitals in 2022 and 2023, the average wait time for the 25 most common procedures was 51 days for publicly funded patients and 24 days for private health insurance patients (AIHW, 2023b). In this context, public subsidies to private health insurance premiums and to private hospitals contribute to inequities in the funding and utilization of services and inefficiencies in funding models through the separation of risk pools (Duckett, 2022).

TABLE 57.3 PROPORTION OF PEOPLE 15 YEARS AND OVER THAT DELAYED OR DID NOT USE SELECTED HEALTH SERVICES WHEN NEEDED DUE TO COST IN THE LAST 12 MONTHS

INDEX OF RELATIVE SOCIOECONOMIC DISADVANTAGE	DENTAL PROFESSIONAL (%)	MEDICAL SPECIALISTS (%)	PRESCRIBED MEDICATION (%)	GP (%)	AFTER-HOURS GP (%)	HOSPITALS (%)
First quintile (most disadvantage)	26.1	12.9	10.2	7.9	5.8	5.4
Second quintile	22.2	12.4	8.3	7.7	2.9	4.3
Third quintile	17.7	10.5	8.2	6.6	5.3	1.1
Fourth quintile	15.9	9.1	6.8	7.0	4.8	4.2
Fifth quintile (least disadvantage)	11.1	8.7	5.4	5.9	2.8	1.2

Source: Adapted from Australian Bureau of Statistics. (2023). *Key statistics*. https://www.abs.gov.au/statistics/health/health-services/patient-experiences/2022-23

Third, there are concerns regarding the equity and efficiency of primary care. Recently, the freezing of the level of MBS reimbursements for 10 years (2013 through 2023) by the federal government led to a decline in bulk billing and GP visits per person, with a greater decline in more disadvantaged areas (Mudiyanselage et al., 2023), creating concern regarding the financial accessibility of primary care. The federal government has increased MBS payments since 2023 which has led to an increase in bulk billing. Only GPs can be reimbursed for most items on the MBS, which also constrains the overall accessibility and efficiency of the system, given the shortage of GPs and the wider availability of cadre, such as nurse practitioners, that could be paid at a lower rate. This is on top of existing inefficiencies associated with the fee-for-service payment model.

Fourth, there is a significant rural and urban divide with respect to the accessibility of care similar to economic disadvantage noted previously (Australian Bureau of Statistics, 2024c). In primary care, this is exacerbated by the lack of GPs in rural and remote areas. First Nations people are often found to have relatively poorer access to health services than non-Indigenous Australians in relation to need for a range of reasons, including barriers such as availability, cost, and a lack of culturally appropriate health services.

Fifth, with the split between primary and specialist/hospital care, including their clinical training programs, location of facilities, funding models, and stewardship (with the federal government responsible for primary care, and state governments for hospitals), challenges have arisen with respect to the coordination of care (Duckett, 2022), with significant emphasis placed on the role of the GP as the coordinator of care. However, this is limited by both the demand for GPs and the workforce shortage already noted.

HEALTHCARE PRACTICES

Australia possesses a broad range of allied healthcare professionals who provide a range of healthcare services. In general terms, the Australian Government recognizes allied health professions that have a university qualification accredited by a national accreditation body, clear national entry-level competency standards and assessment processes, autonomy of practice, and a clearly defined scope of practice (Australian Government, Department of Health and Aged Care, 2023).

The larger allied health professions include physiotherapy, psychology, pharmacy, occupational therapy, social work, and osteopathy. These practitioners work in a variety of public and privately funded settings, including public and private hospitals, private clinical practices, residential aged care facilities, community care centers, schools, and disability services. Some are covered by Medicare and others by private insurance funds, Department of Veterans Affairs, National Disability Insurance Scheme, Workcover and Transport Accident Commission (Australian Government, Department of Health and Aged Care, 2023). Complementary and alternative therapies are estimated to be used by up to two thirds of people in Australia. Some of the more popular therapies include acupuncture, homeopathy, naturopathy, and herbal medicine. Many of these therapies are used alongside conventional medicines or treatments and are predominantly offered in the private sector (Victorian State Government Department of Health, 2021).

CONCLUSION

Australia's healthcare system is among the best in the world. Australia's universal healthcare scheme, Medicare, has been in existence since 1984 and provides free or low-cost access to most healthcare services to Australian and New Zealand citizens and some overseas visitors. There are, however, complex challenges to the public healthcare system including providing equitable health care to regional and remote areas and an aging population, increasing rates of chronic disease, rising OOP expenses, and inequality in access to health services and hospital wait times. Of particular concern is the disproportionate disease burden and lower life expectancy experienced by Australia's First Nations people in comparison to non-Indigenous Australians. Long-term initiatives to close the health and life expectancy gap between Aboriginal and Torres Strait Islander peoples and non-Indigenous Australians within a generation have had mixed results. As you reflect upon this chapter, consider what Australia can do to make healthcare more equitable and affordable.

CASE STUDY: ABORIGINAL COMMUNITY CONTROLLED HEALTH ORGANISATIONS

ACCHOs were established to address the health needs of First Nations people as they were not being met through mainstream services (The National Aboriginal Community Controlled Health Organisation [NACCHO], 2024a). ACCHOs first emerged in the 1970s and a national body (National Aboriginal and Islander Health Organisation [NAIHO]) followed in 1976 to support local ACCHOs. In 1992 this became NACCHO (NACCHO, 2024d). The NACCHO network now consists of 145 ACCHOs and 550 clinic sites, and provides services to over 400,000 people each year (NACCHO, 2024b). Each ACCHO is autonomous, with its own locally elected Board of Management which ensures the ACCHO is run appropriately and serves the community where it is based. There are also state and territory bodies for ACCHO networks. ACCHOs receive state and federal funding for their services and reinvest any revenue back into the communities they serve (NACCHO, 2024b).

ACCHOs provide comprehensive, holistic primary health services to First Nations people including a mix of large, multifunctional services to small clinics in remote areas, and outreach and mobile services. The majority of the workforce is comprised of First Nations people (NACCHO, 2024c). ACCHOs have repeatedly demonstrated effectiveness in improving access to, and uptake of, health services when compared to mainstream services (AIHW, 2023a). Due to community engagement and trust, First Nations people's response to the COVID-19 pandemic in Australia has been recognized as one of the most successful in the world (NACCHO, 2024c). Success has been seen beyond health services with evidence indicating ACCHOs have been effective in addressing the social and structural determinants of health (Pearson et al., 2020). The NACCHO network also forms a critical employment sector and employs more First Nations people than any other sector (AIHW, 2023a). This has been supported through broader education reform that has doubled the number of First Nations people registered as GPs and midwives between 2013 and 2021 (AIHW, 2023a).

Despite these successes, major funding gaps persist. A recent analysis estimated the funding shortfall to be $2.86 billion ($3,250 per First Nations person; NACCHO, 2024b). The funding gap is recognised as a key challenge in the reach and ability of ACCHOs to tackle the health inequalities experienced by First Nations people.

LEARNING ACTIVITIES

CourseConnect

To access self-assessment questions and interactive, competency-based learning activities for this chapter, visit www.springerpub.com/courseconnect. See inside front cover and tear-out for CourseConnect details.

REFERENCES

The Aboriginal Heritage Office. (2024). *A brief Aboriginal history*. https://www.aboriginalheritage.org/history/history/

Australian Bureau of Statistics. (2021a). *Aboriginal and Torres Strait Islander people: Census*. https://www.abs.gov.au/statistics/people/aboriginal-and-torres-strait-islander-peoples/aboriginal-and-torres-strait-islander-people-census/2021

Australian Bureau of Statistics. (2021b). *Cultural diversity: Census*. https://www.abs.gov.au/statistics/people/people-and-communities/cultural-diversity-census/latest-release

Australian Bureau of Statistics. (2022). *2021 Census shows changes in Australia's religious diversity*. https://www.abs.gov.au/media-centre/media-releases/2021-census-shows-changes-australias-religious-diversity

Australian Bureau of Statistics. (2023a). *Australia's population by country of birth*. https://www.abs.gov.au/statistics/people/population/australias-population-country-birth/jun-2023

Australian Bureau of Statistics. (2023b). *Population projections, Australia*. https://www.abs.gov.au/statistics/people/population/population-projections-australia/2022-base-2071

Australian Bureau of Statistics. (2023c). *Record high net overseas migration driven by temporary visa holders in 2022–23*. https://www.abs.gov.au/media-centre/media-releases/record-high-net-overseas-migration-driven-temporary-visa-holders-2022-23

Australian Bureau of Statistics. (2023d). *Aboriginal and Torres Strait Islander life expectancy*. https://www.abs.gov.au/statistics/people/aboriginal-and-torres-strait-islander-peoples/aboriginal-and-torres-strait-islander-life-expectancy/latest-release

Australian Bureau of Statistics. (2024a). *Geography of Australia. Position and area*. https://www.abs.gov.au/ausstats/abs@.nsf/Previousproducts/8826A00C209DDB02CA2573D200106A75?opendocument

Australian Bureau of Statistics. (2024b). *National, state and territory population*. https://www.abs.gov.au/statistics/people/population/national-state-and-territory-population/dec-2023

Australian Bureau of Statistics. (2024c). *Patient experiences*. https://www.abs.gov.au/statistics/health/health-services/patient-experiences/2022-23

Australian Bureau of Statistics. (2024d). *Life expectancy*. https://www.abs.gov.au/statistics/people/population/life-expectancy/latest-release

Australian Competition and Consumer Commission. (2023). *Report to the Australian Senate for the period 1 July 2022 to 30 June 2023 on anti-competitive and other practices by health insurers and providers in relation to private health insurance*. https://www.accc.gov.au/system/files/Private%20Health%20Insurance.pdf

Australian Government Actuary. (2021). *Life tables by relative socio-economic advantage and disadvantage—A microdata approach to resident sub-group tables*. Centre For Population, The Australian Government. https://population.gov.au/sites/population.gov.au/files/2021-12/sgm-paper3.pdf

Australian Government, Australian Institute of Health and Welfare, & National Indigenous Australians Agency. (2021). *Tier 2 determinants of health: 2.08 income.* https://www.indigenoushpf.gov.au/measures/2-08-income

Australian Government, Department of Climate Change, Energy, the Environment and Water. (2013). *Planning and management of urban and peri-urban wetlands in Australia—Fact sheet.* https://www.dcceew.gov.au/water/wetlands/publications/planning-and-management-urban-and-peri-urban-wetlands-australia-fact-sheet

Australian Government, Department of Health and Aged Care. (2019). *The Australian health system.* https://www.health.gov.au/about-us/the-australian-health-system#:~:text=It%20is%20jointly%20run%20by,state%20and%20territory%2C%20and%20local.&text=care%20in%20Australia-,Australia's%20health%20system%20is%20one%20of%20the%20best%20in%20the,life%20expectancies%20in%20the%20world

Australian Government, Department of Health and Aged Care. (2023). *About allied health care.* https://www.health.gov.au/topics/allied-health/about

Australian Government Productivity Commission. (2024a). *Socio-economic outcome area 5: Aboriginal and Torres Strait Islander students achieve their full learning potential.* https://www.pc.gov.au/closing-the-gap-data/dashboard/se/outcome-area5

Australian Government Productivity Commission. (2024b). *Socio-economic outcome area 8: Strong economic participation and development of Aboriginal and Torres Strait Islander people and communities.* https://www.pc.gov.au/closing-the-gap-data/dashboard/se/outcome-area8

The Australian Institute of Aboriginal and Torres Strait Islander Studies. (2022). *Australia's first peoples.* https://aiatsis.gov.au/explore/australias-first-peoples

Australian Institute of Health and Welfare. (2022). *Australia's children.* https://www.aihw.gov.au/reports/children-youth/australias-children

Australian Institute of Health and Welfare. (2023a). *Cultural safety in health care for Indigenous Australians: Monitoring framework.* https://www.aihw.gov.au/reports/indigenous-australians/cultural-safety-health-care-framework/contents/summary

Australian Institute of Health and Welfare. (2023b). *Elective surgery access.* https://www.aihw.gov.au/reports-data/myhospitals/intersection/access/eswt

Australian Institute of Health and Welfare. (2023c). *Health expenditure Australia 2021–22.* https://www.aihw.gov.au/reports/health-welfare-expenditure/health-expenditure-australia-2021-22/contents/summary

Australian Institute of Health and Welfare. (2024a). *Aboriginal and Torres Strait Islander health performance framework: Summary report.* https://www.indigenoushpf.gov.au/report-overview/overview/summary-report

Australian Institute of Health and Welfare. (2024b). *Australia's health 2024: Data insights: The ongoing challenge of chronic conditions in Australia.* https://www.aihw.gov.au/reports/australias-health/chronic-conditions-challenge

Australian Institute of Health and Welfare. (2024c). *Australia's health 2024: In brief.* https://www.aihw.gov.au/reports/australias-health/australias-health-2024-in-brief/summary

Australian Institute of Health and Welfare. (2024d). *Diet.* https://www.aihw.gov.au/reports/food-nutrition/diet

Australian Institute of Health and Welfare. (2024e). *Size and sources of the health gap for Australia's First Nations people 2017–2019.* https://www.aihw.gov.au/reports/australias-health/health-gap-2017-2019

Australian Institute of Health and Welfare. (2024f). *Use of Medicare services and pharmaceuticals by mental health patients in Australia over the last decade.* https://www.aihw.gov.au/reports/australias-health/mental-health-patients

Breadon, P., & Geraghty, J. (2024). *Sickly sweet: It's time for a sugary drinks tax.* Grattan Institute.

Callander, E. J. (2023). Out-of-pocket fees for health care in Australia: Implications for equity. *Medical Journal of Australia, 218,* 294–297. https://doi.org/10.5694/mja2.51895

Darwin, L, V. S., Vollert, E., & Blustein S. (2023). *Intergenerational trauma and mental health.* Australian Institute of Health and Welfare, Australian Government. https://www.indigenousmhspc.gov.au/getattachment/6f0fb3ba-11fb-40d2-8e29-62f506c3f80d/intergenerational-trauma-and-mental-health.pdf?v=1309

Deadly Story. (2024). *Frontier wars.* https://deadlystory.com/page/culture/history/Frontier_wars

Duckett, S. J. (2022). *The Australian health care system.* Oxford Oxford University Press.
The Foundation for Alcohol Research and Education. (2024). *Pricing and taxation.* https://fare.org.au/policy/pricing-taxation/#:~:text=FARE%20is%20calling%20for%20reform,supports%20public%20health%20and%20wellbeing
Institute for Health Metrics and Evaluation. (2024). *Australia.* https://www.healthdata.org/research-analysis/health-by-location/profiles/australia
Mudiyanselage, S. B., Dona, S. W. A., Abimanyi-Ochom, J. & Watts, J. J. (2023). Impact of the Medicare benefits schedule rebate (MBSR) freeze on general practice (GP) use: Multivariable regression analysis. *BMC Health Services Research, 23,* 588. https://doi.org/10.1186/s12913-023-09569-3
The National Aboriginal Community Controlled Health Organisation. (2024a). *Aboriginal community controlled health organisations (ACCHOs).* https://www.naccho.org.au/acchos/#:~:text=What%20is%20the%20history%20of,and%20accessible%20primary%20health%20care
The National Aboriginal Community Controlled Health Organisation. (2024b). *Annual report 2022–23.* https://cahs.net.au/wp-content/uploads/2024/02/Aboriginal-Health-Annual-Report-2022-2023-Print-min-1.pdf
The National Aboriginal Community Controlled Health Organisation. (2024c). *Key facts.* https://www.naccho.org.au/app/uploads/2022/11/NACCHO_KeyFacts_infographics_A4_221115.pdf
The National Aboriginal Community Controlled Health Organisation. (2024d). *Our story.* https://www.naccho.org.au/our-story/
Parliament of Australia. (2024). *Infosheet 20 - The Australian system of government.* https://www.aph.gov.au/About_Parliament/House_of_Representatives/Powers_practice_and_procedure/00_-_Infosheets/Infosheet_20_-_The_Australian_system_of_government
Pearson, O., Schwartzkopff, K., Dawson, A., Hagger, C., Karagi, A., Davy, C., Brown, A., & Braunack-Mayer, A., & Leadership Group Guiding the Centre for Research Excellence in Aboriginal Chronic Disease Knowledge Translation and Exchange. (2020). Aboriginal community controlled health organisations address health equity through action on the social determinants of health of Aboriginal and Torres Strait Islander peoples in Australia. *BMC Public Health, 20,* 1859. https://doi.org/10.1186/s12889-020-09943-4
UN Development Programme. (2024). *Australia Human Development Index.* https://hdr.undp.org/data-center/specific-country-data#/countries/AUS
UNSW & Australian Council of Social Service. (2024). *Inequality in Australia.* https://povertyandinequality.acoss.org.au/inequality/#:~:text=People%20in%20the%20highest%2020,which%20are%20from%202019%2D20
The Victorian Public Sector Commission. (2024). *Aboriginal and Torres Strait Islander culture and history.* https://vpsc.vic.gov.au/workforce-programs/aboriginal-cultural-capability-toolkit/aboriginal-culture-and-history/
Victorian State Government Department of Health. (2021). *Complementary therapies.* https://www.health.gov.au/topics/allied-health/about
Wilkinson, A. L., Scollo, M. M., Wakefield, M. A., Spittal, M. J., Chaloupka, F. J., & Durkin, S. J. (2019). Smoking prevalence following tobacco tax increases in Australia between 2001 and 2017: An interrupted time-series analysis. *Lancet Public Health, 4,* e618–e627. https://doi.org/10.1016/s2468-2667(19)30203-8
World Bank Group. (2023). *Data: Australia.* https://data.worldbank.org/country/australia?view=chart
World Health Organization. (2022). *The global health expenditure database.* https://apps.who.int/nha/database

CHAPTER 58

PAPUA NEW GUINEA

Janell Kayla Atkins, James Giallella, Katelyn Lee, Luke Orgo, and Thomas Foley

GEOGRAPHY AND POPULATION

The **Independent State of Papua New Guinea** is an island country located in the southwestern Pacific Ocean, encompassing the eastern half of New Guinea and several offshore islands and islets. Papua New Guinea is one of the largest island nations in the world with a total surface area of 462,840 square kilometers (287,595 square miles; Jackson & Standish, 2019). It is also the second most populated country in Oceania. In 2023, the population of Papua New Guinea was approximately 10.39 million people (UN Data Portal, n.d.). It includes four regions (the Highlands, Islands, Momase, and Southern Regions), 20 provinces, an Autonomous Region (Bougainville), and a National Capital (**Port Moresby**). Port Moresby is the largest city in Papua New Guinea and has a population density of roughly 1,500 residents per square kilometer (0.6 square miles). In comparison, the population density of Papua New Guinea in its entirety was 21.7 people per square kilometer (0.6 square miles) in 2023 (Jackson & Standish, 2019).

Papua New Guinea has a young and fast-growing population compared to other countries in the region. In 2023, the annual growth rate was 2.31% (U.S. Census Bureau, n.d.). The median age was 22.3 years. Nearly 44% of the population was younger than 20 years and less than 4% of the population was 65 years or older. In addition, the birth rate during 2023, which was 24.6, was much higher than the regional birth rate in Oceania, which was 15.2 (UN Data Portal, n.d.). Figure 58.1 is the age pyramid of Papua New Guinea in 2023, displaying a country with a high birth rate and minimal population aging. Rapid population growth and aging on the island nation makes providing basic health and education services difficult (UN Development Programme, 2024).

CULTURE

Most ethnic groups in Papua New Guinea are indigenous to the area, and PNG has one of the most diverse Indigenous populations in the world. While there are thousands of distinct tribes with their own traditions, a majority of the native population is classified as **Melanesian**; that is, people Indigenous to the Melanesian subcontinent of Oceania. On some of the outlying islands, there are small groups of Micronesians, the Indigenous people of the Micronesian subcontinent, and Polynesians, the Indigenous people of the Polynesian subcontinent. In Papua New Guinea, there are also small nonnative populations such as people who are from Australia, New Zealand, China, Britain, the United States, and the Philippines. Because of its diversity, there are more than 800 languages spoken in Papua New Guinea; however, it recognizes several official languages. **Tok Pisin**, also called Melanesian Pidgin or Neo-Melanesian, is used in everyday contexts and is the most widely spoken language. Tok Pisin is a creole language combing Indigenous languages, German, and English. English is the main language of government and is spoken by approximately 2% of the population (Jackson & Standish, 2019).

Christianity is the main religion, with more than 90% of Papua New Guineans practicing Christianity. The most common forms of Christianity in Papua New Guinea are Catholicism, Lutheranism, Seventh-Day Adventism, Pentecostalism, and the United Church. A small minority of the population is Muslim or members of the Baha'i Faith. Although nonnative faiths are widespread in Papua New Guinea, much of the population still adheres to and promotes traditional

FIGURE 58.1 Age distribution of Papua New Guinea in 2023.

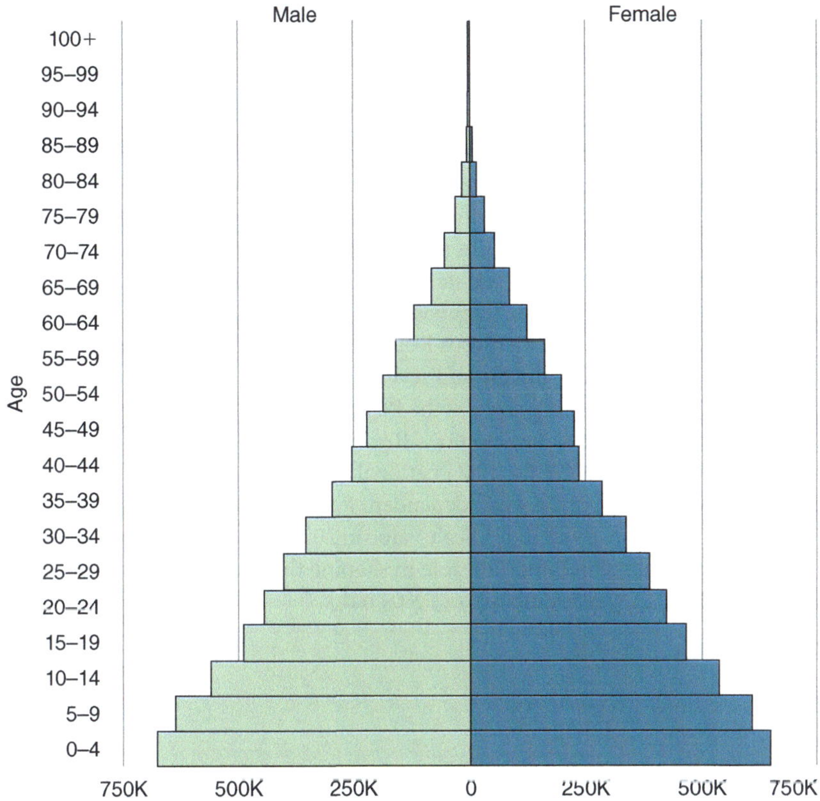

Source: U.S. Census Bureau. (n.d.). *International database*. https://www.census.gov/data-tools/demo/idb/#/dashboard?menu=countryViz&CCODE=PG&CCODE_SINGLE=PG&subnat_map_admin=ADM1&measures=GR&TREND_RANGE=1990

beliefs and practices, referred to as **kastom**, such as Indigenous religions, magic, art, ceremonies, and economics (Central Intelligence Agency [CIA], 2024).

BRIEF COUNTRY HISTORY

The first inhabitants of Papua New Guinea can be traced back to about 50,000 years ago, likely originating from East and Southeast Asia. The first ancient migrations occurred around the same time as Australia and Papua New Guinea was one of the first land masses after Africa and Eurasia to be populated by modern humans. These first inhabitants were largely isolated from each other because of the land's geography, leading to rich ethnic and linguistic diversity (BBC, 2018; CIA, 2024; Embassy of PNG, n.d.).

During the 19th century, the northern and southern parts of the land were colonized separately, with Germany colonizing the north and Britain colonizing the south. "German New Guinea" was established in 1884 by a German charter company due to Europe's need for coconut oil until it was taken over by the German government itself in 1899. "Papua" was put under a British protectorate in 1884, becoming "British New Guinea," then annexed in 1888. British New Guinea was transferred to the newly independent Commonwealth of Australia in 1906, becoming the Territory of Papua. Australian forces occupied German New Guinea during World War I and the League of Nations granted Australia a mandate rule of the area in 1921. The territories of Papua and New Guinea were governed separately from each other. During this modernization period, millions of Indigenous people lived away from the effects of colonization due to geographic barriers, as seen in

1933 when a gold expedition led to the discovery of mountain valley inhabitants who had been living unchanged for thousands of years. Only certain regions of the principal island had interacted or been colonized by Europeans, a key reason why there is such significant Indigenous diversity in modern day Papua New Guinea (BBC, 2018; CIA, 2024; Embassy of PNG, n.d.).

During World War II, Japanese forces invaded and occupied New Guinea in 1941 and Papua in 1942. Allied victories pushed the Japanese out of the area and, after the war, the two territories combined into one administration, becoming the country of Papua New Guinea. While the administration was unified, it was still under the authority of Australia. Papua New Guinea would achieve independence in 1975 with Sir Michael Somare serving as its first prime minister. Papua New Guinea became a Constitutional Monarchy and a member of the British Commonwealth of Nations. Italso joined the United Nations and became an observer state of the Association of Southeastern Asian Nations (ASEAN) in 1975 (BBC, 2018; CIA, 2024; Embassy of PNG, n.d.).

Shortly after gaining independence, separatist from Bougainville Island began fighting for their own right to self-governance. In 2002, Bougainville and several nearby smaller islands were granted some degree of self-governance by being recognized as the Papua New Guinea Autonomous Region of Bougainville. In 2019, the people of the Autonomous Region of Bougainville voted in favor of complete independence; however, as of 2024, the PNG national government has not recognized the Bougainville desire to be fully independent. Newly independent PNG faces several policy, infrastructure, and economic challenges. Their Human Index Scale value in 2022 was 0.57, one of the lowest in the world. Their complex history plays an important role in shaping the challenges that Papua New Guinea faces today (BBC, 2018; CIA, 2024; Embassy of PNG, n.d.).

HEALTH OUTCOMES

LEADING CAUSES OF DEATH

Papua New Guinea continues to face health challenges shaped by its geography, cultural diversity, and resource constraints. Reliable documentation for cause of death data is severely lacking due, in part, to insufficient civil registration in many areas, resulting in quality issues and a poor understanding of causes of deaths (Kitur et al., 2019; Pham et al., 2023). The estimated leading causes of death in Papua New Guinea during 2021 were COVID-19, stroke, heart disease, lower respiratory infections, chronic obstructive pulmonary disease (COPD), diabetes, neonatal disorders, tuberculosis (TB), and congenital defects. Mortality from neonatal disorders and communicable diseases such as lower respiratory infections, diarrheal diseases, and TB have been decreasing while mortality from noncommunicable conditions such as heart disease, COPD, and diabetes have been increasing (Institute for Health Metrics and Evaluation [IHME], n.d.). Figure 58.2 is a comparison of the leading causes of death in Papua New Guinea during 2011 and 2021.

MENTAL HEALTH

In Papua New Guinea, mental health is an underaddressed issue. Stigma and limited resources hinder the ability to receive quality mental healthcare. Common mental health conditions include depression, anxiety, and substance use disorders. These mental health disorders are exacerbated by poverty, domestic violence, and community unrest. Although there are a few specialized facilities where mental health professionals are available, many mental health disorders in Papua New Guinea are undiagnosed and untreated. Traditional beliefs and practices often replace modern approaches to mental health (Eves & Lusby, 2018).

INFECTIOUS DISEASE

Infectious diseases in Papua New Guinea are highly prevalent. Common infectious diseases in the country are TB, malaria, HIV, and diarrheal diseases. Diarrheal diseases are common due to the lack of safe drinking water in many rural and urban areas, as they rely on surface water, wells,

FIGURE 58.2 Leading causes of death in Papua New Guinea, 2011 and 2021.

Cause	2011 rank	2021 rank	Change in deaths per 100K, 2011–2021
COVID-19	–	1	↑ +83.9
Stroke	2	2	↓ −0.4
Ischemic heart disease	3	3	↑ +1.6
Lower respiratory infections	1	4	↓ −29.5
COPD	4	5	↑ +1.3
Diabetes	7	6	↑ +3.6
Neonatal disorders	5	7	↓ −0.3
Diarrheal diseases	6	8	↓ −8.8
Tuberculosis	8	9	↓ −5.8
Congenital defects	9	10	↓ −3.1

● Communicable, maternal, neonatal, and nutritional diseases ● Noncommunicable diseases

COPD, chronic obstructive pulmonary disease.

Source: Institute for Health Metrics and Evaluation. (n.d.). *Papua New Guinea*. https://www.healthdata.org/research-analysis/health-by-location/profiles/papua-new-guinea

and springs that are potentially contaminated. The lack of improved sanitation has led to open defecation and exposure to waterborne diarrheal diseases (UNICEF, 2023). Incidences of TB are among the highest in the Pacific region with multidrug-resistant cases posing challenges in developing effective treatments. Malaria also continues to affect the area, especially in lowland and coastal areas. While morbidity from malaria is extremely high in Papua New Guinea, prevention methods such as insecticide-treated nets have been helping to reduce transmission rates during the 21st century. Vaccination programs and international aid have improved coverage for diseases like measles and polio. Papua New Guinea has the highest HIV/AIDS prevalence rate in the Pacific, making up about 95% of the reported HIV cases within the region. Organizations such as UNAIDS and the World Health Organization (WHO) have been supporting the introduction of the dipivefrine ring for HIV prevention for women at high risk of HIV infection (UNAIDS, 2024).

NONCOMMUNICABLE DISEASES

Noncommunicable diseases (NCDs) in Papua New Guinea have been increasing along with economic development driven by urbanization and social transitions. Development has led to the **nutrition transition** phenomenon, which is a switch from traditional diets and active lifestyles to diets reliant on processed, high-energy dense foods and increased sedentariness. The high rates of cardiovascular diseases and diabetes are linked to the nutrition transition and limited healthcare access. Chronic respiratory diseases have been linked to the smoking culture and air pollution from indoor cooking fires. Some research suggests a variation in risk based on ethnic origin, lifestyle, and living environment. For example, urban dwelling populations of any ethnic origin are more at risk of developing an NCD than their rural peers. The Wanigela people of Port Moresby, the nation's highly dense capital city, have one of the highest rates of diabetes recorded in the entire pacific (Pulford, 2015). Efforts to address NCDs remain limited due to the funding constraints and limited infrastructure (IHME, n.d.).

LIFE EXPECTANCY AND INFANT AND MATERNAL MORTALITY

During 2023, life expectancy at birth in PNG was 63.74, which was well below the regional Oceania average of 79.15 years. PNG also has notably high infant and maternal mortality. In

2023, the infant mortality rate in PNG was 32.2 infant deaths per 1,000 live births, which was more than double the rate in all of Oceania (UN Data Portal, n.d.). High infant mortality in PNG is driven by infections, malnutrition, and lack of skilled birth attendants. The maternal mortality ratio for PNG in 2020 was 191.8 maternal deaths per 100,000 live births (UN Population Fund, n.d.). Infections, obstructed labor, and hemorrhages are primary causes of maternal mortality in PNG (WHO, 2024).

DETERMINANTS OF HEALTH

SOCIOECONOMIC FACTORS

Papua New Guinea experiences significant health disparities due to social, economic, and environmental determinants. The country's unique cultural diversity and limited infrastructure play crucial roles in shaping health outcomes. Papua New Guinea's economy relies heavily on the natural resources that are extracted from mining and agriculture, yet poverty continues to be a widespread problem. It has a gross domestic product (GDP) of approximately $26.7 billion as of 2023, with a per-capita GDP of $3,000, indicating significant income inequality (World Bank Group, n.d.). Poverty rates are also at a high with nearly 35% of the population living below the national poverty line. This disparity has particularly affected rural areas, where 40% of people struggle to afford necessities, compared to 27% within urban areas (UNICEF, 2023). These disparities continue to hinder access to adequate healthcare, food, safe drinking water, and education. The country struggles with low literacy rates and school attendance. Papua New Guinea has a literacy rate of approximately 64% with lower rates among the rural populations that make up about 86% of the population. There is also low literacy among women, especially rural women, who struggle to achieve equitable educational attainment. Many children drop out of the education system early due to financial burdens and inadequate infrastructure. Only 35% of Papua New Guineans have completed primary school. Low literacy and school attendance limits public health education efforts and campaigns for disease prevention, as it becomes difficult to spread information through methods that require reading comprehension (UN Data Portal, n.d.).

High unemployment rates among the youth and women are another cause for concern. Unemployment limits stability and access to healthcare services in Papua New Guinea (World Bank Group, 2023). With a formal unemployment rate around 6%, many rely on **subsistence farming**, where farmers grow crops and raise livestock for their own consumption to meet individual and community needs.

SOCIAL JUSTICE

Papua New Guinea faces numerous social justice challenges that exacerbate health inequalities. Malnutrition among children contributes to stunted growth and increased susceptibility to infections (IHME, n.d.). Gender-based violence is pervasive with over 60% of women experiencing domestic abuse at home (Eves & Lusby, 2018). Survivors of family violence are often unable to seek help due to social stigma. In provinces like Hela, many women do not seek help because the economy is male dominated, meaning that a women would lose financial support if her husband were prosecuted. If a woman seeks safety, her family may not take her back if they did not approve of the marriage or because doing so would require returning a bride price that has already been spent. With few shelters or formal safe houses, many survivors of domestic violence are often left with no place to go. Papua New Guinea has sought to adopt new legal reforms and policies to combat the growing rate of gender-based violence with the support of outside organizations such as WHO (Abay, n.d.).

ENVIRONMENTAL FACTORS

Papua New Guinea also faces several significant environmental challenges that affect its communities. Deforestation and land degradation driven by logging and mining tend to lead to loss of livelihoods and biodiversity. Rising sea levels due to climate change threaten coastal communities with unpredictable weather patterns that affect food security. Earthquakes, volcanic activity, tsunamis, heatwaves, and flooding also pose threats to the well-being of Papua New Guineans and disrupt access to healthcare and basic needs (Jackson & Standish, 2019). These environmental challenges often exacerbate the existing challenges in healthcare and malnutrition in the community.

HEALTHCARE

TRADITIONAL, COMPLEMENTARY, AND INTEGRATED HEALTHCARE

Due to the decentralized nature of the healthcare system, several differing healthcare practices are utilized throughout the nation. Modern medical practice dominates primary care (Grundy et al., 2019) and continues to experience development within Papua New Guinea through reforms in health education and administration. Vaccinations cover approximately half the population against common communicable diseases such as tetanus, TB, rubella, diphtheria, and pertussis (WHO, 2024).

Despite modernizing medical education and practices, many primary care facilities within Papua New Guinea lack proper funding and, thus, adequate resources to administer quality healthcare (Grundy et al., 2019). In areas where modern healthcare is inaccessible, people often rely on traditional herbal medicine based on a variety of plants local to the region. Despite the vast diversity of herbal medicine, four plant-based medicines are shared throughout Papua New Guinea: *Alstonia scholaris* (L.) R.Br., *Cassia alata* L., *Passiflora foetida* L., and *Zingiber officianale* Roscoe. Papua New Guineans use these plants to treat a variety of illnesses, from psychiatric diseases to malaria (Koch et al., 2015).

HEALTHCARE EDUCATION

Healthcare training within Papua New Guinea is administered by the government and Church Health Services (CHS). There are eight schools of nursing in Papua New Guinea. Three of the nursing schools are owned by the government with each offering a 3-year diploma in general nursing. Among the CHS-owned nursing schools, four provide a nursing program diploma and one offers a 4-year undergraduate bachelor program in nursing. Papua New Guinea has two medical schools: the University of Papua New Guinea School of Medicine and Health Sciences and the Divine Word University Faculty of Medicine and Health Sciences. Both schools provide education in a wide range of disciplines including oral, dental, rural, and environmental health and physiotherapy, pharmacy, medical imaging, and health management. Community health work is also provided at a certificate level within 12 of the nation's provinces. Given the impact of infectious diseases and infant mortality in Papua New Guinea, health education prioritizes programs on immunization, communicable disease control, reproductive health, and child health. Healthcare education in Papua New Guinea faces human resource and information technology challenges, preventing many new graduates from receiving the proper instruction needed to address prevailing health issues (Grundy et al., 2019).

Despite persistent educational issues, 21st-century reforms to improve healthcare instruction have been initiated, many of which were enacted by the CHS as part of their continuous quality improvement (CQI) process (Schuele & MacDougall, 2022). Recent reforms are intended to improve the implementation of healthcare directed toward the prevention, diagnosis, and treatment of diseases common to Papua New Guinea such as TB, malaria, and HIV (Chen et al., 2024).

HEALTHCARE GAPS

Despite efforts by the government and the CHS to improve healthcare, Papua New Guinea struggles with geographic, financial, and infrastructural constraints. As a result, several major healthcare gaps persist. Factors contributing to these healthcare gaps require continued investigation due to the nuances of a decentralized population (Schuele & MacDougall, 2022). The healthcare work shortage is a leading cause of the gaps in primary care within Papua New Guinea (Grundy et al., 2019). Primary care is centered around aid posts to support its large rural population (Schuele & MacDougall, 2022), but, despite efforts to provide rural healthcare, approximately one out of every four rural aid post experienced understaffing in the past decade. In fact, staffing Papua New Guinea's primary healthcare facilities is considered the greatest need within the nation's healthcare system. Many well-trained healthcare providers are lost to the private healthcare sector or to healthcare employers in other countries, which further impedes the ability of Papua New Guinea's primary care system to adequately meet the needs of the people (Grundy et al., 2019).

Poor investment in primary care also affects the facilities, especially the aid posts. Approximately half of all aid posts report a lack of basic necessities such as electricity, year-round water supply, refrigeration, and toilets. To cover financial constraints, some primary care facilities make patients pay for services otherwise deemed free by the government. Due to geographic barriers within Papua New Guinea, financial protection against such acts is not enforced by the government. The illegal procurement of healthcare fees prevents many impoverished rural inhabitants from receiving adequate healthcare within primary care facilities (Grundy et al., 2019).

CONCLUSION

Papua New Guinea is a diverse Pacific island nation with over 800 languages and 1,000 Indigenous tribes. With limited access to adequate healthcare, clean water, and sanitation, the population experiences significant morbidity and mortality from preventable communicable diseases. Public health efforts, such as vaccination initiatives and the dipivefrine ring for women, have decreased morbidity and mortality from infectious diseases during the 21st century; however, economic expansion and urbanization have introduced phenomena like the nutrition transition, resulting in increased incidences of and deaths from NCDs such as heart disease and diabetes.

The Papua New Guinea healthcare system faces several challenges, such as lack of funding for primary healthcare training and facilities. Rural aid posts lack resources such as electricity, refrigeration, and toilets. Many Papua New Guineans rely on traditional healthcare practices such as herbal medicine. Efforts from outside organizations such as WHO and UNAIDS, in collaboration with the Papua New Guinea government, work to introduce preventive measures to combat prevalent diseases; however, with the onset of lifestyle and economic changes, the nation's healthcare system is facing multiple health-related crises that require public policy reforms and increased funding to public sector faciltities to increase access to quality primary healthcare in rural areas.

LEARNING ACTIVITIES

CourseConnect

To access self-assessment questions and interactive, competency-based learning activities for this chapter, visit www.springerpub.com/courseconnect. See inside front cover and tear-out for CourseConnect details.

REFERENCES

Abay, N. A., Kuehnast, K., Peake, G., & Demian, M. (n.d.). *Addressing gendered violence in Papua New Guinea: Opportunities and options*. https://www.usip.org/sites/default/files/2024-03/sr-528_addressing-gendered-violence-papua-new-guinea-opportunities-and-options.pdf

BBC News. (2018). *Papua New Guinea profile—Timeline*. https://www.bbc.com/news/world-asia-15593238

Chen, J., Davies, A., Tran, P., Gronau, R., Rangan, A., Allman-Farinelli, M., Porykali, S., Oge, R., & Porykali, B. (2024). Health and nutrition promotion programs in Papua New Guinea: A scoping review. *Nutrients, 16*(13), 1999. https://doi.org/10.3390/nu16131999

Central Intelligence Agency. (2024). *Papua New Guinea—The world factbook*. https://www.cia.gov/the-world-factbook/countries/papua-new-guinea/#people-and-society

Embassy of Papua New Guinea. (n.d.). *History of PNG*. http://en.png.or.jp/about-png/history-of-png/

Eves, R., & Lusby, S. (2018). *Do no harm: The relationship between violence against women and women's economic empowerment in Bougainville*. Department of Pacific Affairs.

Grundy, J., Dakulala, P., Wai, K., Maalsen, A., & Whittaker, M. (2019). Independent State of Papua New Guinea: Health system review. *Health Systems in Transition, 9*(1). https://www.who.int/publications/i/item/9789290226741

Institute for Health Metrics and Evaluation. (n.d.). *Papua New Guinea*. https://www.healthdata.org/research-analysis/health-by-location/profiles/papua-new-guinea

Jackson, R. T., & Standish, W. (2019). Papua New Guinea: Culture, history, and people. *Encyclopedia Britannica*. https://www.britannica.com/place/Papua-New-Guinea

Kitur, U., Adair, T., Riley, I., & Lopez, A. D. (2019). Estimating the pattern of causes of death in Papua New Guinea. *BMC Public Health, 19*(1), 1322. https://doi.org/10.1186/s12889-019-7620-5

Koch, M., Kehop, D. A., Kinminja, B., Sabak, M., Wavimbukie, G., Barrows, K. M., Matainaho, T. K., Barrows, L. R., & Rai, P. P. (2015). An ethnobotanical survey of medicinal plants used in the East Sepik province of Papua New Guinea. *Journal of Ethnobiology and Ethnomedicine, 11*, 79. https://doi.org/10.1186/s13002-015-0065-8

Pham, B. N., Jorry, R., Silas, V. D., Okely, A. D., Maraga, S., & Pomat, W. (2023). Leading causes of deaths in the mortality transition in Papua New Guinea: Evidence from the Comprehensive Health and Epidemiological Surveillance System. *International Journal of Epidemiology, 52*(3), 867–886. https://doi.org/10.1093/ije/dyac232

Pulford, J., Rarau, P., Vengiau, G., & Gouda, H. (2015). *Non-communicable diseases and associated risk factors in the Hiri, Karkar and Asaro integrated health and demographic surveillance sites*. https://www.pngimr.org.pg/wp-content/uploads/2019/05/Report-on-Non-Communicable-diseases-associated-risk-factors-in-the-Hiri-Karkar-and-Asaro-integrated-health-and-demographic-surveillance-sites.pdf

Schuele, E., & MacDougall, C. (2022). The missing bit in the middle: Implementation of the Nationals Health Services Standards for Papua New Guinea. *PloS One, 17*(6), e0266931. https://doi.org/10.1371/journal.pone.0266931

UN Data Portal. (n.d.). *UN Population Division data portal: Interactive access to global demographic indicators*. United Nations. https://population.un.org/dataportal/home

UNAIDS. (2024). *Papua New Guinea*. https://www.unaids.org/en/regionscountries/countries/papuanewguinea

UNICEF. (2023). *Papua New Guinea: Update on the context and situation of children*. https://www.unicef.org/media/152186/file/Papua-New-Guinea-2023-COAR.pdf

UN Development Programme. (2024). *2024 UNDP regional human development report: Pacific snapshot*. https://www.undp.org/pacific/publications/2024-pacific-snapshot-asia-pacific-human-development-report

U.S. Census Bureau. (n.d.). *International database*. https://www.census.gov/data-tools/demo/idb/#/dashboard?menu=countryViz&CCODE=PG&CCODE_SINGLE=PG&subnat_map_admin=ADM1&measures=GR&TREND_RANGE=1990

World Bank Group. (n.d.). *World Bank open data*. https://data.worldbank.org/

World Bank Group. (2023). *Policy reforms necessary to ensure equal economic opportunities for all Papua New Guineans*. https://www.worldbank.org/en/news/press-release/2023/07/10/policy-reforms-necessary-to-ensure-equal-economic-opportunities-for-all-papua-new-guineans

World Health Organization. (2024). *Papua New Guinea data*. https://data.who.int/countries/598.

PART XV: Global Health Moving Forward

CHAPTER 59

GLOBAL HEALTH MOVING FORWARD: OVERVIEW

Thomas Foley, Ammcise Apply, and Mary Hu

INTRODUCTION

While many factors will influence global health moving forward, this section focuses on several key topics that are essential to mitigating preventable morbidity and mortality, promoting health equity, and protecting the quality of life of global citizens. The issues are climate change, infectious diseases, mental health, population aging, and forced migration.

CLIMATE CHANGE

Climate change is driven by human activities like fossil fuel combustion and deforestation. As global temperatures rise, the health of vulnerable communities is disproportionately affected by extreme weather events, heatwaves, air pollution, and vector-borne diseases (Intergovernmental Panel on Climate Change [IPCC], 2021). Climate-induced changes in rainfall patterns and rising sea levels threaten food security and clean water access, increasing malnutrition and waterborne diseases, especially in low-income regions (Garbe et al., 2020). Moreover, extreme weather events such as floods, hurricanes, and droughts not only displace populations but also disrupt healthcare infrastructure, limiting access to essential services. Mental health is increasingly impacted with rising levels of anxiety, depression, and posttraumatic stress linked to climate-induced displacement and the uncertainty of future environmental conditions (Cissé et al., 2022). Mitigating the health impacts of climate change requires comprehensive strategies that include reducing greenhouse gas emissions, enhancing healthcare system resilience, and addressing health disparities through global cooperation (Watts et al., 2021).

INFECTIOUS DISEASES

Despite significant advances in medical sciences and public health, infectious diseases continue to pose grave threats to global health (Baker et al., 2022). Globalization and barriers to vaccinations have facilitated the spread of several infectious agents worldwide. Rapid mass travel and low vaccination rates promote the spread of infectious diseases from isolated areas, quickly becoming regional and global threats. Newly emerging strains of viruses, novel pathogens, low vaccination rates, and antibiotic resistance are among many challenges to the prevention and control of infectious diseases. Infectious diseases remain a devastating cause of preventable childhood mortality, particularly within low-income countries. Communicable infectious diseases also result in significant mortality among the immunocompromised, older adult population, and the unvaccinated. Preventing the spread of infectious diseases is of utmost importance to protecting vulnerable populations and ensuring the health of the global community. The Centers for Disease Control and Prevention (CDC) **Framework for Preventing Infectious Diseases** includes robust infectious disease surveillance, laboratory detection, epidemiologic investigation, high-impact interventions, and sound public health policies (CDC, 2011).

POPULATION AGING

By 2050, there will be an estimated 1.8 billion older adults in the world, which is more than three times the number of older adults in 2000. This change will mean that by 2050 one in six individuals will be 65 years old or older (UN Data Portal, n.d.). The demographic shift toward an older population has profound implications for healthcare, the economy, and social structures. Older populations have higher incidences of chronic diseases that require increased needs for social services, long-term care, and financial resources. These needs put additional pressure on already struggling global healthcare infrastructures, requiring significant investment in healthcare. Countries across the world will need to focus on reforming policies to protect older individuals such as funding palliative care, building senior centers, making urban environments age friendly, and preventing elder mistreatment (Multidisciplinary Digital Publishing Institute [MDPI], n.d.).

MENTAL HEALTH

Mental health disorders such as depression, anxiety, and schizophrenia are increasingly recognized as important aspects of global health, contributing to significant social and economic burdens, particularly in low- and middle-income countries. The World Health Organization (WHO) estimates that mental health disorders will result in economic losses of $16 trillion by 2030 as they are closely linked to reduced productivity, increased healthcare costs, and higher mortality rates. Sociocultural factors such as gender, caste, and socioeconomic status play a significant role in shaping mental health access and outcomes, highlighting the need for culturally responsive care models (Gupta & Coffey, 2020). Recent shifts from deficit-based approaches to a capability approach emphasize empowering individuals and communities to improve mental well-being, a framework that aligns with broader global health goals of fostering resilience and self-determination (Anand, 2021). This includes building mental health systems that incorporate local knowledge and traditions that will not only reduce the treatment gap, but also empower individuals to take control of their mental health.

FORCED MIGRATION

The number of forcibly displaced people has been significantly increasing over the past several decades, reaching 100 million for the first time in 2022. People who are forcibly displaced include several distinct categories such as refugees, internally displaced people, stateless people, and asylum seekers. Forcibly displaced people are in need of protection as they leave their homes largely due to persecution, war and conflict, human rights violation, instability, climate change, and natural disasters (United Nations High Commissioner for Refugees [UNHCR], 2024). The UNHCR promotes three solutions to protect refugees: voluntary repatriation, resettlement, and local integration. The global community, however, should act to mitigate the rapid rise in people who are forcibly displaced by addressing the underlying conditions of forced migration, which include human rights violations, political instability, war, socioeconomic inequities, and climate change.

CONCLUSION

On November 15, 2022, the world's population reached 8 billion. By 2100, the world's population is predicted to be greater than 10 billion (United Nations, n.d.). To protect the quality of life of our large and growing global population, the global community must be prepared to mitigate communicable diseases, find novel ways to promote mental health and the health of an aging population, slow down the rapid pace by which our world is warming while building climate change resilience, and address the underlying causes of forced migration while protecting the rights of those who are displaced. The following chapters describe climate change, infectious diseases, mental health, population aging, and forced migration in greater detail. It is imperative to understand what causes these issues, the populations most affected by these issues, and how we can mitigate their effects.

LEARNING ACTIVITIES

CourseConnect

To access self-assessment questions and interactive, competency-based learning activities for this chapter, visit www.springerpub.com/courseconnect. See inside front cover and tear-out for CourseConnect details.

REFERENCES

Anand, P. (2021). Wellbeing in public policy: Contributions based on Sen's capability approach. *LSE Public Policy Review, 2*(2), 2. https://doi.org/10.31389/lseppr.49

Baker, R. E., Mahmud, A. S., Miller, I. F., Rajeev, M., Rasambainarivo, F., Rice, B. L., Takahashi, S., Tatem, A. J., Wagner, C. E., Wang, L. F., Wesolowski, A., & Metcalf, C. J. E. (2022). Infectious disease in an era of global change. *Nature Reviews. Microbiology, 20*(4), 193–205. https://doi.org/10.1038/s41579-021-00639-z

Centers for Disease Control and Prevention. (2011). *A CDC framework for preventing infectious diseases: Sustaining the essentials and innovating for the future.* https://stacks.cdc.gov/view/cdc/11695

Cissé, G. R., McLeman, H., Adams, P., Aldunce, K., Bowen, D., Campbell-Lendrum, S., Clayton, K. L., Ebi, J., Hess, C., Huang, Q., Liu, G., McGregor, J., Semenza, & Tirado, M. C. (2022). Health, wellbeing, and the changing structure of communities. In H.-O. Pörtner, D.C. Roberts, M. Tignor, E.S. Poloczanska, K. Mintenbeck, A. Alegría, M. Craig, S. Langsdorf, S. Löschke, V. Möller, A. Okem, B. Rama (Eds.), *Climate change 2022: Impacts, adaptation and vulnerability. Contribution of Working Group II to the Sixth Assessment Report of the Intergovernmental Panel on Climate Change* (pp. 1041–1170). Cambridge University Press. https://doi.org/10.1017/9781009325844.009

Garbe, J., Albrecht, T., Levermann, A., Donges, J. F., & Winkelmann, R. (2020). The hysteresis of the Antarctic ice sheet. *Nature, 585*, 538–544. https://doi.org/10.1038/s41586-020-2727-5

Gupta, A., & Coffey, D. (2020). Caste, religion, and mental health in India. *Population Research and Policy Review, 39*(6), 1141. https://doi.org/10.1007/s11113-020-09585-9

Intergovernmental Panel on Climate Change. (2021). *Climate change 2021: The physical science basis.* https://www.ipcc.ch/report/ar6/wg1/

Multidisciplinary Digital Publishing Institute. (n.d.). *Population aging: An emerging research agenda for sustainable development.* https://www.mdpi.com/journal/socsci

United Nations. (n.d.). *Global issues: Population.* https://www.un.org/en/global-issues/population

UN Data Portal. (n.d.). *UN Population Division data portal.* https://population.un.org/dataportal/home/

United Nations High Commissioner for Refugees. (2024). *Refugee statistics.* https://www.unrefugees.org/refugee-facts/statistics/

Watts, N., Amann, M., Arnell, N., Ayeb-Karlsson, S., Belesova, K., & Berry, H. (2021). The 2021 report of *The Lancet* countdown on health and climate change: Code red for a healthy future. *The Lancet, 398*(10311), 1619–1662. https://doi.org/10.1016/S0140-6736(21)01787-6

CHAPTER 60

CLIMATE CHANGE

Pamela Mischen

THE CLIMATE IS CHANGING

Climate change refers to long-term shifts in temperature, precipitation patterns, and other climatic variables that occur over decades or longer periods. While the Earth's climate has changed over its 4.5 billion–year history, the climate change of concern now is **anthropogenic** (i.e., human-caused) climate change. The rapid climate change we are experiencing now is primarily driven by activities that release greenhouse gases (GHGs) such as carbon dioxide (CO_2), methane (CH_4), and nitrous oxide (N_2O) into the atmosphere. These gases trap heat from the sun, leading to a gradual increase in global temperatures, a phenomenon known as **global warming.**

The primary sources of GHG emissions include burning fossil fuels for energy, industrial processes, agriculture, forestry, land-use changes, transportation, and buildings. The impacts of climate change are wide ranging and can affect various aspects of the environment, ecosystems, and human societies. Some of the key impacts of climate change include rising temperatures, melting ice caps and glaciers, extreme weather events, disruption of ecosystems, agricultural and food insecurity, and increased morbidity and mortality.

The Intergovernmental Panel on Climate Change (IPCC) Sixth Assessment Report (AR6) provides a comprehensive overview of the current effects of climate change across various regions and sectors (IPCC, 2021). The report confirms that the Earth's climate is warming rapidly, with each of the past four decades being successively warmer than any preceding decade since 1850. Global surface temperature was approximately 1.09°C higher during 2011 to 2020 when compared with during 1850 to 1900. Global mean sea level increased by 0.2 meters (8 inches) between 1901 and 2018. Additionally, the AR6 states that it is "virtually certain" that the ocean temperature has risen since the 1970s, the Greenland ice sheet has lost mass since the 1990s, and there has been acidification of the global surface ocean. Other changes deemed "very likely" are Arctic Sea ice loss since 1979, Antarctic Ice Sheet mass loss since the 1990s, reduction in Northern Hemisphere springtime snow cover since 1950, and the retreat of glaciers. Nearly all regions of the world have seen an increase in hot extremes, the majority of the regions in the Northern Hemisphere have seen an increase in heavy precipitation events, and regions in North and South America, Europe, Asia, Africa, and Australia have seen increases in agricultural and ecological drought (Figure 60.1).

Current projections indicate that we could pass 2 degrees of warming over preindustrial levels as early as mid-century with 3 degrees of warming by 2100. At 2 degrees, there is a very high probability of having an ice-free Arctic in the summer (Neiderdrenk & Notz, 2018), which is bad for climate systems around the globe. Losing Arctic sea ice could shift the jet stream, leading to more climate variability (Stendel et al., 2021). At the other pole, 2 degrees of warming puts the West Antarctic Ice Sheet in jeopardy (Garbe et al., 2020). Losing this ice sheet would result in a 5-meter (almost 16.5-foot) rise in sea levels. Away from the poles, the warming will reduce water availability for 129 million people in South Asia who are substantially dependent on seasonal meltwater from glaciers (Biemans et al., 2019).

In addition to these impacts on the cryosphere (frozen parts of the earth), 2 degrees of warming will result in an increase in heat waves. It is expected that Europe will experience summers as hot

FIGURE 60.1 Observed change in hot extremes, heavy precipitation, and drought.

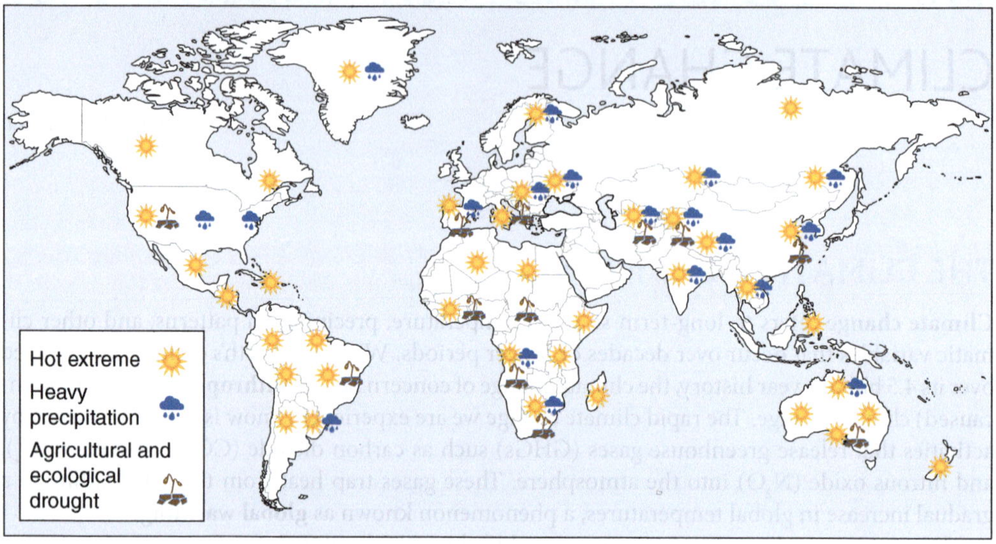

Source: Adapted from Intergovernmental Panel on Climate Change. (2023). *Sixth assessment report (AR6)*. https://www.ipcc.ch/report/ar6/syr/downloads/report/IPCC_AR6_SYR_LongerReport.pdf

as in 2003, which caused tens of thousands of excess deaths, at least once every 2 years (King & Karoly, 2017).

A warmer atmosphere causes more evaporation. Therefore, there will be an increase in global precipitation. However, this precipitation will not fall evenly upon the Earth. It is expected that in East Asia and Northern India there will be an increase in monsoon intensity as global warming increases from 1.5 to 2 degrees (Mondal et al., 2022). Furthermore, nearly 123% more people will experience extreme precipitation events in the Indus River Valley (Zhao et al., 2021). While South Asia is likely to see an increase in precipitation, eastern and southern Africa is likely to see a decrease. Increasing aridity is likely to extend droughts from an average of 2.9 months to 3.2 months, resulting in 410 million more people exposed to drought conditions (Liu et al., 2018). Frighteningly, the Amazon region could experience the greatest reduction in precipitation, putting at risk this biodiverse and carbon-rich area of the world (Lehner et al., 2017).

At 3 degrees of warming, all of these effects intensify. Three degrees of warming is hotter than any time in the last 3 million years—that is, in all of human history. The collapse of the West Antarctic Ice Sheet is a virtual certainty under 3 degrees of warming (DeConto et al., 2021). Furthermore, Greenland could see a 25% to 50% reduction in ice, resulting in another 2- to 4-meter rise in sea levels (Noël et al., 2021). The melting will not happen all at once; it could take hundreds of years. However, once the process starts, it is irreversible. While sea level rise does not happen all at once, it is also not a linear and gradual increase. High tides and storm surges could push seawater inland rapidly. With an increasing intensity of tropical storms, New York City is likely to experience the equivalent of Superstorm Sandy (a large and extremely damaging tropical cyclone that hit New York City as a Category 1 hurricane in October 2012) twice per year by the end of the century (Rasmussen et al., 2018).

Changes in precipitation will likely result in a 187% increase in land burned by wildfire in Mediterranean Europe (Turco, 2018). The Mediterranean region will also see a decrease in streamflow by about 35% (Marx et al., 2018). Heat will make daytime agricultural activity difficult in much of the world. It is estimated that in sub-Saharan Africa and Southeast Asia, 3 degrees of warming could reduce labor capacity in agriculture by 30% to 50% (de Lima et al., 2021). Small landholders who do not have air-conditioned tractors are likely to suffer the most. Food crops are also impacted by heat. It is anticipated that with 3 degrees of warming, global corn and soybean yields could be reduced by one half to two thirds and rice and wheat yields by one quarter to one third just as the global population is peaking at 10 to 11 billion people (IPCC, 2021).

In a 3-degree world, the dieback of the Amazon is much more likely. **Dieback** (progressive death of roots, trees, crops, and woody plants), along with a significant thawing of permafrost, could release even more GHGs into the atmosphere in the form of both CO_2 and the more problematic methane. Methane is more than 20 times better at trapping heat in the atmosphere than CO_2. These ecological changes could result in a **positive feedback loop** (a process in which an initial disturbance creates a chain of events that increase in intensity and exacerbate instability) that pushes the Earth past 3 degrees of warming to a near-apocalyptic 4 degrees (Lynas, 2020).

HUMAN IMPACT ON CLIMATE CHANGE

The science has moved beyond speculation regarding the primary cause of climate change. It is scientific fact that human contribution is the central cause. With that, what countries are the most responsible? Three ways to determine which countries are "most responsible" for climate change are to consider total historical emissions, annual current emissions, and annual per-capita emissions (Table 60.1). Some countries, particularly industrialized nations with long histories of fossil fuel consumption and industrialization, have significantly higher cumulative emissions of GHGs. Historically, countries such as the United States, European nations, and countries with large industrial sectors like China have contributed the most to cumulative emissions. A second way is to consider current emissions. Countries with high levels of current emissions of GHGs are also significant contributors to climate change. China has recently overtaken the United States as the largest emitter of GHGs, followed by India and Russia. These countries have large populations,

TABLE 60.1 SELECT ANNUAL, CUMULATIVE, AND PER-CAPITA EMISSIONS

COUNTRY	ANNUAL TOTAL GHG EMISSIONS (MILLION METRIC TONS)	CUMULATIVE CO_2 EMISSIONS (MILLION METRIC TONS)	PER CAPITA GHG EMISSIONS (METRIC TONS)
China	13,944	260,619	9.8
United States	6,002	426,919	17.7
India	4,047	59,740	2.9
Russia	2,290	119,291	15.8
Brazil	2,248	17,177	10.4
Indonesia	2,127	15,712	7.7
Japan	1,094	67,734	8.8
Mexico	953	21,119	7.5
Iran	935	19,853	10.6
Saudi Arabia	811	17,596	22.3
Canada	782	34,613	20.3
Germany	739	93,986	8.9
South Korea	646	19,529	12.5
Vietnam	619	5,023	6.3

CO_2, carbon dioxide; GHG, greenhouse gas.

Source: Adapted from Our World in Data. (n.d.). *CO_2 and greenhouse gas emissions*. https://ourworldindata.org/co2-and-greenhouse-gas-emissions

robust economies, and high levels of industrial activity, transportation, and energy consumption. However, these numbers mask the impact of population and wealth. Although China emits more GHGs than the United States as a whole, the United States and other wealthy nations have much higher per-capita emissions—17.7 versus 9.8 metric tons per person—and India, although coming in third in current annual GHG emissions has a per-capita emissions rate of only 2.9 metric tons per person.

CLIMATE CHANGE IMPACTS THE VULNERABLE

Importantly, those who are most vulnerable to climate change are those who have contributed the least to it. People living in poverty, including those in informal settlements, rural areas, and Indigenous communities, often lack access to adequate housing, healthcare, clean water, and sanitation. They are disproportionately affected by climate change impacts such as extreme weather events, food insecurity, water scarcity, and displacement (Hallegatte et al., 2020). Children and older adults are more susceptible to the health effects of climate change, including heat-related illnesses, respiratory problems from air pollution, and malnutrition (Ebi et al., 2021; Halldén et al., 2021). They may also face increased risks of injury, displacement, and mental health issues associated with extreme weather events and environmental degradation.

In addition to children, older adults, and those living in poverty, several populations are particularly vulnerable to the impacts of climate change. Women and girls often bear a disproportionate burden of climate change impacts due to gender inequalities and social norms. They may face increased risks of poverty, food insecurity, and water scarcity, as well as greater challenges in accessing healthcare, education, and economic opportunities. Women are also more likely to be affected by gender-based violence and displacement during climate-related disasters (Thurston et al., 2021). People with disabilities may face additional barriers and challenges in adapting to climate change impacts, including limited mobility, communication difficulties, and access to information, services, and support networks (Marshall et al., 2020). They may also be at greater risk of injury, displacement, and social exclusion during climate-related disasters. Climate change can exacerbate existing drivers of migration and displacement, such as environmental degradation, natural disasters, and conflict. Migrant and displaced populations are often more vulnerable to the impacts of climate change due to limited access to resources, social networks, and legal protections (Mazhin et al., 2020). They may also face discrimination, exploitation, and marginalization in host communities. People living in coastal areas and small island states are particularly vulnerable to sea-level rise, storm surges, coastal erosion, and saltwater intrusion. These communities face risks to infrastructure, livelihoods, food security, and cultural heritage, as well as increased exposure to climate-related disasters such as hurricanes, floods, and tsunamis. Farmers, pastoralists, and rural communities are highly dependent on climate-sensitive sectors such as agriculture, forestry, and fisheries for their livelihoods and food security. Climate change impacts such as changes in temperature, precipitation, and extreme weather events can disrupt agricultural production, reduce crop yields, and exacerbate food insecurity in rural areas.

CLIMATE CHANGE ADAPTATION

It is critical that the world takes steps to adapt to climate change. Regardless of what we do now to cut emissions, we have committed the world to a certain level of climate change. Adaptation involves implementing strategies and actions to reduce the vulnerability of human and natural systems to the impacts of climate change, build resilience, and cope with its effects. Current and future climate risks and vulnerabilities must be identified and assessed. Effective adaptation requires the involvement of diverse stakeholders, including government agencies, local communities, civil society organizations, businesses, academia, and Indigenous peoples. Enhancing the adaptive capacity of individuals, communities, institutions, and ecosystems is essential for coping with the impacts of climate change. Nature-based solutions, such as ecosystem restoration, conservation, and sustainable land management, can enhance resilience to climate change impacts and provide multiple cobenefits for people and nature (Seddon et al., 2020). Climate-resilient infrastructure and buildings are essential for reducing vulnerability to climate-change impacts such as flooding, storms, heatwaves, and sea-level rise, as is water management to accommodate changing precipitation patterns, droughts, floods, and water scarcity. Strengthening disaster risk reduction and early warning systems reduces the impacts of climate-related disasters such as hurricanes, floods, droughts, and wildfires. To adapt to the health impacts of climate change, healthcare systems, disease surveillance and monitoring, public health preparedness and response, and measures to protect vulnerable populations from heatwaves, air pollution, vector-borne diseases, and other climate-related health risks must be enhanced. Diversifying livelihoods, promoting sustainable livelihood options, and providing social protection measures can help reduce vulnerability to climate-change impacts, particularly among rural and marginalized populations. This includes supporting alternative income-generating activities, promoting climate-smart agriculture, and implementing social safety nets and insurance schemes. Finally, climate change adaptation must be incorporated into national and local policies, plans, and strategies.

Climate Change Mitigation

Although climate change is already occurring and we need to learn to adapt to it, climate change's ultimate severity is still within our control. Climate change mitigation must therefore be a top priority for individuals, communities, and nations. First and foremost, we must reduce GHG emissions. This includes transitioning to renewable energy sources such as solar, wind, and hydroelectric power, increasing energy efficiency, phasing out fossil fuel subsidies, and implementing policies to limit emissions from industries, transportation, agriculture, and buildings. We must also protect forests, wetlands, and other natural ecosystems to sequester CO_2 from the atmosphere and preserve biodiversity. Sustainable land management practices, such as reforestation, afforestation, agroforestry, and sustainable agriculture, can enhance **carbon sinks** (which are anything that absorbs more carbon from the atmosphere than it releases; e.g., plants, the ocean, soil) and reduce emissions from land-use change and deforestation. Improving energy efficiency in buildings, industries, transportation, and appliances can reduce energy consumption and associated emissions. This includes adopting energy-efficient technologies, building codes, and vehicle standards, as well as promoting public transportation, biking, and walking.

Providing financial resources, technology transfer, and capacity-building support to developing countries is crucial to enable them to mitigate and adapt to climate change effectively. Addressing climate change requires collective action and cooperation among countries, regions, cities, businesses, civil society organizations, and individuals. International agreements such as the Paris Agreement (a legally binding international treaty on climate change adopted in 2015 at the United Nations' Climate Change Conference in Paris, France) provide a framework for countries to work together to limit global warming and adapt to its impacts.

Finally, climate action must be guided by principles of equity, justice, and inclusivity to ensure that vulnerable communities, marginalized groups, and future generations are not disproportionately affected by climate change. This includes addressing social and economic inequalities, ensuring access to climate information and resources, and engaging diverse stakeholders in decision-making processes.

CLIMATE CHANGE AND PUBLIC HEALTH

In 2003, more than 70,000 excess deaths were recorded in Europe, the hottest summer on record (Robine et al., 2008). That was until the temperature record was broken in 2019, and again in 2022. The 2022 European heat wave resulted in 61,672 excess deaths (Ballester et al., 2023). In May 2016, a record high was set in Ragathan, India, of 51°C (123.8°F), possibly the third-highest temperature ever recorded globally (World Weather Attribution, 2016).

Additionally, the IPCC has indicated that there is high or very high confidence in the following statements (Cissé et al., 2022):

- There will be an increase in communicable diseases, particularly those that are vector borne such as malaria, dengue fever, chikungunya, Zika, Japanese encephalitis, and Rift Valley fever.
- Heavy rainfall and higher than normal temperatures will result in an increase in cholera and other gastrointestinal diseases.
- Longer summer seasons with high air and water temperatures will result in food-borne diseases.
- There will be a detrimental impact on mental health.
- There will be an increase in malnutrition, particularly in low- and middle-income countries.

The health impacts of climate change will not be borne equitably and will vary by region. For instance, heat and dangerous wet-bulb temperatures (the combination of temperature and humidity at which the human body cannot cool itself and results in death in a matter of hours) will be most likely in the Persian Gulf, the Indus River Valley, eastern coastal India, Pakistan, northwest India, the shores of the Red Sea, the Gulf of California, and coastal Venezuela and Guyana. Tropical cyclones will likely result in displacement in east and southeast Asia, the Caribbean, the Bay of Bengal, and southeast Africa.

Climate change and natural disasters will effect the ability of governments to continue to fund health and wellness initiatives. *Reuters News & Media* reports that climate change could cost $38 trillion per year by 2050 due to impacts on farming, infrastructure, productivity, and health (Alkousaa, 2024). With such outlays, government budgets will be strained, especially in developing nations where help will be needed most.

CONCLUSION

Climate change is happening now and will intensify before it ameliorates. How much worse climate change becomes depends on the actions of governments, communities, and individuals. Time is of the essence, and technology innovations are necessary. Climate change will impact health directly through heat, tropical storms, wildfires, and changing precipitation patterns. It will impact health indirectly through food insecurity, limited funding for public health, and migration. There is no place on Earth that will be totally immune to the direct and/or indirect impacts of climate change; however, some people and places will fare worse than others. Action must be taken now to mitigate and adapt to the changing climate.

LEARNING ACTIVITIES

CourseConnect

To access self-assessment questions and interactive, competency-based learning activities for this chapter, visit www.springerpub.com/courseconnect. See inside front cover and tear-out for CourseConnect details.

REFERENCES

Alkousaa, R. (2024). *Climate change damage could cost $38 trillion per year by 2050, study finds*. Reuters. https://www.reuters.com/business/environment/climate-change-damage-could-cost-38-trillion-per-year-by-2050-study-finds-2024-04-17/

Ballester, J., Quijal-Zamorano, M., Méndez Turrubiates, R. F., Pegenaute, F., Herrmann, F. R., Robine, J. M., Basagaña, X., Tonne, C., Antó, J. M., & Achebak, H. (2023). Heat-related mortality in Europe during the summer of 2022. *Nature Medicine*, 29, 1857–1866. https://doi.org/10.1038/s41591-023-02419-z

Biemans, H., Siderius, C., Lutz, A.F., Nepal, S., Ahmad, B., Hassan, T., von Bloh, W., Wijngaard, R. R., Wester, P., Shrestha, A. B., & Immerzeel, W. W. (2019). Importance of snow and glacier meltwater for agriculture on the Indo-Gangetic Plain. *Nature Sustainability, 2*(7), 594–601. https://doi.org/10.1038/s41893-019-0305-3

Cissé, G., McLeman, R., Adams, H., Aldunce, P., Bowen, K., Campbell-Lendrum, D., Clayton, S., Ebi, K. L., Hess, J., Huang, C., Liu, Q., McGregor, G., Semenza, J., & Tirado, M. C. (2022). Health, wellbeing, and the changing structure of communities. In H.-O. Pörtner, D. C. Roberts, M. Tignor, E. S. Poloczanska, K. Mintenbeck, A. Alegría, M. Craig, S. Langsdorf, S. Löschke, V. Möller, A. Okem, B. Rama (Eds.), *Climate change 2022: Impacts, adaptation and vulnerability, the Working Group II contribution to the Sixth Assessment Report of the Intergovernmental Panel on Climate Change* (pp. 1041–1170). Cambridge University Press. https://doi.org/10.1017/9781009325844.009.

DeConto, R. M., Pollard, D., Alley, R. B., Velicogna, I., Gasson, E., Gomez, N., Sadai, S., Condron, A., Gilford, D. M., Erica L Ashe, E. L., Kopp, R. E., Li, D., & Andrea Dutton, A. (2021). The Paris Climate Agreement and future sea-level rise from Antarctica. *Nature, 593*, 83–89. https://doi.org/10.1038/s41586-021-03427-0

de Lima, C. Z., Buzan, J. R., Moore, F. C., Baldos, U. L., Huber, M., & Hertel, T. W. (2021). Heat stress on agricultural workers exacerbates crop impacts of climate change. *Environmental Research Letters, 16*(4), 044020. http://doi.org/10.1088/1748-9326/abeb9f

Ebi, K. L., Vanos, J., Baldwin, J. W., Bell, J. E., Hondula, D. M., Errett, N. A., Hayes, K., Reid, C. E., Saha, S., Spector, J., & Berry, P. (2021). Extreme weather and climate change: Populations health and health system implications. *Annual Review of Public Health, 42*, 293–315. https://doi.org/10.1146/annurev-publhealth-012420-105026

Garbe, J., Albrecht, T., Levermann, A., Donges, J. F., & Winkelmann, R. (2020). The hysteresis of the Antarctic Ice Sheet. *Nature, 585*, 538–544. https://doi.org/10.1038/s41586-020-2727-5

Halldén, D. H., Andersson, C, Nilsson, M., Ebi, K. L., Friberg, P., & Alfvén, T. (2021). Climate change and child health: A scoping review and expanded conceptual framework. *The Lancet Planetary Health, 5*(3), e164–e175. https://doi.org/10.1016/S2542-5196(20)30274-6

Hallegatte, S., Vogt-Schilb, A., Rozenberg, J., Bangalore, M., & Beaudet, C. (2020). From poverty to disaster and back: A review of the literature. *Economics of Disasters and Climate Change, 4*, 223–247. https://doi.org/10.1007/s41885-020-00060-5

Intergovernmental Panel on Climate Change. (2021). *Climate change 2021: The physical science basis. The Working Group I contribution to the sixth assessment report of the Intergovernmental Panel on Climate Change*. Cambridge University Press. https://doi.org/10.1017/9781009157896

King, A., & Karoly, D. J. (2017). Climate extremes in Europe at 1.5 and 2 degrees of global warming. *Environment Research Letter, 12*(11), 114031. http://doi.org/10.1088/1748-9326/aa8e2c

Lehner, F., Coats, S., Stocker, T. F., Pendergrass, A. G., Sanderson, B. M., Raible, C. C., & Smerdon, J. E. (2017). Projected drought risk in 1.5°C and 2°C warmer climates. *Geophysical Research Letters, 44*, 7419–7428. https://doi.org/10.1002/2017GL074117

Liu, W., Sun, F., Lim, W. H., Zhang, J., Wang, H., Shiogama, H., & Zhang, Y. (2018). Global drought and severe drought-affected populations in 1.5° and 2°C warmer worlds. *Earth System Dynamics, 9*(1), 267–283. https://doi.org/10.5194/esd-9-267-2018

Lynas, M. (2020). *Our final warning: Six degrees of climate emergency*. 4th Estate.

Marshall, J., Wiltshire, J., Delva, J., Bello, T., & Masys, A. J. (2020). Natural and manmade disasters: Vulnerable populations. In A. J. Masys, R. Izurieta, & M. R. Ortiz (Eds.), *Global health security. Advanced sciences and technologies for security applications*. Springer. https://doi.org/10.1007/978-3-030-23491-1_7

Marx, A., Kumar, R., Thober, S., Rakovec, O., Wanders, N., Zink, M., Wood, E. F., Pan, M., Sheffield, J., & Samaniego, L. (2018). Climate change alters low flows in Europe under global warming of 1.5, 2 and 3°C. *Hydrology and Earth System Sciences, 22*(2), 1017–1032. https://doi.org/10.5194/hess-22-1017-2018

Mazhin, S.A., Hamidreza, K., Mehrdad, F., Mohsen, A., & Mohsen, P. (2020). Migration health crisis associated with climate change: A systematic review. *Journal of Education and Health Promotion, 9*(1), 97. https://doi.org/10.4103/jehp.jehp_4_20

Mondal, M., Huang, J., Wang, Y., Su, B., Kundzewicz, Z. W., Jiang, S., Zhai, J., Chen, Z., Jing, C., & Jiang, T. (2022). Change in extreme precipitation across South Asia for each 0.5˚C of warming from 1.5˚C to 3.0˚C above pre-industrial levels. *Atmospheric Research, 266*, 105961. https://doi.org/10.1016/j.atmosres.2021.105961

Niederdrenk, A. L., & Notz, D. (2018). Arctic sea ice in a 1.5°C warmer world. *Geophysical Research Letters, 45*, 1963–1971. https://doi.org/10.1002/2017GL076159

Noël, B., van Kampenhout, L., Lenaerts, J. T. M., van de Berg, W. J., & van den Broeke, M. R. (2021). A 21st century warming threshold for sustained Greenland ice sheet mass loss. *Geophysical Research Letters, 48*, e2020GL090471. https://doi.org/10.1029/

Rasmussen, D. J., Bittermann, K., Buchanan, M. K., Kulp, S., Strauss, B. H., Kopp, R. E., & Oppenheimer, M. (2018). Extreme sea level implications of 1.5°C, 2.0°C, and 2.5°C temperature stabilization targets in the 21st and 22nd centuries. *Environmental Research Letters, 13*(3), 034040. https://doi.org/10.1088/1748-9326/aaac87

Robine, J. M., Cheung, S. L., Le Roy, S., Van Oyen, H., Griffiths, C., Michel, J. P., & Herrmann, F. R. (2008). Death toll exceeded 70,000 in Europe during the summer of 2003. *Comptes Rendus Biologies, 331*(2), 171–178. https://doi.org/10.1016/j.crvi.2007.12.001

Seddon, N., Smith, A., Smith, P., Key, I., Chausson, A., Girardin, C., House, J., Srivastava, S., & Turner, B. (2020). Getting the message right on nature-based solutions to climate change. *Global Change Biology, 27*(8), 1518–1546. https://doi.org/10.1111/gcb.15513

Stendel, M., Francis, J., White, R., Williams, P. D., & Woolings, T. (2021). The jet stream and climate change. In T. M. Letcher (Ed.), *Climate change* (3rd ed., pp. 327–357). Elsevier.

Thurston, A. M., Stöckl, H., & Ranganathan, M. (2021). Natural hazards, disasters and violence against women and girls: A global mixed-methods systematic review. *BMJ Global Health, 6*, e004377. https://doi.org/10.1136/bmjgh-2020-004377

Turco, M., Rosa-Cánovas, J. J., Bedia, J., Jerez, S., Montávez, J. P., Llasat, M. C., & Provenzale, A. (2018). Exacerbated fires in Mediterranean Europe due to anthropogenic warming projected with non-stationary climate-fire models. *Nature Communications, 9*, 3821. https://doi.org/10.1038/s41467-018-06358-z

World Weather Attribution. (2016). *Record high temperatures in India, 2016*. https://www.worldweatherattribution.org/india-heat-wave-2016/

Zhao, J.-T., Su, B.-D., Mondal, S. K., Wang, Y.-J., Tao, H., & Jiang, T. (2021). Population exposure to precipitation extremes in the Indus River Basin at 1.5°C, 2.0°C and 3.0°C warming levels. *Advances in Climate Change Research, 12*(2), 199–209. https://doi.org/10.1016/j.accre.2021.03.005

CHAPTER 61

COMMUNICABLE DISEASES

Keri A. Mastro Dwyer and Wesley D. Kufel

INTRODUCTION

Infectious diseases are illnesses caused by pathogens such as bacteria, viruses, fungi, and parasites (Cleveland Clinic, 2025; Suffoletto, 2024; Table 61.1). Transmission of pathogens to a susceptible host may occur from an infected person, an infected vector, or a contaminated object/reservoir (Tulchinsky & Varavikova, 2014; van Seventer & Hochberg, 2017). Communicable diseases are infectious diseases that are considered to be contagious or capable of being transmitted from one individual, or species, to another (Pennsylvania Department of Health, n.d.; Suffoletto, 2024). When the rapid transmission of a pathogen occurs within a population, it is considered to be an **epidemic** (Antia & Halloran, 2021). If the communicable disease spreads worldwide, it is then referred to as a pandemic. Compared to an epidemic or a pandemic, the **endemic** state refers to the prevalence of a pathogen being considered maintained or stable, typically at a lower prevalence.

IMPLICATIONS OF COMMUNICABLE DISEASES: MODERN-WORLD THREATS DESPITE HISTORICAL PROGRESS

As evidenced by the coronavirus disease 2019 (COVID-19) pandemic caused by the severe acute respiratory syndrome (SARS)-CoV-2 strain, infectious diseases pose a modern challenge in the 21st century, despite significant advances in medical sciences and innovations in public health (Tulchinsky & Varavikova, 2014). For example, influenza pandemics also remain a modern worldwide challenge, with new virus strains continuing to emerge.

Despite these ongoing concerns, historical progress of addressing various communicable diseases exemplifies adaptation to and mitigation of these ever-evolving threats. The eradication of smallpox occurred in 1977. Although the World Health Assembly has declared polio a candidate for eradication, significant challenges remain to reach this goal (Centers for Disease Control and Prevention [CDC], 2024; Tulchinsky & Varavikova, 2014). Factors such as ongoing conflicts and competing health priorities serve as barriers to achieving vaccination of all children in countries with wild poliovirus, such as Afghanistan and Pakistan (CDC, 2024). In some other countries, poliovirus variants present an additional concern. Variant outbreaks present a threat when there are insufficient childhood vaccination rates against polio. Similarly, although measles-associated mortality has significantly decreased, outbreaks occur where immunization lags or vaccination hesitancy exists (Tulchinsky & Varavikova, 2014).

Examples of other infectious diseases that continue to raise particular concern are HIV, tuberculosis, malaria, dengue, and infections caused by antibiotic-resistant pathogens (superbugs). HIV emerged in the 1980s and rose to a global pandemic, leading to millions of lives lost. Despite immense advancements in medicine and pharmaceuticals, HIV remains a major global health issue. Malaria and tuberculosis continue to be significant global causes of morbidity and mortality, particularly in developing countries, due to their high prevalence and significant geographic overlap between endemic regions (Bijker et al, 2023). There is grave concern regarding the global spread of dengue fever due to climate change and subsequent mosquito growth in warmer and wetter environments (CDC, 2024). Antibiotic-resistant infections are considered a substantial public health threat to modern global populations (Tulchinsky & Varavikova, 2014). Although

TABLE 61.1 INFECTIOUS DISEASES BASED ON ETIOLOGIC PATHOGEN

Examples of viral infections	Examples of fungal infections
• COVID-19 • Influenza • Respiratory syncytial virus • Rotavirus and norovirus gastroenteritis • Viral hepatitis (e.g., A, B, C, D, E) • Herpes simplex virus • Poliomyelitis • Human immunodeficiency virus • Smallpox (*eradicated*)	• Candidiasis • Ringworm • Fungal nail infections • Mold infections
Examples of bacterial infections	**Examples of parasitic infections**
• Strep throat • Pneumonia • Tuberculosis • Sexually transmitted infections • *Clostridioides difficile* • Urinary tract infections • Skin and soft tissue infections • Osteomyelitis • Lyme disease	• Malaria • Toxoplasmosis • Giardiasis • Pinworms/hookworms

Source: Adapted from Cleveland Clinic. (2025). *Infectious diseases*. https://my.clevelandclinic.org/health/diseases/17724-infectious-diseases

various medicinal advancements, including the continued development of antibiotics and vaccinations, have allowed for a reduction in the burden of communicable diseases, factors such as the overuse or inappropriate overprescribing of antibiotics contribute to antibiotic-resistant infections (Cleveland Clinic, 2025). **Antibiotic resistance** occurs when bacteria develop mutations, thereby making established antibiotics less or no longer effective. Antibiotic-resistant infections are challenging to treat and are more commonly life-threatening. There have been increased, widespread efforts toward **antimicrobial stewardship**, which involves initiatives to advocate for the optimal use of antibiotics. Antimicrobial stewardship programs assist with counteracting the emergence of potential antibiotic-resistant infections.

IMPACT OF GLOBALIZATION: SPREAD OF COMMUNICABLE DISEASES AND MITIGATION FACTORS

Globalization has facilitated the spread of several infectious agents worldwide. Rapid mass travel promotes the spread of infectious diseases from isolated areas, quickly becoming worldwide threats. Newly emerging strains of viruses, novel pathogens causing chronic diseases, and antibiotic resistance are among many challenges for infection control, requiring ongoing political, financial, and scientific support. Sanitation, food safety control, and vaccines are all examples of preventive measures that have decreased the burden of communicable diseases (Box 61.1), in addition to treatment measures such as antimicrobials. However, the dynamic nature of infectious diseases poses ever-present challenges.

VULNERABLE POPULATIONS: DISPROPORTIONATE IMPACT OF COMMUNICABLE DISEASES

Communicable diseases pose significant morbidity and mortality threats to current populations across the globe (Tulchinsky & Varavikova, 2014). The impact of these diseases is most

BOX 61.1 Preventive Measures: Communicable Diseases

Preventive measures to mitigate the spread of communicable diseases:

- vaccinations
- safe food handling/ingestion
- handwashing
- covering the nasal/oral regions when sneezing or coughing
- safe sex practices
- social/physical distancing
- avoidance of contact with/ingestion of potentially contaminated water
- use of approved repellents to avoid ticks and other bugs
- disinfection of surfaces

Source: Adapted from Cleveland Clinic. (2025). *Infectious diseases*. https://my.clevelandclinic.org/health/diseases/17724-infectious-diseases

detrimental to developing, lower-income countries. Examples of impacts include hindered economic growth and reduced survival rates, especially with regard to the pediatric population. Middle- and high-income industrialized countries also face severe challenges, including significant health and economic concerns.

Communicable infectious diseases remain a devastating cause of childhood mortality, particularly within developing countries across the globe. These infectious diseases also have a significant impact on patients who are immunocompromised or immunosuppressed due to taking immunosuppressive medications or having immunosuppressive conditions (Cleveland Clinic, 2025; Tulchinsky & Varavikova, 2014). Other particularly vulnerable populations for communicable diseases include the geriatric population, individuals traveling to geographic areas that increase exposure to pathogens that are foreign to their homeland, and those who are unvaccinated against common infectious diseases (Cleveland Clinic, 2025). Infectious diseases disproportionately affect these vulnerable populations, posing a significant global burden and impacting public health systems, as well as economies, worldwide (van Seventer & Hochberg, 2017).

MONITORING SYSTEMS: SYSTEMATIC APPROACHES TO THE PREVENTION OF AND RESPONSE TO OUTBREAKS OF COMMUNICABLE DISEASES

"A changing world requires changing science to evaluate future risks from infectious disease" (Baker et al., 2022, p. 203). The CDC, the national public health agency of the United States, established *A CDC Framework for Preventing Infectious Diseases; Sustaining the Essentials and Innovating for the Future* (https://stacks.cdc.gov/view/cdc/11695). This framework offers guidance for improving the ability to prevent known infectious diseases, as well as the recognition and mitigation of emergent threats, through an adaptable U.S. public health system (CDC, 2011; Tulchinsky & Varavikova, 2014). It includes important components in these efforts: strong public health fundamentals, such as infectious disease surveillance, laboratory detection, epidemiologic investigation, high-impact interventions, and sound health policies (CDC, 2011).

Innovative technological advancements are critical for implementation, particularly in the areas of surveillance and data collection (Baker et al., 2022). Innovative uses of surveillance include using serology strategies or various surveillance platforms, including genomic surveillance platforms, to better understand pathogen spread.

Serologic surveys detect the presence of **antibodies**, which are produced following the presence of an **antigen**, a foreign substance that elicits the immune response. The detection of exposure to multiple pathogens is now possible, due to recent advancements. Serologic surveys have been used during the COVID-19 pandemic to track population exposure, although performance characteristics of these surveys may vary based on multiple factors.

Genomic surveillance systems offer the ability to track and characterize the emergence of new, unique pathogenic variants and were used during the COVID-19 pandemic. The data retrieved from these surveillance systems contributed to the rapid development of vaccines and diagnostics. While there are efforts in place to establish national and international genomic surveillance networks, various barriers, such as resource limitations, have limited the global expansion of these systems.

Innovative techniques such as the use of artificial intelligence (AI) and machine learning are gaining attention and have been considered tools for assessing answers to public health questions. Although using such tools to perform predictions across areas such as viral emergence poses incredible benefit potential, these uses have limitations and drawbacks such as microbiological complexities and high expense (Holmes, 2013). Machine learning may be used to leverage unique, high-volume data streams for information related to learning about population-level drivers of disease transmission (Baker et al., 2022). However, given ever-changing demographic, technological, and environmental factors, more traditional models may be more feasible for use in predicting future outcomes. Future work is warranted in aiming to optimize the integration of AI and machine learning approaches in order to rapidly and accurately assess the public health landscape, as well as anticipate prospective challenges.

IMPORTANCE OF ADVOCACY AND INVESTMENT IN GLOBAL HEALTH EFFORTS

Newly emerging infectious disease threats, as well as new variants of diseases with resistance to current therapeutics, pose immense challenges to 21st-century public health. The need for coordination between public health organizations and health systems, in addition to informed engagement from policymakers, is critical to the employment of innovative strategies to advance public health initiatives. Multidisciplinary clinical teams of providers, particularly those who are specialized in infectious diseases, work in interprofessional collaboration with other clinicians to establish and implement evidence-based medicine in order to prevent, treat, and mitigate the spread of communicable diseases. Policy decisions that support evidence-based practices are important for protecting patients, healthcare providers, and communities (Infectious Disease Society of America [IDSA], n.d.).

Investment in areas of global infectious disease response and research is also vital to the ongoing advancement of public health betterment. For example, the IDSA is a trusted leader in advancing international and national policies, as well as facilitating investments in global health security.

CONCLUSION

Infectious diseases result in significant morbidity and mortality throughout the world. Preventing the spread of infectious diseases is of the utmost importance to public health. The vast diversity of microbes, combined with their ability to evolve in settings of changing populations, environments, practices, and technologies, creates ongoing threats to global public health (Tulchinsky & Varavikova, 2014). Prevention strategies and vigilance with ongoing healthcare advancements and modernized surveillance systems are of critical importance to the health and well-being of populations across the world.

LEARNING ACTIVITIES

CourseConnect

To access self-assessment questions and interactive, competency-based learning activities for this chapter, visit www.springerpub.com/courseconnect. See inside front cover and tear-out for CourseConnect details.

REFERENCES

Antia, R., & Halloran, M. E. (2021). Transition to endemicity: Understanding COVID-19. *Immunity, 54*(10), 2172–2176. https://doi.org/10.1016/j.immuni.2021.09.019

Baker, R. E., Mahmud, A. S., Miller, I. F., Rajeev, M., Rasambainarivo, F., Rice, B. L., Takahashi, S., Tatem, A. J., Wagner, C. E., Wang, L. F., Wesolowski, A., & Metcalf, C. J. E. (2022). Infectious disease in an era of global change. *Nature Reviews. Microbiology, 20*(4), 193–205. https://doi.org/10.1038/s41579-021-00639-z

Bijker, E. M., Deshpande, S., Salgame, P., & Song, R. (2023). Malaria and tuberculosis co-infection—A review. *Oxford Open Immunology, 4*(1), iqad008. https://doi.org/10.1093/oxfimm/iqad008

Centers for Disease Control and Prevention. (2024, May 16). *About global polio eradication*. https://www.cdc.gov/global-polio-vaccination/about/index.html#:~:text=Vaccines%20have%20stopped%20the%20spread,where%20immunization%20rates%20are%20low

Centers for Disease Control and Prevention. (2011). *A CDC framework for preventing infectious diseases; sustaining the essentials and innovating for the future*. https://stacks.cdc.gov/view/cdc/11695

Cleveland Clinic. (2025). *Infectious diseases*. https://my.clevelandclinic.org/health/diseases/17724-infectious-diseases

Holmes, E. C. (2013). What can we predict about viral evolution and emergence? *Current Opinion in Virology, 3*(2), 180–184. https://doi.org/10.1016/j.coviro.2012.12.003

Infectious Diseases Society of America. (n.d.). *Infection and prevention control*. https://www.idsociety.org/policy--advocacy/infection-prevention-and-control/

Pennsylvania Department of Health. (n.d.). *Communicable diseases*. https://www.health.pa.gov/topics/HealthStatistics/CommunicableDiseases/Pages/Communicable%20Diseases.aspx

Suffoletto, D. (2024, May 24). *Infectious diseases*. Public Health-Dayton & Montgomery County. https://www.phdmc.org/news-features/infectious-diseases

Tulchinsky, T. H., & Varavikova, E. A. (2014). Communicable diseases. *The New Public Health*, 149–236. https://doi.org/10.1016/B978-0-12-415766-8.00004-5

van Seventer, J. M., & Hochberg, N. S. (2017). Principles of infectious diseases: Transmission, diagnosis, prevention, and control. *International Encyclopedia of Public Health*, 22–39. https://doi.org/10.1016/B978-0-12-803678-5.00516-6

CHAPTER 62

POPULATION AGING

Gurpreet Singh and Thomas Foley

INTRODUCTION

A population refers to the number of individuals living in a specific geographic area or belonging to a community. Demographers study these populations by examining a variety of factors like size, density, distribution, and vital statistics such as birth rates, death rates, and migration patterns. **Population aging** occurs when the median age of a population rises over time, usually due to a combination of lower birth rates, increased life expectancy, and the aging of large groups of individuals (Smith, 2021). When large groups of people age, like the **baby boomers** (people born from 1946 to 1964 during the mid-20th century, post-World War II baby boom), they significantly contribute to the increase in the median age of the population (World Health Organization [WHO], 2024). Advances in healthcare and living standards have led to people living longer, increasing the number of older individuals in the population. This chapter explores the trends, implications, and innovations associated with population aging.

KEY FACTORS IN POPULATION AGING

DECLINING FERTILITY RATES

The global total fertility rate (TFR) has significantly declined from 4.84 live births per woman in 1951 to 2.23 live births per woman in 2021. While fertility rates are declining on a global scale, there are regions of the world where fertility rates are still exceptionally high. Low-income regions with young median ages and low life expectancy from birth, such as much of Sub-Saharan Africa, tend to have extremely high fertility rates when compared to high-income countries with older median ages and greater life expectancy. High-income countries that experience low fertility and greater life expectancy and median ages, such as Japan, tend to experience significant workforce shortages (GBD 2021 Fertility and Forecasting Collaborators, 2021; United Nations, 2019).

LIFE EXPECTANCY

From 2000 to 2023, global life expectancy at birth increased from 66.4 years to 73.2 years, adding nearly 7 years to the life cycle (UN Data Portal, n.d.). Consequently, healthy life expectancy (HALE) also rose by approximately 8%, increasing from 58.3 years to 63.7 years. Interestingly, this change in HALE was not due to a decline in years lived with disability—it was due to lower mortality rates (WHO, 2024).

AGING OF LARGE BIRTH COHORTS

Population demographics are significantly impacted by the aging of large birth cohorts such as baby boomers born in the post-World War II era. As this group of individuals aged, the proportion of the total population comprised of older adults (adults age 65 and older) rapidly increased, leading to increased chronic disease comorbidities and significant stresses on healthcare, social service, and economic systems (Multidisciplinary Digital Publishing Institute [MDPI], 2023; WHO, 2024).

MIGRATION

Migration patterns also influence population aging. When younger individuals move to urban areas for better opportunities, it creates a population with a higher proportion of older adults in vulnerable rural areas. This shift can accelerate the aging process of the remaining population and create unique challenges in the provision of adequate healthcare and social services (Smith, 2021).

POPULATION AGING TRENDS

By 2050, there will be an estimated 1.8 billion older adults in the world, which is more than three times the number of older adults during 2000. This change will mean that, by 2050, one in six individuals will be 65 or older, compared to one in 14 in 2000 (UN Data Portal, n.d.). Aging trends, however, vary across the regions of the world. While Europe and North America have the highest proportions of older adults, Asia is rapidly aging. It is expected that by 2050, more than 24% of the total population of Asia will be 60 years or older, which is double the percent from 2019. Latin America and the Caribbean are home to the fastest aging populations. In both Latin America and the Caribbean, the proportion of the population that is 60 and older is expected to increase from 12% in 2019 to 25% by 2050. Although Africa is relatively young, there will be a significant increase in its older population, rising from 5% in 2019 to 9% by 2050 (United Nations, 2019; WHO, 2024).

IMPLICATIONS OF AGING FOR POLICIES AND ECONOMICS

The demographic shift toward an older population has profound implications for healthcare, the economy, and social structures. Older populations have higher incidences of chronic diseases such as congestive heart failure, diabetes mellitus, renal failure, cirrhosis of the liver, glaucoma, osteoporosis, sarcopenia, and dementia. Chronic diseases require increased need for healthcare, social services, long-term care, and financial resources (Centers for Disease Control and Prevention [CDC], n.d.; WHO, 2024). Aging populations that require more specialized attention raise the need for better and significantly more long-term care facilities and care services. This increased need puts additional pressure on already struggling healthcare infrastructure globally and requires significant investment in healthcare models, facilities, and training (MDPI, 2023).

As the population ages, the retiree population will increase and the workforce will shrink, which consequently will result in global straining of government aid, pension, and social security systems. The aging workforce could lead to labor shortages, necessitating policies to retain and integrate older workers (International Labour Organization, 2021). Older individuals typically have higher savings but lower consumer spending, affecting economic dynamics. Some economists suggest focusing on well-being rather than just gross domestic product (GDP) growth to mitigate these impacts (Harvard Business Review, 2020).

Population aging can change family structures, requiring more adult children to care for their older adult parents and more elder family members caring for their grandchildren, increasing the burden on informal caregivers and necessitating supportive policies (UNICEF, 2019). Keeping older adults active and engaged is essential. Addressing **ageism** (discrimination based on age) and creating age-friendly environments can enhance quality of life and provide life purpose for older adults (Barbaccia et al., 2022). **Age-friendly** environments are physical and social spaces that promote the health, independence, and quality of life of people as they age. Countries across the world will need to focus on reforming policies to protect older adults such as funding palliative care, building senior centers, and preventing elder mistreatment (Organisation for Economic Co-operation and Development, 2021). Making urban environments more age-friendly is crucial, including improving public transportation, housing, and community spaces to support older adults (WHO, 2024).

INNOVATIONS IN HEALTHCARE SERVICES FOR OLDER ADULTS

As the global population ages, healthcare innovations are increasingly focused on meeting the unique needs of older adults. Key advancements include:

- *Telehealth and remote monitoring*: Telehealth has paved the way for better accessibility by providing opportunities to receive healthcare services remotely, especially for older adults who would otherwise be unable to access services. Remote tracking of vital signs and chronic health conditions has significantly improved the timing of early interventions and prevented many undesirable outcomes (WHO, 2024).
- *Geriatric care management*: Personalized care plans, coordinated services, and regular health assessments by specialized healthcare professionals focus on preventive care and managing multiple health conditions common in older adults (National Institute on Aging, n.d.).
- *Assistive technologies*: Advances in assistive technologies like hearing aids, mobility scooters, smart-home systems, and wearable health monitors have significantly enhanced older adults' ability to live independently (Fotteler et al., 2022).
- *Chronic disease management programs*: Programs designed to manage conditions like diabetes, heart disease, and arthritis are vital for reducing hospital admissions and improving quality of life (WHO, 2024).
- *Mental health services*: Addressing mental health issues such as depression, anxiety, and cognitive decline is essential for older adults. Services include telepsychiatry, online counseling, and cognitive training apps (National Institute of Mental Health, n.d.).
- *Palliative care and hospice*: **Palliative care** provides relief from symptoms and stress of serious illnesses, crucial for maintaining quality of life for older adults facing chronic or terminal conditions. **Hospice** is an extension of palliative care in which the patient is in the terminal phase of a disease and has less than 6 months to live. Hospice, like palliative care, focuses on mitigating and abating pain and on quality of life. Both palliative care and hospice are person-centered approaches that respect the autonomy and preferences of the patient and family members (WHO, 2024).
- *Community-based health programs*: Community-based programs offer health services within local environments, fostering community engagement and reducing isolation (CDC, n.d.).
- *Innovation in medications and therapies*: Pharmaceutical advancements, including personalized medicine and regenerative therapies, are essential for managing age-related diseases. These innovations offer more effective treatments tailored to the needs of individual older adults (National Institutes of Health, 2021).

ORGANIZATIONS ADDRESSING AGING AND ITS EFFECTS

Many organizations around the world are dedicated to addressing the impacts of population aging. These organizations work interprofessionally across a breadth of aging factors such as healthcare, policy development, social inclusion, and research. The following are examples of key organizations making significant contributions in the field of aging:

- *World Health Organization (WHO)*: A specialized agency of the United Nations, WHO focuses on international public health. It's efforts in aging include promoting healthy aging, developing policies and strategies to meet the needs of older adults, and conducting research on age-related health issues (WHO, 2024).
- *International Federation on Ageing (IFA)*: The IFA is a private organization that focuses on the quality of life of older individuals on a global scale. The IFA aims to influence policies

and practices related to aging by collaborating with governments and other agencies in the private sector. Some of the key focus areas of the IFA include discrimination against older adults, health and well-being, income, and resources (IFA, n.d.).

- *HelpAge International*: Promoting the rights and wellness of older individuals is among the top priorities of HelpAge International, which is a leading global network for healthy aging. Some of the primary focus areas of HelpAge are to advocate for policies to improve quality of life, direct support through health services, and inclusion of older adults in developing humanitarian projects. HelpAge additionally supports research and disseminates results regarding issues related to aging (HelpAge International, n.d.).
- *Alzheimer's Disease International (ADI)*: The ADI represents over 100 Alzheimer associations worldwide and has been instrumental in supporting individuals with Alzheimer and other forms of dementia, raising awareness, influencing policies, and advancing dementia research. The ADI also provides resources to other Alzheimer associations globally (ADI, n.d.).
- *Global Coalition on Aging (GCOA)*: GCOA promotes healthy aging by modulating how global leaders approach and respond to aging and the needs associated with aging. GCOA fosters collaborations with businesses, policymakers, and stakeholders to support healthy aging and leverage the variety of economic opportunities for an aging population. The coalition focuses on innovation in healthcare, age-appropriate workplaces, and resources for retirement (GCOA, n.d.).
- *National Institute on Aging (NIA)*: The NIA is one of the largest scientific entities that conducts and supports research in the United States, as well as worldwide. The breadth of NIA research is vast and includes the biology of aging and healthy aging (NIA, n.d.).
- *European Innovation Partnership on Active and Healthy Ageing (EIP on AHA)*: The EIP on AHA is an initiative by the European Commission aimed at increasing the average healthy lifespan of Europeans. It brings together stakeholders from different sectors to foster innovation in aging and health, focusing on integrated care, fall prevention, and the use of technology to support older adults (EIP on AHA, n.d.).
- *United Nations Program on Ageing*: The United Nations Program on Ageing helps raise awareness about global aging and challenges and opportunities that accompany aging. This program advocates for policies and programs that support older individuals and focuses on social inclusion, socioeconomic conditions, and the rights of older adults (United Nations, n.d.).
- *World Economic Forum (WEF)*: The WEF addresses aging through its Global Agenda Council on Ageing, bringing together experts from various fields to discuss and develop strategies for tackling the challenges and opportunities of global aging. The WEF focuses on workforce aging, retirement systems, and the potential for older adults to contribute to society (WEF, n.d.).

CONCLUSION

Population aging has profound effects on society due to several challenges and unique opportunities associated with it. In this global shift, where older adults are accounting for a greater percentage of the total population, several forthcoming challenges may result in a scarcity of resources, challenges with healthcare, and stress on economic systems. Addressing the needs of the rapidly increasing older population is essential to protect quality of life and population health. Several key areas that require our attention include promoting healthy aging through lifestyle changes and prevention, investment in innovative technology for healthcare, and infrastructure building to create more age-friendly care and communities for older adults. Supporting economic and social policies that protect older adults and their caregivers can pave the way for healthy aging and enhance their quality of life on a global scale.

REFERENCES

Alzheimer's Disease International. (n.d.). *Alzheimer's Disease International*. https://www.alzint.org/

Barbaccia, V., Bravi, L., Murmura, F., Savelli, E., & Viganò, E. (2022). Mature and older adults' perception of active ageing and the need for supporting services: Insights from a qualitative study. *International Journal of Environmental Research and Public Health, 19*(13), 7660. https://doi.org/10.3390/ijerph19137660

Centers for Disease Control and Prevention. (n.d.). *Centers for Disease Control and Prevention*. https://www.cdc.gov

European Innovation Partnership on Active and Healthy Ageing. (n.d.). *European Social Network*. https://www.esn-eu.org/european-innovation-partnership-active-and-healthy-ageing

Fotteler, M. L, Mühlbauer, V., Brefka, S., Mayer, S., Kohn, B., Holl, F., Swoboda, W., Gaugisch, P., Risch, B., Denkinger, M., & Dallmeier, D. (2022). The effectiveness of assistive technologies for older adults and the influence of frailty: Systematic literature review of randomized controlled trials. *JMIR Aging, 5*(2), e31916. https://doi.org/10.2196/31916

GBD 2021 Fertility and Forecasting Collaborators. (2021). Global fertility in 204 countries and territories, 1950–2021, with forecasts to 2100: A comprehensive demographic analysis for the Global Burden of Disease Study 2021. *The Lancet, 403*(10440), 2057–2099. https://doi.org/10.1016/s0140-6736(24)00550-6

Global Coalition on Aging. (n.d.). *Global Coalition on Aging*. https://globalcoalitiononaging.com/

Harvard Business Review. (2020). *How GDP metrics mask well-being in older populations*. https://hbr.org/2020/03/how-gdp-metrics-mask-well-being-in-older-populations

HelpAge International. (n.d.). *HelpAge International*. https://www.helpage.org/

International Federation on Ageing. (n.d.). *International Federation on Ageing*. https://ifa.ngo/

International Labour Organization. (2021). *World employment and social outlook: Trends 2021*. https://www.ilo.org/global/research/global-reports/weso/trends2021/lang--en/index.htm

Multidisciplinary Digital Publishing Institute. (2023). *Population aging: An emerging research agenda for sustainable development*. https://www.mdpi.com/journal/socsci

National Institute of Mental Health (n.d.). *Older adults and mental health*. https://www.nimh.nih.gov/health/topics/older-adults-and-mental-health

National Institute on Aging. (n.d.). *National Institute on Aging*. https://www.nia.nih.gov/

National Institutes of Health. (2021). *Advances in regenerative medicine*. https://www.nih.gov/news-events/news-releases/advances-rnihegenerative-medicine

Organisation for Economic Co-operation and Development. (2021). *Pensions at a glance 2021: OECD and G20 indicators*. https://www.oecd.org/publications/pensions-at-a-glance-19991363.htm

Smith, J. (2021). The impact of demographic changes on society. *Demography Journal, 58*(3), 215–232.

UN Data Portal. (n.d.). *UN population division data portal*. United Nations. https://population.un.org/dataportal/home/

United Nations. (2019). *World population prospects 2019: Highlights*. https://population.un.org/wpp/Publications/Files/WPP2019_Highlights.pdf

UNICEF. (2019). *The changing family structure and its impact on family care*. https://www.unicef.org/reports/changing-family-structure

World Economic Forum. (n.d.). *Global agenda council on ageing*. World Economic Forum. https://www.weforum.org/publications/global-agenda-council-ageing-2012-2014/

World Health Organization. (2024). *Aging and health*. https://www.who.int/news-room/fact-sheets/detail/ageing-and-health

CHAPTER 63

MENTAL HEALTH

Diya Mariam Chacko, Rituparna Chakraborty, and G. S. Prakasha

INTRODUCTION

Mental health is more than just the absence of mental illness; it is also the state of an individual's cognitive, behavioral, and emotional well-being and ability to function within the social environment (World Health Organization [WHO], 2022). Mental health has become an important focus in public health and sustainable development. There is a significant need to make mental health care accessible and deal with the sociocultural and economic consequences of depleting mental health. The World Economic Forum estimates trillions of dollars in economic loss due to mental, neurologic, and substance use conditions between 2011 and 2030 (Chisholm et al., 2023).

COMMON MENTAL HEALTH DISORDERS

More than 300 million people across the world suffer from anxiety disorders, including 58 million children and adolescents (WHO, 2022). **Anxiety** disorders are characterized by excessive fear and worry and related behavioral disturbances. Symptoms often result in significant distress or significant impairment in functioning.

According to WHO (2022), approximately 280 million people were reported to have depression, including 23 million children and adolescents. **Depression** is marked by severe emotional challenges in everyday life. Approximately 40 million people were reported to have experienced **bipolar disorder** with alternating depressive episodes and periods of manic symptoms. A depressive episode often involves an individual experiencing a depressed mood (feeling sad, irritable, or empty) or a loss of pleasure in activities previously enjoyed. Manic symptoms may include euphoria, increased activity, and heightened self-esteem. People with depression and bipolar disorder are at an increased risk of suicide. Approximately 720,000 people die by suicide every year, and suicide is the third leading cause of death globally among 15- to 29-year-olds (WHO, 2022).

Schizophrenia impacts approximately 24 million people globally (WHO, 2022), who will have, on average, 10 to 20 years shorter life expectancy compared with people without schizophrenia. **Schizophrenia** is characterized by significant impairments in perception and cognitive functioning and changes in behavior. Symptoms of schizophrenia include persistent delusions, hallucinations, disorganized thinking, highly disorganized behavior, and extreme agitation.

CULTURE AND SOCIAL LOCATION

Individuals from different cultures make meaning of their experiences based on cultural perceptions of "normal" (Rathod et al., 2018), which shape their subjective understanding of mind and behavior. Aspects of social location such as gender, age, race, and ethnicity are identified markers of discrimination and are found to be associated with multiple psychological and developmental disorders. In India, for example, caste is one of the significant intersectional factors impacting mental health (Gupta & Coffey, 2020). Although mental health research (Chu et al., 2022) has highlighted power dynamics concerning issues such as gender, caste, and socioeconomics as related to mental health, research mainly focuses on epidemiologic data. Therefore, a deeper understanding of cultural contribution in shaping psychosocial experiences remains.

The case study in Box 63.1 is an example of how culture contributes to a person's state of wellness. This case study highlights the need to understand the social locations unique to various cultural contexts. Globally, psychiatry and psychology have largely ignored the cultural complexities of the "local." Even the curriculum training of mental health practitioners in countries like India still strongly focuses on Western techniques and models, with potential gaps in addressing local problems and developing plausible solutions.

DEFICIT-BASED APPROACH VERSUS CAPABILITY APPROACH

A **deficit-based approach to mental health** historically shapes research within the mental health space (Ness et al., 2020). This perspective emphasizes an individual's problems and attempts to formulate solutions for those problems. However, focusing on "deficits" overlooks the experiences of communities and individuals and the multiple contributors to an individual's problems. Such interventions fail to address problems holistically and may lead to negative client experiences and behaviors. Diagnostic manuals allow practitioners to efficiently describe client symptoms and possible prognoses. However, classifying individuals based only on diagnostic manuals risks possible **stigmatization**, which means to hold discriminatory attitudes toward mental illness or to characterize it as disgraceful (American Psychiatric Association [APA], 2022).

There is a need to shift to a capability-based approach, focusing on individual and community strengths and capabilities to promote mental health. Anand (2021) mentions Amartya Sen's previously proposed capability-based approach as a less restrictive approach to welfare economics. When applied to mental distress, this approach offers a conceptual framework that challenges the dominance of the medical model. The **capability-based approach to mental health** states that individuals have the inherent capacity and strength to address their problems. Such an approach allows practitioners and communities to recognize sources of discrimination as well as create safe spaces for individuals to reconnect with society after experiencing mental health difficulties. The understanding that every individual has the inherent capacity and existing strength to resolve their problems encourages individuals to make meaningful changes independently.

MILESTONES IN GLOBAL MENTAL HEALTH

The *Diagnostic and Statistical Manual of Mental Disorders (DSM-5-TR*; APA, 2022*)*, a U.S. classification system for diagnosing mental disorders, and the *International Classification of Diseases (ICD*; WHO, 2025) statistical code numbers have gained international interest since the publication of the *DSM-III* in 1980. Present collaboration between the APA and WHO allows the formulation of a common research base through revisions in the *DSM-5-TR* and the *ICD-11*. An

BOX 63.1 Case Study: R. V., a PhD Student in India

A male PhD student, R. V., who belonged to the Dalit community,[a] died by suicide after college officials attempted to expel him after denying him a scholarship that was promised to him and other students. The university reported R. V. as a "troubled" individual who was undergoing personal issues that were the reason for suicide, rather than caste-based discrimination. R. V.'s depression was stated as the reason for the suicide, failing to address the underlying structural and systemic violence that led to his psychologic distress (Sukumar, 2016).

[a]Members of the Dalit community are considered to be "untouchables." They are viewed as being beneath the caste system in India and are considered to be among the most oppressed people globally. They are forced into occupations that often involve unsafe and unhygienic conditions and are also denied access to education, property ownership, and often a minimum wage (Momen & Shahen, 2024).

organizational framework has been formulated by grouping disorders into similar clusters based on shared pathophysiology, genetics, and so on (First et al., 2021).

The *DSM-5-TR* includes significant revisions in terminologies for some mental health disorders. Terminologies are changed for various reasons, such as to address misclassifications, to mitigate stigmatization that can arise from labeling, and to improve understanding of etiological factors. Previous classification terms "substance abuse and substance dependence" are now placed under the category of "substance use disorder." The chapter name has been changed to "substance-related and addictive disorders" to include the term "addictive," matching a proposed *ICD-11* naming convention, which refers to the inclusion of gambling disorder as a behavioral syndrome.

Specifiers and subtypes in the manual provide the various phenomenological presentations of a disorder. The number of specifiers and subtypes in the *DSM-5-TR* has been increased to include recent attempts to dimensionalize disorders (Regier et al., 2013). For example, within the depressive disorders and bipolar and related disorders category, a specifier of "with mixed features" replaces the diagnosis of bipolar I mixed episodes in the *DSM-IV*, given that mixed states of major depressive and manic episodes are much more common and may have specific treatment implications.

The COVID-19 global pandemic caused noteworthy changes in bringing about new adaptive challenges and contributing to unexplored areas of mental health concerns. Digital psychiatry gained prominence during the pandemic. Although virtual platforms have increased mental health care accessibility (Strudwick et al., 2020), there are several challenges regarding use of digital psychiatry such as differential internet access, language and cultural barriers, and privacy concerns. A collaborative approach with stakeholders like practitioners, service users, and researchers may be required to ensure inclusivity in telepsychiatry services. Social media platforms have played a major role in reducing the stigma around mental health conversations. Influencers sharing their experiences of mental health struggles have further encouraged conversations on a global scale and helped spread awareness of the importance of mental health. However, social platforms have come with unintended consequences, such as an increase in self-diagnosis. One therapist has commented, "I've had clients come in stating that their behavior is because of their anxious attachment. They also mention seeing [videos on social media] that have helped identify their mental health disorders or even identify someone else in their lives as a narcissist." Such self-diagnosis and labeling of others based on limited information could have harmful consequences.

The attempt to oversimplify mental health conversations to fit into short-form media has led to an increase in false or incomplete information sharing. Therapists mention that although social media has allowed a shift from the history of silence and stigma, it has also given rise to a concern about "therapy speak," which refers to the usage of therapy terminology in everyday lives (Morgan, 2023). This may trivialize the experiences of individuals suffering from severe mental health symptoms. Moving forward, there is a clear need for mental health practitioners to consider the real impact of social media on their clients and assess the usage of terminology discussed in sessions and its application in their daily lives.

NEED FOR A CONTEXTUAL MODEL OF MENTAL HEALTH

There is a need to develop and promote context within the understanding of mental health and the practice of mental health care. Arnett (2008) assessed six premier APA journals and revealed that 95% of the research published in these journals was conducted on people from either the United States or Europe, with 77% of the U.S. samples being people of European descent. Even in the United States, there are significant social factors that influence the perception of mental health and the practice of mental health care.

Boyd, a senior psychologist for the Chickasaw Nation in Oklahoma and a member of the Cherokee Nation, mentions the importance of learning the values and communication styles of American Indian communities when providing mental health care. She states that interpersonal interactions and behaviors among those from some American Indian cultures can be falsely perceived as symptoms of autism spectrum disorder. For example, some American Indian children may avoid eye contact or pause before answering questions. In Western culture, "normal" functioning among children is associated with prompt answering, so American Indian children may be misdiagnosed with disorders. Boyd further discusses an account of a male American Indian client who showed symptoms of anxiety. The client mentioned that the birds and squirrels around him helped him understand his illness. Providers diagnosed the client with schizophrenia when he attempted to find meaning and comfort in ways that aligned with his culture (Stringer, 2023).

Boyd's case highlights that the current definitions of "normal" or "abnormal" are based on global Western norms and personality structures. Conventional psychotherapy techniques and diagnoses were developed for the problems manifested in certain aspects of Western culture. This case also emphasizes that the psychologic markers of well-being based on conventional models do not necessarily match the worldviews of Indigenous peoples. Indigenous worldviews need to be considered interdependent systems in which the natural environment and the community are connected to wellness. The **contextual model of mental health** allow us to understand the systemic hierarchies prevalent in different contexts.

NARRATIVE THERAPY

Narrative therapy is an alternative to conventional psychotherapy approaches. It allows clients to deconstruct their current experience, empowers them as authors of their own lives, and aids in reconstructing their identity with hopes and expectations. Thus, narrative therapy allows one to externalize the problem, using previously neglected stories. This allows the client to see their story as a new narrative rather than a problem-saturated perspective (Ghavibazou et al., 2022). Box 63.2 shows an example of using narrative therapy within a contextual model approach.

GAPS IN MENTAL HEALTH SERVICES AND APPROACHES TO ADDRESS GAPS

The global mental health treatment gap is slightly more than 50%, but the gap in low-income countries is nearly 90% (Wainberg et al., 2017). These countries have insufficient resources to provide intervention services. Moreover, mental health care services are usually concentrated in densely populated urban areas within a country, indicating an uneven geographic distribution of mental healthcare resources.

The global mental health (GMH) field started focusing on mental health equity and justice by using interdisciplinary approaches to treat populations worldwide (Petagna et al., 2023). For example, WHO developed the Mental Health Gap Action Programme Intervention Guide (mhGAP-IG) to address the existing gap. The mhGAP-IG comprises user-friendly, diagnosis-specific clinical guidelines for providing evidence-based practice (EBP). The guidelines are devised for use by nonspecialized healthcare providers based on contextual needs.

BOX 63.2 Experience Sharing by S. P., a Narrative Therapist

During her practice, S. P. found the models she was trained in, like cognitive behavioral therapy (CBT) and dialectical behavior therapy (DBT), to be individual-focused and to tend to separate the individual from the context. Using narrative therapy, S. P. can help her clients see themselves as belonging to a community. Instead of altering "irrational beliefs" to cope, the client can choose how to go about their beliefs. S. P. gives an example of a female client who found it hard to connect with men because of her negative beliefs about them. Instead of focusing on changing those beliefs, S. P. attempted to place those beliefs and the client's experiences in the structural context, understanding the client's history of oppression and survival. Such contextualization of beliefs allows the client to feel validated, and the focus then becomes less about making the person change and more about helping them see that there is more to the story than what is visible to them.

The effective implementation of EBP remains a major challenge in low-income countries due to shortages of mental health workers, lack of research funding, and mental illness stigma. Currently, significant funding is used on centralized institutions that often isolate clients from their families and support systems. Instead, mental health resources should be available and accessible in the community as a step toward social justice. For example, in 2005, the National Rural Health Mission launched the Accredited Social Health Activists (ASHA) program in India to incorporate community involvement in mental health services. The ASHA program has become one of the world's largest community health worker programs. The extensive knowledge and understanding of the local communities help ASHA workers encourage and improve community participation in mental health programs. ASHA community workers have adequate training and provide psychosocial assistance in the community, especially in times of significant crisis (Sivakumar et al., 2022).

Compared with physical illness, mental illness is significantly associated with stigma. The constant fear of discrimination and loss of relationships becomes an obstacle for those who have mental illness to seek treatment, and more so for marginalized communities (Qin & Hsieh, 2020). In India, being diagnosed with ADHD almost becomes a comorbidity for individuals from the LGBTQIA+ community, as being viewed as "nonnormative" is often labeled as being "deviant." A therapist can only wholly understand experiences when complex dynamics are conceptualized within their unique context. Box 63.3 offers an example of a person who feels stigmatized by a mental health disorder diagnosis.

There is also an apparent need for more diversity in clinical research. Collaboration of clinicians and services in community settings enables community-focused approaches and a clear description of the roles and responsibilities of each stakeholder for a particular action (Isaacs & Mitchell, 2024). Although WHO recommends community-based psychiatric rehabilitation, the limited number of psychosocial rehabilitation centers makes a community-based approach challenging. Community-based rehabilitation is a multidimensional approach that improves patients' quality of life. It has also been found to be a feasible option for low- and middle-income countries as it can be effectively delivered by trained healthcare workers (Saha et al., 2020).

CONCLUSION

Promoting global mental health includes increasing mental health care access equity, using contextual and capability-focused mental health approaches, destigmatizing mental illnesses, and addressing the underlying causes of mental health disorders. India's ASHA program is a good example of how to promote mental health at the community level. Integrating similar programs that address the forementioned issues is essential to increasing global mental wellness and mitigating global incidences of common mental health disorders such as depression, anxiety, bipolar disorder, and schizophrenia.

BOX 63.3 Client Description of Mental Health Stigma From Field Research

"Ever since my therapist diagnosed me with ADHD (attention-deficit/hyperactivity disorder), I feel like this label has made life a little more difficult. I identify as bisexual, so I have always found it tough not just to make sense of my sexuality but also to relate to people from the LGBTIA+ community. I guess that had something to do with my ADHD. But now, knowing this diagnosis is somehow making things more difficult."

LEARNING ACTIVITIES

CourseConnect

To access self-assessment questions and interactive, competency-based learning activities for this chapter, visit www.springerpub.com/courseconnect. See inside front cover and tear-out for CourseConnect details.

REFERENCES

American Psychiatric Association. (2022). *Diagnostic and statistical manual of mental disorders (DSM-5-TR)*. https://doi.org/10.1176/appi.books.9780890425787

Anand, P. (2021). Wellbeing in public policy: Contributions based on Sen's capability approach. *LSE Public Policy Review, 2*(2), 2. https://doi.org/10.31389/lseppr.49

Arnett, J. J. (2008). The neglected 95%: Why American psychology needs to become less American. *The American Psychologist, 63*(7), 602–614. https://doi.org/10.1037/0003-066X.63.7.602

Chisholm, D., Lee, Y. Y., Baral, P. P., Bhagwat, S., Dombrovskiy, V., Grafton, D., Kontsevaya, A., Huque, R., Kalani Okware, K., Kulikov, A., Marahatta, K., Mavunganidze, P., Omar, N., Prasai, D., Putoud, N., Tsoyi, E., & Vergara, J. (2023). Cross-country analysis of national mental health investment case studies in sub-Saharan Africa and Central, South and South-East Asia. *Frontiers in Health Services, 3*, 1214885. https://doi.org/10.3389/frhs.2023.1214885

Chu, W., Wippold, G., & Becker, K. D. (2022). A systematic review of cultural competence trainings for mental health providers. *Professional Psychology: Research and Practice, 53*(4), 362–371. https://doi.org/10.1037/pro0000469

First, M., Gaebel, W., Maj, M., Stein, D., Kogan, C., Saunders, J., Poznyak, V., Gureje, O., Lewis-Fernández, R., Maercker, A., Brewin, C., Cloitre, M., Claudino, A., Pike, K., Baird, G., Skuse, D., Krueger, R., Briken, P., Burke, J., Lochman, J., Evans, S., Woods, D., & Reed, G. (2021). An organization- and category-level comparison of diagnostic requirements for mental disorders in ICD-11 and DSM-5. *World Psychiatry, 20*(1), 34–51. https://doi.org/10.1002/wps.20825

Ghavibazou, E., Hosseinian, S., Kivi, H., & Ale Ebrahim, N. (2022). Narrative therapy, applications, and outcomes: A systematic review. *SSRN Electronic Journal, 2*(4). https://doi.org/10.2139/ssrn.4119920

Gupta, A., & Coffey, D. (2020). Caste, religion, and mental health in India. *Population Research and Policy Review, 39*, 1119–1141. https://doi.org/10.1007/s11113-020-09585-9

Isaacs, A. N., & Mitchell, E. K. L. (2024). Mental health integrated care models in primary care and factors that contribute to their effective implementation: A scoping review. *International Journal of Mental Health Systems, 18*(1), 5. https://doi.org/10.1186/s13033-024-00625-x

Momen, M. N., & Shahen, M. A. (2024). Dalits and their territorial rights in India. *World Affairs, 187*(1), 118–122. https://doi.org/10.1002/waf2.12010

Morgan, E. (2023). "That's triggering!": Is therapy-speak changing the way we talk about ourselves? *The Observer*. https://www.theguardian.com/society/2023/aug/20/triggered-toxic-narcissist-are-you-fluent-in-therapy-speak

Ness, O., Davidson, L., Oute, J., & von Heimburg, D. (2020). Recovery, social inclusion, and the capability approach in mental health. In J. N. Lester & M. O'Reilly (Eds.), *The Palgrave Encyclopedia of Critical Perspectives on Mental Health* (pp. 1–8). Springer International Publishing. https://doi.org/10.1007/978-3-030-12852-4_53-1

Petagna, M., Marley, C., Guerra, C., Calia, C., & Reid, C. (2023). Mental health gap action programme intervention guide (mhGAP-IG) for child and adolescent mental health in low- and middle-income countries (LMIC): A systematic review. *Community Mental Health Journal, 59*(1), 192–204. https://doi.org/10.1007/s10597-022-00981-3

Qin, X., & Hsieh, C. R. (2020). Understanding and addressing the treatment gap in mental healthcare: Economic perspectives and evidence from China. *Inquiry: A Journal of Medical Care Organization, Provision and Financing, 57*, 46958020950566. https://doi.org/10.1177/0046958020950566

Rathod, S., Gega, L., Degnan, A., Pikard, J., Khan, T., Husain, N., Munshi, T., & Naeem, F. (2018). The current status of culturally adapted mental health interventions: A practice-focused review of meta-analyses. *Neuropsychiatric Disease and Treatment, 14*, 165–178. https://doi.org/10.2147/NDT.S138430

Regier, D. A., Kuhl, E. A., & Kupfer, D. J. (2013). The *DSM-5*: Classification and criteria changes. *World psychiatry: Official Journal of the World Psychiatric Association (WPA), 12*(2), 92–98. https://doi.org/10.1002/wps.20050

Saha, S., Chauhan, A., Buch, B., Makwana, S., Vikar, S., Kotwani, P., & Pandya, A. (2020). Psychosocial rehabilitation of people living with mental illness: Lessons learned from community-based psychiatric rehabilitation centres in Gujarat. *Journal of Family Medicine and Primary Care, 9*(2), 892–897. https://doi.org/10.4103/jfmpc.jfmpc_991_19

Sivakumar, T., Kumar, C. N., & Thirthalli, J. (2022). Role of accredited social health activists in treatment of persons with severe mental illness in the community. *Indian Journal of Psychiatry, 64*(1), 102–105. https://journals.lww.com/indianjpsychiatry/fulltext/2022/64010/role_of_accredited_social_health_activists_in.16.aspx

Stringer, H. (2023). *Continuing education. The healing power of Native American culture*. APA Moniter. https://www.apa.org/monitor/2023/2023-10-monitor.pdf

Strudwick, G., Sockalingam, S., Kassam, I., Sequeira, L., Bonato, S., Youssef, A., Mehta, R., Green, N., Agic, B., Soklaridis, S., Impey, D., Wiljer, D., & Crawford, A. (2021). Digital interventions to support population mental health in Canada during the COVID-19 pandemic: Rapid review. *JMIR Mental Health, 8*(3), e26550. https://doi.org/10.2196/26550

Sukumar, N. (2016). "Red Sun in the Blue Sky": Rohith Vemula's Utopian Republic. *Social Change, 46*(3), 451–457. https://doi.org/10.1177/0049085716654819

Wainberg, M. L., Scorza, P., Shultz, J. M., Helpman, L., Mootz, J. J., Johnson, K. A., Neria, Y., Bradford, J. E., Oquendo, M. A., & Arbuckle, M. R. (2017). Challenges and opportunities in global mental health: A research-to-practice perspective. *Current psychiatry reports, 19*(5), 28. https://doi.org/10.1007/s11920-017-0780-z

World Health Organization. (2022). *World mental health report: Transforming mental health for all*. https://www.who.int/publications/i/item/9789240049338.

CHAPTER 64

FORCED MIGRATION

Dilli R. Gautam, Jenny K. Nielsen, and Johnathan D. Tremblay

OVERVIEW OF GLOBAL REFUGEE CRISIS

The number of displaced people has been steadily rising over the last several decades. In 2022, for the first time, there were more than 100 million forcibly displaced persons worldwide (Box 64.1). Climate change, COVID-19, and a global recession have affected the factors that cause people to flee, the living conditions of those who have fled, and the sentiments of the countries that host them.

A large percentage of the global refugee population originates from a small number of countries, primarily located in Asia and Africa, including Syria, Afghanistan, and South Sudan (Fransen & de Haas, 2022); however, there are ongoing displacement crises on every continent. For example, there were more than 5 million refugees from Ukraine in 2022 (UN High Commissioner for Refugees [UNHCR], 2025). Refugees fleeing conflict and persecution face severe challenges, such as being turned away at international borders or left stranded in dangerous areas like the Sahara Desert. As highlighted by Fransen and de Haas (2022), most refugees from Asia and Africa remain within their regions, often in neighboring countries, although the average distance between refugees' origin and destination countries has increased in recent years.

The health and well-being of refugee populations are further strained by emerging global threats such as climate change and pandemics. Refugees are highly vulnerable to climate-sensitive exposures due to their insecure living conditions and lack of resources, which put them at heightened risk for health inequities (Albahsahli et al., 2023). Furthermore, the COVID-19 pandemic exacerbated existing health disparities for refugees and asylum seekers, limiting access to healthcare, increasing misinformation, and compounding mental health challenges in overcrowded camps and shelters (El Arab et al., 2023).

While war and conflict remain the primary drivers of forced displacement, the rising impacts of climate change and pandemics are likely to exacerbate the refugee crisis in coming years. Addressing these interconnected challenges will require sustained global efforts to protect vulnerable populations and adapt to the evolving nature of forced migration.

LEGAL DEFINITIONS AND CATEGORIES OF REFUGEES

While persecution and protection for those fleeing violence have existed for several centuries, formal international protections were first implemented by the League of Nations after World War I

BOX 64.1 Worldwide Displacement in 2022[a]

In 2022, approximately 110 million people were forcibly displaced worldwide (twice the number displaced in 2013), including

- 35.3 million refugees displaced across borders—76% live in low- and middle-income countries;
- 62.5 million internally displaced people—58% of all displaced people; and
- 5.4 million asylum seekers.

[a]Data regarding forcibly displaced people as of May 2023.

Source: Adapted from UN High Commissioner for Refugees. (2023). *Five takeaways from the 2022 UNHCR global trends report.* https://www.unrefugees.org/news/five-takeaways-from-the-2022-unhcr-global-trends-report/

(Jaeger, 2001). The protections that exist today were enshrined by the United Nations in the 1951 Convention Relating to the Status of Refugees. In both situations, a need was recognized due to a large number of displaced persons in Europe following the World Wars (Jaeger, 2001).

The 1951 convention defines a **refugee** as a person who, "owing to a well-founded fear of being persecuted for reasons of race, religion, nationality, membership of a particular social group or political opinion, is outside the country of their nationality and is unable or, owing to such fear, is unwilling to avail themself of the protection of that country" (Convention Relating to the Status of Refugees, 1951). In addition to providing this definition for protection, the convention and its 1967 Protocol also outlined the core protections refugees are entitled to, such as protection from **nonrefoulement** (forced return home). These documents created the UNHCR and laid the framework for its work, including the three durable solutions models, which are discussed in greater detail in subsequent sections.

Only 30% of displaced persons worldwide have been granted refugee status by the UNHCR. To understand the complexity of the displacement crisis and its future directions, a distinction must be made between refugee status and other displacement categories (UNHCR, 2025):

- ***Asylum seeker***: An asylum seeker is individual who is seeking protection, but whose claim has not been determined legally. Not all asylum seekers will be granted asylum protections.
- ***Asylee***: An asylee is an individual who has been granted asylum by a specific country. They must have met the criteria and proven to authorities a well-founded fear of persecution. Asylum is recognized only in the country where it is granted.
- ***Internally displaced person** (IDP)*: An IDP is an individual who has been forced to leave their home but has not crossed an international border. They are still within their home country and are not eligible for refugee status or protections.
- ***Stateless person***: A stateless person is an individual who is not a citizen of any country, typically because their citizenship was revoked for reasons related to religion or membership to a political group.
- ***Migrant***: A migrant is an individual who is moving from place to place, either within their country or across borders, but *was not* forced to leave due to persecution or violence. Migrants typically move for economic reasons in search of a better life.
- ***Climate refugees***: Climate refugees are individuals who have been forced to leave their home due to climate change. The term is not officially recognized under international law, and current statutes do not qualify climate refugees for protection.

Beyond these large categories, there are many other statuses that those seeking humanitarian protection may have. Individual countries have their own immigration systems that may or may not grant legal protection to certain groups. For example, the United States granted "parole" to individuals it evacuated from Afghanistan in August 2021 during the U.S. troop withdrawal; parole status allowed these Afghans to legally remain and work in the United States for 2 years while applying for asylum.

An individual's access to services is greatly influenced by their legal status. While refugees are vulnerable, refugee status does allow them to access services that those without legal protected status, like asylum seekers and IDPs, cannot. Until official status is granted by a government or the UNHCR, individuals are not guaranteed access to food assistance, healthcare, or a path to permanent residence and the stability and safety it brings. The number of those without official protected status, including asylum seekers and climate refugees, has significantly increased over the past few decades, calling into question how those individuals will find safety and security.

CAUSES OF FORCED DISPLACEMENT

OVERVIEW

The factors that force a person to flee from their country can vary; however, the greatest drivers of forced displacement are political instability, economic hardship, and environmental changes

(UNHCR, 2025). When developing effective policies and interventions to ameliorate the global refugee crisis, policymakers must acknowledge and understand how these factors are interrelated and exacerbated by one another.

POLITICAL INSTABILITY AND CONFLICT

Political instability and conflict are the primary causes of forced displacement (UNHCR, 2025). In regions plagued by civil wars and authoritarian regimes, millions of people are forced to flee their homes without promise of return. In Afghanistan, decades of conflict and a recent resurgence of an oppressive political regime have created desperate conditions for many of its citizens. The conflict alone directly resulted in thousands of deaths, and the resulting destruction of infrastructure further exacerbated poor living conditions (Smith, 2024). Then, in 2021, the United States officially completed its withdrawal of military operations and the Taliban returned to power; many Afghans were targeted by theocratic laws or faced retaliation by the restored regime. Additionally, the Taliban's inability to administer a functioning state and their draconian laws for women have resulted in many fleeing the country (Smith, 2024).

Perhaps the direst modern example of state political power forcing the displacement of a population is the Rohingya crisis in Myanmar. In the Rakhine region of Myanmar, the government employed an official military campaign that created conditions similar to an open-air prison for the Rohingya ethnic group (Amnesty International, 2024). Under current government policies, the Rohingya have been subject to direct military brutality and ethnic cleansing campaigns. The conditions in Myanmar have resulted in the displacement of more than 700,000 Rohingya Muslims to Bangladesh (Amnesty International, 2024).

ECONOMIC AND SOCIAL DRIVERS

Restriction from economic engagement or direct prohibition from use of public resources, as well as political disenfranchisement, are other drivers of displacement. Groups of people in some countries are legally classified as second-class citizens due to either government corruption or ethnic discrimination, subjecting them to desperate levels of poverty, unemployment, and lack of access to resources compared with fully recognized citizens (Migration Data Portal, 2024). This type of migration, while only sometimes classified as a refugee movement, is significant and often results in large numbers of people moving across borders in search of economic mobility and stability (UNHRC, 2025).

Those forced into leaving their countries under these conditions may be uniquely vulnerable to human trafficking. For example, in 2022, Qatar was accused of employing modern-day human slavery in the construction of the "Aspire Zone," a series of multiple stadiums for the FIFA World Cup. Construction companies in Qatar were accused of using predatory recruiting tactics in economically disadvantaged countries such as Bangladesh, India, and Nepal (Consunji et al., 2022). Many laborers from these countries were forced to work long hours in incredible heat, with limited food and water, which in some cases resulted in death (Page & Warden, 2022). From 2010, when construction on World Cup facilities began, to 2022, an estimated 6,500 laborers died due to unsafe working conditions, substandard shelter and accommodations, and extreme heat (Page & Warden, 2022).

ENVIRONMENTAL AND CLIMATE CHANGE–DRIVEN DISPLACEMENT

In recent years, climate change has become an increasingly prominent topic in the conversation of forced migration. Severe droughts causing famine or fire, rising sea levels, and increasingly frequent extreme weather events such as typhoons, hurricanes, and tornadoes have already made certain places where people once lived uninhabitable. In the United States, many communities on the Gulf Coast are losing residents after hurricanes, with people choosing not to rebuild but instead to move elsewhere within the country (Hennighausen & James, 2024). Similarly, forest fires have been driving residents in California to move to other states. These new intercountry migration trends in the United States are still being analyzed, including their impacts on the housing market, gentrification, and collateral displacement (Hennighausen & James, 2024).

Populations in countries like Bangladesh, whose neighboring countries face similar threats of increasing inclement weather, have fewer options for destinations where they can find relief from climate issues (Duque, 2024). Additionally, small island nations in the Pacific, such as Tuvalu, experience erosion conditions, which can destroy significant land mass and endanger biodiversity on the island (Islam et al., 2022). Populations such as the Tuvaluans cannot be easily relocated to nearby countries, and international law, as of 2024, does not recognize "climate refugees" in any capacity. The United Nations and other international agencies acknowledge worrisome trends and conditions, but have yet to rise to a level of action through new laws or policies to address direct climate change–based displacement (UN Development Programme, 2023).

THE THREE DURABLE SOLUTIONS AND REFUGEE RESETTLEMENT

In line with its mandate of protecting refugees, the UNHCR promotes **three durable solutions** for long-term safety and security for those with refugee status: voluntary repatriation, local integration, and resettlement (UNHCR, 2003).

- *Voluntary repatriation*: If the situation in their country of origin has stabilized, a refugee may decide to return home. The UNHCR oversees many repatriation programs to ensure that the choice to return home is free from coercion and based on accurate information. Per humanitarian law, refugees should never be forced to return.
- *Resettlement*: The UNHCR facilitates resettlement to third countries when a refugee may have specific needs that cannot be addressed in a country of asylum or is not safe in the country of asylum. Countries around the globe, including the United States and Canada, have agreed to admit refugees referred by the UNHCR and grant them permanent residence. The UNHCR has determined that 7% of refugees worldwide are in need of third-country resettlement, but only 1% of refugees worldwide are resettled each year (UNHCR, 2025).
- *Local integration*: When returning home or being resettled to a third country is not possible, refugees may integrate into the country of asylum to which they have fled. This is a gradual process that starts with host countries granting basic rights to displaced populations, such as right to work, access to healthcare and education, and right to freely travel. The scope and pace with which local integration can proceed depends on the host country's political and economic situations and their ability and willingness to integrate refugees.

The UNHCR does not promote one solution over the others as its preferred method for addressing forced displacement. Likewise, refugees are not presented with each option and given a choice among the three (UNHCR, 2023). Which pathway a refugee travels is determined by many factors, including the geopolitical context of the crisis causing displacement, the situation in the country of asylum, and the refugee's individual health needs. Each individual crisis has unique challenges, and the UNHCR often takes a targeted approach using all three solutions to manage each crisis.

The timeline for resettlement to a third country also varies widely based on context, not only in the country of asylum but also in the host country. Host countries set their own policies for the number of individuals they will resettle each year; these capacities frequently shift with political administration changes. Each host country also has its own procedure for completing its screening process before approval for departure, with different requirements and timelines. Once a refugee's case has been accepted by a host country, which they rarely have the ability to influence, it cannot be transferred to another country. The exception is when refugees apply for reunification with family members in a host country.

HEALTH AND LIVING CONDITIONS IN COUNTRIES OF ASYLUM

Access to clean water, adequate sanitation, and the provision of healthcare are critical in refugee camps, but significant gaps persist. According to the UNHCR, only 35% of refugees in Ethiopia and 55% in the Democratic Republic of Congo have access to basic drinking water services. Water, sanitation, and hygiene (WaSH) infrastructure remains underfunded and highly vulnerable to climatic events like floods, which further disrupt access (UNHCR, 2025). Refugees receive, on average, 15 to 20 liters (4 to 5 gallons) of water per person per day, barely meeting international standards, while women and children often shoulder the burden of fetching water, increasing risks of gender-based violence (Harvey et al., 2020; UNHCR, 2023).

Sanitation facilities are often inadequate, leading to open defecation in some camps and increasing spread of waterborne diseases such as cholera. A study analyzing multiple refugee camps revealed that access to improved sanitation is uneven across different regions, with many refugees lacking facilities that ensure hygiene privacy and protection (Cronin et al., 2008). In Bangladesh's Cox's Bazar and Uganda's Nakivale Camp, poor water quality and limited sanitation result in a high prevalence of diseases, further burdening healthcare services (Cronin et al., 2008; UNHCR, 2023).

In addition, overcrowding is a pressing challenge in large camps like Zaatari in Jordan and Dadaab in Kenya, where resources are stretched beyond capacity. In protracted situations, where displacement lasts years, infrastructure deteriorates, leaving refugee populations in precarious conditions. Overcrowded camps exacerbate mental health issues, leading to increased anxiety, depression, and trauma-related disorders. Mental health services remain underdeveloped in many refugee settings, with limited integration into primary healthcare (Harvey et al., 2024; UNHCR, 2023).

Furthermore, healthcare access varies significantly based on the policies of host countries. Some countries, like Uganda, actively integrate refugees into national health systems, improving access to essential services, including maternal and child health programs (UNHCR, 2016). Conversely, countries with weaker healthcare infrastructures often rely on ad hoc clinics within camps, resulting in fragmented care that fails to meet refugees' long-term health needs (UNHCR, 2023). Integrated healthcare services are crucial, as camps that depend solely on humanitarian agencies face challenges in sustaining care over time, especially during funding shortages (Harvey et al., 2024).

Women and children are among the most vulnerable in refugee camps. The prevalence of gender-based violence increases in overcrowded conditions, while reproductive health services are often limited. Refugee women in Uganda, for example, face anemia rates above 40%, driven by poor nutrition and inadequate healthcare (UNHCR, 2016). Maternal care services are critical, yet many camps fail to provide consistent access to antenatal care and emergency obstetric services, increasing risks of maternal mortality (UNHCR, 2025).

Children also face severe health challenges, with stunting and malnutrition being widespread due to limited food diversity and contaminated water sources. Addressing these issues requires a multisectoral approach involving both healthcare and nutrition support. In Uganda's refugee settlements, nearly 72% of children younger than 5 years suffer from anemia, which highlights the need for integrated health interventions (UNHCR, 2016).

FUTURE TRENDS IN DISPLACED POPULATIONS AND RECOMMENDATIONS FOR IMPROVING PROTECTION

Recent studies confirm that climate change, conflict, and socioeconomic instability will continue to drive global displacement in coming decades. Climate-induced migration is expected to increase significantly, with projections suggesting that, by 2050, as many as 216 million people could be displaced globally due to environmental degradation (UNDP, 2023). Climate change is not only triggering sudden displacements through extreme weather events like floods and hurricanes, but also forcing gradual migrations as livelihoods deteriorate in regions affected by drought or rising sea levels. The COVID-19 pandemic further intensified the vulnerabilities of displaced populations by disrupting mobility and straining resources, revealing the fragile nature of existing support systems for migrants (Mendez et al., 2024).

To address these challenges, policymakers must advocate for expanding legal frameworks to recognize displacement caused by climate change. Current conventions, such as the 1951 Refugee Convention, do not cover individuals displaced by environmental factors, necessitating reforms to bridge these gaps (Ionesco et al., 2017). The **Global Compact for Safe, Orderly, and Regular Migration (GCM)** offers a platform for cooperation, emphasizing sustainable solutions that integrate refugees into national systems, particularly healthcare and education (UNHCR, 2025). Nongovernmental organizations and host communities also play vital roles by offering grassroots solutions, but long-term success requires enhanced international cooperation, improved funding mechanisms, and climate-resilient strategies to sustainably support displaced populations (Mendez et al., 2024; UNDP, 2023).

LEARNING ACTIVITIES

CourseConnect

To access self-assessment questions and interactive, competency-based learning activities for this chapter, visit www.springerpub.com/courseconnect. See inside front cover and tear-out for CourseConnect details.

REFERENCES

Albahsahli, B., Dimitrova, A., Kadri, N., Benmarhnia, T., & Rousan, T. A. (2023). Implications of climate-related disasters on refugees' health: A case study of resettled Syrian and Iraqi refugees in San Diego, California. *Research Square*, rs-3392999. https://doi.org/10.21203/rs.3.rs-3392999/v1

Amnesty International. (2024). *Myanmar's apartheid against the Rohingya*. Amnesty International UK. https://www.amnesty.org.uk/myanmar-apartheid-against-rohingya

Consunji, R., El-Menyar, A., Hirani, N., Abeid, A., Al-Thani, H., Hardan, M. S., Chauhan, S., Kasem, H., & Peralta, R. (2022, December 5). Work-related injuries in Qatar for 1 Year: An initial report from the work-related injury unified registry for Qatar. *Qatar Medical Journal*. https://pmc.ncbi.nlm.nih.gov/articles/PMC10100584/

Cronin, A. A., Shrestha, D., Cornier, N., Abdalla, F., Ezard, N., & Aramburu, C. (2008). A review of water and sanitation provision in refugee camps in association with selected health and nutrition indicators—The need for integrated service provision. *Journal of Water and Health, 6*(1), 1–13. https://doi.org/10.2166/wh.2007.019

Duque, M. C. (2024, September 4). *Climate change in Bangladesh shapes internal migration and movement to India*. https://www.migrationpolicy.org/article/bangladesh-india-climate-migration#:~:text=By%20205 %2C%20the%20World%20Bank,it%20is%20difficult%20to%20track

El Arab, R. A., Somerville, J., Abuadas, F. H., Rubinat-Arnaldo, E., & Sagbakken, M. (2023). Health and well-being of refugees, asylum seekers, undocumented migrants, and internally displaced persons under COVID-19: A scoping review. *Frontiers in Public Health, 11*, 1145002. https://doi.org/10.3389/fpubh.2023.1145002

Fransen, S., & de Haas, H. (2022). Trends and patterns of global refugee migration. *Population and Development Review, 48*(1), 97–128. https://doi.org/10.1111/padr.12456

Harvey, P., Adams, J., & Biran, A. (2020). Social and geographic inequalities in water, sanitation, and hygiene access in 21 refugee camps and settlements in Bangladesh, Kenya, Uganda, South Sudan, and Zimbabwe. *International Journal for Equity in Health*. https://equityhealthj.biomedcentral.com/articles/10.1186/s12939-020-01318-2

Hennighausen, H., & James, A. (2024, October 1). Catastrophic fires, human displacement, and real estate prices in California. *Journal of Housing Economics*. https://www.sciencedirect.com/science/article/abs/pii/S1051137724000421

Ionesco, D., Mokhnacheva, D., & Gemenne, F. (2017). *The atlas of environmental migration*. Routledge. https://www.routledge.com/The-Atlas-of-Environmental-Migration/Ionesco-Mokhnacheva-Gemnne/p/book/9781138022065

Islam, S. N., Reinstädtler, S., Reza, M. S., Afroze, S., & Azad, A. K. (2022, July 3). *Climate change versus livelihoods, heritage and ecosystems in small island states of the Pacific: A case study on Tuvalu—Environment, development and sustainability*. SpringerLink. https://link.springer.com/article/10.1007/s10668-022-02367-7#citeas

Jaeger, G. (2001). On the history of the international protection of refugees. *IRRC Septembere, 83*(843), 727–737.

Mendez, M., Pastor, M., & Lesaca, A. C.(2024). *Climate change, migration, and health disparities at and beyond the US-Mexico border*. JAMA Network Open. https://jamanetwork.com

Migration Data Portal. (2024, June 20). *Forced migration or displacement*. Migration Data Portal. https://www.migrationdataportal.org/themes/forced-migration-or-displacement#:~:text=While%0there%20were%2059.5million,12%20years%20(ibid.)

Page, M., & Warden, M. (2022, November 30). *Qatar World Cup chief publicly admits high migrant death tolls*. Human Rights Watch. https://www.hrw.org/news/2022/11/30/qatar-world-cup-chief-publicly-admits-high-migrant-death-tolls

Smith, G. (2024, August 14). *Afghanistan three years after the Taliban takeover*. Crisis Group. https://www.crisisgroup.org/asia/south-asia/afghanistan/afghanistan-three-years-after-taliban-takeover

UN Development Programme. (2023). *Climate change, migration and displacement: Policy solutions for sustainable development*. https://www.undp.org

UN High Commissioner for Refugees. (2003). *Framework for durable solutions for refugees and persons of concern*. https://www.refworld.org/policy/strategy/unhcr/2003/en/35014

UN High Commissioner for Refugees. (2016). *Food security and nutrition assessment in refugee settlements*. https://data.unhcr.org/en/documents/details/63358

UN High Commissioner for Refugees. (2023). *Health in camps and settlements*. UNHCR Emergency Handbook. UNHCR. https://emergency.unhcr.org

UN High Commissioner for Refugees. (2025). *Global report 2024*. https://www.unhcr.org/publications/global-report-2024

GLOSSARY

1947 Partition of India	Following World War II, the British Raj was dissolved in 1947 and the region was partitioned into separate nations: India and East and West Pakistan. The 1947 Partition of India displaced millions of people along Hindu and Muslim religious lines, leading to violence, refugee crises, and social inequities that continue to impact the region today.
2020 Global Gender Gap Index	The Global Gender Gap Index is a report published by the World Economic Forum that measures gender-based disparities across countries in areas such as economic participation, education, health, and political empowerment; the 2020 edition ranked countries based on their progress toward gender equality.
2021 Seema Hospital project	Built in 2021 at a cost of $92 million, the Seema Hospital is one of few newer facilities in Iraq with high quality healthcare resources. It has 161 beds and oncology, radiotherapy, and burn centers.
Aboriginal Community Controlled Health Organisations	An Australian-based community health organization that offers primary care services under a different provider payment model with salaried general practitioners and no to minimal fees
Abuja Declaration	The Abuja Declaration is a commitment made by African Union member states in 2001 to allocate at least 15% of their annual budgets to improving healthcare services across the continent.
Accreditation Canada	Accreditation Canada is a nonprofit organization that evaluates and accredits healthcare organizations in Canada based on their adherence to national standards of quality and patient safety.
Ad valoreum tax	Value-based tax
Adolescent birth rate	The number of births per 1,000 women aged 15 to 19 in a given year, used as an indicator of reproductive health and gender equality among youth
Advanced practice registered nurses (APRNs)	Highly trained nurses with advanced education (e.g., nurse practitioners, nurse anesthetists) who can provide a wide range of healthcare services, including diagnosing and prescribing medications
African Union	A pivotal center for African diplomacy, shaping the continent's political landscape and fostering cooperation among nations
Age dependency ratio	Ratio of those who are too young or too old to work to those who are of working age
Age-friendly	Inclusive and accessible, respectful of individual needs, and addressing the wide range of capacities across the life span

Ageism	Prejudice, discrimination, and stereotyping based on age, often older age
Aging index	Represents the number of older individuals (65+) per 100 persons younger than 15 years old within the population
Anma and Shiatsu	Traditional Japanese massage therapies; *Anma* uses kneading and rubbing techniques, while *Shiatsu* involves applying pressure to specific points to balance energy flow and improve health.
Anthropogenic	Human-caused
Antibiotic resistance	When bacteria develop mutations, it makes established antibiotics less or no longer effective
Antibodies	Proteins produced by the immune system following the presence of an antigen
Antigen	A foreign substance that elicits the immune response
Antimicrobial stewardship	Initiatives to advocate for the optimal use of antibiotics
Antiretroviral therapy (ART)	A treatment for HIV that uses a combination of medications to suppress the virus, helping individuals live longer, healthier lives and reducing the risk of transmission
Anxiety	Excessive fear and worry and related behavioral disturbances
Archipelagos	Island chains
Ashura	Approximately 60% of the Muslim population in Iraq is Shia, a sect of Islam that practices various religious observances such as the annual remembrance of Ashura, which has been commemorated for more than 1,000 years and maintains a prominent occurrence in Iraq. Ashura signifies a time of mourning for the martyrdom of Prophet Muhammad's grandson Hussein ibn Ali.
Asana	Physical posture in yoga
Association of Southeast Asian Nations (ASEAN)	An intergovernmental organization formed in 1967 and made up of 10 member states: Indonesia, Malaysia, Philippines, Singapore, Thailand, Brunei, Vietnam, Lao PDR, Myanmar, and Cambodia
Asylee	An individual who has been granted asylum by a specific country
Asylum seeker	An individual who is seeking protection but whose claim has not been determined legally
Autonomous regions	Areas like Tibet and Xinjiang that have a higher concentration of ethnic minorities and are granted limited self-governance under the Chinese constitution
Baby boomer	People born from 1946 to 1964 during the post–World War II, mid–20th-century "baby boom"
Baghdad	The smallest governorate in Iraq, spanning 673 square kilometers; it is the capital and the most populated region with around 7.2 million inhabitants

Bengali	National language of Bangladesh
Beveridge model	A single-payer, universal health servces system financed by the government via taxes
Bhojpuri	A Hindi dialect spoken in the Republic of Trinidad and Tobago
Biomedicine	A system of medical practice based on the application of biological and physiological principles, using scientific methods to diagnose, treat, and prevent disease
Birth rate	The number of live births per thousand of population per year
Bismarck model	A multipayer universal health coverage system primarily financed by employer and employee contributions, which are referred to as sickness funds
Brain drain	Refers to the emigration of educated or skilled professionals from one country to another, often in search of better opportunities, which can negatively impact the workforce in their home country
Bridgetown	Capital of Barbados
British East India Company (BEIC)	During the Colonial period, the BEIC, which acted on behalf of the British Crown, became the dominant power in the Indian peninsula.
British Raj	Official British rule over most of South Asia, which was known as the British Raj, began in 1857 after a failed rebellion against the British East India Company.
Bulk billing	Refers to payment mechanism. If the patient is not charged an out-of-pocket fee, the general practitioner or medical provider will "bulk bill" Medicare for provision of the services.
Burmese	The official language of Myanmar
Bush medicine	Traditional plant/herbal medicine of the Republic of Trinidad and Tobago
Capability-based approach to mental health	Approach that understands that individuals have the inherent capacity and strength to address their problems; allows practitioners and communities to recognize sources of discrimination as well as create safe spaces for individuals to reconnect with society after experiencing mental health difficulties
Capitation	A payment model where providers receive a fixed amount per patient for a specified period, regardless of how many services the patient uses
Carbon sinks	Anything that absorbs more carbon from the atmosphere than it releases—for example, plants, the ocean, and soil
Central Asia	The least populated Asian subregion, comprising five countries: Tajikistan, Uzbekistan, Kazakhstan, Turkmenistan, and Kyrgyzstan
Cerebrovascular disease	A group of conditions affecting blood flow to the brain, including strokes and aneurysms, which can lead to brain damage or neurologic impairments

Chhaupadi	Traditional practice, observed by many in western parts of Nepal, where menstruating women and girls are secluded outside their homes in makeshift huts or livestock sheds. During their periods, females are considered impure, and are refrained from participating in daily activities (including going to school or work) and banned from touching family members or things in the house. This discriminatory practice obstructs women and girls' access to education, healthcare, community, and safety.
Children's Health Insurance Program (CHIP)	A U.S. program that provides low-cost health coverage to children in families who earn too much to qualify for Medicaid but cannot afford private insurance
Chinese Communist Party (CCP)	The ruling political party of China since 1949, founded in 1921, which led the communist revolution and established the current socialist state
Chinese Revolution of 1911	Also known as the Xinhai Revolution, this uprising overthrew the Qing Dynasty and ended over 2,000 years of imperial rule in China, leading to the establishment of the Republic of China
Chronic-care capitation	A capitation model specifically designed for managing long-term care of patients with chronic conditions, offering providers a fixed payment per patient to manage all related care
Citizens Health Insurance	A public health insurance system in Japan designed for self-employed individuals, retirees, and others not covered by employer-based insurance, providing access to medical care through contributions and subsidies
Climate change	Long-term shifts in temperature, precipitation patterns, and other climatic variables that occur over decades or longer periods
Climate refugee	An individual who hase been forced to leave their home due to climate change
Colloquial language	Informal/conversational and common lanuage dialect
Colonialism	Practice of acquiring political control over the Indigenous people of an area
Communicable diseases	Infectious diseases considered contagious or capable of being transmitted from one individual or species to another; examples include COVID-19, influenza (flu), measles, tuberculosis, syphilis, HIV, dengue, malaria, polio, cholera, and shingles
Community and family care model	A holistic approach to healthcare that emphasizes the role of families and communities in promoting health, preventing disease, and providing care. It integrates community-based services with family support systems to ensure accessible, culturally appropriate, and continuous care tailored to local needs.
Community health	Field of study and practice that focuses on improving the health and well-being of defined populations or communities

Community health centers (CHCs)	Centers that are crucial for delivering primary healthcare services, particularly in rural and underserved areas; they provide essential services like immunizations, maternal and child health, and treatment of common illnesses, often on a sliding fee scale.
Community hospitals	Local, smaller hospitals that provide basic healthcare services to the surrounding community, often with a focus on accessibility
Community-based health insurance (CBHI) program	Nonprofit health financing mechanism in which members of a community pool their resources to cover healthcare costs, typically on a voluntary basis
Contextual model of mental health	Model that allows understanding of the systemic hierarchies prevalent in different contexts
Cradle of civilization	A term used to describe regions where the earliest complex societies and cultures emerged, such as Mesopotamia, Ancient Egypt, the Indus Valley, and Ancient China
Cultural competency	The ability of healthcare providers to appropriately care for diverse populations while responding to each patient's beliefs, practices, and values
Dalits	The so-called "lower" castes of Nepal
Deficit-based approach to mental health	Perspective that emphasizes an individual's problems and attempts to formulate solutions for those problems
Democratic People's Republic of Korea	The official name for North Korea, established in 1948 in the northern part of the Korean Peninsula, governed by a centralized, authoritarian regime
Demographic	Statistical data relating to the population and particular groups within it, such as age, gender, income, or education
Demographic transition	The shift from a younger to an older population
Demographic window of opportunity	Opens in a country when the ratio is 60 dependents or less to every 100 working-age people
Depression	Severe emotional challenges in everyday life, often involving a depressed mood (feeling sad, irritable, or empty) or a loss of pleasure in activities previously enjoyed
Desertification	Process by which fertile land degrades due to lack of water; it damaged 70% of land in 2023, further affecting crops, the populations who reside in those arable regions, and the number of displaced persons
Determinants of health	The factors that influence health, such as behavioral, biological, economic, environmental, political, and social
Dieback	Loss of tree cover and biodiversity due to climate change, deforestation, and changing precipitation patterns

Dietary energy supply adequacy	Measures the dietary energy consumed against the country's average dietary energy requirement. Computed at the national level, this indicator considers variations in how sex, age, and height are distributed between different countries as people of the same sex, age, and height are estimated to have the same energy requirement.
Digital Quality of Life Index	Assesses internet affordability, quality, infrastructure, security, and e-government by country
Directly controlled municipalities	Major cities such as Beijing, Shanghai, Tianjin, and Chongqing that are governed directly by the central government and have the same administrative level as provinces
District Health Management Teams (DHMTs)	Teams who manage healthcare governance at the district level in Uganda
Divine healer	A divine healer is a spiritual practitioner who believes in using prayer, rituals, or divine intervention to heal physical or mental ailments, often within a religious or cultural context.
Doi Moi	Economic reforms initiated in Vietnam in 1986 known as Renovation
Double burden of disease	Prevalance of both communicable and noncommunicable diseases
Dragon Boat Festival	A traditional Chinese holiday celebrated in Taiwan and other regions, featuring dragon boat races and eating sticky rice dumplings (zongzi), held on the fifth day of the fifth lunar month
Endemic	The prevalence of a pathogen being considered maintained or stable, typically at a lower prevalence
Epidemic	When the rapid transmission of a pathogen occurs within a population
Epidemiologic transition	The shift from communicable to noncommunicable disease mortality
Epidemiologists	One who studies the occurrence, distribution, and determinants of health and disease to make evidence-based decisions and recommendations that are intended to improve community and population-based health outcomes
Episode-of-care	A bundled payment model covering all the services a patient receives for a specific condition or treatment over a set time period
Etiology	Causes
European Health Insurance Card (EHIC)	Tool that allows citizens of the European Union (EU) to receive healthcare when traveling within the EU
Expanded Programme on Immunisation (EPI)	Initiative in Barbados preventing morbidity and mortality from common vaccine-preventable diseases—primary vaccine coverage target of 95%
Fee-for-service	A payment model where healthcare providers are paid separately for each service or procedure performed

Fenceline communities	Communities located near industrial facilities, often exposed to environmental hazards such as pollution, which can harm their health.
Fertile Crescent	Region in West Asia from which arose cradles of civilizations such as the Sumerians of Mesopotamia. Landmark developments that emerged in the Fertile Crescent include agriculture, farming, the use of irrigation, and writing.
Food swamp	An area with an abundance of fast food and junk food outlets, contributing to poor dietary habits and higher rates of obesity and related diseases
Forcibly Displaced Myanmar Nationals (FDMNs)	Refugee population found in Bangladesh
Framework for Preventing Infectious Diseases	A structured public health strategy created by the U.S. Centers for Disease Control and Prevention that outline policies, surveillance systems, education, vaccination, and emergency response measures to prevent and control the spread of infectious diseases
French patois	A dialect spoken in the Republic of Trinidad and Tobago, also known as Creole
G7 nations	A group of seven of the world's most advanced economies—Canada, France, Germany, Italy, Japan, the United Kingdom, and the United States—that collaborate on global economic and political issues
Gender Inequality Index (GII)	A composite measure developed by the United Nations to reflect gender-based disparities in reproductive health, empowerment, and economic status. It highlights the loss in human development due to inequality between female and male achievements.
Gender-affirming care	Social, behavioral, medical, and/or physiological services that focus on understanding and validating an individual's gender identity
Global Compact for Safe, Orderly, and Regular Migration (GCM)	A platform for cooperation, emphasizing sustainable solutions that integrate refugees into national systems, particularly healthcare and education
Global Fund	An international financing organization that mobilizes and allocates resources to fight HIV/AIDS, tuberculosis, and malaria, supporting programs in countries with high disease burdens
Global health	A multidisciplinary field that seeks to improve health and achieve equity (fairness and justice) in health for all people worldwide
Global warming	Greenhouse gases such as carbon dioxide, methane, and nitrous oxide in the atmosphere trap heat from the sun, leading to a gradual increase in global temperatures.
The Golden Triangle	The mountainous region of eastern Myanmar, northwestern Thailand, and northern Loas
Greater Antilles	Consists of six major island nations in the northern region of the Caribbean Sea: Cuba, the Cayman Islands, Jamaica, Haiti, the Dominican Republic, and Puerto Rico

Group of Twenty (G20)	The G20 is an international forum of 19 countries and the European Union that brings together the world's major economies to discuss and coordinate global economic policy, financial stability, and sustainable development.
Gulf War	War triggered in 1990 by Saddam Hussein's invasion of Kuwait
Gupta Empire	The Classical Period saw the rise and spread of the Gupta Empire that brought urban, religious, artistic, agricultural, scientific, and technological innovations.
Hakeems	Traditional healers of Pakistan
Han Dynasty	A major Chinese dynasty that ruled from 206 BCE to 220 CE, known for consolidating imperial power, expanding territory, and advancing culture, technology, and trade, including along the Silk Road
Health disparity	A health disparity is a difference in health outcomes caused and/or exacerbated by health inequities.
Health equity	A fair and just state in which all people can achieve their full health potential
Health inequities	Structural differences in the opportunity for people to achieve full health potential
Health maintenance organizations (HMOs)	Managed care plans that provide healthcare services through a network of doctors and hospitals, typically requiring referrals from a primary care physician
Health reforms	Systematic changes in policies, regulations, and structures within a healthcare system to improve accessibility, quality, efficiency, and equity in healthcare services. These reforms may involve financing, service delivery, workforce management, and governance.
Health Savings Account (HSA)	A tax-advantaged savings account used to pay for qualified medical expenses, often paired with high-deductible health plans
Health systems	The organized structures and processes through which health services are delivered, financed, and governed to meet a population's health needs
Health transition	Societal shift from a high level of physical activity to increased sedentariness (too much time being seated) and from traditional, well-balanced whole food diets to highly processed, calorie dense, and nutrient deficient diets. The health transition occurs along with the demographic transition, which is the shift from a younger to an older population, and the epidemiologic transition, which is a shift from communicable to noncommunicable disease mortality.
Health Unit Management Committees (HUMCs)	Committees that support District Health Mangement Teams in Uganda with community involvement
Healthcare	The effort to maintain or improve a person's physical, mental, or emotional well-being. It includes the prevention, diagnosis, treatment, and management of illnesses, injuries, and other health issues.

Healthcare delivery	The provision of healthcare services
Healthcare financing	The management of money to cover the health needs of people within the system
Healthcare insurance	A contract that specifies how services will be paid under a health plan
Herbal medicine	Refers to the use of plant-based substances and extracts for therapeutic purposes, often relying on traditional knowledge or cultural practices
Herbalist	Practitioner who uses plants and natural remedies to treat illnesses and promote health, often based on traditional knowledge and practices
High-deductible health plans (HDHPs)	Insurance plans with lower premiums but higher deductibles, requiring the policyholder to pay more out-of-pocket before insurance coverage kicks in
Hikmat	Traditional medicine used in Pakistan
Hospice	An extension of palliative care in which the patient is in the terminal phase of a disease and has less than 6 months to live
Hospitals	Healthcare facilities that provide inpatient, outpatient, emergency, and surgical care
Hu Huanyong Line	A demographic line drawn by Chinese geographer Hu Huanyong in 1935 that divides China into a densely populated eastern region and a sparsely populated western region
Human Development Index (HDI)	Metric developed by the United Nations that considers the performance of a country in three main achievement areas: life expectancy at birth, knowledge/literacy rate, and standard of living quality (gross domestic product [GDP] per capita)
Independent State of Papua New Guinea	A sovereign country in the southwestern Pacific, occupying the eastern half of the island of New Guinea, known for its cultural and linguistic diversity and independence from Australia in 1975
Indigenous Languages Development Act	A Taiwanese law enacted to preserve, promote, and revitalize the languages of Taiwan's Indigenous peoples, recognizing them as national languages
Indigenous peoples	The original inhabitants of a region, including First Nations, Métis, and Inuit in Canada, each with distinct cultures, languages, and histories
Indus Valley Civilization	One of the world's earliest urban civilizations
Infant mortality rate (IMR)	The number of infant deaths (before the first birthday) per 1,000 live births
Infectious diseases	Illnesses caused by pathogens such as bacteria, viruses, fungi, and parasites
Informal care	Unpaid caregiving, often provided by family members or friends, to individuals with chronic illnesses or disabilities

Integrated care systems	Alliances comprised of National Health Services institutions, representatives from local government, and private bodies involved in heathcare care charged with improving overall population health and improving efficiency
Integrated Mosquito Vector Management	Barbados program employing a multisectoral strategy to prevent and control arboviral diseases including the endemic Dengue fever transmitted by the *Aedes aegypti* mosquito
Internal market	Competitive market in the National Health Service established by Margaret Thatcher
Internally displaced person	An individual who has been forced to leave their home but has not crossed an international border
International health	A field that traditionally emphasizes the health needs of low- and middle-income countries and the role of developed nations in addressing these issues through aid and technical support
Iran–Iraq war	War arising from jurisdictional conflicts between Iraq and Iran from 1980 until 1988
Iraq War	War that began due to Iraq's noncompliance with UN resolutions and the United States goal of ending Saddam Hussein's presidency based on claims that Iraq possessed weapons of mass destruction and had links to terrorism
Judo therapists	Licensed practitioners in Japan whose use techniques derived from traditional Japanese martial arts to treat musculoskeletal injuries, often involving manual therapy, joint manipulation, and rehabilitation
Junta	Group ruling a country after taking it over by force
Kalinago Caribs	Indigenous people of Barbados arriving from South American in the mid-1200s
Kangaroo care	Promotes skin-to-skin contact between mothers and infants, especially important for babies with preterm and low birth weight
Kastom	A term used in Melanesia, especially in Papua New Guinea and Vanuatu, to describe traditional customs, beliefs, and cultural practices passed down through generations
Kay Manmito	Mother's House at the University Hospital in Mirebalais, Haiti; serves women with at-risk pregnancies and provides free maternal–child health education, resources like food and blankets, and a kangaroo care center
Kurdistan	Region in northern Iraq where the the Kurds, the second largest ethnic group (approximately 17%) in Iraq, primarily reside
Las Fallas	A regional festival in Valencia, Spain, held in March
Lesser Antilles	An arc of islands along the eastern boundary of the Caribbean Sea that are located north off of mainland Venezuela
Life expectancy at birth	The average number of years a newborn can expect to live

Lifestyle-related diseases	Chronic illnesses, such as diabetes, heart disease, and certain cancers, that are primarily caused by unhealthy habits like poor diet, lack of exercise, smoking, and excessive alcohol use
Lightwave Health Information Management System (LHIMS)	LHIMS is a digital health management platform in Ghana designed to improve healthcare delivery by efficiently managing patient data, hospital processes, and medical records.
Lokahi	Hawaiian term meaning harmony, unity, or balance, often used in the context of holistic health and well-being
Los Barbados	"The bearded ones" in Portuguese—origin of Barbados' name
Lucayan Archipelago	Group of islands located in the western area of the northern Atlantic Ocean, north of Cuba and southeast of Florida. Includes the Bahamas and Turks and Caicos
Lunar New Year	Also known as Chinese New Year, it marks the start of the lunar calendar and is celebrated with family reunions, feasts, and cultural festivities
Malaria	A life-threatening disease caused by *Plasmodium* parasites, transmitted to humans through the bites of infected mosquitoes, leading to fever, chills, and severe complications if untreated
Martial law	A period in Taiwan's history (1949–1987) when the government imposed strict military control, limiting civil liberties and political freedoms under the Kuomintang (KMT) regime
Maternal mortality ratio (MMR)	The number of maternal deaths per 100,000 live births
Medicaid	A U.S. government program providing healthcare coverage to low-income individuals and families
Medical Aid Program	South Korean government-funded program that offers healthcare coverage to low-income individuals who cannot afford contributions to the National Health Insurance
Medical and Dental Council of Nigeria (MDCN)	The regulatory body responsible for overseeing the practice of medicine and dentistry in Nigeria, ensuring that practitioners meet professional standards and ethics
Medical Benefits Scheme (MBS)	The type and level of reimbursement for each fee-for-medical-service from the Australian government via Medicare
Medical Care Act	A 1966 Canadian law that laid the foundation for the country's publicly funded healthcare system, establishing the principle of universal coverage for hospital and physician services
Medicare (Australia)	Australia's universal, tax-based, public national health insurance system, which finances care for all by public and private providers
Medicare (U.S.)	A federal health insurance program for people aged 65 and older, and some younger people with disabilities

Melanesian	Refers to the people, cultures, and geographic region of Melanesia, which includes Papua New Guinea, Fiji, Solomon Islands, Vanuatu, and New Caledonia
Mental health	The state of an individual's cognitive, behavioral, and emotional well-being and ability to function within the social environment
Mental morbidity	A metric of mental illness that adjusts for demographic factors (e.g., age distribution, regional differences) in a population, providing a more representative estimate of how many people are affected by mental illness
Mestizo	A term traditionally used in Latin America to describe a person of mixed European (typically Spanish) and Indigenous ancestry. It reflects both cultural and racial blending that emerged during the Colonial period.
Mid-Autumn Festival	A major lunar holiday in Taiwan focused on family gatherings, moon gazing, and eating mooncakes, celebrated on the 15th day of the eighth lunar month
Migrant	An individual who is moving from place to place, either within their country or across borders, but was not forced to leave due to persecution or violence. Migrants typically move for economic reasons in search of a better life.
Ministry of Health and Population (MoHP)	Egyptian ministry that oversees the public healthcare system, which includes a network of hospitals, primary care clinics, and specialized facilities
Ministry of Health and Wellness (MHW) of Barbados	The administrative and regulatory authority for the provision of public healthcare services in Barbados
Mobile clinics	Healthcare units that travel to provide medical services in underserved or remote areas, often using vans or buses equipped with medical equipment and staff
Mortality rates	Mortality rates refer to the frequency or number of deaths in a given population, typically expressed per 1,000 or 100,000 individuals within a specific time frame.
Moxibustionists	Practitioners of moxibustion, a traditional East Asian therapy involving the burning of mugwort (moxa) on or near the skin to stimulate acupuncture points and promote healing
My Health Bank	A digital health platform in Taiwan that allows individuals to access their personal medical records, prescriptions, and healthcare utilization history online
Narrative therapy	An alternative to conventional psychotherapy approaches that allows clients to deconstruct their current experience, empowers them as authors of their own lives, and aids in reconstructing their identity with hopes and expectations

National Cancer Plan	Initiative created in Barbados to address factors such as patient education, risk factor reduction, screening, and a clinical pathway review for the cancers of epidemiologic concern
National Council for Traditional Healers and Herbalists Associations	Council established by the Ugandan government to regulate and integrate traditional practices in modern healthcare
National fee schedule	A standardized list set by the government in Japan that specifies the reimbursement rates for medical procedures, services, and medications under the national health insurance system
National Health Insurance (NHI) Committee	A governing body that oversees Taiwan's National Health Insurance system, including decision-making on coverage, reimbursement, and policy implementation
National Health Insurance (NHI) Family Physician Integrated Care Projects	Initiatives in Taiwan aimed at strengthening primary care by encouraging patients to register with family physicians who coordinate comprehensive and continuous healthcare services
National Health Insurance (NHI) MediCloud System	A cloud-based system in Taiwan's ational Health Insurance program that provides real-time access to patients' medical data for healthcare providers, improving treatment safety and efficiency
National health insurance model	A single-payer universal health coverage system that combines elements of the Beveridge and Bismarck models
National Health Insurance Scheme	A government-run program in Ghana designed to provide affordable and accessible healthcare services to citizens by pooling funds from contributors to cover medical expenses
National Health Insurance Service	South Korea's single-payer public health insurance system that provides coverage to nearly the entire population through mandatory contributions
National Health Service (NHS)	Government-owned and -operated health system in the United Kingdom that is free to patients at the point of service
National Institute for Health and Clinical Excellence (NICE)	United Kingdom regulatory body charged with assessing clinical interventions for effectiveness and recommending them for inclusion within National Health Service institutions
National Long-Term Care Insurance (NLTCI) for the Elderly Act	A South Korean law enacted in 2008 that provides long-term care services and support to older adults who need assistance with daily activities due to age or illness
National Referral Hospitals	Hospitals in Uganda that provide specialized care

Naturopathic doctors	Healthcare providers who focus on natural remedies and treatments, such as herbs, nutrition, and lifestyle changes, to promote healing and prevent disease
Neglected tropical diseases	Infectious diseases that include malaria, tuberculosis, and HIV/AIDS
Neonatal mortality	The newborn mortality period during the first 28 days of life for a given year
Nepali	Official language of Nepal
Net migration	Difference between the number of people who come into a region and the number who leave the region
New Innovative Medical Education Initiative (NIMEI)	Initiative that aimed to accelerate the production of healthcare professionals in Ethiopia through a shorter medical program
Noncommunicable diseases (NCDs)	Long-lasting diseases that are not directly transmitted from one person to another
Nonrefoulement	Forced return home
Nutrition transition	A shift in dietary patterns, often seen in developing countries, from traditional diets high in fiber and low in fat to more processed foods high in sugar, fat, and animal products, often leading to increased rates of obesity and chronic diseases
One-Child Policy	A Chinese government policy implemented from 1979 to 2015 that restricted most families to having only one child to control population growth
Palliative care	Care that provides relief from symptoms and stress of serious illnesses, crucial for maintaining quality of life for older adults facing chronic or terminal conditions
Pandemics	Global outbreaks
Parasuicide	An act of self-harm that mimics suicide—the aim is not to kill oneself.
Paris Agreement	An internationally enforced treaty designed to address climate change and global warming
Parliamentary constitutional monarchy	A form of government where a monarch acts as the ceremonial head of state within the limits of a constitution, while elected officials in a parliament hold legislative power and govern the country
Parliamentary democracy	Form of government where the prime minister is the leader and the president is head of state
Partitioning of the Ottoman Empire	Following World War I, the defeated Ottoman Empire was partitioned into several new separate nations that included diverse people and territories with conflicting views.
Patient Protection and Affordable Care Act of 2010 (ACA)	U.S. healthcare reform law aimed at expanding health insurance coverage, reducing healthcare costs, and improving the quality of care

People's Republic of China	The official name for mainland China, established in 1949 by the Chinese Communist Party under Mao Zedong after defeating the Nationalist forces in the Chinese Civil War
Pharmaceutical Benefits Scheme (PBS)	The type and level of reimbursement for each fee-for-pharmaceutical-service from the Australian government via Medicare
Pharmacopeia	An official publication listing recognized drugs, their formulations, standards for purity and dosage, and guidelines for preparation and use, used as a reference for medical and pharmaceutical practice
$PM_{2.5}$	Fine particulate matter found in the atmosphere that is 2.5 micrometers or smaller and can be deeply absorbed into the lungs and cause substantial health risks
Polyclinic	Community-based ambulatory center
Population aging	When the median age of a population rises over time, usually due to a combination of lower birth rates, increased life expectancy, and aging of large groups of individuals
Port Moresby	The capital and largest city of Papua New Guinea, located on the southeastern coast of the island of New Guinea
Port of Spain	Capital city of the Republic of Trinidad and Tobago
Positive feedback loop	When the product of a reaction leads to an increase in that reaction
Precision medicine	The practice of medicine that uses an individual's genetic profile to guide decisions made regarding the prevention, diagnosis, and treatment of disease
Preferred provider organizations (PPOs)	A type of health plan that offers more flexibility in choosing healthcare providers and does not require referrals for specialists
Prevention of Mother-to-Child Transmission (PMTCT) program	The PMTCT program aims to prevent the transmission of HIV from an HIV-positive mother to her child during pregnancy, childbirth, or breastfeeding through testing, treatment, and counseling.
Primary healthcare	A community-based approach to health that provides accessible, affordable, and comprehensive services, including prevention, treatment, and health promotion. It serves as the first point of contact in the healthcare system, addressing most health needs and coordinating further care when necessary
Primary prevention	Preventing the onset of disease or illness
Private for-profit hospitals	Hospitals operated by private entities or corporations, where profits are distributed to shareholders or owners
Private nonprofit hospitals	Hospitals operated by nonprofit organizations, reinvesting any profits back into patient care and community services

Private sectors	Includes privately owned hospitals, pharmacies, labs, and clinics that operate for profit, often charging more while purportedly providing better services than public hospitals
Public health system	A network of organizations, institutions, and resources that work collectively to promote, protect, and improve the health of populations through disease prevention, health education, policymaking, and access to healthcare services
Public hospitals	Hospitals funded and operated by government agencies, often serving a broad demographic including low-income populations
Public sector	A government-managed system that provides services at no or minimal cost
Purchaser–provider split	Part of the national health system's internal market which separates those who purchase healthcare services from those who provide healthcare services
Qinghai-Tibetan Plateau	A high-altitude region in western China known as the "Roof of the World," characterized by harsh climates and low population density
Queen Elizabeth Hospital (QEH)	Barbados' lone accredited public acute, secondary, and tertiary care institution
Redlining	A discriminatory practice where services like housing or loans are denied to residents in certain neighborhoods, often based on racial or ethnic composition
Refugee	A person who, due to a well-founded fear of being persecuted for race, religion, nationality, membership in a particular social group, or political opinion, is outside the country of their nationality and is unable to avail themselves of the protection of that country
Regenerative therapies	Replacing or "regenerating" human cells, tissues, or organs to restore or establish normal function
Regional health authorities (RHAs)	Agencies responsible for delivering public healthcare services in the Republic of Trinidad and Tobago
Regional referral hospitals	Regional hospitals offering tertiary care across regions in Uganda
Registered nurses (RNs)	Healthcare professionals who provide patient care, administer medications, and educate patients on health management, typically requiring a nursing degree and licensure
Republic of China	The government founded after the 1911 revolution, which initially ruled mainland China until 1949 and now governs Taiwan and some nearby islands
Republic of Korea	Official name for South Korea, a democratic nation in East Asia established in 1948 following World War II and the division of Korea. It is known for its advanced economy, high-tech industries, and universal healthcare system

Republic of Trinidad and Tobago (T&T)	A twin-island country in the Caribbean region with a unique societal structure, traditions, history, and religious backgrounds that influence health and healthcare practices
Rohingya refugees	Refugees primarily from the Rakhine region of Myanmar
Salud Mesoamerica Initiative	A public–private partnership aimed at improving maternal, child, and reproductive health for the poorest populations in Central American countries. It provides results-based funding and technical support to strengthen healthcare systems and reduce health disparities in the region.
Schizophrenia	Significant impairments in perception and cognitive functioning and changes in behavior; symptoms include persistent delusions, hallucinations, disorganized thinking, highly disorganized behavior, and extreme agitation
Scramble for Africa	African colonization by Belgium, England, France, Germany, Italy, and Portugal
Scratching	A Southeast Asian traditional medicine process in which the skin is deliberately broken by an object such as a coin
Secondary prevention	Screenings for early detection and subsequent health education, lifestyle, and pharmaceutical interventions to abate disease progression
Semashko model	A state-run healthcare system originally developed in the Soviet Union, characterized by centralized planning, government-funded services, and universal access, with an emphasis on preventive care and hospital-based treatment
Semiautonomous special administrative districts	Regions like Hong Kong and Macau that are part of China but operate with a high degree of political and economic independence under the "one country, two systems" principle
Shalyapahartrika	Ancient indian branch of medicine specializing in surgery
Shinto	The traditional religion of Japan centered around the worship of kami (spirits or deities), nature, and ancestral reverence, emphasizing rituals and harmony with nature
Siddha	Over 10,000 year old medicinal system practiced in South India
Single-payer healthcare system	A system in which a single public or government entity finances healthcare services for all citizens, typically through taxes, rather than relying on multiple private insurers
Small island developing state (SIDS)	A group of small island countries noted for shared sustainable development and challenges that include geographic isolation, frequency of natural disasters, limited resources, and growing populations
Social protection	Policies and programs designed to reduce poverty, vulnerability, and social exclusion by providing support such as cash transfers, healthcare, unemployment benefits, and social insurance. It aims to enhance well-being and resilience, especially for disadvantaged groups.

Sociodemographic Index	A composite measure that reflects a region's level of development using income per capita, educational attainment, and fertility rates
Southern African Development Community (SADC)	SADC is a regional organization comprising 16 Southern African countries, aimed at promoting economic development, political stability, and cooperation, including efforts to improve public health and combat diseases.
Stateless person	An individual who is not a citizen of any country, typically because their citizenship was revoked for reasons related to religion or membership to a political group
Stigmatization	To discriminate by characterizing as disgraceful
Subsistence farming	A type of agriculture where farmers grow food primarily to feed themselves and their families, with little or no surplus for trade
Sumer	One of the world's original civilizations in the Mesopotamia region of the Fertile Crescent; Sumerians are credited with some of the earliest developments in written language, mathematics, astronomy, time keeping, architecture, and urban planning.
Suriyanamaskaaram	Popular Indian practice where one performs a set of yoga asanas early in the morning facing the direction of sunrise
Syncretism	The attempted union of diverse tenets or practices, especially in philosophy or religion
T&T Ministry of Health	Leading authority with responsibility for supervising the Republic of Trinidad and Tobago's entire health system
Taino Arawaks	Indigenous people of Barbados arriving from South American in 800 CE
Taiwan Diagnosis-Related Groups (TW-DRGs)	A payment system under Taiwan's National Health Institute that classifies hospital cases into groups to standardize reimbursement rates based on diagnosis and treatment complexity
Tertiary prevention	Treating an existing disease to prevent further disease progression and reduce the risk of severe complications associated with the disease
Three durable solutions model	Voluntary repatriation, local integration, and resettlement
Tigris–Euphrates	Rivers that flow through parts of Turkey, Syria, and Iraq and have provided irrigation and allowed for the early growth of civilization in those exceptionally dry areas
Tok Pisin	A widely spoken creole language in Papua New Guinea that developed from English and is one of the country's official languages
Traditional Chinese medicine (TCM)	A holistic system of medicine that includes herbal remedies, acupuncture, and other practices developed over thousands of years in China
Traditional medicine/traditional healthcare	The knowledge, skills, and practices based on theories, beliefs, and experiences indigenous to different cultures, used for maintaining health and treating illnesses

Tutela	In some healthcare systems, especially in South America, a *tutela* is a legal mechanism allowing patients to demand immediate medical treatment when their right to health is threatened or denied.
Unani	Traditional Muslim medicine originating from Greece
UNICEF	UNICEF (United Nations International Children's Emergency Fund) is a UN agency that works globally to promote and protect the rights and well-being of children, focusing on health, education, nutrition, and emergency relief.
Universal coverage model	The universal coverage model ensures that all individuals, regardless of income or status, have access to essential healthcare services, typically funded by the government to guarantee equitable access for everyone.
Universal Health Insurance (UHI)	Government program launched in 2019 to provide comprehensive healthcare coverage to all Egyptians by 2032
Universal Healthcare (UHC) Service Coverage Index	Measurement of how well countries provide essential health services
Urban Employee Basic Medical Insurance	A public health insurance program in China covering urban workers, funded by both employers and employees
Urban healthcare	Healthcare that is provided to people living in urban areas with focus on improving the quality of life and well-being of people living in cities
Urban–Rural Resident Basic Medical Insurance	A unified health insurance scheme in China covering unemployed urban residents and rural populations
Urdu	One of the two major languages of Pakistan (the other being English)
Vertical transmission	Mother-to-child disease transmittion
Village Health Teams (VHTs)	The lowest level of Uganda's health system
Vulnerable populations	Groups of people who face a higher risk of harm due to factors such as economic disadvantage, health disparities, disability, age, or social exclusion
West Asia	Often referred to as the Middle East, the second least populated Asian subregion
Yuans	The five main branches of government in Taiwan's constitutional system, based on Sun Yat-sen's theory of separation of powers, which include the Executive Yuan, Legislative Yuan, Judicial Yuan, Examination Yuan, and Control Yuan—each with distinct functions in governance and administration
Zakat	Annual charitable contribution obligated by the Islamic faith
ZEF Agreement	Includes a pledge to stop gas flaring by 2030, in Iraq

INDEX